Sexual Rehabilitation of the Spinal-Cord-Injured Patient

Sexual Rehabilitation of the Spinal-Cord-Injured Patient

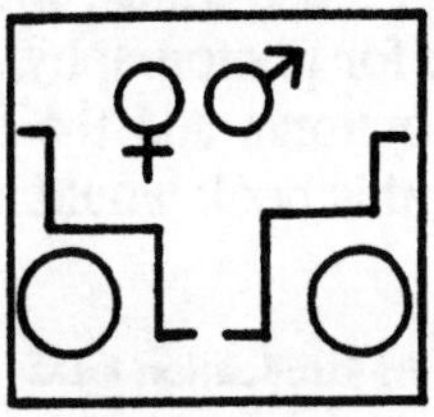

Edited by

Jose Florante J. Leyson
MD, FACS, FICSEP, FICP, ACS, AASECT

Director, Center for Sexual Dysfunctions and Neurourology
Clinical Chief, Spinal Cord Injury Service
VA Medical Center, East Orange, New Jersey
Chief of Surgery, 322nd US Army General Hospital,
Picatinny Arsenal, Dover, New Jersey

Humana Press • Clifton, New Jersey

Dedication

This book is warmly dedicated to my patients' unswerving courage to live and love; to the volunteers who participated in the research data gathering; to my parents, Gertrudes and Leon, who gave me life and taught me to love and be sensual; and to my beloved wife, Karen, whom I love most of all.

Acknowledgments

The Editor is indebted to the Dept. of Veterans Affairs (VA) Medical Center, East Orange, NJ; the administrative support of Drs. Boston F. Martin and Arthur S. Cytryn; the clinical assistance of Dr. Joseph Seebode; the technical critique of Dr. Andrew Sporer; the secretarial assistance of Ms. Jean Rich; the Medical Media service, Chief; the late Stanley Schwartz for art and illustrations; Joe Jones for graphics; Jack Ficarra and Harry Kubasek for photography; the contributors for their colorful and vibrant contributions; and the Publisher, without whose patience and understanding this book would not have been possible.

Library of Congress Cataloging-in-Publication Data

Sexual rehabilitation of the spinal-cord-injured-patient edited by
Jose Florante J. Leyson.
p. cm.
Includes index.
ISBN (invalid) 0-89603-145-5
1. Spinal cord—Wounds and injuries—Patients—Rehabilitation.
2. Spinal cord—Wounds and injuries—Patients—Sexual behavior.
3. Sex counseling. I. Leyson, Jose Florante J.
[DNLM: 1. Sex. 2. Sex Counseling. 3. Spinal Cord Injuries--rehabilitation. WL 400 S518]
RD594.3.S49 1990
617.4''8203—dc20
DNLM/DLC
for Library of Congress 90-4685
CIP

Crescent Manor
PO Box 2148
Clifton, NJ 07015

Printed in the United States of America.

Preface

G. Blasius first described the anatomic aspects of spinal cord injury (SCI) in 1666. Until that time, society had totally ignored the physically disabled, let alone allowed them to mingle socially and sexually.

The military mortality rate between 1814–1914 was estimated to be 50–80%, although sexual and sociocultural implications were not addressed. In a 1928 novel, *Lady Chatterley's Lover,* D. H. Lawrence strongly reflected the sexual concerns of a paraplegic who had been labeled impotent. The modern management of SCI was initiated by Monroe and Guttman in 1943, but with heavy emphasis on physical and urological rehabilitation and only superficial attention to sexual dysfunctions. H. W. Horne et al. started the investigation of SCI infertility problems in 1950. It was not until 1960 that Bors and Comarr collaborated on a study that classified the types of sexual dysfunctions in relation to neurological levels of lesions following spinal cord trauma.

Normal (nondisabled) sexuality came of age during the past two decades. This was highlighted by the 1966 publication of W. Masters', *Human Sexual Response*. However, the topic of sexuality in physically challenged (handicapped) persons remains largely taboo in our present society.

There are an estimated 10–12 million SCI persons worldwide. In America, there are approximately 1.2–1.5 million SCI victims, with an annual incidence of 12,000–15,000, or one every 35 minutes. The visibility of SCI persons was enhanced when the United Nations declared 1980–1990 as the decade of disabled persons. Furthermore, the enactment into law, in July, 1990, of the *American Disabilities Act,* pointed out the handicapped person's right to the fullest pursuit of happiness. Since the release in 1974 of K. Heslinga's *Not Made of*

Stone, only a handful of books on medical sexuality for the disabled have been published.

This book has three major objectives:

1. to provide thorough and comprehensive coverage of disabled persons' sexuality *in all sexual orientations;*
2. to introduce new terminologies and theories, to redefine certain sexual dysfunctions, and to describe updated treatment formats; and
3. to present research and innovations that may stimulate further investigations into disabled sexuality during the next decade.

The first part of this book defines new sexual terminology and describes the full spectrum of SCI sexual challenges.

The second half of the book deals with a variety of diagnostic and therapeutic sexual innovations, AIDS implications, and cosmic sexology.

Finally, the Appendix lists international sexual referral centers and information organizations.

This book differs greatly from other published works because it refocuses on the psychoemotional aspects of sexuality, and reminds us that sexuality is one of the most intense of all human emotions.

Jose Florante J. Leyson

Contents

Contributors

Michael A. Alexander, MD • Alfred I. du Pont Institute of the Nemours Foundation, Wilmington, DE

Jack Dahlberg, MA • Dalhberg and Associates, Rehabilitation Consultants, Denver, CO

Kowit Danviriyasup, MD • VA Medical Center, Long Beach, CA

Ananias C. Diokno, MD, FACS • William Beaumont Hospital University of Michigan Hospital, Ann Arbor, MI

Myron G. Eisenberg, PhD • VA Medical Center, Hampton, VA and Eastern Virginia Medical School, Norfolk, VA

Robert T. Francoeur, PhD, ACS • Fairleigh Dickinson University, Madison, NJ

Dorothea D. Glass, MD • VA Medical Center and University of Miami, Miami, FL

Rachel J. Harris, PhD • University of Miami School of Medicine, Miami, FL

Jay B. Hollander, MD, FACS • William Beaumont Hospital, Ann Arbor, MI

Beverly Hotchner, PhD, ACS, AASECT • Deaconness Medical Center, St. Louis, MO

Joanne M. James, MA • Private practice, Berthoud, CO

Sofjan Lamid, MD • Private practice, Harvey, LA

Jose Florante J. Leyson, MD, FACS, FICS, FICSEP, FICP, ACS, AASECT • University of Medicine and Dentistry, Newark, NJ, and VA Medical Center, East Orange, NJ

J. Keith Light, MD, FACS • Baylor College of Medicine, Houston, TX

Eli F. Lizza, MD, FACS • University of Medicine and Dentistry, Newark, NJ

Jeffrey L. Marks, MD • Baylor College and University Hospital, Houston, TX

Shirley McCluer, MD • University of Arkansas for Medical Sciences, Little Rock, AR

Edward J. McGuire, MD, FACS • University Hospital, University of Michigan, Ann Arbor, MI

Robert J. Neumann, PhD • Cardinal Stritch College, Waukesha, WI

Concetta J. Panzarino, MA • Center for Autonomous Living and Recreation Through the Arts and Agriculture and Disabled Lesbian Alliance, Monticello, NY

Warren R. Procci, MD, FACP • Harbor University of California and Los Angeles Medical Center, Torrance, CA

Domeena C. Renshaw, MD, FACP • Loyola University of Chicago, Maywood, IL

James F. Sagala, MS • VA Medical Center, East Orange, NJ

W. Ronald Skowsky, MD, FACP • University of Florida Health Science Center, Jacksonville, FL

Andrew Sporer, MD, FACS • University of Medicine and Dentistry, Newark, NJ and VA Medical Center, East Orange, NJ

Roberta Trieschman, PhD • RBT Associates, Scarsdale, AZ

Wouter H. Verduyn, MD • Covenant Rehabilitation Center and University of Iowa, Iowa City, IA

Robert L. Winer, MD, FACP • VA Medical Center, Long Beach, CA and University of California, Irvine, CA

Beverly Whipple, PhD, RN, ACS, AASECT • Rutgers State University of New Jersey, Newark, NJ and Thomas Jefferson University, Philadelphia, PA

1

Historical and Sociocultural Perspectives in Human Sexuality

Robert T. Francoeur

Introduction

The terms "sex," "sexual," and "sexuality" are seldom defined with precision in the professional literature. Their meaning is generally left to a reader's intuitive understanding. The term *sex* may be used to indicate male or female anatomy, the general distinction between male and female genders or between distinctive masculine and feminine behaviors attributed to the two genders, to activities leading to orgasm (*8,9*), or to penile/vaginal intercourse and reproduction. *Sexual* and *sexuality* are used with equal imprecision, referring to the sexual organs, to functions of sexual organs, to sexual drives, or to instincts. Gender, gender identity, and gender roles, on the other hand, have precise definitions derived from recent conceptualizations in psychosexual research. *Gender* usually indicates the equivalent of male or female anatomic sex. *Gender identity* refers to one's personally experienced sexual identity, a persistent individual self-awareness of being either male or female without regard to how or with whom one expresses this identity. *Gender role* involves everything one says or does to indicate his/her gender identity to others (*11*).

Sexual Rehabilitation of the Spinal-Cord-Injured Patient
Edited by J.F. Leyson, © 1990 The Humana Press, Inc.

Historical Aspects

This difference between common imprecisions in the usage of sexual terms and the clarity of gender terms reflects a historic ambivalence. Sex in western Christian thought has been viewed through the lens of a pervasive negative dualism in which one's good rational spirit/soul is opposed by one's evil, emotional, and passionate body, of which sex is a major component. Traditionally, sex has been justified by reproduction and limited to married partners. This religious view has been reinforced culturally and economically by men's need to control women and their sexuality in order to protect the legitimate inheritance of property acquired by males. Until the shift from an agrarian to urban culture, the advent of effective, inexpensive contraceptives, and the economic liberation of women in the past century, everything associated with sex and sexual activities was viewed as some kind of "monster in the groin," which had to be carefully restrained lest it run rampant and destroy society (*3*).

In this context, the sexuality and sexual needs of physically handicapped persons have been traditionally ignored or denied. For example, in 1982, an Indiana quadriplegic male was denied the right to marry in a Catholic church until he could prove his ability to engage in procreative coitus. Such proof was a "Catch-22 requirement," since it would entail a sinful act of fornication. After considerable media coverage, the regional Bishop allowed the man to marry without proof of potency. If sex is justified solely by reproductive capacity and limited to married couples, then those persons we feel should not marry because they cannot successfully carry out penile/vaginal coitus and those we judge incapable of reproducing or raising children are best handled by denying their sexual nature and needs. Children, teenagers, and older persons have traditionally been subject to this defensive desexing process. The physically handicapped have been traditionally included in this "asexual" group by their families and by health professionals. Not only might the physically handicapped have problems consummating a marriage or reproducing, but they also violate our prevailing cultural image in which only young, able-bodied persons seem to be capable of engaging in sex.

In the 1970s, a new perspective emerged, and sex education was introduced into medical school curricula while sex research began exploring the sexual needs and expressions of the disabled and other such minorities. Alex Comfort stated:

> "The disabled *are* people, and people are sexual. Much of our sense of personhood comes from our ability to play a sexual role. The disabled share with the rest of us the misfortune of living in a society that has traditionally avoided and censured sex, but this hits the disabled harder than others. They have been subjected, like the old (and children), to castrating black magic. . . Virtually nobody is too disabled to derive some satisfaction and personal reinforcement from sex—with a partner if possible, alone if necessary. When a disabled person is unable to enjoy sex, the greatest obstacle to enjoyment usually isn't the difficulty or impossibility of making particular movements, but the social contention that sex consists of putting the penis in the vagina and that all the remaining range of human and mammalian sexual responses—oral, manual, and skin stimulation—are abnormal. Human sex is widely versatile and hardly limited to the genitalia." (2)

Sociocultural Perspectives

Traditional definitions of sexuality and sexual attitudes have been summarized by Francoeur and Francoeur (*4*) as patriarchal with active males and passive females, sex role stereotyped, obsessed with genital performance and female virginity, accepting sexually exclusive monogamy or sexual abstinence as the only life-styles for adults, and fearful of sex, emotions, nudity, and the body. Many social factors in the twentieth century have radically altered this definition, with clear options for the disabled. Along with the contraceptive technologies, economic liberation of women, and rural-to-urban shift, other social factors that combine to redefine sex and sexual relations are our increasing life expectancy, reduced family size (less infant and maternal mortality), the liberalizing and permission-giving media reports of new life-styles, increased mobility and leisure, and tendencies to delay marriage and accept premarital sex.

In these new definitions, we find new paradigms for gender and gender roles. Gender and gender identity are no longer viewed as static all-or-nothing realities, but as expressions in a lifelong psychosexual developmental process. This process begins with the union of egg and sperm, and the establishment of chromosomal gender in the *XX* or *XY* chromosomes. These genetic elements turn a pair of undifferentiated primordial gonads into either ovaries or testes, which produce their appropriate balance of male and female steroid hormones. The balance of these hormones and their threshold levels then direct internal and external male development with female anatomy developing independent of the steroid hormones. At birth, a male or female gender is assigned to the neonate's anatomy. As the infant grows and explores his or her sexual identity, social scripting and the emerging personal identity work together to fix a firm gender identity by age 3 (*12*).

The emergence of sexual orientation expands this process of becoming a sexual person during the erotic maturation of adolescence. Kinsey's dualistic tension of a ratio between heterosexual and homosexual experiences and fantasies was a useful conception from the late 1800s through the 1970s. However, research into gender orientation and psychosexual identity indicates this operational conception is now obsolete (*3*). In its place, we have Stayton's "panerotic potential paradigm," which rejects Freud's negative polymorphous perversity for a positive image of each person having the potential to reach out in unlimited ways to meet his or her needs for physical communication, sensual contact, and erotic nurturance. We can fulfill our need for nurturance in relations with persons of the same or other gender, in the sensuality and eroticism of nature, music, and art, in the sensual eroticism of our own bodies, and finally in the eroticism and nurturance of mysticism and religion (*14*).

In this psychosexual developmental process we each experience, in our own unique way, a new flexibility emerges that *degenitalizes the traditional view.*

The popularist surveys of Hite and others (*5,6*) indicate the emergence, especially among women, of a new definition of sexuality that is clearly degenitalized or "de-coitalized."

> "There is no reason why physical intimacy . . . should always consist of 'foreplay' followed by intercourse and male orgasm; and there is no reason why intercourse must always be a part of heterosexual sex. Sex is intimate physical contact for pleasure; to share pleasure with another person (or just alone). You can have sex to orgasm, or not to orgasm, genital sex, or just physical intimacy—whatever seems right to you. There is never any reason to think the 'goal' must be intercourse, and to try to make what you feel fit into that context. There is no standard of sexual performance 'out there' against which you must measure yourself (or others). . . . You are free to explore and discover your own sexuality, to learn or unlearn anything you want, and to make physical relations with other people, of either sex, anything you like." (*5*) (Fig. 1)

With the advent of this new awareness, neologisms have been developed to express and emphasize this broader and more accurate

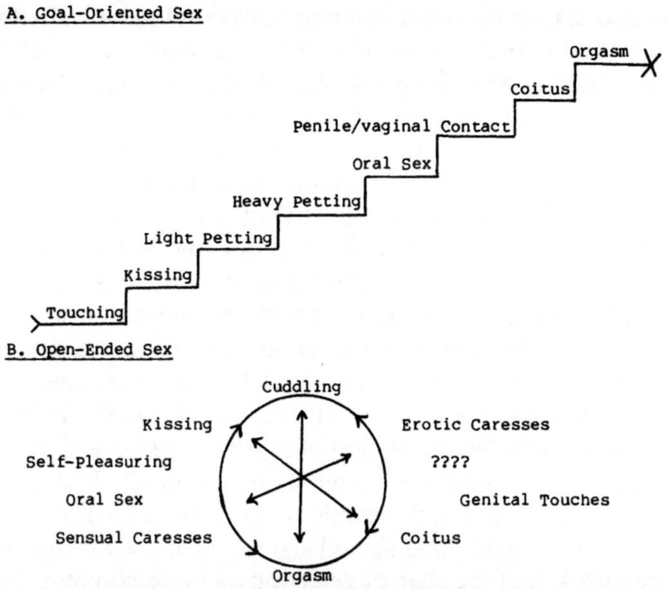

Fig. 1. A comparison of goal-oriented sexual experiences with an open-ended model of sexual expressions. (A) Goal-oriented sexual experiences progress from superficial physical intimacy through a series of progressively more intimate experiences to the climax or ultimate goal of all sexual intimacies, coital intercourse, and orgasm. (B) Nongoal-oriented sexual experiences are open to any outcome that is mutually acceptable, pleasurable, and nurturing.

meaning in a society that is still not comfortable with the new definitions. Leyson has suggested "sexual celebration" instead of sexual intercourse, since sexual activity encompasses not only coitus in the goal-oriented model, but also a wide range of noncoital, erotic expressions, sensuality, and romanticism—music, lights, wine, and other erotic–sensual stimuli. In the open-ended model (Fig. 1), the skin replaces the penis and vagina as the main erotic "organ," encouraging the exploration of the hidden frontiers of personal and interpersonal pleasuring.

A second part of this new definition leads to a rejection of the traditional gender dichotomy of masculine and feminine sexual roles and behaviors. The traditional masculine/feminine conception was that of two opposing gradients or poles. If a woman was truly feminine, she suppressed any behavior and attitude society labeled masculine. The reverse held for a male who had to deny any putatively feminine traits to which he might be inclined. The new view proposes that every sexual person has the potential to express a basic mixture of what has been characterized as masculine and feminine behavioral patterns. In this view, masculinity and femininity are relatively independent but related axes, rather than existing opposite poles of a single dimension. Psychologists now use the term androgynous to express the dynamic balance of *yin* and *yang*, Jung's *animus* and *anima*, the poetic and the rational, the emotional and the intellectual, the feminine and masculine that are part of every person's sexual nature (*13*) (Fig. 2).

In 1948 and 1953, Alfred Kinsey documented the varieties of American sexual behaviors in detailed interviews of a predominantly middle class white group of men and women, most with some college education (*8,9*). These essential behavioral data were complemented by the physiologic work of Masters and Johnson with their work on behavioral treatments for sexual dysfunctions (*10*). In the 1970s, Helen Singer Kaplan added the dimension of sexual aversion and lack of sexual desire to our categories of sexual dysfunction (*7*). In documenting the many psychological and organic origins for sexual dysfunctions, Kaplan and others highlighted altered and negative body image, negative social pressures, and the fear of rejection as three common causes of dysfunction among the able-bodied. These three factors are encountered more frequently by the disabled who seek to continue their sexual relations after the onset of a chronic disease or disabling condition. Persons born with a disabling condition or disease often suffer even more from these factors, since they have never experienced sexual intimacy without this problem and have often been desexed as children because of the reactions of their families, educational system, and society to their disabilities.

The first specialized spinal cord injury (SCI) treatment center was opened in 1944 at Stoke Mandeville Hospital in England under the direction of Sir L. Guttman (*1*). In the 1950s and 1960s, A. E. Comarr initiated the scientific study of the effects of SCI on sexual functioning. Considered by many to be the father of SCI sexual rehabilitation in the USA, Comarr pioneered the classification of male erectile dysfunctions according to clinical findings of reflex status. However, it was not until 1970 that the Rehabilitation Services Administration, an agency of the Federal US Government, formalized a model for support services of the SCI patients in Phoenix, Arizona. It was not until the mid 1970s that male SCI-related sexual dysfunctions were considered a medical problem treatable at the Veterans Administration SCI Centers, where Leyson later initiated the study of female SCI sexual dysfunctions with vaginal myography, thermography, and pressure gradients.

As new health care professionals and the general populations became more aware of the dimensions of sexual needs and relationships among

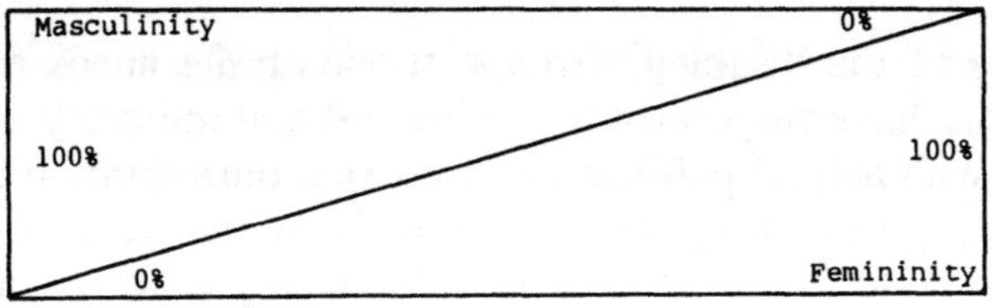

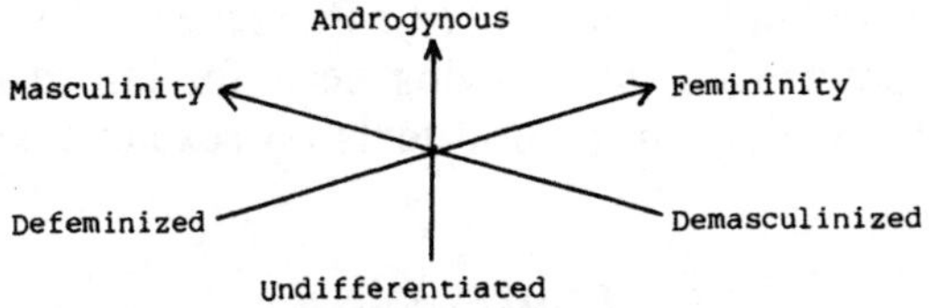

Fig. 2. The traditional model and a new paradigm for masculine/feminine development. The first diagram presents masculinity and femininity as two opposing poles of development. The second model shows these two as different and relatively independent axes, in which moving along either axis does not of necessity prevent development along the other axis. One can, in fact, combine the two axes in an androgynous balance.

the able-bodied population in the 1960s and 1970s, disabled persons were being drawn into the sexual revolution along with everyone else. The civil rights movement created an awareness of the political power of organized minorities that speak out to challenge traditional images, be they ethnic minorities, women, or the gay population.

In 1975, Alex Comfort stressed two factors in the recognition of the handicapped as sexual persons. First, the handicapped have to reject the idea that they are not potentially sexual persons and are, therefore, unattractive to anyone as a sexual partner. The second step is effective militancy—doing something about it. Here the most liberating strategy is open discussion. For couples with a disablement problem, the most helpful first step is discussion with other individuals or couples who share the problem and counseling of each other. In institutions, despite the embarrassment of the staff, patients should demand that the matter be talked out, that privacy be available, that "sexual segregation" be ended, and that disabled children be given adequate sex education and helped to realize their sexual potential. The able-bodied have projected their embarrassment on the disabled; now the disabled are learning to ignore red faces and speak out (2).

The growing participation of disabled persons in the sexual revolution of the 1970s was reinforced by the movement in government funding to deinstitutionalize care of the handicapped and return them to the social mainstream. The growing number of spinal cord injured veterans of the Korean and Vietnam Wars likely added to the militancy for sexual rights of the disabled. Groups servicing the needs of particular populations have responded to the interest and militancy of their constituents with helpful publications on sexual rehabilitation and specific disabilities produced by the American Heart Association, Paralyzed Veterans' Association of America, the Multiple Sclerosis Society of Canada/USA, the United Ostomy Association, the Sister Kenny Institute, and several rehabilitation centers (*13*). Publishers of health care texts have also acknowledged the growing need for information with the publication of a variety of general texts on sexuality and disability.

Conclusion

The deconstruction of traditional sex-related definitions was a necessary preliminary to the recognition of the sexual rights and needs of the disabled. The new degenitalized and nongoal-oriented definitions of sex, the androgenous views of gender roles, and the panerotic potential conception of sexual outlets create a congenial environment in which SCI persons and others with physical disabilities can assert and express their sexuality. The introduction of urodynamics (pressure studies of the urethra and urinary bladder) and refinements of urological vesicourethral operations (sphincterotomy) have made urinary rehabilitation most effective with minimal or no postsurgical sexual impairment. The acceptance and utilization of clean intermittent catherization has made the Foley catheter obsolete, and "sexual celebration" less cumbersome, more hygienic, and enjoyable. Penile prostheses and artificial urinary sphincter implantations can provide an erect penis and urinary continence during any sexual/sensual activity. In addition, militancy and rejection of desexing negative body images by the disabled have combined with changing social conditions and a growing recognition among health professionals of the importance of sexual self-image and expression to create a more holistic view of human sexuality, rehabilitation, and health care.

References

1. Anon. (1983) Bringing research into effective focus: *Rehab. Brief.* Statistical Findings at the Regional Spinal Cord Injury System **6**, 1–4.
2. Comfort, A. (1975) Foreword, in Mooney, Cole, and Chilgren, *Sexual Options for Paraplegics and Quadriplegics* (Little Brown, Boston).
3. Francoeur, R. T. (1982) *Becoming a Sexual Person* (Wiley, New York), pp. 3–41; 511–527; 662–697.

4. Francoeur, R. T. and Francoeur, A. K. (1974) *Hot and Cool Sex: Cultures in Conflict* (Harcourt Brace Jovanovich, New York).
5. Hite, S. (1976) *The Hite Report* (Macmillan, New York).
6. Hite, S. (1981) *The Hite Report on Male Sexuality* (Knopf, New York). p. 365.
7. Kaplan, H. S. (1979) *Disorders of Sexual Desire and Other Concepts and Techniques in Sex Therapy* (Brunner Mazel, New York).
8. Kinsey, A. C., Pomeroy, W. B., and Martin, C. E. (1948) *Sexual Behavior in the Human Male* (Saunders, Philadelphia).
9. Kinsey, A. C., Pomeroy, W. B., Martin, C. E., and Gebhard, P. H. (1953) *Sexual Behavior in the Human Female* (Saunders, Philadelphia).
10. Masters, W. and Johnson, V. (1970) *Human Sexual Response* (Little Brown, Boston).
11. Money, J. and Erhardt, A. (1972) *Man and Woman, Boy and Girl* (Johns Hopkins University, Baltimore).
12. Money, J. and Tucker, P. (1975) *Sexual Signatures: On Being a Man or Woman* (Little Brown, Boston).
13. Reinisch, J. M. and Sanders, S. A. (1984) Hormonal influences on sexual development and behavior, in *Sex and Gender: A Theological and Scientific Inquiry*, Moraczewski, A., ed. (Pope John Center, St. Louis).
14. Stayton, W. R. (1980) A theory of sexual orientation: The universe as a turn-on. *Topics Clin. Nursing.* **1:4**, 1–7.

2

Cross-Cultural and Religious Perspectives

Robert T. Francoeur

Introduction

Two interacting sources and energies mold an individual's development and experiences as a sexual person. On the endogenous side, emerging psychobiologic sexual identity develops from the synergisms of genes, hormones, anatomy, body self-image, and gender identity. On the exogenous side, the individual experiences a constant bombardment of social scripting (*3*). Together, these two forces of sources create the unique realities of sexual identity and experience.

The conceptions, attitudes, and values that become part of a person's developing sexual nature come from many years of interaction with family, friends, peers, and society. One's sexual identity, attitudes, and values arise from the social scripting experienced as individuals breathing a cultural air particular to a social environment. Though vital factors in any such environment, the religious and ethnic elements have often, until recently, been ignored or overlooked by health professionals and sexual counselors. In dealing with the sexual rehabilitation of SCI patients, ethnic and religious factors can frequently be hidden inhibitors.

Able-bodied individuals who are functioning well in their social milieu have little need to be aware of the ethnic and religious influences that affect their sexual attitudes, values, and behavior patterns. This changes when a sexual dysfunction arises and intervention by a second party is sought. The second party may or may not share the same set of subconscious ethnic and religious attitudes and values about what may or may not be acceptable in sexual behaviors and relationships. If intervening health professionals are not aware of possible radical dif-

Sexual Rehabilitation of the Spinal-Cord-Injured Patient
Edited by J.F. Leyson, © 1990 The Humana Press, Inc.

ferences between their sexual values and attitudes and those of their patients, the hoped-for return to normal sexual functioning may be thwarted. When a disabled person is faced with adjusting his or her sexual expressions to the limitations of a physical handicap, these same unspoken religious and ethnic attitudes, expectations, and values about sex and disability may be important factors in the success of any specific intervention.

Before discussing these factors, I must comment on two types of intervention in the sexual rehabilitation of SCI patients and other persons with physical disabilities. When the disability arises after adolescence, the patient usually has had some sexual relationships, including intercourse. A patient with this type of background experience can be given specific sexual information. However, the situation is quite different for someone who has been physically disabled from birth or early childhood.

As mentioned in Chapter 1, such patients have often been treated as asexual children by their families and society, even though they may now be in their late teens or 20s. This desexing occurs even more frequently when the person has grown up in a residential institution. For these patients, even panel discussions on sexual relations and the disabled can be very traumatic and frightening. It is bad enough when a parent who has never mentioned sex suddenly sits down with a 15-year-old son or daughter to explain the facts of life in a few minutes. The desexed, congenitally disabled person may have a similar reaction to a health professional who suddenly recognizes the patient's sexual rights and needs. However, the need to adjust and compensate for a physical disability compounds the patient's fears.

Ethnic Factors

Although the United States is the most ethnically diverse nation in history, the importance and richness of this diversity is veiled by referring to it as "the American melting pot." The pressure to relinquish cultural variations and conform to a single middleclass Anglo-European caucasian cultural system dominated American values until challenged by the civil rights movements of the 1960s and 1970s. As new waves of Cuban, Haitian, Oriental, Islamic, and other immigrants arrived, they were met by the growing militancy of Blacks, Puerto Ricans, and Mexican-Americans. The American "melting pot" was slowly replaced by the realities of diverse ethnic groups fighting with pride to retain their traditions.

"Having seriously changed group relationships in American society, the ethnic identity movements of the 1960s and 1970s should have also had profound impact on the way professionals practiced in the field of mental health" (*5*). But this new consciousness has had an uneven, halting, and controversial impact. A 1968 National Consultation on Ethnic America at Fordham University led to a new ethnotherapy and important breakthroughs in mental health work with Blacks, Jews, and Italians. Still, little can be found in the literature documenting the powerful impact of ethnocultural factors on sexual attitudes, expectations, and values in sexual counseling. In 1983, *Ethnicity and Family Therapy* edited by McGoldrick, Pearce, and Giordano (*7*) and *Contemporary Families and Alternative Lifestyles: Handbook on Research and Theory* edited by Macklin and Rubin (*6*) focused on ethnic factors in marital therapy and research. Scattered among chapters on 20 some American ethnic groups are many references to sexual attitudes and different patterns of male–female relationships that can come into play during sexual rehabilitation. For a full picture, one needs to study these two texts. However, some useful generalizations can be made here.

Some may argue that ethnic generalizations do more harm than good. However, counselors and health professionals can use relatively simple ethnic paradigms, while maintaining an openness to new experience as they work with individuals and couples in an ethnic group. As McGoldrick et al. urge, "We hope readers will move past the stereotypes, using them as starting points from which to learn more" (*7*).

A first generalization, well documented in the literature, suggests that persons with limited education and living in a lower socioeconomic culture frequently view sex and sexual relations in very traditional genital terms as simple coitus with a minimum of fore- and afterplay and oriented primarily to male enjoyment. Since male performance pressures are high, the ability of a male to have an erection whenever desired and intercourse whenever a partner is available becomes a dominant value. Prosthetic penile implants may be very therapeutic psychologically, though the male has little or no sensation during coitus. At the same time, oral sex, masturbation, and erotic massage may be totally unacceptable as an alternative to coitus even without sensation. Males who engage in such alternatives are often viewed with disdain as "not manly" or "unable to do it the way real men should" (*13*).

An impotent working-class SCI male who suggests oral sex as an alternative may place his wife in a uncomfortable dilemma. Cunnilingus may be tolerated because it involves the husband "doing to the passive wife." Fellatio may trigger a strong reaction from the wife, as Rubin reports:

> "How do I know he won't think I'm cheap?"—(is) a question asked over and over again, an issue that dominates these women and their attitudes toward their own sexuality. Some husbands reassure them. Such reassurances remain suspect, however, partly because it's so hard for these women to move past the fears of their own sexuality, with which they have been stamped, and partly because some men are not without their own ambivalence about it. As long as men distinguish between the girls they marry and the girls they use, many women will remain unconvinced by their reassurances and wary about engaging in sexual behaviors that seem to threaten their "good girl" status (*8*).

If a working-class woman refuses to engage in oral sex with her SCI partner, she may be labeled "frigid" and unsympathetic. If she agrees, her partner may consciously or unconsciously react by putting her in the same category as the bar girls and prostitutes he may know. One black SCI woman reported to this author a custom indicative of the variety of ethnic responses to oral sex. In rural Georgia, she reported, persons who engage in oral sex always bring their own dishes, cups, and silverware when going out to eat. If they use a dish of a person who does not engage in oral–genital sex, that dish is broken because it has been "contaminated." The more educated the disabled person is and the higher his or her socioeconomic level, the more open he or she should be to suggestions commonly made to physically disabled persons for whom coitus is not feasible.

A few other examples will help illustrate the diversity of ethnic reactions to sexual matters that the reader can pursue in original sources. With Chinese couples, health professionals should approach sex with "extreme discretion" and not until good rapport has been established. Mention of sexual topics during the holidays or when a woman is pregnant "would be serious breaches of acceptable behavior" and likely to bring the family "bad luck" (*7*). Since, in the Portuguese culture, "a woman's sexuality is seen as powerful, even magical, though unconscious," a female health professional, especially a single woman, needs a cross-sex cotherapist to be effective with a Portuguese male. Even then, direct eye contact between a female therapist and the patient may be considered rude or a sexual overture (*7*). Despite open bantering about sexual matters in the family circle, a Polish male who expresses concern or anxiety about his sexual adjustment to a disability would be implying a need for emotional reassurance and support from his wife, which would be totally inappropriate and unacceptable (*7*).

Religious Factors

Until the early 1960s, any discussion of correlations between sexual values and attitudes and religious traditions could be easily set within a denominational framework. Roman Catholics followed the Vatican statements and positions; Episcopalians were in a more liberal sexual tradition; Methodists, Congregationalists, and Lutherans were somewhere between the Roman Catholics and Episcopalians. Jews were quite liberal, except in the small hassidic and conservative communities.

In a burst of ecumenical dialog, the Second Vatican Council and parallel confessional meetings in the Protestant churches in the 1960s altered all this. A new alignment emerged that focused, not along the old denominational lines, but along diverging cosmologic or philosophic orientations. As a result, a radical split can now be found within each church group. On one end of the spectrum are those who hold a fixed old-world view, in which creation was completed in the beginning with male–female sex roles and heterosexual monogamy. Under this view, premarital sex and adultery are legally proscribed, and there are strong positions on the procreative role of sex and an ascetical tradition necessary to maintain superiority of the spirit over the body, its emotions, and its sexual drives.

On the other end of the spectrum are those who hold a process or evolutionary view of human nature in which sexuality is an ongoing creation to be completed with human cooperation in the future. There is a much more flexible and egalitarian view of male/female relations and roles in this view. Our sexuality becomes a positive, natural, creative energy that permeates everything we do. Its goal is interpersonal communion. Noncoital and nonprocreative sexual activities can express the incarnation of divine love because sex is viewed as a diffused, degenitalized, sensual embodiment—a kind of positive "polymorphic perversity"—Stayton's "panerotic potential" (*9*). Thus, a variety of primary and secondary or satellite relationships, genital and nongenital, intimate and passing, become acceptable with the religious covenant and life (*2*).

Both the fixed-world view and the process view can be found within the divisions of the Protestant, Catholic, Jewish, and Islamic traditions. The authors of the liberal Presbyterian work-study document on sexuality (*11*) are very much in agreement with the liberal view of the Catholic Theological Society Report on human sexuality (*4*) and the United Church of Christ statement (*10*). On the other end of the spectrum, there is considerable agreement and convergence in the official

Vatican views of sexual behavior and relationships, the Protestant Moral Majority, Eastern Orthodox, and hassidic Jews (*1*). Alternatives to coital sexual expression and to heterosexual exclusive monogamous marital relations that could be suggested to SCI persons as part of their sexual rehabilitation might be quite acceptable to persons with a religious view rooted in the process perspective and totally unacceptable to others of the same denomination who hold a fixed-world view. Suggesting, for example, that an SCI patient explore just what he or she can do sexually with a surrogate partner might be acceptable for a patient holding a process-oriented religious view and be rejected outright by a second person holding a purely religious fixed-world view, regardless of denominational affiliation.

This new alignment of Judaeo–Christian religious views of sexuality and relationships parallels the results of Yankelovich's analysis of 40 years of changing American values (*12*). This analysis revealed that 20% of Americans are basically unchanging in their traditional views of male–female relations and marriage values, 17% are definitely committed to change and new values, and 63% are caught between these two ends of the spectrum, changing but still not fully committed to the new values and lifestyles. Older persons in the lower socioeconomic group with a limited education and those living in rural areas more often fell into the traditionalist group, which rejects any change in sexual values or relations.

Islamic religious views also appear to fit this dichotomy in world views. Fundamentalists in Pakistan and Iran are strongly patriarchal in their repression of female sexuality and homosexuality, whereas more liberal Islamic traditions pursue paths found in liberal Judaeo–Christian traditions. A similar dichotomy between Hindu celibate asceticism and the Tantric celebration of sexuality as a path to the divine may or may not be linked with the fixed vs process world views found in western culture. As yet, the possible effects of sexual values in Shintoism, Buddhism, and other eastern religions on sexual therapy and rehabilitation have not been thoroughly explored.

Conclusion

The generalizations on ethnic and religious factors in sexual attitudes and values offered here should be taken as *open-ended starting points* by the health professional working with a particular patient. If the professional is sensitive to the possible importance and variations these factors can have in the rehabilitation process, the mutual objectives of patient and professional may be more readily achieved. As sociological researchers and health professionals become more aware of these issues, one can expect to find much more helpful and specific information in the literature on these factors in the years ahead.

References

1. Francoeur, R. T. (1982) *Becoming a Sexual Person*, pp. 661–698. Wiley, New York.
2. Francoeur, R. T. (1983) Religious reactions to alternative lifestyles, in *Contemporary Families and Alternative Lifestyles: Handbook on Research and Theory*, pp. 387–394 (Macklin, E. and Robin, R., eds.) Sage, Beverly Hills, CA.
3. Gagnon, J. and Simon, W. (1973) *Sexual Conduct: The Social Origins of Human Sexuality* (Aldine, Chicago).
4. Kosnick, A., Carroll, W., Cunningham, A., Modras, R., and Schulte, J. (1977) *Human Sexuality: New Directions in American Catholic Thought* (Paulist Press, New York).
5. Levine, I. M. (1983) Introduction, in *Ethnicity and Family Therapy* (McGoldrick, M., Pearce, J. K., and Giordano, J., eds.) Guilford Press, New York.
6. Macklin, E. and Rubin, R. (1983) *Contemporary Families and Alternative Lifestyles: Handbook on Research and Theory* (Sage, Beverly Hills, CA).
7. McGoldrick, M., Pearce, J. K., and Giordano, J. (1983) *Ethnicity and Family Therapy* xvi, 398–403, 426–427, 537, (Guilford Press, New York).
8. Rubin, L. B. (1977) Sexual liberation and marital strain in the working class. *Sexual Med. Today.* **Sept.**, 19–25.
9. Stayton, W. R. (1980) A theory of sexual orientation: The universe as a turn-on. *Topics Clin. Nursing.* **1**, 4, 1–7.
10. United Church of Christ, Board of Home Ministries: Human Sexuality: A Preliminary Study. The Eleventh General Synod.
11. United Presbyterian Church in the U.S.A. (1970) Sexuality and the Human Community (UPC Press, Philadelphia).
12. Yankelovich, D. (1982) *New Rules: Searching for Self-Fulfillment in a World Turned Upside Down* (Random House, New York).
13. Yorburg, B. (1974) *Sexual Identity: Sex Roles and Social Change.* (Wiley, New York).

3

Female Sexuality

Beverly Whipple

Introduction

We are all sexual beings from the day we are born to the day we die. How we choose to express our sexuality depends on a number of complex factors that affect many aspects of our lives. The term sexuality refers to the totality of a being—to human qualities, and not just the genitalia and their function. It includes all of the qualities—biological, psychological, emotional, social, cultural, and spiritual—that make people who they are. People have the capacity to express their sexuality in any of these areas. An expression of the psychological aspect, for example, is the person's inner self-concept—I am a man or I am a woman, or I am "half a man," or I am no longer attractive. By viewing sexuality holistically, the health care provider can better understand how a spinal cord injury can affect a person's total health (*48*).

Women in our society have been considered passive receptors of male sexual expression. Prior to the research of the past three decades, it had been denied that women had sexual needs and sexual responses. This may account for the paucity of research concerning female sexual response, as well as the paucity of research concerning spinal-cord-injured women. Most of the literature cited in the references tells us that the major research related to sexual function and spinal cord injury has involved male samples (*49*). We are told that "the neurophysiological and neuroanatomic basis of the female orgasm have not yet been studied and one must rely on inferences from the male in this area" (*29*).

When we talk about female sexuality and "normal" female sexual response, we must keep in mind that the information that is being disseminated is based on a limited number of studies done with a

Sexual Rehabilitation of the Spinal-Cord-Injured Patient
Edited by J.F. Leyson, © 1990 The Humana Press, Inc.

volunteer population of usually white, middle-class, college-educated, able-bodied women. This biased sample may affect the knowledge we have to date, or it may turn out to be representative. Only more research with samples from different races, cultures, and physical abilities will support or reject these data. Although the information that will be disseminated in this chapter is based on the average response patterns of the samples tested, it must be kept in mind that each person, whether able-bodied or with a disability, is a unique individual capable of a variety of sexual responses. To say that a person must fit into a monolithic pattern of the one "right, healthy, and normal way to respond" will help to limit that person's responses as well as limit the effectiveness of the health professional in providing information and counseling.

Anatomy, Physiology, and Sexual Response Cycles in the Female

When considering the anatomy and physiology of sexual response, we must consider the total body as the sex organs and not just the genitals. Special sexual as well as more subtle stimuli can trigger erotic feelings and physiological responses. Tactile stimuli, such as gentle kissing and caressing, seem to be more potent erotic stimuli for women in our culture that are visual stimuli (*29*). Many women are unaware of the changes that are taking place in their bodies in response to stimuli and deny that they are sexually aroused. It is easy to understand a woman's unawareness of the changes taking place in her body because many of a woman's specific sexual reactions are internal, and also because women have been culturalized to be passive and deny their sexual feelings.

Little was known about the physiology of sexual response before Masters and Johnson published their pioneering research in 1966 (*34*). They found that two principal physiological changes take place—vasocongestion and myotonia. Vasocongestion is the congestion of tissues and blood vessels, usually venous vessels, and was said to occur first in response to sexual stimulation. Myotonia, increased muscle tension, was the second physiological response to occur with sexual stimulation (*34*). Perry and Whipple (*39*), using a combination probe that included a vaginal myograph and a photoplethysmograph, found that measurable contractions of the orgasmic platform muscles preceded vasocongestion. They hypothesize that vasocongestion follows myotonia (*39*). Whatever the sequence of events, vasocongestion and myotonia are believed to be responsible for the changes observed during the sexual response cycle.

Using direct observation and measurement of the changes that occurred with sexual stimulation, Masters and Johnson reported their findings using arbitrarily chosen phases. They divide that sexual response cycle into four phases: excitement, plateau, orgasm, and resolution (*34*). These phases correspond to the levels of sexual arousal and describe the typical responses. Excitement results from any source of physical and/or psychological stimulation. The intensity of this phase can increase with increased stimulation, or be interrupted or ended by distracting stimuli. The plateau phase follows excitement if adequate stimulation is continued. This phase can also be affected by distracting stimuli. Orgasm, the involuntary climax of sexual tension, involves only a few seconds of the sexual response cycle. During orgasm, vasocongestion and myotonia are released. There is a great deal of variation in the subjective and objective reports of female orgasm. Resolution is the phase in which there is a return to the unaroused state. Females have the capacity for multiple orgasms during any point in the resolution phase.

Although Masters and Johnson (*34*) state that females are capable of great variation in both the intensity and duration of orgasmic experience, they describe three of the most prevalent patterns (Fig. 1). In pattern 1, the woman experiences multiple orgasms and then a resolution phase. In pattern 2, there is a nonorgasmic cycle in which several peaks are recorded in the plateau phase and a longer resolution phase occurs. Pattern 3 shows a cycle in which the woman's excitement is interrupted or distracted, although an orgasm occurs followed by a rapid resolution phase.

The specific physiological changes observed and reported by Masters and Johnson (*34*) during the various phases are well known. During the excitement phase of the human sexual response cycle, there is an appearance of vaginal lubrication, which occurs 10–30 s after the onset of sexual stimulation. Vaginal lubrication occurs because of vasocongestion in the walls of the vagina. This leads to moisture seeping across the vaginal lining in a process called transudation. Early in this stage, the amount of vaginal lubrication may be so small that it is not noticed. However, the amount usually increases with further stimulation. The glans clitoris becomes tumescent or enlarged, and the clitoral shaft increases in diameter and elongates. The inner two-thirds of the vagina expand, while the cervix and uterus are pulled upward and the labia majora flatten and move apart. The labia minora may enlarge in diameter. The nipples typically become erect during this phase as a result of contractions of small muscle fibers. Later in the excitement phase, the veins in the breasts become more visible as a result

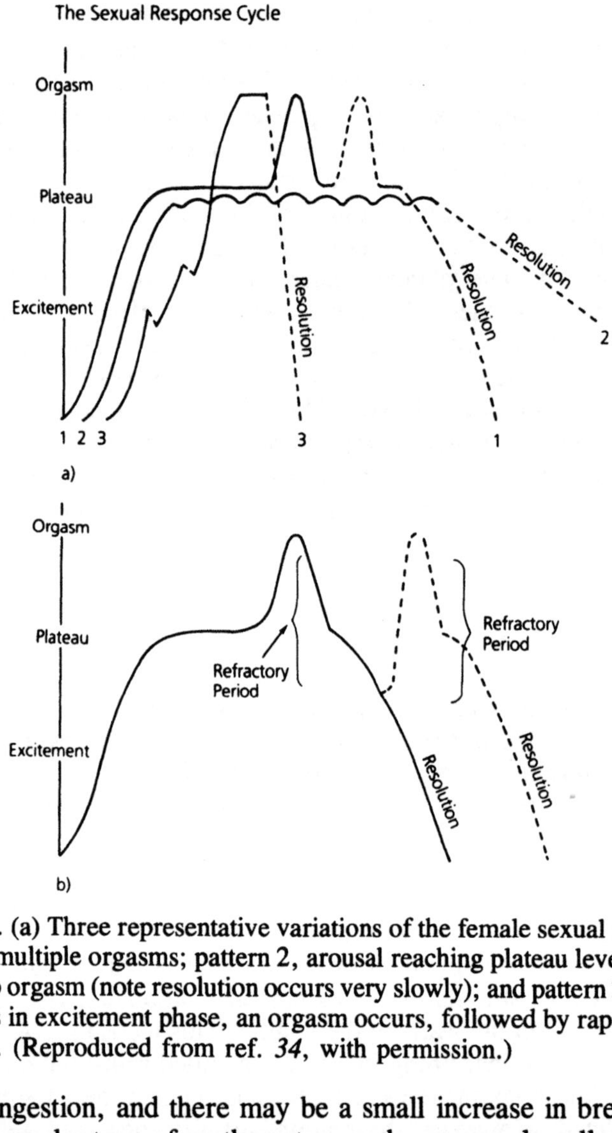

Fig. 1. (a) Three representative variations of the female sexual response: pattern 1, multiple orgasms; pattern 2, arousal reaching plateau level without going on to orgasm (note resolution occurs very slowly); and pattern 3, several brief drops in excitement phase, an orgasm occurs, followed by rapid resolution phase. (Reproduced from ref. *34*, with permission.)

of vasocongestion, and there may be a small increase in breast size. A maculopapular type of erythematous rash, commonly called the sex flush, may first appear over the epigastrium either late in the excitement phase or early in the plateau phase. This sex flush then spreads rapidly over the breasts and then on the anterior chest wall (Fig. 2).

During the plateau phase, vasocongestion in the outer third of the vagina causes the tissues to swell. This reaction, called the "orgasmic platform" by Masters and Johnson, causes a narrowing of the introitus

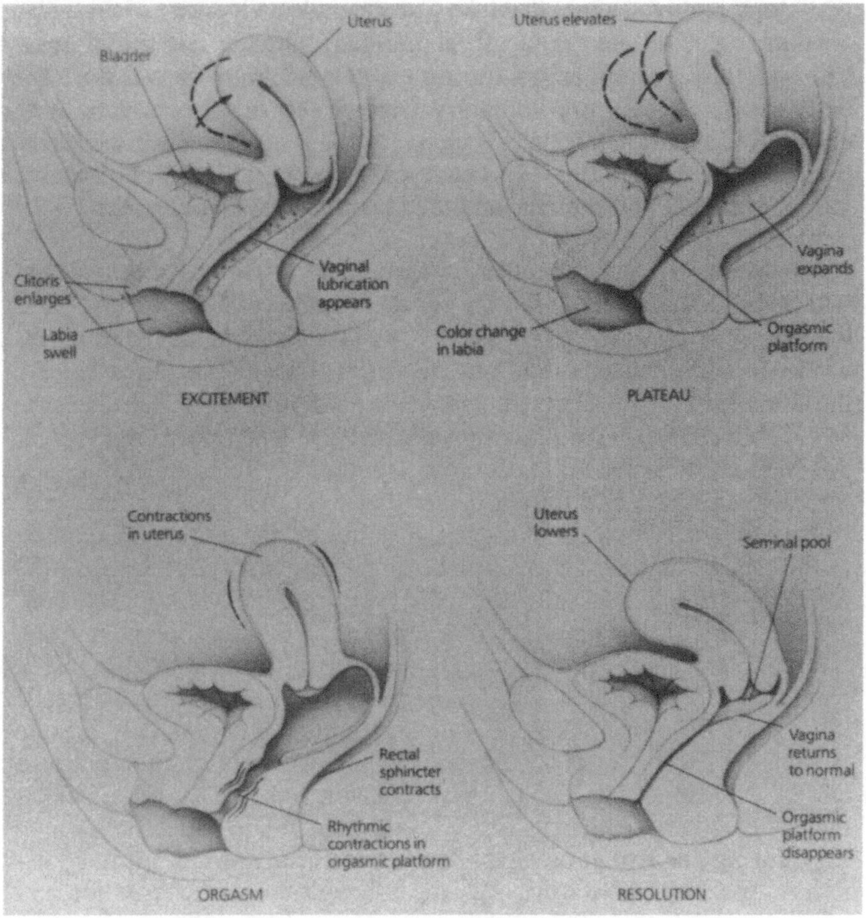

Fig. 2. Changes during the female sexual response. (Reproduced from ref. *34*, with permission.)

of the vagina. During this phase, the inner two-thirds of the vagina expand slightly more in size as the uterus becomes more elevated. Vaginal lubrication may diminish some during this phase. The clitoris retracts underneath the clitoral hood. The clitoris does not lose sensation during this change. In both nulliparous and multiparous women, the labia majora continue to become engorged. However, this is more pronounced in the multipara. The labia minora undergo a color change from bright red to a deep wine color. The areolae of the breast continue to swell, and the nipple erection usually becomes obscured. There is a further increase in breast size.

Other bodily changes that take place include an increase in muscular tension, especially in the facial, abdominal, buttock, and thigh areas. The sex flush, which began during excitement, may spread over the body. Some women use voluntary vaginal and rectal contractions to enhance stimulation during this phase. Hyperventilation occurs, along with a heart rate of 100–175 beats/min. The systolic blood pressure may increase 20–60 mmHg, and the diastolic pressure elevates 10–20 mmHg.

If effective sexual stimulation continues, a point may be reached where the body suddenly discharges its accumulated sexual tension in the orgasmic phase. Physiologically, certain changes may take place. There are simultaneous rhythmic muscular contractions of the uterus, the outer third of the vagina (the orgasmic platform), and the anal sphincters. The first few contractions are intense and close together at 0.8-second intervals. As the orgasm continues, the contractions may diminish in force and duration, and occur at less regular intervals. Respiratory rates may go as high as 40/min, and the pulse may increase to 110–180 beats/min. The systolic blood pressure may be elevated 30–80 mmHg and the diastolic 20–40 mmHg. According to Masters, Johnson, and Kolodny (*35*), women often describe an orgasm as beginning with a momentary sense of suspension, quickly followed by an intensely pleasurable feeling that usually begins at the clitoris and spreads throughout the pelvis. They do state that orgasms vary not only for one person at different times, but also for each individual (*35*). Though maintaining that "an orgasm is an orgasm is an orgasm" (*35*), they do allow that, subjectively, orgasms are felt and interpreted differently.

During the resolution phase, the clitoris returns to its normal position within 5–10 s after the orgasm, although the vasocongestion and tumescence of the clitoris dissipate more slowly. There is rapid detumescence of the orgasmic platform. The labia and vaginal wall return to their normal color and size. There is a reversal of the sex flush and a decrease in breast size. The respiratory rate, pulse rate, and blood pressure return to normal levels. A film of perspiration may appear. If there has been considerable excitement but orgasm has not occurred, resolution takes a longer time. Females are capable of being multiorgasmic and may go onto having more orgasms, depending on effective sexual stimulation and the person's interest.

Other researchers reported data that differ from Masters and Johnson's response cycle. Kaplan (*29*) developed a model that divides the response pattern into two stages: excitement and orgasm. During excitement, the sexual responses result primarily from vasocongestion controlled by the parasympathetic nervous systems. Vaginal lubrication is mediated by acetylcholine, a secretion of the parasympathetic nervous system. Orgasm and the rhythmic contractions are controlled by the release of norepinephrine secreted by the nerves in the sympathetic division of the autonomic nervous system. Francoeur feels there are both conscious and reflective controls over sexual responses (*21*).

Singer (*43*) criticized Masters and Johnson's selection of research subjects who could achieve orgasm by masturbation of the clitoris. He felt that his provided biased data in terms of interpreting that there was only one kind of female orgasm. He felt that women who were capable of achieving orgasm from vaginal stimulation alone should also be evaluated. The Singers proposed three types of orgasm: vulval, uterine, and blended (*44*). They call the "normative" orgasm of Masters and Johnson a vulval orgasm, characterized by involuntary, rhythmic contractions of the orgasmic platform. The uterine orgasm is defined by contractions of the uterus itself, and not by contractions of the orgasmic platform. They state that the uterine orgasm includes apnea and is caused by buffeting of the uterus. Support for their contention that stronger uterine contractions occur in the uterine orgasm came from Cyril and Beatrice Fox (*19*). The Singers' third type of orgasm is called blended, and is a combination of uterine and vulval. "It is characterized by contractions of the orgasmic platform, but the orgasm is subjectively regarded as deeper than a vulval orgasm" (*43*).

The hypotheses of Singer and Fox are partially supported by the work of Perry and Whipple (*38,40*). They have reported that there is a sensitive area within the anterior wall of the vagina about halfway between the back of the pubic bone and the cervix along the course of the urethra, which swells when stimulated and is reported by research subjects as being the "trigger point" for their deeper orgasms (*30,40*). Perry and Whipple have named this sensitive area the Grafenberg spot in honor of Ernst Grafenberg, who in 1950 described its existence and association with an orgasmic explusion of fluid from the urethra. Grafenberg (*22*) noted that stimulation of this area does not elicit contractions of the pubococcygeus muscle, but rather contractions of the upper vaginal barrel and the uterus itself.

Using a vaginal myograph to measure EMG readings of the pubococcygeus muscle (orgasmic platform) and a uterine myograph to measure EMG of the cervix of the uterus, Perry and Whipple (*38*) were able to record EMG levels from two ends of the vagina simultaneously, something which had not been previously done by researchers who used a single intravaginal or intrauterine electrode. They were able to determine that stimulation of the clitoris provided muscle response patterns different from stimulation of the area of the Grafenberg spot. They also observed that manual stimulation of the Grafenberg spot to the point of orgasm showed an absence of a "tenting" effect (the ballooning out of the vagina and elevation of the uterus that occurs with clitoral stimulation). In response to Grafenberg spot stimulation, the vagina collapses and exerts great pressure against the palpating finger or penis. The cervix is pressed firmly in the vagina. The introitus of the vagina often gapes, as if to release the stimulator (*38*). Perry and Whipple call this the A-frame effect to show the difference that results from Grafenberg spot stimulation as compared to clitoral stimulation. Clitoral stimulation leads to an elevation of the uterus, whereas stimulation of the area of the Grafenberg spot leads to a descent of the uterus. Muscular contractions from clitoral stimulation are stronger in the area of the pubococcygeus muscle or orgasmic platform. Muscular contractions from Grafenberg spot stimulation are stronger in the uterus and upper part of the vagina (*38*) (Fig. 3).

The theories of Masters and Johnson (*34*) and Kaplan (*29*) describe one reflexive pathway in sexual response. In women, it includes the clitoris as its major source of stimulation, the pudendal nerve as its pathway, and the major part of the pubococcygeus muscle (or "orgasmic platform") as the major manifestation of myotonic buildup and discharge in orgasm (*39*). According to Perry and Whipple, this single-reflex model is unable to account for the awareness of the separation of emission or ejaculatory inevitability from ejaculation, in either males or females. However, Kaplan divided ejaculation into two phases (*29*) that can be expanded to explain the processes in both sexes (*40*).

Perry and Whipple (*39*) hypothesize that there is a second pathway that included the Grafenberg spot as its major source of stimulation, the pelvic plexus as its major pathway, and the musculature of the uterus, the bladder, the urethra, and the paraurethral glands as its major myotonic manifestation. When this second nerve pathway is properly conditioned, ejaculation in females is likely to occur. Ejaculation from the urethra does occur in most men and in a smaller percentage of women (*40*). Involvement of the uterus may account for the subjective feeling of a deeper or uterine orgasm (*38,39*).

The fluid expelled from the urethra in women was examined by Addiego et al. (*1*) and by Belzer et al. (*6*), and found to be different in chemical composition from urine samples from the same subjects. The ejaculate specimens were higher in tartrate-inhibited acid phosphatase and glucose, and lower in urea and creatinine than were the urine specimens. It has been hypothesized that this fluid is different from urine. Perry and Whipple also found that women who claim to ejaculate have much stronger voluntary contractions of their pelvic muscles than do

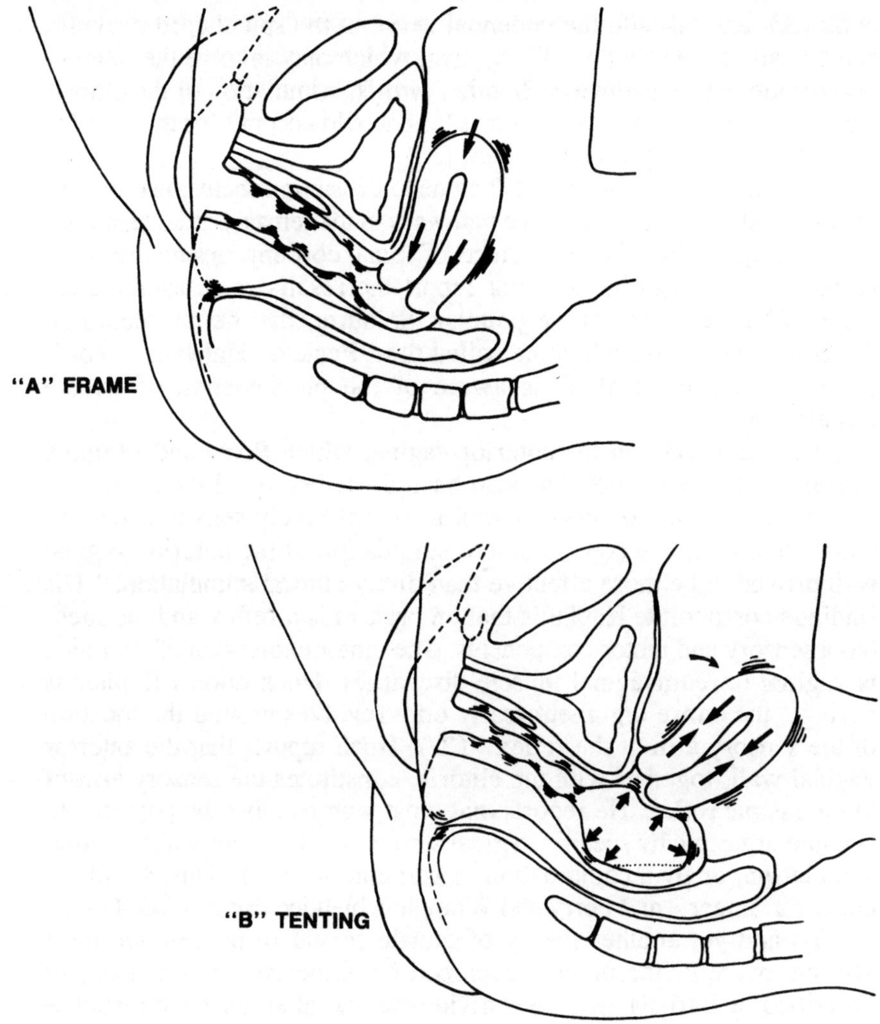

Fig. 3. (A) Response from Grafenberg spot stimulation. (B) Response from clitoral stimulation. (Illustrations by Stephen Z. Cohen.)

women who do not ejaculate. They were concerned that these women were being diagnosed and treated as having urinary stress incontinence, when the only time they lost this fluid from the urethra was during orgasm (*40*). Further research is underway concerning this phenomenon and many studies have been undertaken.

Perry and Whipple also proposed an explanation for the blended orgasm based on their research. The fact that the pelvic nerve, which comes off the hypogastric plexus, and the pelvic plexus partially overlap at S2, S3, and S4 with the pudendal nerve in the spinal cord provides some basis for the "blended" orgasm, which may involve the interaction of both nerve pathways. In other words, stimulation of the clitoris and the Grafenberg spot at the same time would account for the blended orgasm reported by many women (*38*).

In France, Tordjman (*46,47*) came to the same conclusion concerning the existence of two reflexive pathways in the female sexual response. His findings are based on the effects of spinal cord injuries on orgasmic responses, although he does not report the results of measurements. He also has reported, in the popular literature, that he too identified the Grafenberg spot, which he called the "Facie de Haleban." Tordjman also reports that he is aware of the phenomenon of female ejaculation.

This sensitivity in the anterior vagina, which Perry and Whipple call the Grafenberg spot, has also been described by Hoch (*27*), who has found the anterior vaginal wall to be extremely sensitive and excitable and that, "in some women, stimulation of the anterior vaginal wall proved to be more effective than direct clitoral stimulation." His findings corroborate Kaplan's that an orgasm is a reflex and, as such, has a sensory and motor components. The motor expression of the reflex is vaginal (circumvaginal muscle discharge). Hoch quotes Kaplan as saying "the entire argument really only revolves around the location of the sensory arm of the reflex" (*27*). Hoch reports that the anterior vaginal wall, together with the clitoris, constitutes the sensory arm of the orgasmic reflex. He reports that most women have the potential to become orgasmic by specific vaginal stimulation (anterior wall), clitoral stimulation, or by a combination of stimulations (*27*). This would account for Singer's and Perry and Whipple's blended orgasm (*40,43,44*).

To add yet another theory of female sexual responses, we must also be aware of the model developed by Zilbergeld and Ellison, as described by Barbach (*3*). They divide the sexual arousal and response cycle into five parts: desire, arousal, physiological readiness, orgasm, and satisfaction.

This author believes that there is not enough research data to determine completely what is happening in the female body during sexual response and orgasm. Many definitions of orgasm must be considered. When discussing changes that may occur in a woman's orgasmic response caused by a spinal cord injury, we must be aware of, when speaking of orgasm, whether we are referring to the area stimulated, the area in which the orgasm is perceived, or the physiological and anatomical changes that take place in the body. We must realize that we may not be considering all aspects of a woman's response pattern if we are questioning the reports of a woman who has a spinal cord injury and judging her to be having a phantom orgasm because there is no accompanying series of regular pelvic contractions. The response may be in another area of the body. Bohlen (*8*), whose research on orgasm showed that "results from our laboratory fail to reveal any simple correlations between the level of perceived pleasure and amount of physiologic change during arousal and orgasm," also said that some researchers have been forcing the definition of orgasm to conform to a narrow physiologic mold, rather than listening to what women say is an orgasm. He asks if:

> perhaps we are like the man who lost his keys in the street at night. Yet, he looked only under the street lamp because there he can search thoroughly. Sex researchers are limiting their examination of orgasm to the objective physiologic changes that they can measure, and in turn using these changes to define orgasm. In doing so, they are ignoring the actual issue that brings attention to orgasm in the first place—the fact that it feels good. Should we be searching for the keys wherever they are instead of where we can presently measure most carefully?

Before we can look at the response patterns of women with spinal cord injuries and try to classify their responses, it is important to realize that women are capable of experiencing a variety of orgasmic responses, and that a woman's experience cannot be denied or negated because it does not fit into a monolithic model developed as the "normal" sexual response pattern. The present author feels that a disservice has been done to able-bodied women and women with a disability by not listening to what they are saying feels pleasurable to them. As Singer said, "there is no single correct, definitive, or supremely normal kind of female orgasm. Some people differ in so many aspects of their being, one should expect variability in their modes of sexual satisfaction as well" (*43*).

Alterations in the Neurophysiology of the Sexual Response Post Spinal Cord Injury

After reviewing the literature available (*4,5,7,9,10,12,17,23–25, 28,33,37,41,42*), one could come to the conclusion that women with spinal cord injuries are capable of menstruating, conceiving, and giving birth. However, one might wonder, after reading the current literature, whether women with a disability have any libido. Then one might judge whether, when women with spinal cord injuries do engage in sexual intercourse, it is in the supine position and for the purpose of procreation, certainly not for their own enjoyment. Does the lack of research and failure to acknowledge women with spinal cord injuries as sexual beings result from the smaller number of women who have spinal cord injuries, and thus the smaller number of research subjects available? Or does the lack of research occur because most researchers are male and, thus, are more interested in male sexual responses? Or is it because women often assume the passive role in sexual intercourse, so that this is judged to be normal? To quote one reference, "Paraplegic women, because their role can be passive, may enjoy intercourse and be perfectly capable of satisfying their mate. Little is known about their capacity for orgasm, however, because the majority of clients with paraplegia are men . . ." (*7*). Whatever the reason, most references state that female response patterns will have to be extrapolated from the research concerning male responses.

Woods (*49*) does this and describes the neurophysiology in terms of Masters and Johnson's sexual response cycle. During the excitement phase, physiological stimuli are transmitted by ascending sensory pathways and/or psychic impulses by descending motor pathways. The clitoris appears to be the focal receptive point for sensual stimuli, especially tactile ones. The afferent fibers of the pelvic and pudendal nerves convey impulses to the sacral cord, where synapses with parasympathetic efferent nerves to the pelvis evoke reflex erectile responses in the clitoris. Reflex centers in the brain may be activated by psychic stimuli, which in turn creates vaginal lubrication and clitoral erection. Local reflexes important in orgasms are thought to be integrated into the lumbar and sacral regions of the cord.

During the plateau phase, as excitement intensifies, the parasympathetic impulses stimulate Bartholin's gland to secrete mucus immediately inside the vaginal introitus. Contraction of the perineal musculature in the female during orgasms is thought to be caused by impulses from visceral afferent pathways, which eventually reach efferent fibers of the hypogastric nerves (Fig. 4) (*49*). In other words, the somatic, parasympathetic, and sympathetic nervous systems all influence sexual function. Obviously, an injury to the spine can affect two or more of these systems and their associated sexual functions. Yet even with complete "clinically" severing of the spinal cord, sexual responses are still possible for most women with spinal cord injuries.

There have been a few subjective and objective studies done to determine whether women who have a spinal cord injury do indeed experience orgasm. Bregman and Hadley (*10*) interviewed 31 spinal cord injured

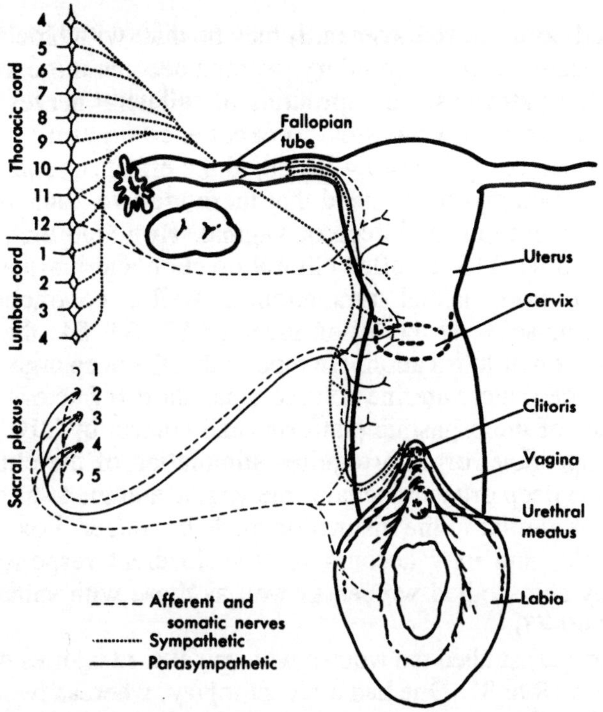

Fig. 4. Neurologic bases of female sexual response. (Reproduced from ref. *49*, with permission.)

women, all of whom had had at least one sexual experience since their injuries. Twenty-seven reported having had intercourse. "Most subjects' descriptions of orgasm were very similar to those of able-bodied women as reported by Kinsey and associates and Masters and Johnson." Three of the subjects reported orgasms that were not different from those before their injuries. Some subjects found certain sexual positions to be more pleasurable than others, such as the woman on top, the woman lying on her back with legs up and back, or the couple facing each other, while she sat on his lap and they moved in a rocking position (*10*). These positions are the same as those mentioned by women who enjoy orgasm from stimulation of their Grafenberg spot. This may be because of the nerve pathways that are intact. Methods of physical stimulation enjoyed most by the subjects were body massage, rubbing each other's genitals, oral–genital intercourse, and sucking the woman's breast. Bregman and Hadley (*10*) state that it is interesting to note how much potential people still have to experience orgasm and sexual pleasure, despite the fact that significant parts of their bodies are sensationless and motionless. It is concluded that satisfactory sexual adjustment can be achieved for many spinal-cord-injured women. It may be that, with blocking of one pathway because of the cord injury, women become more aware of or develop other pathways, i.e., sprouting of collateral nerves (regrowth of surviving neuronal processes) to experience orgasm.

In France, Tordjman (*46,47*) studied the effects of spinal cord injuries on women and determined that there are two kinds of orgasm: superficial or clitoral, and deep or vaginal. He found that, when the lesion was above T10, a reflex clitoral erection and lubrication could be observed during sexual stimulation, as well as contractions of the perivaginal muscles. If the lesion included S2, S3, S4, there was no clitoral erection or lubrication. He reports that the deep orgasm has different characteristics: uterine contractions, short refractory phase, no contractions of the orgasmic platform, and control by T10, T11, and L1. The superficial orgasm requires stimulation of the clitoral area, whereas, the deep orgasm includes the vagina and the total body (*47*). This again is similar to the distinction made by Singer, Fox, and Perry and Whipple, and may account for the different response patterns reported by able-bodied women as well as those with spinal cord injuries (*20,40,43*).

Leyson (*31*) studied ten women with spinal cord injuries whose ages ranged from 18 to 81. One had a recent injury, whereas two had acute and seven had chronic spinal cord lesions. He used an EMG urodynamic anal probe, both anally and vaginally, to measure the results of stimulation of the anterior vaginal wall and the clitoral area. The results showed that two acute and two chronic complete sacral-cord-injured women complaining of anorgasmia showed no spike potentials. Four of the women with incomplete and recovering lesions revealed increased EMG potentials, which coincided with their genital sensations and orgasmic experiences. He also studied temperature change and degree of wetness. It would be helpful for researchers to study EMG while using a photoplethysmograph and thermography at the same time to obtain more accurate assessments (*20*). It would also be useful to know what the orgasmic response pattern of the women was before injury. In other words, did they have orgasms and from what form of stimulation? From the limited research that has been done, it seems that women who have had a spinal cord injury (SCI) are capable of experiencing sexual pleasure.

Implications for Sex Counseling and Therapy

Although the information disseminated here is based on data demonstrating what people can do, it must be remembered that each person, able-bodied or with a disability is a unique individual capable of a variety of sexual responses. It is also important to be aware that we do not label people according to a certain medical diagnosis. A label such as disabled or handicapped (physically-challenged) implies that all people so labeled have the same needs. This negates the individual who is a unique person; a person first who happens to have a problem such as a spinal cord injury. It is important to keep this in mind, so that counseling will be given to the person and not to the disability.

An individual who is counseling clients and their significant others must be aware that some health-care providers make value judgments on clients whose beliefs or practices do not meet with their standards of acceptable behavior. Many times, they are unaware that they are making value judgments. It is important for the counselor to be aware of and accept the patient's own feelings and value system before offering any counseling.

It is also important to consider what the health care provider views as the goal of sexual expression and experiences. Often in our technological society, we think that sexuality consists only of genital expression. According to Timmers et al. (*45*), there are two attitudes. The most common is goal-directed, which can be compared to climbing a flight of stairs. The first step is touching, leading to the next step of kissing, the next to caressing, then to vagina/penis contact, which leads to the final step of intercourse and orgasm. The goal both partners have in mind is orgasm. If the sexual experience does not lead to a fulfillment of the goal, then problems result. Another way to look at sexual experiences is pleasure or nongoal-directed expression. This can be conceptualized as a circle, with each expression of the circle considered an end in itself. Whether the experience is kissing, self-touching, oral sex, holding, intercourse, touching, manual sex, and so on, each is an end in itself, each is satisfying to the couple, and there is no need to have this form of expression lead to anything else. If the counselor is "genital–orgasm goal directed," he or she may have difficulty suggesting alternative forms of sexual expression to the couple being counseled.

One method that is frequently employed in sex counseling and therapy has been developed by Annon (*2*). It is a conceptual scheme he calls the P-LI-SS-IT model. The four levels are *P*ermission, *L*imited *I*nformation, *S*pecific *S*uggestions, and *I*ntensive *T*herapy. Theoretically, each succeeding level requires increasing degrees of knowledge, training, and skill on the part of the counselor. The model offers guidelines that help the counselor to distinguish problems that can be handled and those that require greater knowledge, training, and skill. This model can be applied when counseling couples or individuals who have a spinal cord injury. Whenever possible, the client's significant other should be included in sexuality counseling or therapy.

One of the most important things any woman with a spinal cord injury needs in sexuality counseling is permission to acknowledge that her sexuality is still an important part of her being. She is still a sexual being; she is not asexual. Applying Annon's (*2*) model, the women may need permission to engage in activities that were normal for her before her injury, such as relating to others, going out socially as well as professionally, enjoying masturbation, oral sex, and intercourse. Her partner may need permission to acknowledge and accept her as a sexual being.

Limited information provides clients with specific factual information directly relevant to their particular sexual concerns. This information may be disseminated through reading material, talking about sexual enhancement, or attending a sexual attitude reassessment workshop (*26*). Discussions of feelings of self-esteem as well as society's view of a person in a wheelchair will help to provide the client with insight into these areas.

Specific suggestions mark the level that requires the counselor not only to be able to give permission and limited information, but also give accurate neurological, physical, and psychological information. Suggestions can be given about various forms of sexual stimulation, including vibrators. Women can be told that people have orgasms from sensory input to areas of the body other than the genitals. The area around the injury and just above it can become very erogenous and/or hypersensitive for some people. Some authors have suggested that people with spinal cord injuries have "phantom" or "para" orgasms (*36,42*). However, Knight is quoted as saying, "The human being is too complex in his or her repertoire of physical and psychic responses to discredit any experience as 'phantom' " (*11*). If a woman, with or without a cord injury, says that she feels satisfied, feels a sense of release, and that she has had an orgasm, it should be accepted and acknowledged.

The last step of Annon's (*2*) model is intensive therapy. Intensive therapy is a highly individualized treatment program that is necessary when permission, limited information, and specific suggestions are not sufficient to meet the client's goals. This will be discussed later in this book.

Accepting each person as a unique individual and a sexual being who happens to have a disability will help your clients to see and accept themselves as unique sexual beings with many abilities to build upon.

Conclusion

We know that people with spinal cord injuries are sexual beings. We also know that people with injuries have altered or no sensation in certain areas. We also know that women with spinal cord injuries report experiencing orgasm. How are these orgasms achieved? Are there any new avenues or unidentified neurotransmitters present or released in and around the traumatized spinal segments? Can secondary anorgasmia be restored pharmacologically in SCI women? Are humoral elements involved? Are there new compensatory mechanisms that have been developed or have these compensatory mechanisms always been present? Are circumvaginal muscle contractions in women feasible by direct pudendal–pelvic nerve or lumbosacral segment stimulation as they are in animal research? (*50*) These concerns help us to recognize and acknowledge the need for more research concerning the sexuality and sexual response of women and women with spinal cord injuries.

Acknowledgments

The author gratefully acknowledges the assistance of George Sellmer, Karen Comisky, and Frank Addiego in the revision of this manuscript.

References

1. Addiego, F., Belzer, E. G., Comolli, J., Moger, W., Perry, J. D., and Whipple, B. (1981) Female ejaculation: a case study. *J. Sex. Res.* **17**, 13–21.
2. Annon, J. S. (1976) *The Behavioral Treatment of Sexual Problems. Brief Therapy.* (Harper & Row, New York).
3. Barbach, L. (1982) *For Each Other* (Doubleday, New York).
4. Baxter, R. T. (1978) Sex counseling and the SCI patient. *Nsg. 78* **8**, 46–52.
5. Becker, E. F. (1978) *Female Sexuality Following Spinal Cord Injury.* Cheever, Bloomington, Il.
6. Belzer, E. G. Whipple, B., Moger, W. (1984) Comments regarding "Female ejaculation: a case study." *J. Sex. Res.* **20**, 403–406.
7. Billings, D. M. and Stokes, L. G. (1982) *Medical Surgical Nursing* (The C V Mosby Co., St Louis).

8. Bohlen, J. G. (1981) State of the science in sexual physiology research. Presented at the Society for the Scientific Study of Sex, New York City, New York, November 21.
9. Bregman, S. (1975) *Sexuality And The Spinal Cord Injured Woman* (Sister Kenny Institute, Minneapolis).
10. Bregman, S. and Hadley, R. G. (1976) *Sexual adjustment and feminine attractiveness among spinal cord injured women.* Arch. Phys. Med. Rehabil. **57**, 448–450.
11. Bullard, D. G. and Knight, S. E. (1981) *Sexuality and Physical Disability.* (The C V Mosby Co., St Louis).
12. Campling, J. (1981) *Images of Ourselves: Women With Disabilities* (Routledge and Kegan Paul, Boston).
13. Caparulo, F. and Caparulo, B (1979) Sexuality and the handicapped: Whose problem is it? *SIECUS Report* **7**, 1 & 5.
14. Cole, T. M. and Cole, S. S. (1982) How physical disabilities affect sexual health. *Med. Aspects of Human Sexuality* **16**, 136–151.
15. Cole, T. M. and Cole S. S. (1976) The handicapped and sexual health. *SIECUS Report* **4**, 1–10.
16. Cornelius, D. A., Chipouras, S., Makas, E., and Daniels, S. M. (1982) *Who Cares? A Handbook On Sex Education and Counseling Services for Disabled People* (University Park Press, Baltimore).
17. Eisenberg, M. G. and Rustard, L. C. (1976) Sex education and counseling program on a spinal cord injury service. *Arch. Phys. Med. Rehabil.* **57**, 135–140.
18. Fox, C. A. (1976) Some aspects and implications of coital physiology. *J. Sex. Marital Ther.* **2**, 205–213.
19. Fox, C. A. and Fox, B. (1971) A comparative study of coital physiology, with special reference to the sexual climax. *J. Reprod. Fertil.* **24**, 319–336.
20. Fox, C. A., Wolff, H. S., and Baker, J. A. (1970) Measurement of intra-vaginal and intra-uterine pressures during human coitus by radio-telemetry. *J. Reprod. Fertil.* **22**, 243–251.
21. Francoeur, R. T. (1982) *Becoming a Sexual Person* (John Wiley & Sons, New York).
22. Grafenberg, E. (1950) The role of the urethra in female orgasm. *Int. J. Sexol.* **3**, 145–148.
23. Griffith, E. R. and Trieschmann, R. B. (1975) Sexual functioning in women with spinal cord injury. *Arch. Phys. Med. Rehabil.* **56**, 18–21.
24. Hale-Harbaugh, J., Norman, A. D., Bogle, J. and Shaul, S. (1978) *Within Reach: Providing Family Planning Services to Physically Disabled Women* (Human Sciences Press, New York).
25. Hanlon, K. (1975) Maintaining sexuality after spinal cord injury. *Nsg. 75* **5**, 58–62.
26. Held, J. P., Cole, T. M., Held, C. A., Anderson, C., and Chilgren, R. A. (1975) Sexual attitude reassessment workshops: effect on spinal cord injured adults, their partners and rehabilitation professionals. *Arch. Phys. Med. Rehabil.* **56**, 14–18.

27. Hoch, Z. (1980) The sensory arm of the female orgasmic reflex. *J. Sex Educat. Ther.* **6**, 4–7.
28. Isaacson, J. and Delgado, H. E. (1974) Sex counseling for those with spinal cord injuries. *Social Casework* 622–627.
29. Kaplan, H. S. (1979) *The New Sex Therapy* (Brunner/Mazel, New York).
30. Ladas, A., Whipple, B., and Perry, J. D. (1982) *The G Spot and Other Recent Discoveries About Human Sexuality* (Holt, Rinehart and Winston, New York).
31. Leyson, J. F. J. (1983) Electromyographic (EMG) urodynamic anal probe as a diagnostic tool in the management of sexual dysfunctions in female spinal cord injured patients. *J. Am. Paraplegia Soc.* **6**, 79–80.
32. Leyson, J. F. J. (1982) Intravaginal temperature recording as an adjuctive tool in the diagnosis of sexual dysfunctions in female spinal cord injured patients. Paper presented at American Association of Sex Educators, Counselors and Therapists, New York City, March, 13–15.
33. Leyson, J. F. J. (1979) Counseling the female spinal cord injured patient. *Med. Aspects of Human Sexual Response* **13**, 59–60.
34. Masters, W. and Johnson, V. (1966) *Human Sexual Response* (Little, Brown and Co, Boston).
35. Masters, W., Johnson, V., and Kolodny, R. C. (1982) *Human Sexuality* (Little, Brown and Co, Boston).
36. Money, J. (1960) Phantom orgasm in the dreams of paraplegic men and women. *Arch. Gen. Psychiatry* **3**, 373–382.
37. Mooney, T. O., Cole, T. M. and Chilgren, R. A. (1975) *Sexual Options for Paraplegics and Quadriplegics* (Little, Brown and Co, Boston).
38. Perry, J. D. and Whipple, B. (1982) Multiple components of the female orgasm, in *Circumvaginal Musculature and Sexual Function* (B. Graber, ed.) S Karger, New York.
39. Perry, J. D. and Whipple, B. (1982) Vaginal myography, in *Circumvaginal Musculature and Sexual Function* (B. Graber, ed.) S Karger, New York.
40. Perry, J. D. and Whipple, B. (1981) Pelvic muscle strength of female ejaculators: Evidence in support of a new theory of orgasm. *J. Sex. Res.* **17**, 22–39.
41. Romano, M. E. (1975) Sexuality and the disabled female, *Accent on Living, Inc.*, Bloomington, IL.
42. Sex Education, Counseling and Therapy For The Physically Handicapped (1979) American Association of Sex Educators, Counselors and Therapists, Washington, D.C.
43. Singer, I. (1973) *The Goals of Sexuality* (Schocken, New York).
44. Singer, J. and Singer, I. (1978) Types of female orgasm, in *Handbook of Sex Therapy* (LoPiccolo, J. and LoPiccolo, L., eds.) Plenum, New York.
45. Timmers, P. O. (1976) Treating goal-directed intimacy. *Social Work.* 401–402.
46. Tordjman, G. (1980) New realities in the study of the female's orgasms. *J. Sex Educat. Ther.* **6**, 22–26.

47. Tordjman, G. Nouvelle acquisitions dans l'étude des orgasmes feminins (1979) *Contracept Fertil. Sex* **7**, 215–222.
48. Whipple, B. and Gick, R. (1980) A holistic view of sexuality-Education for the health professional. *Topics in Clinical Nursing* **1**, 91–98.
49. Woods, N. F. (1979) *Human Sexuality in Health and Illness* (The C V Mosby Co., St. Louis).
50. Pacheco, P., Martinez-Gomez, M., Whipple, B., Beyer, C. and Komisaruk, B. R. (1989) Somato-motor components of the pelvic and pudendal nerves of the female rat. *Brain Research 490*, 85-94.

4
Male Sexuality

Andrew Sporer

Gross Anatomy

Anatomically, the penis is composed of two cavernosa and one spongiosa bodies. The two corpora cavernosa are surrounded by the very strong but elastic tunica albuginea, which gives the erectile corpora cavernosa its firmness. The corpus spongiosum has no true tunica and does not participate in erection, although engorgement is present. The turgidity of the corpus spongiosum is proportional to the rigidity (enlargement) of the corpus cavernosum.

A damaged or diseased tunica albuginea interferes with erection. If the tunica or a fibrotic scar (i.e., Peyronie's disease) is replaced with skin, as is done when the fibrotic scar is removed, the penis will be straight but the erection will be a soft one, making penetration impossible at times. The cavernous sinuses are filled with blood during erection, and the walls of the cavernous sinuses are rigidly contracted.

Penile Blood Supply

The vascular supply to each corpus cavernosum arises from the pudendal artery. The arterial branch to the penis divides into three parts at the level of the urogenital diaphragm to form the deep artery, the dorsal artery of the penis, and the artery of the bulb. The deep artery enters the corpus cavernosum, where it branches off again. The dorsal artery of the penis lies on the corpora with numerous branches anastomosing with the deep penile artery. The artery of the bulb is the main artery of the urethra and the glans penis. The three arterial branches communicate with each other through numerous branches, and

Sexual Rehabilitation of the Spinal-Cord-Injured Patient
Edited by J.F. Leyson, © 1990 The Humana Press, Inc.

all vessels, including the deep dorsal vein, lie under Buck's fascia, the fibrous tissue surrounding the entire penis.

Venous drainage is provided by the superficial and the deep veins. The former lie above the tunica albuginea, form the dorsal vein of the penis, and drain into the saphenous venous system. The deep veins drain into Santorini's plexus.

Nerve Supply and Receptors

The innervation of the penis is threefold: somatic (afferent), sympathetic, and parasympathetic (efferent-autonomic nervous system). The somatic sensory and the somatic motor nerves form the pudendal nerve. The sympathetic system provides modulating fibers, coming from the T1 to L2 segment. Parasympathetic innervation originates from the S2-S4 anterolateral horn cells. Each nerve fiber is composed of many neurofibrils, each with a presynaptic terminal. The terminals are located on the dendrites and cytons of secondary neurons on effector cells. Excitatory and inhibitory stimuli, either norepinephrine or acetylcholine, are released from vesicles located on the terminals.

Neuroreceptors

Receptors are numerous in the genital tract and are usually located on the walls of the capillaries, which are more numerous in the submucosa of the proximal urethra than necessary to meet its physiologic requirements. The receptors are innervated by the sympathetic nervous system, and sympathetic stimuli increase resistance at the level of the posterior urethra. Sympathetic fibers for erection originate at T11 to L2 anterolateral horn cells and, after multiple synapses, enter the pelvic plexus. Postganglionic fibers are long and travel a long way before they reach the pelvic receptors. Moduling sympathetic fibers may arise from high thoracic sympathetic segments.

Parasympathetic fibers (S2-S4) form the nervi erigentes. The role of these nerves is primarily that of vasodilation; their action is mediated by acetylcholine. Atropine, administered before the nervi erigentes are stimulated, will prevent erection.

Principal Neurotransmitters: Alpha- and Beta-Adrenergic, and Cholinergic

Two types of neurotransmitters are present in the genital tract—$\text{alpha}_{1,2}$ and $\text{beta}_{1,2}$. Alpha_1 and beta_1 are probably not involved in the erection process. Norepinephrine is needed to stimulate receptors and, in high doses, stimulates alpha$_2$ receptors. Intravenous or intracorporal alpha$_2$-blocking agents can cause erection. Low doses of norepinephrine (NEP) stimulate the beta$_2$ receptors. Beta$_2$-adrenergic activity predominates in the penis.

High doses of propranolol, a beta$_1$- and -$_2$-adrenergic blocking agent, abolishes erection by its beta$_2$ effect. Interneurons probably connect the sympathetic with the parasympathetic nervous system and are potentially capable of blocking each segment. Although most of the receptors are sympathetically and NEP controlled, recent studies indicate that there are cholinergic fibers in the corpora cavernosa. Stimulation of the sympathetic nerve fibers will increase the norepinephrine content of the corpora cavernosa and corpus spongiosum.

NEUROTRANSMITTERS FOR ERECTION (MISCELLANEOUS). *Substance P.* Substance P is a potent smooth muscle contracting agent with the ability to cause marked vasodilation. This substance is located in the nerves of erectile tissue (*11*). It is also present in the hypothalamus near the orgastic center and in the abdomen. Its role is uncertain at present. Substance P is not mediated by either adrenergic or cholinergic agents, and neurotransmission is probably accomplished by adenosine triphosphate (ATP) and other neuropeptides.

Prostaglandins. The roles of the prostaglandins E_2 and F_2 were proven recently. Prostaglandin E_2 (PGE_2) decreases catecholamine output, thereby indirectly causing vasodilation and modifying the organ response. Prostaglandin F_2 (PGF_2) increases catecholamine output, increases vasoconstriction and the end organ reaction to NEP increases. Prostaglandin may seem to be a coordinator between alpha$_2$ and beta$_2$ responses and between sympathetic and parasympathetic effects. The role of PGE_2 and PGF_2 in accommodating large urine volumes without increasing intravesical pressure is convincing, but their role in erection is not clear (*10*). However, PGF_2 is believed to be responsible for orgasmic bulbocavernosus and ischiocavernosus muscle responses in both men and women.

Vasoactive Peptides. Vasoactive intestinal peptide (VIP) has been found in the corpora cavernosa of estrogen-treated males undergoing gender reassignment surgery (*12*). High concentrations have been described in the walls of the pudendal arteries in penile erectile tissues. These investigators also noted that VIP can exert regulatory control on blood vessels and smooth muscle tone.

Cyclic Adenosine Monophosphate (cAMP). This neurotransmitter may mediate other neuroendocrine secretions, such as prostacyclin and the endorphins, released during sexual activity. Some SCI patients noted a reduction in "arthritic" pains after sex, probably because of the release of brain endorphins. A few SCI patients exhibit lowered blood pressures after frequent sexual encounters. These reductions may be the result of the smooth muscle relaxing effect of circulating prostacyclin after coitus (*8*).

Hormone Control of Erection and the Orgastic Center

Testosterone has long been suspected to play a role in erection and sexual behavior. Castration causes sequential behavior changes in experimental animals that are similar in many respects to those in humans. The time interval between castration and behavioral changes, however, varies in different species. A male rat may mount the female several times, penetrating several times before eventually ejaculating. After ejaculation, the rat rests for many minutes in perfect relaxation before restarting the same pattern of sexual activity. Eventually, he ejaculates four to five times.

After castration, the sequential pattern described changes. First there will be no ejaculation, then less and less penetration, and eventually, even the mounting ceases. When all sexual activity disappears, testosterone can reestablish the male rat's normal sexual pattern. However, return to such activity may take several months. The later testosterone therapy is started after castration, the longer it takes to reestablish normal sexual patterns and the higher the dose of androgen required to obtain results. Apparently, the target cells in which the testosterone receptors are located become less sensitive to the androgen. (This phenomenon, called the receptor hyposensitivity syndrome, probably occurs in elderly men.)

Certain hormone levels are necessary for normal sexual patterns, but increased amounts of androgenic hormone, above basic needs, do not increase sexual activity. In rats, there is no increased mounting, penetration, or ejaculation with increased hormone levels, and the interval between ejaculations does not diminish. Several studies on humans indicated that high levels of testosterone do not help an individual perform intercourse more often than at adequately low androgen levels.

The gonadotropic releasing hormone in the hypothalamus acts on the pituitary to release the luteinizing hormone, which in turn stimulates the interstitial cells (Leydig cells) to produce testosterone. The hormone produced is bound to testosterone-binding globulin and albumin. Only 3% of the circulating testosterone is free (unbound); this is the active hormone. Testosterone metabolism depends on the amount of free hormone; the utilization and output of testosterone diminish with advancing age. However, stimulated by chorionic gonadotropin, the testicle can produce equal quantities of testosterone at any age.

In the brain, testosterone is aromatized to estradiol. This estrogen is required to potentiate the action of testosterone. The combination of estrogen and androgen has long been used in France to treat impotency. The estrogen also acts as a feedback control on the pituitary in the release of luteinizing hormone.

Sexual Centers

Central Sexual Center and Sex Hormones

The orgastic center is located in the brain (*14*), near or in the preoptic anterior hypothalamic area, and is controlled by testosterone. Pellets of androgen implanted in the anterohypothalamic preoptic area (AHPO) of rats can restore up to 80% of the animal's normal sexual behavior and mating pattern; 50% of the animals can ejaculate. Testosterone implants elsewhere in the brain do not restore normal sexual patterns, indicating that leakage after testosterone implantation will not restore normal sexual patterns. Additional testosterone, applied subcutaneously, is even more effective in reestablishing normal sexual behavior, provided brain centers are intact. The high effectiveness of subcutaneous testosterone is probably the result of its peripheral and central effects and of the need for the brain and genitalia to be stimulated simultaneously. Genital stimulation alone will not cause sexual arousal. (*9*).

Actually, testosterone has no effective stimulatory effect on the genitalia. To be effective, the androgen must be transformed to dihydrotestosterone in peripheral tissues, with the help of the 5-alpha-reductase enzyme. Dihydrotestosterone (DHT) is the peripheral stimulating hormone. There are no DHT receptors in the brain, the hormone has no central effect and the peripheral stimulus alone is inadequate to maintain normal sexual patterns. The aromatized testosterone–estradiol is required for stimulus and orgastic (orgasm) control. Interestingly, estradiol (E_2), the aromatized product of testosterone, also potentiates erection by potentiating the activity of testosterone. Also, estrogen enhances the secretion of prolactin, a hormone that, when present in excessive quantity, is associated with impotence.

Prolactin

The pituitary produces prolactin, but its release is inhibited by a prolactin inhibitory factor, a dopamine, present in the hypothalamus. Estrogen therapy depletes this dopamine depot, thereby stimulating the pituitary to increase its release of prolactin. This hormone can be produced in the brain outside the pituitary and in malignant tissue in the abdomen. Levels in men are only slightly below those in women, 5–12 ng/mL. It is not known why this high level of prolactin is present in the healthy male. Hyperprolactinemia, in addition to causing impotence, can cause galactorrhea, hypogonadism and sometimes premature ejaculation.

Neuroendocrine Control

Sexual behavior and changes in potency have been associated with changes in brain serotonin and dopamine levels. The administration of serotonin antagonists enhances sexual activity. Dopamine agonists probably depress the output of prolactin and may indirectly stimulate erection (*7*).

OTHER SEXONEUROENDOCRINE MECHANISMS. The pineal gland has an inhibitory effect on the hypothalamus. Neural pathways from the pineal body originate in the retina and go directly to the pineal body. However, the neural connection is not present after birth, although some sympathetic effect is maintained. The inhibitory effect will prevent the release of gonadotropic releasing hormone, and gonadal function will decrease (*9*). Pineal gland function is depressed by light and stimulated by darkness. A marked loss in sexual activity has been observed in some experimental animals maintained in the dark. However, darkness has not been shown clinically to influence sexual behavior in SCI men.

The adrenal gland does not seem to influence the sexual pattern directly. On the other hand, it may be involved indirectly by producing sex steroids (testosterone precursors) through the stimulation of adrenal androgenic stimulating hormone (AASH). Figure 1a outlines the hormonal interactions modulating male sexual behavior. Figure 1b shows the male sexual response process.

Peripheral (Local) Sexual Center

The peripheral reflex center for erection lies in the lumbosacral area of the spinal cord. The reflex arc may be stimulated by enteroceptive, exteroceptive, and proprioceptive stimuli (*2*). Although the reflex erectile center lies in the lumbosacral cord, some sensory fibers follow or go up with the sympathetic T11-L2 or T12-L2 and enter the spinal cord at a much higher level.

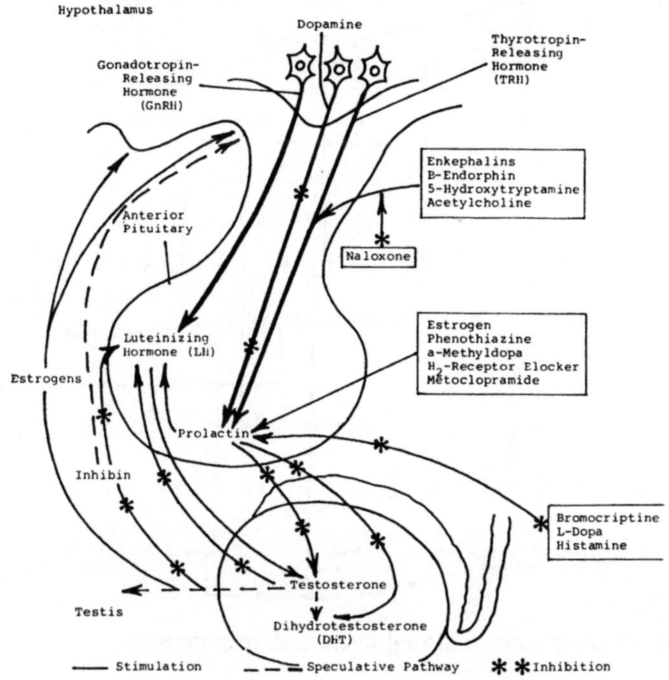

Concepts based from J.D. Horowitz, G.M. Besser, G. Tolis and N.J. Cole. (Modified from Krauss, D.J.: The Physiologic basis of male sexual dysfunction. Hosp. Practice. pp. 209, Feb. 1983).

Fig. 1A. Neuroendocrine pathways and hormonal interactions mediating male sexual behavior.

Vascular Mechanisms

Penile Blood Flow

An increased penile blood flow is required for erection. A 20- to 50-mL increase creates an immediate erection; an additional 15-mL increase above the normal inflow will maintain the erection. Penile blood pressure is essentially the same as systolic blood pressure. If there is an impediment to blood flow, erection will be inadequate. If the penile systolic blood pressure is 40 mmHg less than the systolic pressure, vasculogenic or organic impotence occurs. The inflow and outflow of blood must be regulated, but the regulatory mechanism is not well understood at present. However, blood flow can be increased by 175 mL/min to provide an immediate erection, but this erection will not

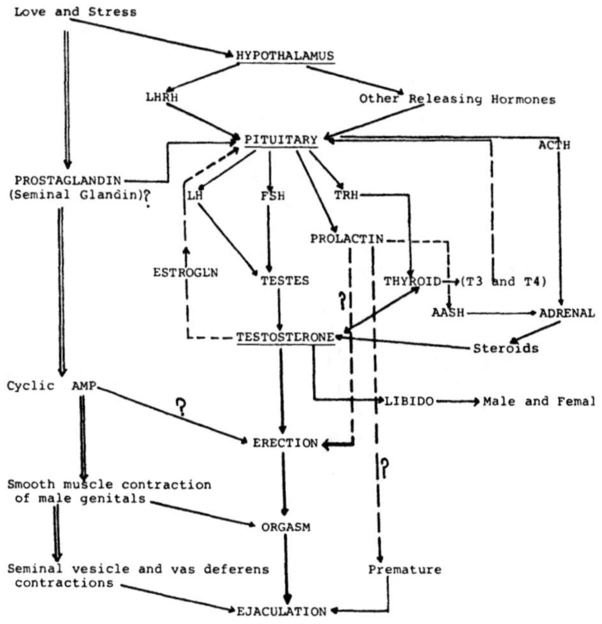

Fig. 1B. Neurohormonal sexual cycle and responses.

be maintained if outflow is not regulated. Venous compression does not regulate outflow. It only causes penile edema, not erection.

A plausible explanation for erection was postulated by Conti (*4*), who observed that the deep penile artery, before it entered the corpus cavernosum, gives off a branch that bypasses the cavernous body to connect directly with the capillary system. In this view, the penile arteries contain "polsters" (Fig. 2), or Edner's pads, which are smooth muscle fibers lying under the arterial lumen intima. During erection (Fig. 3a), the arterial branch bypassing the corpus cavernosum is closed by the "polsters" and all blood goes to the corpora cavernosa, creating an erection. During flaccidity (Fig. 3b), the arteries entering the corpora are closed and all blood, except for the minimal flow required to maintain the viability of the corpora, is shunted to the capillaries. The existence of these "polsters" has been questioned by many investigators (*2*). Some consider them degenerative intimal products and not actively contracting muscles. If the polsters exist, they are sympathetically controlled.

Recent studies further clarified the chain of events that lead to erection and detumescence. The sinusoidal places in the corpora and the afferent arterioli contain smooth muscles. In flaccid state these smooth

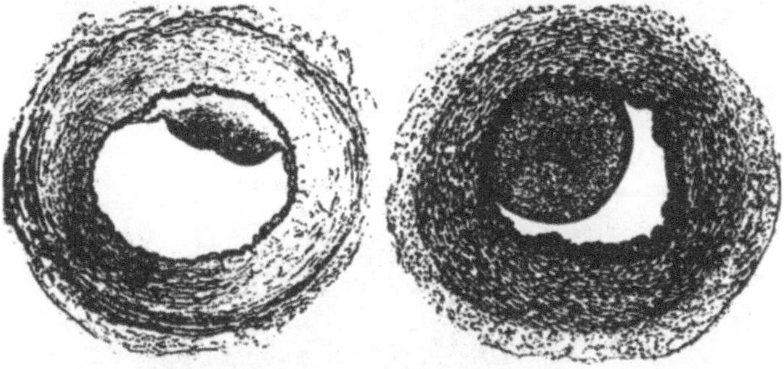

Fig. 2. Microscopic appearance of the penile blood vessels (arterioles and/or venules) with *A*—open or contracted "polsters" and *B*—closed or relaxed "polsters."

muscles are partially contracted, thereby diminishing the lumen of the cavernous sinuses and thus the arterial inflow into the sinuses. The veins in the corpora are placed between the sinusoidal places and under the subtunical area. These subtunical veins communicate with the deep dorsal veins through perforating branches and the lumens of these veins are widely open during flaccidity (*15*). Virag demonstrated that, when a smooth muscle relaxant such as papaverine is injected into the corpora, the smooth muscles relax both in the arterioli and in the sinusoids (*16*).

The overfilled sinuses compress the subtunically placed veinous system, diminishing the veinous outflow, and erection then results.

During detumescence the smooth muscles both in the corpora and arterioli regain their tonus, the compressed veins dilate, and the diminished blood flow results in detumescense. Thus, the vascular aspects of erection involve three stages: (a) arterial vasodilation, (b) venous (indirect) compression, and (c) sinusoidal (corpora cavernosa) cavities relaxation.

Sexual Implications Post-SCI

Patients with T12 lesions have an essentially normal sensation of bladder fullness, but most of those with sacral cord lesions are impotent; only 25% have erections. Two possible explanations are: (a) the thoracic lumbar outflow acts as the stimulus for erection, or (b) the sacral cord has not been destroyed completely.

Dogs with a midthoracic spinal cord transsection have erections if the glans penis is stimulated. If the stimulus is maintained, they may even exhibit a tendency to mount. Reflex erection has been shown to

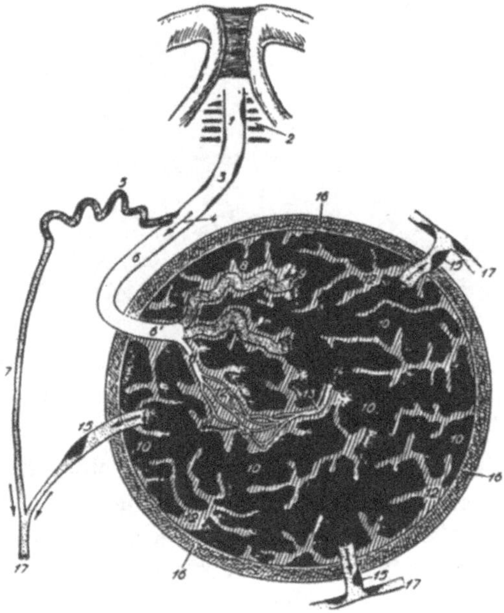

Fig. 3A. Shunt closed—corpus cavernosum fills. Polsters closing lumen in shunt.

recur in rats following implantations of testosterone pellets at different levels of the spinal cord (*5*). Testosterone receptors are found in the spinal cords of rats, but their presence in the human spinal cord has not yet been proven. However, I have observed recurrent erections after testosterone injections in two patients who had had no erections for years after sustaining an injury to the spinal cord at the level of T11.

The sexuality of SCI patients has been studied extensively by Bors and Comarr (*3*), who described the reflex erections in these patients. They proved that mechanically stimulated erections can be maintained long enough to permit penetration and satisfactory intercourse. In a healthy individual, erection is initiated by a psychogenic stimulus; penetration and friction lead to contraction of the bulbocavernosus and ischiocavernosus, which results in ejaculation and orgastic activity. With psychogenic impotence, satisfactory erection cannot be attained; individuals may be able to create an erection by mechanical stimulation (masturbation) and they may even be able to penetrate. However, if psychogenic reinforcement is absent, the erection cannot be maintained.

The psychogenic input may be mental (fantasy), auditory, visual, sensory, or olfactory, carried by fibers that descend from the brain to

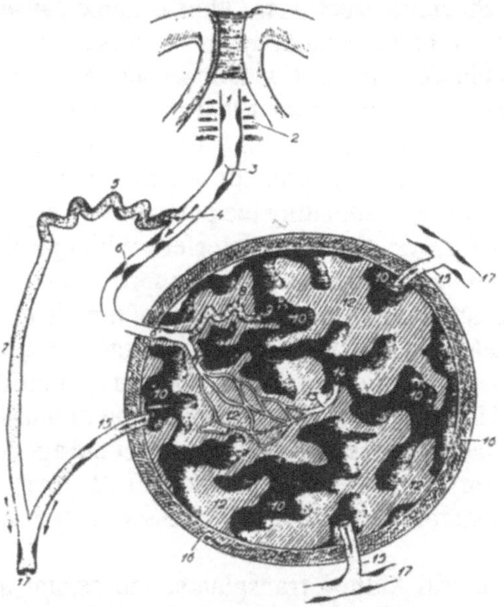

Fig. 3B. Shunt open—corpus cavernosum empty. Polsters closing lumen of artery.

the thoracolumbar and sacral areas of the lateral column. How the psychogenic input acts is not clear, but it has been postulated that a neurohormone transmitter is released that acts on the brain, peripheral spinal center, and genitalia simultaneously (*9*). In most SCI patients, the psychogenic stimulus is absent, especially in those in whom the spinal cord has been completely transsected. These patients have reflex erections that, to a certain extent, are hormonally influenced and induced by the slightest mechanical stimulus. Unless reinforced, they are usually inadequate for penetration. Only by maintaining mechanical stimulation can penetration and satisfactory intercourse be achieved.

Orchiectomy after the spinal cord has been transsected abolishes reflex erections, but they recur with testosterone therapy. Some sensory pathways enter the spinal cord at much higher levels and can stimulate the reflex arc. These fibers travel with the sympathetic chain, entering the spinal cord at the level of a low thoracic segment. Lumbar sympathectomy diminishes reflex erections, but total thoracolumbar sympathectomy abolishes them completely. Diseases that interfere with reflex erections in nonparalyzed individuals affect reflexogenic erections in SCI patients. Sedatives and antihypertensive drugs adversely affect both reflex and psychogenic erections. Other organic causes of impotence should be ruled out before sexual dysfunction is treated in SCI patients.

Just as ejaculation can occur with or without erection, so can orgastic sensation. Heath (*6*) demonstrated that the septal nuclei are responsible for cerebral sexual stimuli and a direct stimulus to this area can cause erection without peripheral stimulation. The same effect can be obtained in animals by stimulating the putamen and adjacent nuclei (*13*). A wide range of medications can interfere with ejaculation potential, abolish erections, and diminish sexual appreciation (*1*).

The sexual activities of more than 40% of uremic patients on dialysis progressively deteriorate. A gonadal dysfunction also appears to develop, and testosterone production has been reported to diminish in para- and quadriplegics. However, we were unable to find diminished testosterone or elevated prolactin levels in 40 patients (average age 39 yr) with complete transsection of the spinal cord above T12. Nor were we able to prove that testosterone levels were depressed in our SCI population 1 yr postinjury.

After successful kidney transplants, the sexual activities of the uremic patients not only improve, but spermatogenesis increases. In SCI patients, renal transplants have a limited indication. Most develop repeated urinary tract infections, and immunosuppressive therapy will make it even more difficult to control these infections. Furthermore, many uremic patients have elevated prolactin levels that must be correlated clinically with the level of their lesions so that management of their sexual problems can be tailored accordingly. SCI patients with diabetic nephropathy have a more compromised erectile function.

Therapeutic Implications

Before rehabilitation, all SCI patients should have a thorough urologic, neurovascular, endocrinologic, and psychological workup. If all results are satisfactory, sexual rehabilitation can begin. A period of depression follows the injury, and this period can last for many months. Worry about the future, financial insecurity, and fears that an asexual life will disrupt family harmony are real problems. Fear of inadequacy hinders the SCI patient's ability and willingness to renew sexual activities. These patients hide their true feelings, refusing to discuss them. If the patient is newly married, the patient's wife often cannot cope with the complex manifestations of these problems. The unmarried youth soon will appreciate the loss of body attractiveness, which perpetuates the depression. Once the injury is stabilized and the patient is ready to face the world in his disabled state, he begins to think about his discharge from the hospital. At this point, sexual rehabilitation should begin.

Unfortunately, sexual therapy at most sexual rehabilitation institutes is very difficlt, because there is no privacy. Also, it is almost impossible to find sexual partners for SCI patients. Consequently, audiovisual material, often perceived as pornographic, is used. Without sexual stimulation to the young, inexperienced individuals, the material may be repulsive. However, with properly and carefully planned sex education, SCI patients soon learn what they can expect and obtain.

A healthy individual enjoys sexual stimuli and orgastic ability. For the paralegic, the lower the SCI, the easier it is to obtain orgastic feeling from touch and caresses. Sexual stimuli are touch, a feeling of caressing, and being caressed; an extensive sexual encounter mostly involving touch can induce some sort of orgastic activity. Comarr has studied this, and found that a fairly high percentage of his patients achieved sexual satisfaction (*3*). We examined and interviewed 50 SCI patients with injuries above T12, at least 4 yr after their injuries. The age range of these patients was 21–55 yr. Only five had attempted intercourse, but only two were able to feel some sexual satisfaction. None were interested in renewing their sexual activities. If they had once had partners, the partners now refused to help. More than half of these patients disliked the audiovisual material and did not consider oral sex a satisfactory substitute. Only three patients in the past 5 yr were able to find a sexual partner. One married and divorced in less than a year, one lives with his girlfriend, and the third plans to marry.

In a different atmosphere, the rehabilitation rate is higher. Comarr (*3*) proved that sexual rehabilitation is possible, but in our experience, the success is very limited and not long lasting. A home-care program by the Veterans Medical Centers ensures better results. Service-connected patients receive an overall tax-free allowance up to $40,000, enabling them to buy a house and/or a car. With financial security, it is hoped that in this new surrounding it will be easier for SCI patients to find companions and establish lasting partnerships.

If erection or maintaining erection is a problem, and if medical sex therapy fails, a penile prosthesis is then indicated. However, such a prosthesis requires additional and more careful penile care. The pressure of a condom could erode penile skin much more readily if compressed against a solid substance such as a prosthesis.

The difficult problem is arousing the partner sexually. Cleansing the SCI patient's bowel, applying the condom, or catheterizing them compromises the partner's sexual drive. Furthermore, sexual activity may induce reflex urination, even after catheterization, and reflex defecation. Intercourse with an indwelling catheter has been advised, attempted, and is feasible, but none of our patients would try it.

Sexual stimulation during foreplay or during actual penetration may initiate a sympathetic crisis among SCI patients with lesions at or above T5. The crisis usually begins with excessive perspiration and headache followed by a rapid rise in blood pressure. The crisis (autonomic hyperreflexia) is milder if the patient has voided before intercourse.

The neurophysiology of erection in healthy and SCI men has recently been reviewed and clarified. In SCI patients, the organic damage is further aggravated by periods of depression, sociofamilial neglect, and the inability to find a suitable sexual partner(s). With sexomedical therapeutic advances, community awareness, and research innovations, it is hoped that sexual rehabilitation in these types of patients will in time become a smoother and more effective process.

References

1. Ban, T. H. A. and Freyhan, F. A., eds. (1980) *Modern Problems of Pharmacopsychiatry. Drug Treatment of Sexual Dysfunction.* (S. Karger. Basil—New York). 15 Vol.
2. Benson, G. S. (1979) Mechanism of human erection, emission and ejaculation. Current concepts. *Sexual Rehabilitation in Urologic Cancer Patient.* (C. K. Hall, Boston).
3. Bors, E. and Comarr, A. E. (1960) Neurologic disturbances of sexual function with special reference to 529 patients with spinal cord injury. *Urol. Surg.* **10**, 191–200.
4. Conti, G. (1952) L'erection du penis humain et ses bases morphologicovasculaire. *Acta Anal.* (Basel) **14**, 17–24.
5. Hart, B. L. and Haugen, C. M. (1968). Activation of sexual reflexes in male rat by spinal implantation of testosterone. *Physiol. Behav.* **3**, 735–742.
6. Heath, R. G. (1975) Brain function and behavior. Emotion and sensory phenomena in psychiatric patient and in experimental animals. *J. Neurol. Ment. Dis.* **160**, 159–168.
7. Krane, R. J. and Siroky, M. B. (1981) Neurophysiology of erection. Male sexual dysfunction, in *The Urologic Clinics of North America.* W. L. Furlow, ed. **8**, 91–102 (W. B. Saunders, Phila., PA).
8. Leyson, J. F. J. and Powell, R. (1979) Sex and pain in Spinal Cord Injury patients. Unpublished clinical observations.
9. MacLean, P. D. (1966) Studies of the cerebral representation of certain basic sexual functions, in *Brain and Behavior.* Gorski, R. A. and Whalen, R. E., eds. Vol. 3 (Univ. of California Press, Berkeley, Los Angeles, CA).

10. Melman, A. and Henry, D. (1979) The possible role of catecholamine of the corpora in penile erection. *J. Urol.* **121**, 419–423.

11. Pickel, V. N., Reis, D. T., and Leeman, S. E. (1977) Ultrastructural localization of substance P in neurons of rat spinal cord. *Brain Res.* **122**, 534–538.

12. Polak, J. M., Mina, S., Gu, J., and Bloom, S. R. (1981) VIP-ergic nerves in the penis. *Lancet* **II**, 217–220.

13. Robinson, B. W. and Mishkin, M. (1968) Penile erection evoked from forebrain structures in Macaca Mulatta. *Arch. Neurol.* **19**, 184–190.

14. Ryan, K. J. et al. (1972) Estrogen formation in the brain. *Am. J. Obstet. Gynecol.* **114**, 454–460.

15. Fournier, G. and Lue, T. (1988) *Vasculogenic Impotence: Physiology, Diagnosis and Treatment, Monographs in Urology* Stanley, T., ed. **9**, 20–31.

16. Virag, R. (1982) Intracavernous injection of papaverine for erectile failure. Letter to the Editor. *Lancet* **2**, 938.

5

Sexuality and Urology

E. J. McGuire

Neural Lesions and Sexual Dysfunction

The peripheral and low central innervations of the genital and lower urinary tracts are similar. Both areas receive sympathetic, parasympathetic, and somatic innervation from identical or adjacent thoracolumbar and sacral cord areas. Major afferent pathways are shared or closely related (*1–3*), and it is not surprising, therefore, that urologic disease processes initiated by neural lesions adversely influence sexual function.

Peripheral Neural Injuries and Specific Sexual Dysfunctions

Improved methods for measuring urodynamic pressure in the urinary bladder internal and external sphincters help to identify specific neural injuries (*4,5*). The ability to localize neural injuries, especially peripheral ones, and the study of associated sexual and genital dysfunction, provide the information needed to predict abnormal sexual function caused by central neural disease processes.

Sympathetic Neural Lesions and Genital Innervation

Injury to the sympathetic innervation of the genital tract at the time of retroperitoneal node dissection has definite effects on the genital system. These effects are somewhat difficult to explain in the light of current knowledge (*6,7*). The center for hyperclosure of the internal sphincter with ejaculation and the center for semen emission into the prostatic urethra lie within the thoracolumbar spinal cord (*3*). The precise peripheral pathway ganglionic synapses of the adrenergic motor fibers

Sexual Rehabilitation of the Spinal-Cord-Injured Patient
Edited by J.F. Leyson, © 1990 The Humana Press, Inc.

concerned with these processes and the afferent reflex limbs serving them have not been established. Urethral smooth sphincter continence function is under sympathetic control. However, loss of urethral smooth muscle closing function does not occur after retroperitoneal lymph node dissection, indicating that hypogastric nerve section is, in fact, a partial denervation. Total loss of urethral smooth muscle closure function, seminal transport, emission, and ejaculation are known to occur after spinal cord infarction and after extensive peripheral sympathetic injury deep in the true pelvis.

Injuries to the sympathetic neural system may be associated with retrograde ejaculation, or with total loss of seminal emission and ejaculation. Erectile function is usually not impaired, nor is the sensation of orgasm, although it may be "altered." Retrograde ejaculation, as an isolated finding, can be reversed by alpha-stimulating agents, e.g., ephedrine. Loss of seminal transport and emission may be restored by the prolonged administration of imipramine hydrochloride. These findings, and the selective nature of the genital abnormalities with sparing of urethral closing function, suggest that these are incomplete neural lesions and that the pathways from the thoracolumbar centers to the vas, seminal vesicle, and urethral preprostatic sphincter, which hypercontracts with ejaculation, are not exclusively through the hypogastric nerves. It is possible, experimentally, to diminish urethral closing pressure by section, but not by eliminating the sympathetic nerves at the inferior mesenteric ganglion (*8*). Stimulation of the hypogastric nerves increases urethral closing pressure and results in the emission of seminal material from the ejaculatory ducts (*9*).

It is probable that an alternative sympathetic pathway involves the sympathetic chain, which descends into the true pelvis along the vertebral column (*10*). Total denervation between the thoracolumbar center and the pelvic plexus, lateral and anterior to the rectum, may require transection of both the hypogastric and the sympathetic chain pathways. Abnormal urethral and genital functions associated with total central or extensive peripheral denervation do not respond to alpha-adrenergic agents (*11*). These findings support the concept of a dual intermediate pathway for the sympathetic innervation of the genitourinary tract.

Erectile Impotence and Urological Disease

Loss of reflex and psychic erections regularly follows radical prostatectomy and cystoprostatectomy. Since the description by Eckhart in 1863 of the nervi erigentes, erection has been known to result from stimulation of the S2-3-4 anterior roots (*1*). These parasympathetic fibers traverse the inferior hypogastric plexus, where they are joined by sympathetic fibers from the superior hypogastric plexus and the sacral sympathetic chain. They then course lateral to the rectum behind and in close relationship to the prostate. In this area, they pierce the urogenital diaphragm and finally enter the corpora cavernosa. Walsh and Donker have recently reported that careful surgical dissection of the posterior aspect of the prostate can preserve these fibers and spare sexual potency (*12*). On the other hand, injury to the pelvic plexus more posteriorly, as for example during an abdominal perineal resection, can induce loss of urethral closing pressure, loss of erection, and presumably seminal emission and ejaculation, although it is difficult to substantiate the genital effects given the urethral sphincter deficit. At this time, too little is known about the correlation between urodynamic findings and sexual function. For example, it is perfectly possible for a hypertonic, areflexic detrusor, which implies a complete neural injury, to coexist with normal erection, ejaculation, and fertility. It is equally possible to find patients with total erectile and ejaculatory impotence with normal vesical and urethral function.

Central Neurologic Injury or Disease and Sexual Dysfunction and Its Relationship to Urinary Tract Disability

Females

Sexual function in females has not been studied as completely as in males, nor have the underlying neurophysiological pathways involved in the sexual function of females been elucidated. Changes in the female genital tract with sexual activity have certain parallels to those in males. These changes include vaginal lubrication, labial swelling, clitoral erection and regression, and a sequence of events at the time of orgasm that is similar, although not identical to that in males, including rhythmic 0.8-s contractions of the pelvic floor musculature (*14*). Radical pelvic surgery, with consequent damage to innervation of the bladder and urethra probably induces changes in sexual function, but data on peripheral neural injuries and sexual dysfunction in females in contrast to males is sparse (*15*). Whether the majority of women who sustain damage to the pelvic plexus lateral to the cervix at the time of radical extirpative surgery experience loss of vaginal lubrication, clitoral erection, and the vascular-mediated responses in the labia and vagina as well as the sensation of orgasm is not known. We know even less about specific changes in sexual function in females with spinal cord injury or disease. To some degree, this is true of our knowledge of male sexual dysfunction after spinal cord injury as well. However, reflex erections in males with upper motor neuron lesions are presumably paralleled by similar changes in females, e.g., reflex vaginal lubrication, which occur during deep sleep cycles. However, only limited studies have been done in spinal injured women. The background information on males with specific injury to peripheral innervation mentioned above provides a framework that can be used to predict findings that might be encountered in patients with specific spinal cord injury or disease at a given level.

Sexual Dysfunction Associated with So-Called Lower Motor Neuron Injuries

Lower motor neuron injuries are expressed typically by flaccid paralysis of the lower extremities and a bladder that cannot contact reflexly, but there is normal closure of the urethral smooth sphincter mechanism, indicating intact sympathetic neural function. Spinal cord injury inducing a lower motor neuron lesion is typically associated with injury to the vertebral column at or below the T12-L1 level. The variable expression of such lesions is well known, and it is not unusual for patients with complete lesions with respect to the bladder to preserve external urethral sphincter activity mediated by alpha-motor neurons originating within the sacral cord and reaching the pelvic floor and external sphincter via the pudendal nerve. Because the thoracolumbar sympathetic innervation of the proximal urethra is spared, proximal urethral closing pressures and function are normal. Patients with lower motor lesions not surprisingly have difficulty achieving erections with stimulation and typically do not experience reflex erections. They are reported to have an incidence of psychogenic erections of about 24% (*13*). It is not clear whether these erections are in fact psychogenics, or whether they are an expression of an incomplete lesion of the sacral cord. As mentioned above, it is possible for patients with total vesical decentralization to manifest normal erectile activity, normal orgasm, and normal ejaculation. The disparity in findings with respect to sexual activity and lower urinary tract function is consistent in SCI patients. In addition, sexual dysfunction in male SCI patients tends to be a topic for discussion, whereas that in female patients is not, since measurable parameters for function and dysfunction are not yet clearly established. Moreover, the absence of sufficient reflex erectile activity to permit intercourse is relatively remarkable and is much more apparent than the subtler changes in female neurophysiologic function, which also result in impaired sexual ability. Emphasis in the United States on management of lower urinary tract dysfunction by achieving low-pressure urinary storage and relying on intermittent catheterization has improved chances for relatively normal sexual function in patients with lower motor neuron lesions (*16*). Management by intermittent catheterization together with anticholinergic agents is associated with a low incidence of chronic urinary tract infection, protection of the urethra from the development of fistulas, and protection of the vas and testicles from repeated episodes of infection. There is some question about whether any specific SCI by itself can induce changes in testicular physiology and seminal transport (*17*). Seminal quality in patients with SCI who have been subjected to stimulation to obtain semen has been poor (*18,19*). Seminal quality declines with time after spinal cord injury. Whether the decline in sperm viability and seminal production is the result of the neural lesion, or related to treatment of the neural lesion, with subsequent development of infection induced by catheter drainage is not yet clearly defined. Prospective studies are currently in progress to determine, in nonhuman primates, whether specific neural lesions induce specific testicular dysfunction as well as dysfunction of the seminal transport system. In view of our knowledge of the profound effect of peripheral neural injuries involving the sympathetic or pelvic neural plexus on erectile function, seminal transport, and ejaculation, it seems very likely that "lower motor neuron lesions" (or lesions of the sacral cord, cauda equina, or the conus medullaris) would be likely to induce changes in sexual function that are neurally mediated and not limited to lack of reflex and psychic erectile activity.

Since patients with so-called lower motor neuron lesions experience a lesser incidence of reflex or stimulative erectile activity than do patients with upper motor lesions, it seems reasonable to assume that a number of such patients will ask to be evaluated for a penile prosthesis. Part and parcel of the evaluation for penile prosthetic surgery should be a detailed exploration of the patient's ability to experience ejaculation and orgasm. Although orgasm may be prevented by damage to sacral sensory fibers or the sacral cord itself, stimulated ejaculation may still be possible. Unfortunately, we have no information on whether complete sacral cord injury results in permanent ablation of ejaculatory function since the precise sensory pathway involved is unknown. Whether some patients with lower motor neuron lesions can experience ejaculation and a kind of orgasm cannot be ascertained from Comarr's data (*13*). We do not know whether these patients had incomplete lesions with sparing of the thoracolumbar center for emission and ejaculation; total destruction of the sacral cord would imply some afferent activity reaching the thoracolumbar spinal cord via sensory fibers that parallel sympathetic fibers. However, the persistence of some pudendal nerve-mediated reflex activity in the external sphincter, and the association of pudendal afferent fibers with persistent ability to achieve orgasm and ejaculation in patients who experience pelvic nerve injury at the time of radical extirpative surgery, suggests that preservation of ejaculation and orgasm following sacral spinal cord or root injuries is the result of the partial nature of the lesion. As mentioned above, total denervation of the bladder is often associated with partial denervation of the external sphincter and pelvic floor. At least as far as the lower urinary tract is concerned, no reflex sensory pathway appears to parallel the sympathetic motor fibers, and all afferent activity essential for reflex bladder storage and evacuation appears to be conveyed by sacral sensory pathways. The interconnections between thoracolumbar genital ejaculatory centers and the sacral cord are complex. Lesions between the sacral cord and thoracolumbar sympathetic outflow would be expected to interfere with ejaculation since that process requires intact pathways between the sacral cord and thoracolumbar centers, unless one postulates the existence of a separate sensory pathway paralleling the sympathetic motor fibers, which seems unlikely. The increasingly severe testicular dysfunction with time following SCI suggests that, in part, the abnormalities of seminal production are related to infection and lower urinary tract dysfunction rather than to the neural abnormality, but definitive information in this area is currently lacking. Since useful erectile activity in patients with complete lower motor neuron lesions tends to be relatively rare, implantation of a suitable penile prosthesis is a reasonable alternative in the treatment of sexual dysfunction. These devices do not interfere with intermittent catheterization, nor is the incidence of urinary tract infection in patients maintained on intermittent catheterization high enough to preclude their use. The major problem with penile prostheses in SCI patients is erosion of the corpora cavernosa. The high incidence of corporal erosion appears to be related to pressure necrosis, and may be related to the use of condom catheter drainage. Nevertheless, the incidence of corporal erosion in patients with upper or lower motor neuron lesions treated with penile prostheses is higher than in patients without SCI. *However, when erosion of the corpora cavernosa occurs with extrusion of the prosthetic device in spinal cord injured patients, it is not associated with the disastrous complications than it is in patients with diabetes, in whom the corpora generally erode as a result of deep-seated penile infection.* Patients with SCI who experience erosion and extrusion of a prosthetic device can usually be reoperated on in 3–6 mo, when a smaller device can be inserted. As a general rule, the smallest diameter device available should be utilized.

High-Pressure Sphincteric Dysfunction and Lower Motor Neuron Lesions

Some patients with lower motor neuron lesions will wish to be maintained on condom drainage. Patients with apparent upper urinary tract dysfunction in whom urethral resistance values are high are not suitable candidates. In such instances, ablation procedures on the external and internal sphincter may be necessary. It should be kept in mind that ablation of internal sphincter resistance by transurethral prostatic resection obviates normal antigrade ejaculation. In addition, external sphincterotomy may be associated with impotence. Reports in the urologic literature indicate that a 12 o'clock external sphincterotomy is safer with respect to erectile function than a 3 and 6 o'clock transection, but the possibility that impotence may occur is not totally obviated by the 12 o'clock incision. It is my feeling that patients with lower motor neuron lesions should be maintained on intermittent catheterization rather than subjected to sphincter ablative procedures if at all feasible. It is not clearly established whether resection of internal and external sphincters, with consequent pooling of urine in the prostatic urethra, leads to an increased incidence of testicular dysfunction because of the reflux of urine down the vas deferens. The occurrence of epididymoorchitis is higher in patients with high pressure detrusor dysfunction associated with high sphincter pressures than it is in patients with lower pressures, but epididymitis and epididymoorchitis occur in both groups.

Females with Lower Motor Neuron Lesions

Most females with lower motor neuron lesions are currently managed by intermittent catheterization with a minimal effect on lower urinary tract function. The avoidance of suprapubic tubes and Foley catheters permits maintenance of a relatively normal genital tract, and sexual intercourse in these patients is quite feasible. Somewhere in the past 10 years of the urologic literature, there is the statement: "there are no impotent females; all they have to do is lie there." This is an inacurrate, sexist, misleading statement but is descriptive of certain attitudinal prejudices of physicians caring for patients with SCI. The visual evidence of a penile erection is relatively dramatic and urologic research, interest, and engineering determination to achieve erection have not been paralleled by similar efforts to normalize female sexual dysfunction following SCI. It would appear from the nature and extent of the neural injuries sustained by females with a sacral cord or cauda equina lesion that sexual dysfunction would be inevitable. If, in fact, vaginal lubrication, swelling of the labia, and clitoral erection are the homologs of male erection, these activities would be expected to be markedly impaired by sacral SCI. Similarly, the sensation of orgasm and the attendant rhythmic contraction of the pelvic floor musculature should be absent in a large percentage of such patients.

Upper Motor Neuron Lesions

Upper motor neuron lesions are associated with lower urinary tract dysfunction, which is frequently related to upper tract deterioration and vesicoureteral reflux, which can ultimately lead to renal failure (*18*). Because of the serious and relatively rapid changes in upper urinary tract function, associated with upper motor neuron lesions, treatment is necessarily vigorous. Detrusor-external sphincter (incoordination) dyssynergia is the most common abnormality of lower urinary tract function in this patient group. Whereas the standard method of therapy has been external sphincterotomy and condom drainage in males, it is now apparent that these methods are necessary only in about one-third of such patients. The remaining two-thirds can be managed satisfactorily by intermittent catheterization and anticholinergic agents (*16*). Thus, the type of management used for lower motor neuron lesions can be applied to most patients with upper motor neuron lesions, avoiding the use of condom drainage, Foley catheters, and suprapubic tubes. Although suprapubic tubes and Foley catheter drainage are to be condemned in view of the 50% incidence of upper urinary tract dysfunction experienced over a 10-year-period, condom drainage has not yet been entirely supplanted by intermittent catheterization. One-third of patients with upper motor neuron lesions will demonstrate detrusor reflex responses that are totally resistant to anticholinergic therapy, and since low-pressure bladder storage activity cannot be induced, intermittent catheterization is not feasible. Typically, such patients have febrile urinary tract infections, elevated residual urine volumes, and an abnormal intravenous pyelogram. In these cases, the only alternative in males is to proceed with external sphincterotomy. As stated earlier, the procedure is associated with the development of erectile impotence in a small but significant number of patients. Incision of the external sphincter at the 12 o'clock position diminishes, but does not eliminate the incidence of erectile impotence.

Reflex erectile activity can be a problem in patients who require condom catheter drainage. A vigorous erection induced by the application of a condom catheter is followed by detumescence and leakage of urine. To avoid the leakage, patients may wrap the condom with tape or place a double-back tape too tightly on the penis. Tight condom drainage encourages the development of bulbous urethral diverticuli and impedes urinary flow. Insertion of a penile prosthesis, which guarantees a certain minimal penile girth, makes it easier to apply the condom and prevents the drainage device from occluding the lumen of the urethra. Reflex erectile activity is a lesser problem in patients with thoracic lesions than in quadriplegics.

Problems in Females

Females with quadriplegia who experience autonomic dysreflexia at the time of intercourse can be treated satisfactorily with a small daily dose of an alpha-blocking agent. Phenoxybenzamine (dibenzyline) was first used in patients with autonomic dysreflexia induced by attempts at intercourse in 1976 (*20*); a dose of 10 mg/d or 1 mg/d of prazosin (Minipres) obviates this complication.

Females with reflex bladder activity that is poorly controlled by anticholinergic agents (and perhaps one-third of the females with SCI fall in this category) are most commonly treated by Foley catheter or suprapubic tube drainage. These methods, while safer in females than in males, are not benign. Erosion of the urethra and gradual fibrosis of the bladder with development of vesicoureteral reflux and intravesical calculi slowly but almost invariably occur. Since irreparable damage to the bladder as a storage reservoir, to the upper urinary tract, and to continence function can be induced by chronic Foley or suprapubic catheter drainage, these methods should be avoided. Alternatives in females with uncontrollable reflex vesical activity are relatively limited. Sacral rhizotomy either surgicially or by the injection of phenol or alcohol has been found useful (*21*). However, intermittent self-catheterization in quadriplegic females is usually impossible. Although some female quadriplegics can perform intermittent self-catheterization, the manipulation and assistance necessary to do so tend to place a heavy burden on the family or other care providers. It is reasonable in such individuals to proceed with construction either of a continent vesicostomy or, as an alternative to sacral rhizotomy, excision of most of the bladder, combined with a cecocystoplasty (*22*). A small segment of ileum can be brought to the skin to facilitate intermittent self-catheterization. These methods place an accessible stoma just below the umbilicus that does not leak and permits the patient to be independent as far as the urinary tract is concerned, even with extremely limited hand function. Although sacral rhizotomy and sacral neurolytic procedures have been avoided in males because of loss of erectile function, no such contraindications have been applied to females. To a degree, the use of sacral rhizotomy and neurolytic procedures in females has been the result of our ignorance of genital functional changes induced by neural lesions. Until more is known about the effect of complete lower motor neuron lesions on female sexual function (or the lack of effect), sacral rhizotomy should be reserved for those patients with intractable autonomic dysreflexia or upper urinary tract changes associated with Foley or suprapubic tube drainage, in whom no other method of therapy offers the same kind of protection to the upper urinary tract. In most of these individuals, an augmentation cystoplasty obviates reflex bladder activity; an ileal segment brought to the skin for intermittent self-catheterization provides continence and independence, but avoids an irreversible neurolytic procedure within the sacral spinal canal. Moreover, Leyson suggested to use Oxybutynin HCL (Ditropan) 5-7½ mg or Imipramine (Trofranil) 50-75 mg orally 1-2 hrs. prior to sexual activity in order to minimize or prevent urinary incontinence during orgasm (*23*).

Intractable Autonomic Dysreflexia

Infrequently, male and female patients with a spinal cord injury have intractable autonomic dysreflexia. In such individuals, neural ablative procedures are occasionally necessary to control a condition that may be life-threatening. Neurolytic procedures directed at the sacral roots or cord can effectively eliminate autonomic dysreflexia. However, such procedures are expensive in terms of functional loss, since reflex bladder activity and reflex erectile or orgastic activity are compromised. Male patients subjected to sacral rhizotomy for the control of autonomic dysreflexia require both sphincterotomy and total ablation of internal sphincter resistance to enable bladder "tap" (Credé) voiding. Credé voiding into a condom catheter, with leakage with transfers or any kind of physical exertion, is a likely consequence of a sacral rhizotomy. Although reflex erectile activity does not interfere with condom application after sacral rhizotomy, the loss of erectile activity may have to be treated with a penile prosthesis.

Long-Term Goals and the Preservation of Sexual Function in SCI Patients

Spinal cord lesions above T10-11 are associated with maintenance of an intact sacral cord and presumably preservation of the thoracolumbar reflex centers for ejaculation and emission. Based on current experimental and clinical knowledge, it would appear that both erection and ejaculation of viable sperm can be induced in patients with complete lesions above the thoracic cord level of T10. Less is known about the theoretical ability to induce similar erectile and ejaculatory activity in patients with lower lesions, but until it is definitely known that such techniques will not have the desired result, it seems reasonable to make every effort to preserve as nearly normal a lower urinary tract as possible, and to avoid neurosurgical and urologic procedures that damage the genital tract. Avoidance of Foley catheters and suprapubic tubes for drainage and either condom catheter drainage or intermittent catheterization in effect would improve the long-term outcome of the upper urinary tract, and preserve a reasonably normal bladder and urethra, as well as a more normal genital tract. The lesser incidence of urinary tract infection with intermittent catheterization and/or condom drainage may be associated with preservation of better seminal quality. At present, intermittent catheterization and suppression of detrusor activity or tone can be used in approximately 80% of SCI patients. In those cases where detrusor external sphincter dyssynergia cannot be medically controlled and low pressure storage not achieved, external sphincterotomy may be necessary and desirable. External sphincterotomy and condom drainage can be facilitated by a penile prostheses, which may improve sexual performance. Nevertheless, sphincter ablative procedures may have a deleterious effect on reflex erection, and as yet we are uncertain about the effect of an external sphincterotomy, or an individual's potential for electrically stimulated erection and ejaculation. Transection of the internal sphincter to improve drainage is necessary only in relatively unusual circumstances. In general, with adequate reflex bladder activity, the internal sphincter will open. If the detrusor contracts poorly or with very low pressure, the internal sphincter may not open. These patients can be better managed by intermittent catheterization than total destruction of internal and external sphincter function and conversion to condom drainage. Permanent ablation of internal sphincter activity after transurethral resection of the prostate often results in retrograde ejaculation. Most patients with detrusor sphincter dyssynergia, who might be considered for an internal and external sphincterotomy because of large residual urines, would theoretically be capable of undergoing successful electrically stimulated erection and ejaculation. Moreoever, persistent residual urine following external sphincterotomy is associated with inadequate, low-pressure detrusor responses. In that case, internal sphincterotomy will destroy part of the genital tract in individuals who would be better managed by intermittent catheterization.

In quadriplegics, autonomic dysreflexia may be induced by attempts to achieve electrically stimulated erection and ejaculation. In many such individuals, autonomic dysreflexia is associated with dyssynergic closure of the internal sphincter at the time of detrusor contraction. Although internal sphincter dyssynergia in quadriplegic patients with autonomic dysreflexia can be satisfactorily treated by transurethral incision or resection of the bladder neck and prostate, alpha-blocking agents, which provide a reversible method of therapy, are preferred. Prolonged $alpha_1$ blockade results in suppressed internal sphincter function and an open bladder neck and prostatic urethra, but the changes are reversible.

Patients with incomplete lesions do not require irreversible methods of therapy. They should be maintained on intermittent catheterization and anticholinergic agents for as long as feasible to allow the lesion to evolve toward normalcy. Preservation of internal and external sphincter function and the avoidance of neurolytic procedures, as well as the preservation of normal bladder storage activity, should be the underlying goal in such individuals until such time as the final effects of neural lesions are clear and fixed. Urologists should preserve, in so far as possible, lower urinary tract function and avoid irreversible drainage or neurolytic procedures in such patients until a clear and demonstrable danger to upper urinary tract function exists.

References

1. Eckhard, C. (1863) Untersuchungen über die erection des penis beim Hund. Beitr. *Anat. Physiol.* **3**, 123.
2. Langley, J. N. (1895) Innervation of pelvic and adjoining viscera. *J. Physiol.* **19**, 85.
3. Newman, H. F. Reiss, H., and Northrup, J. D. (1982) Physical basis of emission, ejaculation and orgasm in the male. *Urology* **19**, 341.
4. Woodside, J. R. and McGuire, E. J. (1979) Urethral hypotonicity after suprasacral spinal cord injury. *J. Urol.* **121**, 783.
5. McGuire, E. J. (1977) Combined radiographic and manometric assessment of urethral sphincter function. *J. Urol.* **118**, 632.
6. Kadia, K. R., Markland, C., and Fraley, E. (1975) Sexual function following high retroperitoneal lymphadenectomy. *J. Urol.* **114**, 237.
7. McGuire, E. J. (1979) Urethral sphincter mechanisms. Urol. Clin. North Am. **1**, 39.
8. McGuire, E. J. and Herlihy, E. (1979) Bladder and urethral responses to sympathetic stimulation. *Invest. Urol.* **17**, 9.
9. Learmouth, J. R. (1931) A contribution to the neurophysiology of the urinary bladder in man. *Brain* **54**, 147.
10. Downie, J. W. (1983) Unpublished observations. Personal communication.

11. McGuire, E. J., Woodside, J. R., Borden, T. A., and Weiss, R. M. (1981) Prognostic value of urodynamic testing in myelodysplastic patients. *J. Urol.* **126**, 205.
12. Walsh, P. C. and Donker, P. C. (1982) Impotence following radical prostatectomy: Insight into etiology and prevention. *J. Urol.* **128**, 492.
13. Comarr, A. E. (1970) Sexual function among patients with spinal cord injury. *Urol. Int.* **25**, 134.
14. Masters, W. H. and Johnson, V. E. (1966) *Human Sexual Response* (Boston, Little, Brown and Co., Boston, Mass.).
15. Woodside, J. R. and McGuire, E. J. (1982) Detrusor hypertonicity as a late complication of a *Wertheim* hysterectomy. *J. Urol.* **127**, 1143.
16. McGuire, E. J. and Savastano, J. A. (1983) Long term follow-up of spinal cord injury patients managed by intermittent catheterization. *J. Urol.* **129**, 775.
17. Leriche, A., Berard, E., Vauzelle, J. L., Minaire, P., Girard, R., Archimbaud, J. R., and Bourret, J. (1977–1978) Histological and hormonal testicular changes in spinal cord patients. *Paraplegia* **15**, 274.
18. Bensman, A. and Kottke, F. J. (1966) Induced emission of sperm utilizing electrical stimulation of the seminal vesicles and vas deferens. *Archives of Phys. Med. and Rehab.* July **47**, 436.
19. McGuire, E. J. and Brady, S. (1979) Detrusor sphincter dyssynergia. *J. Urol.* **121**, 774.
20. McGuire, E. J., Wagner, F. M., and Weiss, R. M. (1976) Treatment of autonomic dysreflexia with *Phenoxybenzamine*. *J. Urol.* **115**, 53.
21. McGuire, E. J. and Morrissey, S. G. (1982) The development of neurogenic vesical dysfunction after experimental spinal cord injury or sacral rhizotomy in nonhuman primates. *J. Urol.* **128**, 1390.
22. Green, D., Mitcheson, H. D., and McGuire, E. J. (1983) Management of the difficult bladder by continent vesicostomy and augmentation ileocecocystoplasty. *J. Urol.* **130**, 133.
23. Leyson, J. F. J. (1989) Biotechnological advances in sexual medicine. Presented at the Assoc. of Phil. Physicians in America, Inc. Annual meeting. July 26-30. St. Louis, MO.

6

Sexuality and the Adolescent

Michael A. Alexander

Introduction

Adolescence, or the "latency period," as Erickson (*6*) describes it, represents a stage of human development in which children leave behind the final phase of childhood. By the end of this latency period, adolescents have, one hopes, developed a sense of mastery and competency in peer relationships. During latency, adolescents should be able to come to grips with the moral attitudes and values of others, and establish their sexual identification firmly (*6,22*). For most children, it represents a stable time in their psychosocial development.

Adolescents and Disability

Several difficulties encountered by disabled preadolescents and their parents have been identified. The patients have had to cope with a number of severe stresses, and many parents have become aware of the inconsistency between how they view their children and the issue of these children's disabilities. Parents see themselves as protectors of the helpless, yet fall prey to feelings of revulsion for the abnormal. They see themselves as inadequate reproducers and child-rearers. They continually feel a social unease as a result of a vicarious stigma. They feel, and

Ed. Note: It is estimated that accidents (mostly vehicular) disable 50,000 children each year in the USA. In third-world countries, spinal cord traumas are chiefly caused by domestic violence and/or projectile (missile) injuries.

Sexual Rehabilitation of the Spinal-Cord-Injured Patient
Edited by J.F. Leyson, © 1990 The Humana Press, Inc.

perhaps rightly know, that in the eyes of many others they are less than normal; they are viewed as being less than whole themselves (*9*). They often develop a pattern of overprotection that impairs their children's development (*3*) and results in decreased social interaction and mobility for the children.

These parental stresses often lead to a type of family behavior that seeks to avoid stressful issues (*23*), and can take the form of ignoring or creating smoke screens. It is obvious that, if the sexuality of their disabled children is stressful to the parents, it becomes an issue they will avoid.

The health care professions are often guilty of fostering in the family a feeling of inadequacy and incompetence by the manner in which they manage families in the clinical setting. Seldom are the children and their families given choices; instead, they must turn to the omnipotent health care provider for answers (*8*).

Disabled children frequently see themselves as extensions of their parents and, consequently, have little vision of themselves in the future. Their lives are complicated by the presence of multiple adult figures, health care providers, and educators. Their capacities for self-assertion, self-determination, and gradual growth away from their families is decreased (*18*).

In their attempts to establish relationships with others, disabled children often receive inappropriate and abnormal feedback from the able-bodied. Their plight is that inappropriate signals are inappropriately received (*18*). For example, the able-bodied actually place a greater physical distance between themselves and the disabled whenever standing or sitting in a group. There is more eye contact between the able-bodied and the disabled. This can delude the handicapped into believing that the able-bodied are really interested and care. Paradoxically, less time is spent in that same interaction between the able and disabled. Finally, the able-bodied will admit to experiencing a high level of discomfort in the presence of the disabled (*28*). In a normal classroom situation, able-bodied children consistently, in testing, show a preferred interest in associating with the able-bodied. They view the physically disabled, but intellectually intact child as ahead of the mentally retarded (*3,19*), but still a poor second choice. Disabled children are intimately aware of their loss of normalcy and mourn that loss. They go on to anticipate failure throughout life (*26*). In discussing themselves, children are able to note that their functional restrictions deprive them of social experiences (*21*). They may become so anxious about facing new social situations that they often set themselves up for failure (*3*).

Disabled adolescents know that the able-bodied barely see them as neighbors and certainly not as potential spouses (*29*). Aware of their embarrassment about feeling different, they develop and use an egocentric and aloof pattern of behavior as a social defense (*14*).

With the onset of adolescence and hormonal changes, teenagers are confronted within an awakening need for psychosexual interaction (*2*). Adolescents have several important tasks to complete during this developmental stage, the major ones among them being to achieve a sense of independence and to acquire a set of social skills that will allow them to function as young adults in both work and social settings. Each must achieve a sense that he/she is a worthwhile person and develop a level of self-esteem that will allow him/her to tolerate the pain of failure and rejection. It is a stage at which the adolescents must develop necessary academic and vocational skills, and achieve an internalized set of guiding norms and values that will withstand the pressures of the outside world. Most importantly, adolescents must adjust to a rapidly changing physique and sexual maturation, and then learn to understand that the physiques they develop will be those they will have for the rest of their lives (*6*).

Disabled adolescents must face some additional difficult issues. Often during this stage of their lives, disabled adolescents begin to experience a decrease in mobility and proficiency in activities of daily living. This often results from an increase in size and obesity, which can occur at this age. These adolescents are keenly aware that at this stage they themselves are noticing more about others and, consequently, that their peers will notice more about them—in short, that their fantasies must now end (*10*).

Coping with their own fears and guilt, and the stigma that comes as a result of their disability can leave these children in a situation where they do not feel positive about their self-worth and can, in fact, leave them programmed for failure (*4,5*). It is fascinating that the very fact of being aware that one is stigmatized can lead to decreased performance in social situations (*7*). In coping with these issues of sexuality, clinicians are confronted by individuals who are limited in their ability to achieve independence as a result of a persistent physical dependence on others. This societal immobility prevents these adolescents from acquiring a set of social skills and impairs their chances for success. Consequently, it is even harder for them to develop visions of themselves as worthwhile individuals. To the realization that their disability affects their ability to develop necessary academic and vocational skills are added self-guilt and stigma, which lead to an increased awkwardness, overcompensation of their egocentric behavior, and social aloofness, all of which place the disabled adolescents at an extreme disadvantage.

Disability and Sexuality

It is well documented that disabled adolescents lag behind other children in knowledge and awareness of sexuality (*1,22,25*). Not only do these children have less information, but the diminished chance for social interaction frequently leaves them with poor judgment when handling matters of sexuality (*25*). At this point, a case history might help to make this clear. "RR" was a 14-year-old, quadriplegic child. On one particular day, he was brought in by both parents who were very upset with the young man. At first, they would not discuss their anger. They finally broke down and gave the following account. Three nights before, they had left RR with a 16½-year-old babysitter while they went to a movie. They returned home to find, in their living room, four members of the church, the babysitter, her parents, and RR waiting for them. It seems that while watching a television program that involved some amount of sexual innuendo, the patient asked the sitter if she would show him her breasts. The patient was totally incapable of helping her in this activity. This so unnerved the sitter that she called her parents who called the elders of the church, setting the scene that the family walked into. In discussing this with the family, several very important issues in the management of this child were made clear. Although the patient had never had the opportunity to view any other nude person, the entire family was most cavalier about being around the patient during his bathing and toileting. At no time had the family or the school provided any information to this young man about sexuality. He had never asked any questions, and they had never offered any information. With all of his other activities and concerns, they had always been honest and forthright in answering questions. It then appeared that this young man, aroused by the television, felt he had a very appropriate question to ask of the babysitter. It was clear that this young man needed a program of lectures to bring his level of knowledge up to that of the able-bodied population. Judging from this case and from the experiences of many others, it is evident that a definite need exists for sexual adjustment counseling for persons with severe disabilities, including children (*27*).

Programs of instruction in sexuality may have to be multilingual for multiracial populations of disabled adolescents. Sex education and value systems should start in the early or prelatency stage. All children need to have available to them the experiences of seeing adults of both sexes acting out their appropriate psychosexual roles. They need to develop an intimacy and closeness to both parents or to suitable substitute adult figures. They must be encouraged in an open and frank manner to acquire the knowledge, awareness, and appropriate specific words, gestures, and questions. Some of the questions asked by patients in a rehabilitation hospital are given in Table 1.

It is an interesting phenomenon of our times that the procreative function of sex is often deferred for 15–20 yr beyond the age at which it most commonly occurred in the past. This postponement has added to the stress of developing a competency in appropriate intersex social activities. As the patient reaches adolescence, specific physical deficits must be addressed, and goals and resources in meeting those goals must be provided. It is at this time that the educator must be careful to work within the constraints of the children's and families' religious beliefs and attitudes regarding birth control, premarital sexual relationships, and masturbation. A guideline questionnaire for parents regarding sex education and relationships is given in Table 2.

With the exception of the Catholic Church, there appears to be universal consensus that masturbation has no deleterious effect on the psychosocial maturation of children (*2,16,20,22,24*). There is a good deal more to the teaching of appropriate sexuality than issue of simply moral concern. Many programs concern themselves with the following important aspects of their sexuality: (a) the adolescents are encouraged always to care for and to be responsible for their own bodies, (b) they are expected to avoid sexual exploitation of others, and (c) they are to remember that they are not only ultimately responsible to others, but to themselves as well (*17*).

Counseling these families and their SCI children involves attention to their most common questions and fears (Tables 1 and 2). The purpose of a sex education program needs to be explained, and reassurances must be given that the aim is not to introduce and start adolescents on the path to sexual debauchery. The family must be led through the issues discussed here until they realize the extent of their children's ignorance of fundamental information. If the families can understand that ignorance of sexual issues amounts to vulnerability and sets the children up for rejection and even worse, exploitation, they are then usually able to accept the importance of such an education program.

There still remains a fair degree of controversy concerning how one guarantees that disabled adolescents can have these meaningful interpersonal relationships. There are those who advocate pairing disabled

Table 1
Common Questions and Fears of Adolescents

Is it normal to masturbate?
Am I masturbating too much?
Do I have homosexual tendencies?
Am I abnormal if I have thoughts involving sex with people I know, even members of my family?
What is a homosexual?
Are my breasts too small?
Is the pill safe?
Is my penis too small?
How can I get birth control without my parents' knowing about it?
How can you tell if you have VD?
Is there something wrong with me if I remain a virgin?
How can you avoid pregnancy?
How can I say "no"?
How can I tell if I'm really in love?
How can I know if I have an orgasm?
Is sexual intercourse painful?
Is oral sex normal?
What about having sex with someone you're not in love with?
Where can I get an abortion?
How can I tell if I'm pregnant?
How can I enjoy sex more?
Why do I have these unexplained erections?

children, rather than attempting to mix them with the able-bodied, because the youngsters will be more likely to have success and experiences the excitement and joys of that phase of development (*11*). It is interesting that these are not, for the most part, the opinions of the disabled themselves, who often feel that being seen with an able-bodied person enhances their own self-image (*12*). Some feel that the handicapped adolescents who rush to avoid other disabled people are unwilling to accept the reality of their less-than-perfect bodies. The point is that there is no correct solution to this controversy. Unfortunately, adolescents are attracted to other adolescents who are unstable and in the middle of their own crises. At this point, there still remain multiple barriers to sociosexual intergrations of the disabled adolescents. These include the disability itself and the subsequent abnormal-normalization as previously discussed. There are the barriers that result from both the vicarious stigma and the "sick role." Society exempts the sick from the obligations of work, school, and social responsibility. However, the "sick" have an obligation to receive help and be appropriately ill

Table 2
Human Growth and Development: Parent Questionnaire

1. What particular issue of sexual development do you find most difficult to talk to your child about?
2. Do you feel you need some kind of help in discussing issues of sexual development with your child?
3. If so, what particular kind of help do you think would be most useful to you?
4. Is your child overly friendly to the point that worries you?
5. Do you think your child will ever want to get married?
6. Do you think your child will ever want to have dates with someone of the opposite sex? If so, will you allow this?
7. If your child wanted to get married, do you think you could ever consider giving your permission?
8. Do you think your child will ever be capable of being a parent to a child?
9. Does your child know where babies come from? (Explanation)
10. Does your child know how babies begin to grow in the mother's body?
11. Does your child know how long babies grow in the mother's body?
12. Does your child know how a baby gets out of the mother's body? (Explanation)
13. Has masturbation been an issue in regard to your child?
14. How have you attempted to handle the issue of masturbation with your child?
15. How have you attempted to handle the issue of menstruation with your daughter? (Where appropriate) What would you tell her if she expressed fears?
16. What would you consider the ideal situation for your son/daughter when he/she reaches the age of 20?
17. Do you think that you will be able to proceed with discussing sexuality with your child?
18. How would you explain what falling in love is like?
19. What religious values, regarding sexuality, do you want to impart to your child?

(*30*). If the disabled are cast in this role, they are viewed as repugnent by the able-bodied when they profess sexual needs. The myth that the disabled are sick is still rampant. There are able-bodied children who actually fear "catching" a physical disability. Other barriers are architecture, transportation, finances, and time (*12*). As one disabled women put it, "Every date is well planned and methodical; casual sex is a fantasy" (*12*). Any and all of these problems alone or in combination can present unsurmountable barriers (*12*).

Blind disabled (SCI) children who are "eager" to understand their changing bodies need help from family or rehabilitation/sex education physicians who will initiate sex education at these patients' first signs of puberty (*30*). Sex education consists of verbal and touching methods, either with inanimate or live models (anatomy, pregnancy, and birth). If the patient is mentally impaired, sex education should be taught as soon as she/he attains a certain level of intelligence, at which time basic (simple) information about sex will be understood. If the patient is an adolescent with a postspinal-cord injury, sex education/counseling can be taught before the first weekend pass (with parental consent). Adolescent SCI sexuality education should consist of topics concerning disability, social sexual issues (dating, love, and sex roles), sexual value systems, pregnancy, fertility/contraception, (sexually) transmitted diseases, anatomy/physiology, and psychosexual (sexual performance) categories. Handicapped children of lesbian and gay parents may need additional psychotherapeutic counseling because they may experience dissonance resulting from an atypical parental role model.

Literature addressed to how the disabled can quickly disarm and engage the able-bodied in meaningful social discourse is just developing. One technique meriting further study is that of simply acknowledging their own disability (*15*). Thus, it seems that to succeed socially the disabled teenager needs to be adroit at putting the able-bodied at ease.

Conclusion

Disabled adolescents must endure the same crises and hardships that their able-bodied counterparts endure. However, many of these crises are made worse by the addition of a disability with its own unique set of problems about which the able-bodied individual has no insight or understanding. The individuals involved in counseling and preparing adolescents for their emerging sexuality must be aware of these issues. They must seek to soften the crisis of adolescence, aware that trauma and pain are something that we have all had to endure.

References

1. Bloom, J. L. (1961) Sex education for handicapped adolescents. *J. School Health* **39**, 363–367.

2. Bradfield, K. (1972) *Life Together: the Situation of the Handicapped* (E. Olofssone Boktryckeri AB Stockholm).

3. Carter, V. E. and Chess, S. (1951) Factors influencing the adaptations of organically handicapped children. *Am. J. Orthopsychiatry* **21**, 827–837.

4. Coulter, D. L. (1980) The unfairness of life for children with handicaps *JAMA* **244**, 1207–1208.
5. Cruickshank, W. M. (1951) The relation of physical disability to fear and guilt feelings. *Child Development* **22**, 291–298.
6. Erickson, E. H. (1964) *Childhood & Society*, 2nd Ed. (W. W. Norton, New York).
7. Farina, A., Allen, J. G., and Brigid, B. (1968) The role of the stigmatized person in affecting social relationships. *J. Pers.* **36**, 169–182.
8. Fox, A. M. (1977) Psychological problems of the physically handicapped. *Br. J. Hosp. Med.* **17**, 479–490.
9. Fraser, B. C. (1980) The meaning of handicap in children. *Child Care Health Dev.* **6**, 83-91.
10. Freeman, R. D. (1970) Psychiatric problems in adolescents with cerebral palsey. *Dev. Med. Child Neurol.* **12**, 64–70.
11. Garret, J. Sex education: a second opinion. *Spec. Educ.* **60**, 16–17.
12. Goldman, F. (1978) Environmental barriers to sociosexual integration: the insiders perspectives. *Rehab. Lit.* **39**, 185–189.
13. Goodman, N., Richardson, S. A., Dornbusch, S. M., and Hastorf, A. H. (1963) Variant reactions to physical disabilities. *Am. Soc. Rev.* **28**, 429–435.
14. Harper, D. C. (1978) Personality characteristics of physically impaired adolescents. *J. Clin. Psychol.* **34**, 97–103.
15. Hastorf, A. H., Wildfogel, J., and Cassman, T. (1979) Acknowledgement of handicap as a tactic in social interaction. *J. Personal. Soc. Psychol.* **37**, 1790–1797.
16. Heslinga, K., Schellen, A. M., and Verkugl, A. (1974) *Not Made of Stone* (Charles C. Thomas, Springfield, Illinois).
17. Kempton, W. (1975) Sex education: a cooperative effort of parent and teacher. *Except. Child* **41**, 531–535.
18. Nigro, G. (1976) Some observations on personal relationships and sexual relationships among lifelong disabled. *Am. Rehab. Lit.* **37**, 328–334.
19. Parish, T. S., Ohlsen, R. L., and Parish, J. G. (1978) A look at mainstreaming in light of children's attitudes toward the handicapped. *Percept. Motor Skills* **46**, 1019–1021.
20. Rhodes, P. (1976) Psychosexual problems of chronic handicapping disease. *Med. J. Australia* **2**, 688–692.
21. Richardson, S. A., Hastorf, A. H., and Dornbush G. (1964) Effects of physical disability on a child's description of himself. *Child Dev.* **35**, 893–907.
22. Robinault, I. P. (1978) Sex, Society and the Disabled (Harper and Row, Hagerstown, Maryland).
23. Rogers, B. M., Hillemeiser, M. M., O'Neill, E., and Slonim, M. B. (1981) Depression in the chronically ill or handicapped school-aged child. *MCN* **6**, 266–273.
24. Rutter, M. (1971) Normal psychosexual development. *J. Child Psychol. Psychiatry* **11**, 259–283.

25. Schlesinger, B. (1976) Sexuality and the physically handicapped. *CMA* **114**, 772–773.
26. Schowalter, J. E. (1979) The chronically ill child, in *Basic Handbook of Child Psychiatry* (Noshpitz, J. D., ed.) **1**, 432–436, Basic Books, New York.
27. Shrey, D. E., Kiefer, J. S., and Anthony, W. A. (1979) Sexual adjustment counseling for persons with severe disabilities: a skill-based approach for rehabilitation professionals. *J. Rehab.* April/May/June, 28–33.
28. Somervill, J. W., Veeder, M. N., Miller, B. E., and Zortman, G. L. (1981) The sex variable and reactions to the physically disabled by eighth grade students. *Am. Cour. Ther. J.* **35**, 48–51.
29. Togonu-Bickersteth, F. (1982) Social distance between self and stigmatized others. *R. Soc Health J.* **102**, 144–149.
30. Welbourne, A. K. (1982) Sexual education of the blind adolescent. *Sexual Med. Today* **6**, 10–14.

7
Psychological Assessment and Therapy for the Spinal-Cord-Injured Patient

M. G. Eisenberg

Introduction

Disorders of sexual function occur frequently in patients with spinal cord injury, but have not until very recently been studied in a systematic fashion. The frequent occurrence of this disorder is clearly related to the fact that the sexual organs are directly controlled by components at all levels of the nervous system, ranging from the peripheral nerves to the cerebral hemispheres. In addition, it must be emphasized that sexuality is not just a biologic function, but also has complex psychological and social aspects. The work of ethnologists, such as Lorenz (*25*), has shown this to be true for most animal species. In humans, this aspect of sexuality appears to be particularly important. Small children, when asked to identify themselves, often respond by saying, "I'm a boy" or "I'm a girl," their gender providing a source of personal identification. Frequently, how well individuals perform sexually determines how much of a "man" or a "woman" they see themselves to be. Given this system of beliefs with respect to the emphasis on sexuality and sexual performance, a great deal of anxiety becomes attached to situations in which sexual behavior is expected. These added meanings and expectations impart considerable importance to sexual behavior and have contributed to the fact that human sexuality consists of much more than reproductive function. These factors may help explain why sexual functions are highly vulnerable to all types of severe and chronic

Sexual Rehabilitation of the Spinal-Cord-Injured Patient
Edited by J.F. Leyson, © 1990 The Humana Press, Inc.

diseases, particularly diseases of the nervous system, which so frequently disrupt motor behavior.

The scarcity of published material on this topic is, therefore, difficult to explain. Supposedly the subject of sex is no longer taboo, yet health care professionals all too often neglect the subject of sexual functioning with their patients. In turn, patients often hesitate to volunteer symptoms related to what is considered a highly personal part of their lives. Changes are occurring however. In a recent bibliographic review of the literature on the general topic of sex and disability, Eisenberg (*8*) notes that, of the 925 papers he found on the subject, over 80% were published since 1960. Now available are journals devoted to the topic of sexuality and medical/physical problems, such as *Medical Aspects of Human Sexuality* and *Sexuality and Disability.*

It was not until the late 1960s and early 1970s that programs designed to introduce the issue of sexual function into rehabilitation began to surface. In fact, because of the increasing freedom with which the general public discussed sexual issues and the heightening awareness of the disabled themselves, the pendulum swung from the belief that sex was not important following disability to the belief that sex was very important following spinal cord injury. In fact, a rehabilitation program was not thought to be comprehensive unless it had a sex education component.

It was not until 1976 that cord injured persons were asked to rate the importance of sexual loss vis-à-vis other major functional losses. Hetrick (*17*) found that, whereas sexual functioning was thought of as being important, use of paralyzed extremities and bowel and bladder control were considered more significant by the cord injured themselves.

A second investigation into the perceived importance of sexual functioning by staff and cord injured patients was conducted by Hanson and Franklin (*16*). They asked 54 paraplegic males and 74 quadriplegics males to rank the importance of various bodily functions to them. First choice received a 1, second choice received a 2, and so on. For persons with paraplegia, use of legs obtained a mean rank of 1.63, control of bowel and bladder ranked 1.83, and normal feeling and use of sex organs ranked 2.53. For persons with quadriplegia, the average rankings were use of arms and hands, 1.31; normal bladder and bowel function, 2.5; legs, 2.65; and sex, 3.54. Time since injury and marital status were not factors in these ratings.

The rehabilitation staff was also asked by Hanson and Franklin to rate the importance they thought the cord injured would attach to various bodily functions. The mean ranks for staff were: arms and hands, 1.62;

sex, 2.5; bowel and bladder function, 2.69; and legs, 3.2. Based on these data, the investigation concluded that they could not support the notion that sex is often the most devastating of all functional losses to men with spinal injury. Two-thirds of the men ranked sex last in order of importance, but the rehabilitation staff consistently overestimated the importance of sexual function to their patients.

The foregoing discussion was presented to help place the issue of sexuality in some perspective. Sex is a primary drive, as are hunger, thirst, and the avoidance of pain. The onset of chronic illness or physical disability, such as spinal cord injury, often affects a person's ability to function "normally" and, equally important, may lead one to reevaluate his/her masculinity or femininity. Self-image may be compromised, and the ability to establish relationships affected. However, sexual identity comprises only one segment of a person's total psychosocial status. Certainly, it is an important dimension, but it is one that must be seen as only one piece of the puzzle—one factor in the constellation comprising a person's "personality." Undue emphasis on sexual issues can run counter to the attitude that functionally intact genitals are not necessary for a successful sexual adjustment to the disability. In addition, an exaggerated emphasis on sexual issues can magnify the importance of penile-vaginal intercourse and minimize the role of open and honest communication in maintaining relationships. This author has seen many hundreds of cord-injured couples who were initially presented as having a "sexual problem." However, relatively quickly into the assessment process, it became abundantly clear that the sexual incompetence of one member of the couple may have been focused upon, but the lack of communication between the two was the major source of problem. Their inability to communicate sexually served as a microcosmic study of their more generalized inability to communicate on a wide range of topics.

Interestingly, the methods used to communicate are used in sexual acts as well. Some use sex as a way of controlling, manipulating, threatening, or withdrawing from others. A thorough sexual history yields much useful data about the total relationship, which can be used in treating the alleged sexual problem and in resolving other problems that are nonsexual in nature.

In summary, whereas sex may not be the most important issue facing the spinal cord injured, as early writers suggested, it is a significant one that often affects an individual's gender identity and ability to establish and maintain relationships. It is, therefore, an area that must be addressed if the person is to function optimally following a spinal cord injury.

Sexual Functioning and Self-Image

The dependent position a person experiences following a spinal cord injury often has a devastating effect on self-concept, and concomitant changes in function and appearance may initiate body image disturbances. Conomy (*7*) studied the disturbances in body image occurring in 18 cord injured patients. He found that body image disorders involved hallucinatory disturbances, including disordered perception of the body in space (proprioceptive body image), of posture and movement, and of somatic bulk, size, and continuity. Patients found these experiences terrifying and feared they were becoming mentally unbalanced. Because of the hospitalization and immobility at an age when able-bodied young adults are actively coping with problems of life, many cord-injured persons experience severe depression, frustration, and anxiety, all expressed by acting-out behavior involving aggression, hostility, and anger. Some of the frustration and testing of limits is expressed through sexually oriented jokes and flirting with staff members. In addition, such remarks and comments are often seen as a means by which the patient is affirming masculinity or femininity and testing out in a safe environment their sexual attractiveness to others. Such sexually oriented comments serve a very real need and should be dealt with in a therapeutic fashion.

Sex role behavior is precipitously interrupted by a spinal cord injury. The role relationship with the sexual partner may be reversed or significantly damaged, with the partner assuming employment and financial responsibilities, but of even greater importance, actual physical care of the cord injured person. A parent–child rather than a husband–wife relationship can easily develop. It is difficult to continue to view someone as being sexually attractive after performing bowel care on him/her.

Following a spinal cord injury, many persons report difficulty maintaining relationships and finding new ones. Cogswell (*6*) studied 36 young adult paraplegics, both male and female, black and white, from a variety of socioeconomic backgrounds. All experienced a marked reduction in their social contacts and frequency in entering community settings, as well as in the number of roles they played. Cogswell also noted that, as SCI persons resumed social relationships, they seldom resumed relationships with pretrauma friends, but rather associated with individuals of lower class status, decidedly younger or older, or less attractive in other ways. They may have terminated relationships because they found it difficult to assist others to adjust to their new status as disabled persons. By forming new relationships, they were able to project themselves as persons of worth. In addition, investigators (*18*) have observed that conflict often exists over the resumption of sexual activity.

In a permanent relationship, one of the partners may wish to resume or attempt sexual activity, whereas the other may fear injury or harm in some way.

One of the most pervasive fears of the cord injured is that the spouse or sexual partner may reject them because they cannot function satisfactorily (*18*). Berkman et al. (*5*) surveyed 148 cord injured outpatients using the Index of Sexual Adjustment, an instrument that measures factors such as adaptation to sexual limitations, partner satisfaction, sexual self-concept, and regularity of sexual contact. They found that high scores on the index were positively correlated with better physical function, higher income, the role of worker and community participant, higher morale, injury at an earlier age, younger current age, and positive attitudes of self-acceptance and independence. It was evident that psychologic and social, as well as physical factors were relevant for sexual rehabilitation.

Of the 148 persons in the Berkman study, 33 reported no sexual relations since injury. Forty-one percent rated their sex relations as satisfactory, 36% indicated they were somewhat satisfied, and 23% stated they were unsatisfied. In contrast, 76% thought their partners were satisfied. Since sexual partners were not interviewed, the accuracy of the reports could not be verified. However, the findings of the study are significant, since they refute the myth that individuals cannot engage in sexual activity after cord injury. Of the group studied, 97% had sexual experiences, and 79% felt they were desirable as partners.

Each of the 31 spinal-cord-injured women interviewed by Bergman and Hadley (*4*) had at least one sexual experience since the injury, not necessarily involving intercourse; however, 27 reported they had intercourse. Sexual adjustment scores were computed on the basis of each subject's stated degree of adjustment, the subject's and her mate's satisfaction with the frequency of the sexual encounters, and the woman's stated degree of pleasure derived from the sexual encounter. Seven women reported their sexual adjustment and satisfaction improved over time; however, the correlation between sexual adjustment scores and time since injury was near zero. Fourteen women who had received some information about sexual ability were not adjusting any better than the 17 who had not received information. However, the women were told only that they could have intercourse, would have normal menstrual cycles, and would be able to have children. They were not told how they could go about having intercourse, and most were not given sexual counseling while in the hospital.

The first sexual experiences after injury appears to be the most psychologically uncomfortable, and much time was needed to get over the fear of rejection experienced by divorced and single women. As women began to feel more secure, their social and sexual relationships improved. Those with poor self-images had more difficulty adjusting sexually. All stressed the importance of being open and honest with sexual partners, and that communication was the key to a healthy relationship.

The quality of the relationship between sexual partners is of the greatest importance in adjusting to other modes of sexual behavior. Empathic understanding on the part of a spouse or sexual partner plays a vital role in the nature of any sexual relationship, but even more so if one has a physical disability. Many of the newly disabled are not married and do not have sexual partners. Their greatest concern is finding mates who are willing to work their problems through with them. For them, the issue of sexual incompatibility is secondary to the social problem of meeting and developing a relationship.

Even though men and women whose lesions are complete have no sensations below the level of the injury, decreasing subjective pleasures of sex, most indicate that the general bodily responses and stimulation above the injury are satisfying. The most significant satisfaction is probably not physiologic, but that of participating in what is one of the most important social experiences.

Psychologic Assessment and Treatment of SCI Patients

If the individual is going through the grieving process and is depressed, little energy will be mobilized for interest in sexual activities. Some patients continue to deny that loss of sexual function is permanent, and are not interested in discussing or learning about alternate sexual life-styles. Other concerns, such as incontinence or financial difficulties, may occupy most of the individual's attention. Identification of the correct time for intervention is essential.

SCI persons, like others, are usually not direct in their requests for information and their expressions of concern about sexuality. Nonverbal behavior indicating signs of depression or sexual acting-out statements such as, "I'm not good for much anymore," or "I wonder why my girlfriend bothers to visit me," may be the first indication that the individual has sexual concerns. The degree of interest in sex must also be assessed. Some become obsessed with sexuality, whereas others sublimate it completely.

Sociologic factors must be considered in the assessment process, including marital status, presence of a girlfriend or boyfriend, and the nature of these relationships. Fears and concerns of the patient and sex partner about sexuality, their attitude about the disability, and forms of sexual activity other than penile–vaginal intercourse must also be evaluated. Religious and sociocultural beliefs about "normal" sexual activity must also be assessed, as should financial problems that may be stressing the relationship and contributing to compromised sexual functioning.

Paramount in the psychological assessment and treatment of the cord injured individual is ascertaining the etiologic basis of the sexual dysfunction, i.e., organic vs functional (psychological). The remainder of this chapter examines the assessment and treatment of sexual problems that are psychogenic in nature. Treatments for such problems are psychologically based, whereas those determined to be organic in origin may require surgical involvement (i.e., penile implants). Definitive diagnosis of the role of organic contributions in erectile dysfunction can be aided by a lengthy interview, a comprehensive physical examination, and a detailed questionnaire that is filled out by clients (*1,23,26*).

Devices that directly measure daytime and nocturnal penile tumescence can also be employed. Good clinicians, however, can usually differentiate organic from psychological origins of poor erections by asking a few simple questions to ascertain the conditions under which the male usually functions. In the event that the dysfunction is organic and a penile prosthesis is being considered, a thorough psychologic evaluation is indicated. However, it is important to understand that most cord injured patients presenting with sexual difficulties have both psychologic and organic features to the dysfunction.

The prevailing view of the best therapeutic approach to sexual dysfunction has undergone considerable change over the past decade. Until recently, sexual dysfunctions were widely accepted as symptoms of a deep-seated personality conflict, reflecting the influence of instinctual drives, maturational changes in focus of sexual responsiveness from the oral to the anal to the genital zone, and crucial early childhood experiences (*12,14*). As such, sexual dysfunction could only be treated through individual insight-oriented psychotherapy requiring "an appointment several times a week for a minimum of eight months" (*2*). Given this viewpoint, it logically follows that most people suffering from sexual dysfunction could not be helped, or, as it has been phrased, "as a mass problem, the question of frigidity is unfortunately not to be solved" (*3*). For the cord injured, the possibility of receiving help was even more remote. Clinicians would assume the dysfunction was organic in nature ("After all, he/she is paralyzed! What do you expect?"), and give little or no thought to the possibility that the dysfunction might be functional (psychological) in nature, arising out of concerns about altered role functions, immobility, reduced sensation, comprised respiratory functioning, and so on.

The general public first became aware of the effectiveness of an alternative approach to the treatment of sexual dysfunction with the publication of Masters and Johnson's *Human Sexual Inadequacy* (*26*). This approach involved brief, time-limited, directive counseling aimed at symptom removal rather than attainment of insight, uncovery of repressions, or resolution of unconscious conflict. Although the direct, symptomatic treatment of sexual dysfunction has recently received much publicity, the roots of this "new" therapy actually go back over 200 years. However, only publication of Masters and Johnson's (*26*) unquestionable data on the effectiveness of the direct approach led to its general acceptance.

The principles of direct treatment of sexual dysfunction were developed for the able-bodied. They are, nonetheless, appropriate for use with the cord-injured whose dysfunction is functional in nature. There are various adaptive prosthetic devices that may also be useful in treatment, but the principles on which psychologic treatment is based are still considered essential if the problem is to be resolved.

Researchers writing on the treatment of sexual dysfunction tend to use different theoretical labels for rather similar therapy procedures. For example, the virtually standardized treatment procedures now used for erectile failure may alternatively be described as

(a) A means of reducing performance demands and the spectator role (*26*)
(b) An in vivo systematic desensitization of anxiety through reciprocal inhibition by sexual arousal (*29*) and
(c) A way of stopping the couple's attempt to voluntarily control an involuntary behavior by using quasihypnotic instructions (*20*), to disrupt a self-maintaining "vicious cycle" of the fear of erectile failure actually causing erectile failure by preventing sexual arousal (*24*), or
(d) Anxiety reduction through specific suggestions based on paradoxical intention or successive approximation (*1*).

With this in mind, it is possible to describe the common elements in various sex therapy programs, avoiding theoretical interpretation and simply focusing on the actual procedures used.

Mutual Responsibility

All sexual dysfunctions are shared disorders; that is, the husband of the inorgasmic cord-injured female should also be viewed as a patient in need of help, as should be the wife of the cord injured male unable to produce an erection sufficiently firm for penetration. Regardless of the cause of the dysfunction, both partners are responsible for future change and the solution of their problems. Some patients will resist the notion of mutual responsibility quite vigorously in a defensive attempt to protect their self-image as sexually adept, or to maintain a position of power and control in the relationship. Reassurance, distinction of "responsibility" from "blame," and prognosis of successful outcome will usually deal with the self-image issue. Use of sexual dysfunction in a power struggle may be an indication for more general marital therapy instead of sex therapy. If reassurance does not eliminate resistance, raising the defensive spouse's anxiety about his/her sexual ability may motivate him/her to enter therapy on an equal basis with his/her spouse. Therapeutic anxiety can be engendered by such statements as, "I agree that your spouse has severe and long-standing sexual problems, but I know from clinical experience that, had you responded differently, he/she could have overcome these difficulties, and sex therapy would never have been necessary" (*21,22*). Involving both spouses is also made easier by using a male–female cotherapy team, which gives each patient someone with whom to identify. Such cotherapy is common in most sex therapy programs, but does not seem to be essential (*20*).

Information and Education

Most patients suffering from sexual dysfunction are ignorant of both basic biology and effective sexual techniques. Sometimes this ignorance can directly lead to the development of anxiety, which in turn produces sexual dysfunction. Many cases of vaginismus seem to be caused by the husband's forceful attempts to accomplish intromission despite his uncertainty about the exact location of the vagina. The wife's anticipation of painful battering about her vaginal introitus directly leads to the involuntary spastic contraction of the vaginal musculature called vaginismus. In direct therapy, the therapist ensures that the patients have accurate knowledge of the sexual cycle through verbal discussion, providing the patients with appropriate reading materials, and the use of educational films. In the case of disability, there exists an abundance of written material developed for a lay audience, which outlines in great specificity options and precautions to observe (*8–11*). In addition, information is available by lecture, books, and films, on the general principles of effective techniques of kissing, manual and oral foreplay, positions of intercourse, and so forth. Although this specific information is not usually sufficient to produce symptom remission, it appears to be necessary for treatment to succeed (*27*).

Attitude Change

Negative societal and parental attitudes toward sexual expression, post-traumatic experiences, and current acute distress combine to make dysfunctional patients approach each sexual encounter with anxiety or, in extreme cases, with revulsion and disgust. Consider for a moment the fear and anxiety experienced by the cord-injured male afraid of having an accidental bowel movement or bladder problem while engaged in sexual activity. The therapist must directly induce attitude change in such patients. Procedures used may involve having the patient read positive materials on sexuality; arranging consultation with sympathetic clergy in the case of negative attitudes; instructing the husband to make it clear to his wife that he will value her more, not less, if she becomes more sexual; having the patient attend lectures or workshops on sexuality and sexual values, which may be offered by local colleges, churches, or social-interest groups; and use of the therapeutic relationship itself. Some authors (*19,21*) suggest that therapists can use their role and relationship to produce attitude change in the patients through self-disclosure about their own enjoyment of sexuality. If the patient has a negative attitude toward sex and a positive attitude toward the therapist, the self-disclosure that the therapist enjoys sex creates cognitive dissonance (*13*) for that patient: "Someone that I like and respect enjoys something I think is reprehensible, immoral, and disgusting." The resolution of this conflict can lead to acceptance of sex as decent, moral, and enjoyable. Alternatively, if such self-disclosure is too extreme or used too early in therapy, the patient may resolve the dissonance by losing respect for the therapist or deciding that the therapist is simply a different type of person.

Eliminating Performance Anxiety

In the culture of the 1980s, with its heavy emphasis on youth, beauty, vigor, and sexual attractiveness, demands for sexual competence and expertise seem to have assumed a larger role in the development of sexual dysfunction. The cord-injured are particularly vulnerable to such societal attitudes. The resulting anxieties can only further compromise their all-too-often marginal sexual status. For therapy to work and the cord injured to function optimally, they must be freed from anxiety about their sexual performance. Patients, regardless of the presenting complaint, are told to stop "keeping score," to stop being so goal-centered on erection, orgasm, or ejaculation, and to focus instead on enjoying the process. For example, the therapeutic procedure of forbidding intercourse in the treatment of erectile failure makes it possible for the patients to enjoy mutual kissing, hugging, body massage, and manual or oral stimulation of the genitals without anxiety about whether erection sufficient for intercourse will occur. Other techniques include reassuring a woman that she need not feel that she must reach orgasm in order to enjoy intercourse or to confirm her husband's belief that he is a good lover for her, and instructing patients that they can each provide sexual satisfaction for each other through manual and oral stimulation, even when they are not capable or desirous of having intercourse. Giving one partner "permission" to masturbate as a legitimate route to sexual satisfaction will also reduce demands for performance in some cases.

Increasing Communication and Effectiveness to Sexual Technique

Dysfunctional couples tend to be unable to clearly communicate their sexual likes and dislikes to each other because of inhibitions about discussing sex openly, excessive sensitivity to what is perceived as hostile criticism by the spouse, inhibitions about trying new sexual techniques, and the incorrect assumption that a person's sexual responsiveness is unchanging, i.e., an activity that is pleasurable on one occasion will always be pleasurable. Accordingly, direct therapy encourages sexual experimentation and open, effective communication about technique and response. Procedures that are used include having the couple share their sexual fantasies with each other, read explicit erotic literature, see explicit sexual movies that model new technique, and train the couple to communicate during their sexual interaction. It is stressed that patients are to ask and tell each other what they would like to do during each particular sexual encounter.

Changing Destructive Lifestyles and Sex Roles

Direct therapy for sexual dysfunction often involves the therapist stepping outside the usual therapeutic posture of responding to the patient and, instead, taking an active, directive, and initiating role with the patient in regard to general lifestyle and sex-role issues. For example, many dysfunctional patients make sex the lowest priority item in their life. Sex occurs only when all career, housework, child-rearing, home management, friendship, and family responsibilities have been met. This usually insures that sex occurs infrequently, hurriedly, and late at night and when both partners are physically and mentally fatigued. In such cases, patients may be instructed to make "dates" with each other for relaxing days or evenings. (*1*). These dates may involve dinner and the theater, a day at the beach, or simply sending the children to the babysitter and spending the night at home. This simple change in itself tends to make sex a more positive experience. Similarly, patients may be advised to disengage from parents or others who are a destructive influence on their sexuality, e.g., overprotective, oversolicitious parents who may foster dependency, or to enter bankruptcy to solve hopeless financial troubles that consume all their emotional energy.

Rigid and unsatisfying sex-role separation is also a major negative influence on many couple's sexual relationship. If a husband and wife spend virtually no time together and have no mutual shared responsibility for the tasks of day-to-day living, it is unlikely that they will find sex to be a rewarding, close, sharing experience. The most common problem of this type involves the "housewife's lament" syndrome. In this syndrome, an educated, intelligent women has given up her career or education to become a homemaker, maid, cook, and nurse to her disabled spouse. Her husband fails to recognize the strain she lives with. She would often like conversation and interaction with her husband. If he is unwilling to help reduce her work load and increase her life satisfaction, a poor and unrewarding sex life is perhaps the best he can hope for in the continuing progress of their relationship. In such cases, it may be necessary for the therapist to take a very active role and, perhaps, suggest that a nurse or aid perform some of the routine nursing care functions, or that someone assist with the cleaning of the house or caring for the children.

Prescribing Changes in Behavior

If there is any one procedure that is the hallmark of direct treatment of sexual dysfunction, it is the prescription by the therapist of a series of gradual steps of specific sexual behaviors to be performed by the patients in their own home. These behaviors are often described as "sensate focus" or "pleasuring" exercises. Typically, intercourse (in some cases "stuffing") is prohibited, as is breast and genital touching.

The patients are told only to examine, discuss, and sensually massage each other's body. The couple's sexual relationship is then rebuilt in a graduated series of successive approximations to full sexual intercourse. At each step, anxiety reduction, elimination of performance demands, and other components described above are used to keep the couple's interactions pleasurable and therapeutic experiences.

Psychologic Evaluation for Penile Prosthesis in Organic Impotence

Remarkable progress has been made in the past two decades in the field of implants for impotent men. Earlier types were "constant erection" or "semirigid," with the use of bone, then the Small-Carrion more flexible silicone implants. Physical complications, including nonhealing, infection, hematoma, fracture of the implant with vigorous thrusting, and erosion at either end, are noted in the literature. Then came the much proclaimed Scott-Bradley flexible "inflatable hydraulic system" penile prosthesis. Candidates clamored for insertion, even at the overall cost (including hospital stay) of around $12,000+.

However, the initial enthusiasm has now been tempered with caution. Questionable and dramatic early results of the Scott-Bradley (inflatable) prosthesis have included the postoperative discovery of an unrecognized exhibitionist. He was in his mid-20s and merely wanted a guaranteed erection on demand. Another failure was an "impotent" middle-age man forced to the "penis doctor" by his angry wife. He was a quadriplegic, unable to inflate the device. It was a surgical success, certainly. To a passive man with a hostile, demanding wife, his "impotence" may be either relief or retaliation. Prediction is difficult in any medical specialty. However, clinical experience and some failures indicate a need for more careful screening of impotent males before referring them for a penile prosthesis (*15*).

Screening Outline for Penile Prosthesis

An assessment of how well a penile prosthesis will meet the needs of a patient should include an evaluation of that patient, his physical functions, personal sexual pattern and attitudes, and the nature of his sexual relationship with his spouse. The screening outline given in Table 1 has been suggested by Renshaw (*28*) and is only one of many available.

Table 1
Screening Outline of Patient Evaluation for Penile Prosthesis

Physical factors

1. Do you have partial erections now?
2. Do you have orgasms now?
3. Do you ejaculate now? (frequency?)
4. Do you masturbate now? (frequency?)
5. Do you ejaculate when you masturbate? (frequency?)
6. Do you have morning erections?

As part of the physical evaluation, nocturbal penile plethysmography can be done to measure sleep erections to differentiate organicity.

Personal sexual patterns and attitudes

1. What does the penile implant mean to you?
2. What do you expect to feel after you have it?
3. Do you expect a climax/ejaculation?
4. Do you expect to masturbate after you have it?
5. How accepting (relieved) or upset (preoccupied) are you about being impotent?

Sexual relationship with spouse (or partner)

The prosthesis is predominantly for giving sexual pleasure to his partner. It does not of itself provide new arousal, ejaculations, or orgasm for the patient. Therefore, the following questions should be asked:

1. What does you partner's sexual enjoyment mean to you?
2. Would you feel satisfied to share her climax?
3. Before becoming impotent, were you concerned with your partner's having an orgasm?
4. Since becoming impotent, what alternative sexual techniques have you employed to provide sexual stimulation for your partner?
5. What was your coital frequency preimpotence?
6. What has been your sex play frequency since the impotence?
7. Is your partner pressuring you to have an implant?
8. What do you think her coital demands will be postimplant?
9. Have you discussed divorce in the past year?
10. Have you thought of or tried marital therapy?

What is important is the comprehensiveness of the interview designed to ascertain previous attempts to remedy the problem and to communicate openly. The patient's willingness to experiment, and his flexibility, sexual attitudes, beliefs, and motivations are also assessed thoroughly.

Renshaw insists that it is essential that the patient be told as clearly and directly as possible that

(a) The implant is predominantly for the male to give pleasure to his partner
(b) The implant does not provide a sensation of arousal but only an artificial erection for the male and
(c) It does not provide ejaculation or orgasm for the male.

Thus, the crucial issue becomes: "Is the male able to enjoy and obtain satisfaction from his partner's sexual arousal." To such a man, it can be exhilarating to once more share closely in his partner's orgasm.

Conclusions

This chapter has investigated the psychological significance of sexual functioning to spinal-cord-injured persons. Because more than 80% of spinal cord injuries occur in males, the bulk of research conducted in this area has focused on male sexual behavior following injury. A review of the literature suggests there may be a constellation of personality factors characteristic of persons most prone to acquiring this type of disability. However, additional empirical research is needed to substantiate this clinical observation. Although loss of sexual function vis-a-vis other major functional losses has been considered by many to be the most significant deficit following injury, recent research suggests this may not be the case. In this increasingly progressive and liberal society, this finding is an important one. Rather than focusing too little on sexuality, as was the case prior to the early 1970s, we may be focusing too much on sexuality and, by so doing, actually encouraging the attitude that intact genital functioning is necessary to establish sexual identity. The assessment and treatment of sexual problems therefore must be conducted in the context of total psychosexual functioning. To concentrate exclusively on sexual problems and ignore problems associated with social functioning may turn out to be an unproductive course to follow. Rather, sexual problems may be more amenable to change by remembering and practicing the adage, "If everything in the living room is all right, problems in the bedroom will work themselves out."

It is hoped that the need for sex therapy will eventually disappear entirely. Perhaps in the future society will come to value sexuality as one of the least destructive and most loving components of the human personality. Persons raised in such a culture would presumably find the idea of "sexual dysfunction" emotionally incomprehensible. It is the responsibility of those of us working in the area of human sexuality to foster this change in our society.

References

1. Annon, J. S. (1974) *The Behavioral Treatment of Sexual Problems*, Vol. 1 (Kapioloni Health Services, Honolulu).
2. Bergler, E. (1947) Frigidity in the female: Misconceptions and facts. *Marriage Hyg.* **1** 16–21.
3. Bergler, E. (1951) *Neurotic Counterfeit Sex.* (Grune and Stratton, New York).
4. Bergman, S. and Hadley, R. (1976) Sexual adjustment and feminine attractiveness among spinal cord injured women. *Arch. Phys. Med. Rehab.* **57**, 448–450.
5. Berkman, A. H., Weissman, R., and Frielich, M. (1978) Sexual adjustment of spinal cord injured veterans living in the community. *Arch. Phys. Med. Rehab.* **59**, 29–33.
6. Cogswell, B. E. (1968) Self-socialization: Readjustment of paraplegics in the community. *J. Rehab.* **Spring**, 11–35.
7. Conomy, J. P. (1973) Disorders of body image after spinal cord injury. *Neurology* **23**, 842–850.
8. Eisenberg, M. G. (1978) Sex and the handicapped: A selected bibliography (Monograph issue) *Rehabil. Psychol.* **25(2)**, 59–113.
9. Eisenberg, M. G. and Falconer, J. (1978) Current trends in sex education programming for the physically disabled: Some guidelines for implementation and evaluation. *Sex. Disabil.* **1**, 6–15.
10. Eisenberg, M. G. and Rustad, L. C. (1976) Development of a sex education and counseling programming on a spinal cord injury service. *Arch. Phys. Med. Rehab.* **57**, 135–140.
11. Eisenberg, M. G. and Rustad, L. C. (1980) *Sex and the Spinal Cord Injured: Some Questions and Answers*; 3rd ed. (US Government Printing Office, Washington, DC).
12. Fenichel, O. (1945) *The Psychoanalytic Theory of Neurosis* (Norton, New York).
13. Festinger, L. (1957) A theory of cognitive dissonance (Stanford University Press, Stanford).
14. Freud, S. (1965) *Standard Edition of the Complete Psychological Works of Sigmund Freud* (Hogarth, London).
15. Gee, W. F. (1977) Ejaculatory difficulties with penile prosthesis. *Med. Aspects Hum. Sex.* **11(2)**, 97.
16. Hanson, R. and Franklin, M. (1976) Sexual loss in relation to other functional losses for spinal cord injured males. *Arch. Phys. Med. Rehab.* **57**, 291–303.

17. Hetrick, W. R. (1967) *Sexuality Following Functional Transaction of the Spinal Cord.* Doctoral dissertation, University of Houston (1967); (University Microfilms, Ann Arbor, Michigan).
18. Hogan, R. (1980) *Human Sexuality: Implications for Nursing Care* (Appleton-Century-Crofts, New York).
19. Jourard, S. M. (1964) *The Transparent Self* (D. Van Nostrand, Princeton).
20. Kaplan, H. (1974) *The New Sex Therapy* (Brunner/Mazel, New York).
21. Lobitz, W. C. and LoPiccolo, J. (1972) New methods in the behavioral treatment of sexual dysfunction. *J. Behav. Ther. Exp. Psychiatry*, **3(4)**, 265–271.
22. Lobitz, W. C., LoPiccolo, J., Lobitz, G., and Brockway, J. (1974) A closer look at "simplistic" behavior therapy for sexual dysfunction: Two case studies, in *Case Studies in Behavior Therapy* Eysenck, J., ed. Routledge & Kegan Paul, London.
23. LoPiccolo, J. and LoPiccolo, L. (1978) *Handbook of Sex Therapy* (Plenum, New York).
24. LoPiccolo, J. and LoPiccolo, W. C. (1973) Behavior therapy of sexual dysfunction, in *Behavior Change: Methodology, Concepts, and Practice* (Hammerlynck, L. A., Handy, L. C., and Mash, E. J., eds.) (Research Press, Champaign, Ill).
25. Lorenz, K. (1970) *Studies in Animal and Human Behavior* (Harvard University Press, Cambridge).
26. Masters, W. H. and Johnson, V. E. (1970) *Human Sexual Inadequacy.* (Little, Brown & Co., Boston).
27. Moore, B. E. (1961) Frigidity in women. *J. Am. Psychoanal. Assoc.* **9**, 571–584.
28. Renshaw, D. C. (1978) Impotence in diabetics, in *Handbook of Sex Therapy* (LoPiccolo, J. and LoPiccolo, L., eds.) Plenum Press, New York.
29. Wolpe, J. (1958) *Psychotherapy by Reciprocal Inhibition* (Stanford University Press, Stanford).

8

Pastoral Approaches to Sexual Dysfunctions

James F. Sagala

Introduction

Modern society has raised many questions about the nature of sex and its role in human life. Many of these questions demand a religious response. As we understand it, human sexuality depends largely on how one looks at the human body and relates it to the totality of communication. Judeo-Christian ethics views human sexuality as a gift of the Creator, reiterated by the redeemer with the message that God speaks in love to all (*2*).

Humans are embodied spirits and spirited bodies. Each is a word spoken by God in a special way, and this word takes on human flesh. The Creator calls us to transform bodily being into a glorification of his name; as quoted from the scriptures: "Then honor God in your body" (*2*) (1 Cor. 6:20). Consequently, to root a vision of sexuality in an adequate theologic framework, I will briefly explore certain psychological, scriptural, and moral themes, and apply these to pastoral counseling as it pertains to the spinal-cord-injured (SCI) patient.

Psychological Basis of Sexuality

Many articles have been written about the relationship between psychology and sexuality. Just as there is a pluralism in theology and philosophy, so there is pluralism in psychology. Among the psychological theories proposed, there is as yet no single acceptable comprehensive approach to sexuality and human development.

Sexual Rehabilitation of the Spinal-Cord-Injured Patient
Edited by J.F. Leyson, © 1990 The Humana Press, Inc.

Since humans are polymorphic, there never will be a single-concept model, or for that matter, a simple method that exhausts our understanding of human nature. Nevertheless, much can be learned about this area of human sexuality from the behavioral sciences. As such, it is generally accepted among most behaviorists of the necessity of having one's physical needs met before one is even capable of socialization and that the physical level is the basis on which all else rests, even the sense of self-interacting in a social world.

That this has a bearing on sexuality is obvious sexual experience is bodily experience. As a result then any discomfort with one's body precludes self-esteem. Any lack of self-esteem blocks advanced human development and therefore spiritual development. So sexuality and spirituality are closely related. Therefore, it seems logical to state that without sexual integration one cannot be a fully functioning person, and only a fully functioning person can be spiritually developed (*3*).

And as such psychological insights are examined, it should be remembered that sexuality can only be understood correctly as a dimension of one's total personality. Since personality is the more basic concept, a sexual person therefore is primarily a sexual "person."

The premise that a person is sexual incorporates a multiplicity of meanings. It can mean that a person becomes a sexually differentiated male or female. It also can denote the person's becoming relational—i.e., individually oriented or socially directed. Sexual existence thus becomes both corporeal and social. Human sexuality, although similar to that of animals in terms of biologic functioning, is not just a mere expression of a primitive nature, but is instead filled with tremendous possibilities beyond the simple potential for procreation (*1*). Thus, sexuality's two dimensions: affective and genital. Our culture, sadly, has too often reduced sexuality to the latter, which is primarily biologic (*2*). Moreover, many people tend to confuse the physical drive for sex with the affective desire for intimacy. They experience sexual desire and equate it with genital satisfaction when, in reality, what they want is closeness. We have been told that the higher need in a person is the need for intimacy and that genital expression is not the initial step in developing a relationship. Instead, it should serve as the means for ever-closer intimacy and the culmination of a person's striving for this closeness (*1*).

The principles next discussed are very important in their application to the counseling attitudes proposed by the pastoral counselor to the SCI patient and to other similarly disabled persons.

Some theorists maintain that genital abstinence is not harmful for self-actualizing people (i.e., those actively seeking to develop their total personalities). Such persons are able to accept genital deprivation, and still be at peace with themselves and their sexual lives. Deprivation, however, becomes pathologic only when a pathogenic occult problem surfaces, e.g., when it is experienced as rejection of the opposite sex, or as inferiority or isolation. In such cases, therefore, the desire for genital sex may deepen the individual's affective needs. Consequently, the significant element in personal development is not genital abstinence of sex, but the individual's attitude toward it (*1*).

Growth can safely be said to be a fact of life. To realize one's sexual identity embodies a lifelong process of spiritual growth and integration. This process is not simply a biologic one; it also involves religious and moral issues. Only against a spiritual backdrop can a person properly see the goal toward which he or she ought to be striving. For this insight, the sacred/ancestral writings (Moslems, Hindus, Shintoists, and others) are of interest.

The Bible and Human Sexuality

Does the Bible provide directives concerning human sexuality in general and sexual behavior in particular? Even though many allusions to sexuality can be found in the scriptures, the Bible is not directly concerned with sexuality as such. Nor are the scriptures intended to be a systematic presentation on sex; they are not a textbook on ethics. One cannot find prefabricated ethical models for sexual behavior in the Bible any more than one can find ethical models for medicine, civil rights, nuclear disarmament, or other moral issues. Still, by permitting one's self to become attuned to the various social and cultural movements represented in scriptural statements, the foundation of an ethical tradition can be found that suggests certain models of behavior (*1*).

It is true that the Bible does not offer simple yes or no answers regarding a code of sexual ethics. Yet, most scholars would agree that sacred scripture in its totality views sexuality as one aspect of human life seen within the context of the whole person and the whole of human life with all of its relationships and responsibilities (*4*).

Pastoral Care

Having laid some groundwork as to the principles involved, I will now attempt to apply them to the practical aspect of ministering to SCI patients.

It strikes me that, in an area as delicate and as important as this, the pastor/chaplain/rabbi needs to prepare in several ways. First, it would be very helpful if the religious counselor would become acquainted with some of the basic physiologic and psychological aspects of spinal cord injury. It is essential to be especially aware of the aspects of the adjustment process to the injury and disability. Then, after becoming familiar with the common concerns and problems of the disabled person, the counselor will have to deal with his/her personal feelings about spinal cord injuries and disabled persons (*1*). More specifically, the counselor will need to deal with his/her own feelings about such problems as the extreme dependency of the SCI patient. The pastoral or religious counselor who reacts against his/her own unconscious tendency toward strong dependency will find it difficult to relate appropriately to patients who need a great deal of support. Finally, the religious counselor must decide what the specific goals and methods of pastoral care will be. The job is not to convert a person to the counselor's values, but to help that person become aware of his/her own inherent unique God-given capacities and values, thus giving the SCI patient's life new meaning (*4*).

I would suggest a methodology of pastoral care that includes (a) comfort, (b) catalysis, and (c) challenge (*4*). Through a *ministry of comfort*, the pastor/chaplain communicates to the patients a genuine acceptance of the patient for who he or she may be. By the counselor's very presence, the SCI patients are reminded that God accepts them, reinforcing the unconditional values and meanings of life still to be lived (*3*).

In the ministry of catalysis, the chaplain functions as a catalyst by attempting, through empathetic questioning, to accelerate the patients' acceptance of their spinal cord disabilities and guiding them to discover a vocational purpose. The counselor also tries to help these patients become aware of their responsibilities and capabilities, using reflection to focus the patients' attention on what they can be or do in the future, rather than on what has been lost (*4*).

Finally, through a ministry of challenge, the SCI patients can be helped to commit themselves to positive values and goals. Chaplains need to establish a warm and understanding relationship with these patients, so as to lead them toward commitment by communicating that what they do in life makes a difference to other people as well as in their own relationship to God (*4*). Thus, ministering to the SCI patient is a challenging task that requires skill as well as concern. An excellent summary of what the Chaplain's task involves follows:

The greatest service the pastor can offer the disabled is to walk with him through the valley of anguish, depression, and anger; to stand at his side in the struggle with confusions and doubts; to work with him toward a new inner balance, as well as toward a realistic acceptance of accommodation of what the future will hold for him/her, and to do all of this in the spirit and as the representative of the community of the faithful (*3*).

References

1. Avento, G. P. (1982) *Sexuality; a Christian View* (Twenty-Third Publications, Mystic, Ct.).
2. Haring, Bernard (1979) *Free and Faithful in Christ—The Truth Will Set You Free.* 2nd Ed. (Seaburg, New York).
3. Helminiak, Daniel A. (1989) "Self-Esteem, Sexual Self-Acceptance and Spirituality." *Journal of Sex Education & Therapy.* **15**, 203–209. (Guilford Press, New York).
4. McEver, D. H. (1972) Pastoral care of the spinal cord injury patient. *Past. Psy.* **23**, 47–56.

9

Psychiatric Evaluation and Treatment Formats

Warren R. Procci

Introduction

The SCI patient is susceptible to a host of psychological difficulties and complications, including sexual dysfunction. However, a discussion of the multiple problems that can befall these individuals is beyond the scope of this chapter. (Interested readers may consult refs. *7* and *18*). The literature concerning the psychological complications of SCI covers a wide range of disciplines, and is contained in variegated journals and widely disparate books. Any attempt to collate this data systematically would require Herculean efforts. The major focus of this chapter is far more modest and specific; that is, to provide an overview of the reactions to physical trauma and to outline an approach to the investigation of sexual dysfunction in these patients.

Psychiatric Reactions to Physical Trauma

The integrity of the body is of crucial importance to just about everyone, not just athletes or physical fitness buffs. Freud made an emphatic point about this. The individual's sense of identity originates from the awareness of the body and its boundaries (*4*). If there is any accuracy in Freud's observation, and undoubtedly there is some, it is obvious that any bodily injury will always cause at least an implicit threat to the individual's sense of identity. The reaction of a given person to physical trauma is, of course, impossible to predict since it is dependent upon so many factors. The extent and location of the injury, the

Sexual Rehabilitation of the Spinal-Cord-Injured Patient
Edited by J.F. Leyson, © 1990 The Humana Press, Inc.

individual's work habits, the athletic and motoric needs, the patient's age, whether or not there is any previous experience with injury, and the individual's characteristic psychologic defenses are just a few among the huge number of variables that must be entered into the equation.

It is of interest that there is a paucity of well-organized data in the psychiatric literature concerning the psychological responses to SCI. An exception is a recent paper by Fullerton et al., who found that 30% of patients experienced a *major* depression following spinal cord injury, generally within the first mo (*5*). Nearly all of these depressions occurred in those subjects with complete cord lesions. Also of interest was the fact that 13% of these patients had prior histories of serious alcoholism. Not surprisingly, 50% of the patients had been actively drinking prior to the time of the accident that produced their disability. Furthermore, 90% of the patients were male and their mean age was 27 years. Clearly, this patient population is a highly select one. Patients with SCI are primarily young males with considerable risk for major psychiatric disturbance.

The reaction to serious physical trauma can be conceptualized as occurring in a series of stages or steps similar to the stages described in dying patients by Kubler-Ross (*10*). It must be kept in mind that it is simplistic to imagine that the adaptation to physical trauma unfolds like a play, with each scene and act the same for each patient. Instead, there is a series of psychological states that most patients will demonstrate at various times in the course of adapting to injury. These stages are familiar to most readers: denial, anger, bargaining, depression, and acceptance. A detailed discussion of these stages is beyond the scope of this chapter, so I will give only a very brief explanation of each. The interested reader is referred to Kubler-Ross' superb description (*10*).

Denial is commonly used to shield and protect individuals from the impact of the injury while other adaptive processes are put to work. Denial will usually diminish and ultimately resolve, but in some individuals, it may become chronic. It must be kept in mind, however, that denial is not necessarily undesirable. For patients unable or unwilling to accept the impact of physical disability fully, some chronic use of denial may be necessary for their well being.

Obviously, *anger* is a frequent occurrence in individuals with serious illness or disability. Just about everyone who is or has been a member of a medical team dealing with the chronically ill or disabled has encountered innumberable hostile patients. The frustrations, limitations, confinements, and irreversibility of serious injury make anger all but inevitable.

Bargaining is characterized by the patient's making certain promises dependent on their achieving some predetermined degree of rehabilitation. Often, patients are willing to make drastic changes if only they will be cured of their injury. Guilt concerning certain unsatisfactory relationships or undersirable parts of their lives frequently underlies bargaining. For example, spinal cord patients with long-standing problems related to alcohol abuse may "promise" to give up drinking completely if they are able to walk again.

Depression, as already noted by Fullerton (*5*), is a serious complication of many spinal cord injuries. This may be the result of the failure of denial or the failure of bargaining. Patients are forced, often reluctantly, to accept the horrendous, inescapable consequences of their injuries.

Generally considered last in any discussion of *adaptation* to physical disability is the stage labeled *acceptance*. Ideally, this represents the end stage of the evolving process of adaptation to chronic illness. In reality, nirvana is never achieved, so many individuals really do not manage to attain a stage of acceptance of their injury. For example, *a substantial number remain fixed in an angry or depressed mode.* Even for those who do achieve some measure of acceptance, it may not be permanent. For a whole host of reasons, one can regress into a state of anger or denial.

The main point of this is that we should be cognizant that psychological responses to physical injury are fluid. Patients may be very labile, with rapid shifts from one mood to another. Naturally, the degree of adaptation to injury has marked implications for the sexual functioning of the chronically disabled. Patients able to achieve a measure of acceptance are obviously more likely to retain some capacity for satisfactory sexual activity than are patients mired in anger or preoccupied with depressive thoughts. It is very important, therefore, to keep clearly in mind that the sexual adjustment of chronically ill individuals may be subject to considerable variation, depending on their level of adaptation at the time sexual functioning is assessed.

Psychiatric Assessment of Sexual Dysfunction

It is a fundamental rule in business that the most dangerous and vulnerable time is during a stage of rapid growth. Notoriously, businesspeople are likely to become overzealous and to extend themselves far beyond what they can realistically handle. Bankruptcy may result.

This is exactly the case with the current state of knowledge concerning the diagnosis and treatment of the sexual dysfunctions. During the past 10 yr or so. There has been an enormous increase in the number of patients coming to physicians for the evaluation of sexual dysfunction. A whole plethora of diagnostic tests has been developed, and more are being developed. There is a vast amount of literature concerned with this subject, and it encompasses many fields, e.g., psychiatry, psychology, neurology, endocrinology, cardiovascular medicine, surgery, obstetrics/gynecology, urology, and so on. If one includes the subspecialties of these fields, the list is virtually endless. Any kind of comprehensive review or even a survey of such broad, complex literature involving many different fields, is far beyond the scope of this chapter.

In my view, the evaluation of sexual dysfunction needs to become a specialty in its own right to contain this rapid growth. Otherwise, we would wind up with completely unchecked and disorganized expansion, perhaps with resultant scientific bankruptcy.

The First Step: Sexual History

Traditional thinking has viewed sexual dysfunction as either organic or psychogenic in nature. This dichotomous thinking is oversimplistic at best, and vague and imprecise at worst. For example, the supposed ratio of psychogenic to organic impotence varies widely from 20:1–1:7, depending on the studies examined (*19*). Quite clearly, this indicates that there are considerable gaps in our knowledge and conceptual understanding of the various sexual dysfunctions. No doubt this results, in part, from the fragmentation involved in studying the subject.

The following approach, which is schematized in Table 1, evolved from work I did while at the University of Southern California School of Medicine and the Los Angeles County/University of Southern California Medical Center. We undertook a 4-yr prospective study of male sexual dysfunction in patients with chronic renal failure (*15*). I make no claims to our approach being a comprehensive evaluation, but I do see it as providing a beginning for the systematic investigation of sexual dysfunction. I also see it as readily applicable to patients with any chronic illness or disability. I should point out that my discussion will emphasize male sexual dysfunction, though female sexual dysfunction will not be ignored. Since most spinal cord injuries are suffered by males (*5*), the limitations of this approach may not be so severe for the purposes of this chapter.

The initial step is a good sexual history. I am assuming that, prior to any psychiatric consultation, the patient will have already received

Table 1
Key Elements in the Evaluation of Psychosexual Functioning

Basic evaluation
Medical history
General physical examination
Neurologic examination
Psychiatric evaluation
Sexual history
Includes psychological evaluation for performance anxiety, depression, and marital discord
Each partner examined separately, then conjointly
Use of standardized psychological tests (e.g., Sexual Interaction Inventory, Derogatis Sexual Functioning Inventory, MMPI)
NPTR, 2 night
Specialized investigations (if NPTR abnormal)
Endocrine
Vascular
Neurologic (for details see last chapter)

a medical history and physical examination, including a thorough neurologic evaluation. Sexual behavior is a very personal, very delicate matter for many people. It will often require a number of consultations before a patient can talk about sexual performance with comfort and, therefore, honesty. I favor discussing sexual performance first with *both* partners individually, since each brings a different perspective and perhaps different information. The nature of the difficulty must be described in detail. Sexual dysfunction is not a wastebasket term. It encompasses a number of very specific conditions, and the clinician must be vigorous in defining the problem precisely. A detailed description of the various sexual disorders is beyond the scope of this chapter, and the interested reader is directed to more specific references (*8,14*). There are any number of very useful paper and pencil sexual history inventories [such as the Sexual Interaction Inventory (*11*) or Derogatis' Sexual Functioning Inventory (2)] that can assist the clinician in systematically acquiring data. It is also very helpful to obtain information concerning general psychological health; standardized psychological tests such as the MMPI can be very useful since they provide information concerning depression, anxiety, and so on. There is an excellent, recent, and thorough review of the use of psychological rating scales in the assessment of sexual dysfunction (*17*).

After each partner has had an opportunity to discuss the problem, I suggest a joint meeting. It is surprising how frequently spouses disagree on the nature of the problem, and the conjoint interview, of course, provides a mechanism whereby such discrepancies can be aired and, one hopes, resolved. The manner in which the couple talks about their sexual difficulty in the conjoint session also provides information concerning the strengths and weaknesses of the relationship.

Throughout this series of interviews, it is essential to be alert for the most likely "psychological" contributors to sexual dysfunction—performance anxiety, depression, and marital discord. Fortunately, there are relatively useful methods of intervening to deal with these conditions, and they can be successfully treated in many cases.

Performance anxiety is perhaps the most common psychological contributor to sexual dysfunction. Put most simply, individuals become so preoccupied and worried about performance, obtaining pleasure, or pleasing the partner, that they are unable to function. Keep in mind that good sexual performance is incompatible with a high level of anxiety. The phenomena is also known as "spectatoring," i.e., individuals are overly concerned about viewing their own performance.

Depression is another common psychological contributor to sexual dysfunction. It can easily be recognized by the depressed mood with its attendant anhedonia, helplessness, and hopelessness. Severe depression also includes sleep disruption and appetite disturbance. The MMPI can often indicate the presence of major depression.

Marital discord is an obvious cause of sexual dysfunction. If two people are out of touch with each other emotionally, it is unlikely they will perform well sexually. Marital discord should be very apparent from a conjoint interview. Psychological testings such as: Beck Depression, Millon Behavioral Health Inventory and Locke-Wallace Marital Adjustment Scale can help determine the couple's suitability for penile prosthesis surgery.

The Second Step: Nocturnal Penile Tumescence/Rigidity (NPTR) Measurement

I recommend the use of NPTR measurement in nearly all cases of male sexual dysfunction, even if a "psychological" contribution appears obvious. As suggested above, it is often simplistic to consider sexual dysfunction as either "organic" or "psychogenic." The picture is very often mixed.

NPTR is a relatively recent addition to the assessment of sexual dysfunction, even NPTR though it has been utilized in the sleep laboratory as a REM correlate for many years. The use of portable NPTR in the evaluation of sexual dysfunction is not yet fully understood (*16*). There are analogous devices to investigate vaginal and clitoral blood flow changes in women, but these are in an even earlier stage of development.

The main value of NPTR lies in its ability to suggest whether or not an organic component is present. Briefly, if the biologic pathways for erection are intact, NPTR should be normal (presuming normal sleep). If there is some compromise in the neuronal or vascular pathways, or the end organ itself, NPTR will be diminished. At this point, there is sufficient experience with normal subjects to establish a basis for comparison. Generally, normal subjects have 3–5 nocturnal erections with rigidity and a maximum change in penile circumference of 25–30 mm (*3*). An erection with a penile circumference change of at least 16–20 mm is required for successful vaginal penetration (*9*).

NPTR can best be investigated in a sleep lab setting. However, this is very expensive, and sleep labs are few in number. In recent years, portable monitors have greatly expanded the utility of NPTR, but obviously without sleep lab data there are some difficulties, though none are insurmountable. The sleep lab setting rules out cases in which an abnormality in sleep pattern produces a lack of REM sleep and an apparent lack of nocturnal erections. This could be erroneously interpreted as the presence of an organic component when lack of REM sleep is really the case. Another problem is that it is possible to confuse an increase in penile circumference without rigidity. The difficulty can be resolved by awakening the subject during what appears to be a maximal erection, and then directly palpating the penis for rigidity. A more specific technique being developed in several laboratories is the use of a 'manometer,' which measures the pressure required to reverse an erection. This gives a quantitative measure of penile rigidity.

If the results of NPTRR testing indicate consistently normal erections of adequate firmness, the subsequent work-up should be redirected toward an even more detailed examination of the various psychological factors discussed above. If indeed there is a problem in this area, the clinician who has already done a thorough history should already have had an idea as to its nature. If NPTR results are consistently abnormal, then more thorough testing is necessary to understand the nature of the organic component. It is of course possible that *both* organic and psychogenic factors may be present. If organic factors are present, NPTR provides no information as to the nature of the disturbance. Thus, we approach the final step in the evaluation, more specific investigations.

The Third Step: Specialized Investigations

Broadly speaking, there are three major biologic areas that can impede sexual performance: endocrine, vascular (*13*), and neurologic. I will not discuss the specialized investigations in these areas, since they are discussed in detail elsewhere in this book. The major purpose of these specialized investigations is to help pinpoint an exact cause of sexual disturbance.

Therapeutic Approaches

A basic tenet of any therapeutic program is that treatment must match diagnosis. Obviously with sexual dysfunction, there are numerous potential therapeutic approaches. I will direct most of this discussion toward the psychological approaches.

The treatment of psychogenically mediated aspects of sexual dysfunction was revolutionized by the work of Masters and Johnson (*12*). Prior to that time, sexual dysfunction was nearly always considered to be the result of neurotic conflict. Resolution of the conflict required intensive psychotherapy with the assumption that, with conflict resolution, there would be remission of sexual dysfunction. The results of this form of treatment were disappointing. Masters and Johnson chose instead to focus on the specific overt behaviors involved in sexual activity and not on unconscious conflict. Their results have been far more encouraging. The basic principle is rather simple, and this approach has been described in detail in a recent review (*1*). Sexually dysfunctional individuals have *learned* bad habits, and both partners are involved. Therefore, both partners must be taken back to the beginning, and they must start over again. Subjects are given a series of exercises in which they are instructed to try to learn what gives their partner physical *pleasure*. They are both actively told *not* to seek orgasm, since preoccupation with orgasm may preclude pleasure. As subjects focus more on what stimulates their partners rather than on their own performance, they naturally begin to move in the direction of a heightened sense of physical pleasure. They are progressively encouraged to expand the "pleasuring" of the partner, moving toward foreplay, then mutual masturbation, and finally coitus. This approach is the treatment of choice for patients in whom "performance anxiety" is a major problem.

For spinal cord patients with incomplete lesions, the physical capacity for sexual response may be intact, but anxiety about performance may be present. Here the approach described above may prove very beneficial. For subjects with complete lesions of the cord, there is often a total lack of the so-called psychogenic component of erections, although the capacity for reflex erections may persist. For these subjects, a different approach is often necessary. I would suggest (as I do with organically impotent renal failure patients), that the couple definitely remain in physical contact with each other. This can be difficult, since there is a tendency for them to withdraw. This only serves to increase their sense of isolation, and it actually makes matters worse. They can still hold, touch, and caress each other, so they can still experience a sense of mutual loving. Perhaps, too, they can be encouraged to interact such that the "intact" partner can remain orgasmic. An injured husband might continue to bring the wife to orgasm, either manually or orally. I would caution clinicians, however, to be very delicate in pursuing this, since many individuals have inhibitions about noncoital sex. *The key element is to help the couple define what is comfortable and right for them, and then to help them pursue it.* For some couples, merely holding each other may be satisfactory.

If depression is present, it must be specifically addressed. If the depression includes an appetite and sleep disturbance, it is most likely a major psychiatric depression requiring intervention with antidepressant medication, usually a tricyclic. If the depression does not include an appetite or sleep disturbance, and seems strongly related to events in the patient's current life or the result of long-standing psychological conflict, psychotherapy is the treatment of choice. For cases in which serious marital discord exists, marital therapy is the treatment of choice, provided the couple wishes to try to salvage their marriage.

Naturally if there is a specific organic contributor to impaired sexual function, an attempt must be made, if possible, to reverse it. For totally irreversible male sexual dysfunction, consideration should be given to the use of penile "implants." I have been quite surprised both by anecdotal responses from patients, as well as from systematically obtained clinical data that suggests that implants (prostheses) are surprisingly well accepted by most couples (*6*). The psychopharmacologic approaches to sexual dysfunctions in SCI patients should be tempered with caution because of the possibility of drug interactions. A majority of patients are taking muscle relaxants, tranquilizers/hypnotics, analgesics, and anticholinergics. Tricyclics may potentiate the effects of most of the aforementioned medications. Drug addicts should be addressed accordingly. Diazepam (Valium) is effective in treating muscle spasms in patients with incomplete lesions. This drug is also frequently used/abused as a tranquilizer and, when given with antipsychotic medications, may precipitate undue muscle weakness or even drowsiness. The dosage of tricyclics should be reviewed periodically with other medications. Pharmacosexology will be discussed in detail in a later chapter of this book.

Women (taking tricyclics) with premenstrual tension syndrome, postacute SCI phase, may experience irritability, depression, or unusual personality changes and so on, several days prior to their periods. During this time, they may be disinterested in sex. However, following the menstrual period, normal sexual responsivity returns.

Conclusions

Spinal cord patients are asked to perform a very difficult task: to adjust to significant alterations in their lifestyles. The loss of body integrity leads to a wide range of emotional responses. There are a series of psychological states that most patients experience: denial, anger, bargaining, depression, and acceptance. These states often require psychological assistance and support.

Sexual dysfunction is one of a number of serious medical complications secondary to spinal cord injury. A wide variety of differing medical disciplines are involved in the comprehensive study of sexual dysfunction: psychiatry, neurology, endocrinology, cardiovascular medicine, surgery, obstetrics/gynecology, urology, and so on. Obviously, the investigation of sexual dysfunction requires special expertise. Such evaluation should include at least: a thorough sexual/psychiatric history; NPTR measurement; and perhaps more specific investigations for organic abnormalities. It is overly simplistic to consider sexual dysfunction as easily classified into "organic" or "psychogenic" types. Significant overlap is frequent. Prescription of therapy can occur only after thorough diagnostic evaluation, since so many different factors may play a role. Individualized approaches are often necessary, since many variables are frequently involved. Basic psychological approaches are derived from the work of Masters and Johnson, but the special needs of these patients make creativity on the part of the clinician a necessity. Depression is a possible complication that often requires specific investigation and treatment. Penile implant surgery is occasionally called for, and in certain cases, it is extremely effective. Psychotropic medication may play a useful adjunctive role.

Prognosis is not always sanguine, so a considerable amount of long-term psychological (or psychiatric) support is mandatory for these patients and their spouses. As already mentioned, this chapter has focused primarily on male patients, since they suffer the majority of serious spinal cord injuries. However, the problems of female patients obviously require equally careful attention.

References

1. Birk, L. (1970) Shifting gears in treating psychogenic sexual dysfunction: medical assessment, sex therapy, psychotherapy and couple therapy. *Psychiatr. Clin. North Am.* **3**, 153–172.
2. Derogatis, L. R. and Melisaratos, N. (1979) The DFSI: A multidimensional measure of sexual functioning. *J. Sex Marital Ther.* **5**, 244–281.
3. Fisher, C., Schiavi, R. C., Edwards, A., Davis, D. M., Reitman, M., and Fine, Y. (1979) Evaluation of Nocturnal Penile Tumescence in the differential diagnosis of sexual impotence: a quantitative study. *Arch. Gen. Psychiatry.* **36**, 431–437.
4. Freud, S. (1923) The ego and the id. *Standard Edition of The Complete Psychological Works of Sigmund Freud.* **19**, 19–27.
5. Fullerton, D. T., Harvey, R. F., Klein, M. H., and Howell, T. (1981) Psychiatric disorders in patients with spinal cord injuries. *Arch. Gen. Psychiatry.* **38**, 1369–1371.
6. Geistenberger, D., Osborne, D., and Furlow, W. (1979) Patient-partner satisfaction. *Urology.* **14**, 583–587.
7. Higgins, G. E. (1978) Aspects of sexual response in adults with spinal-cord injury: a review of the literature, in *Handbook of Sex Therapy* (LoPiccolo, J. and LoPiccolo, L., eds.), pp. 387–410. Plenum, New York.
8. Kaplan, H. S. (1974) *The New Sex Therapy* (Brunner/Mazel, New York).
9. Karacan, I., Sales, P. J., Ware, J. C., Dervennt, B., Williams, R. L., Scott, F. B., Attia, S. L., and Beutler, L. E. (1978) Nocturnal Penile Tumescence and diagnosis in diabetic impotence. *Am. J. Psychiatry.* **135**, 191—198.
10. Kubler-Ross, E. (1969) *On Death and Dying* (MacMillan, New York).
11. LoPiccolo, J. and Steger, J. (1974) The sexual interaction inventory. A new instrument for assessment of sexual dysfunction. *Arch. Sex. Behav.* **3**, 585–595.
12. Masters, W. H. and Johnson, V. E. (1966) *Human Sexual Response.* Little Brown, Co., Boston).
13. Michal V. and Pospichal, J. (1978) Phalloarteriography in the diagnosis of erectile impotence. *World J. Surg.* **2**, 239–248.
14. Munjack, D. J. and Oziel, L. J. (1980) Sexual medicine and counseling in office practice. A comprehensive treatment guide. (Little Brown, Boston).
15. Procci, W. R., Goldstein, D. A., Adelstein, J., and Massry, S. G. (1981) Sexual dysfunction in the male patient with uremia: a reappraisal. *Kidney Int.* **19**, 317–323.
16. Procci, W. R. and Martin, D. J. (1984) Preliminary observations of the utility of portable NPTR. *Arch. Sex. Behav.* **13**, 569–580.
17. Schiavi, R. C., Derogatis, L. R., Kuriansky, J., O'Connor, D., Sharpe, L. (1979) The assessment of sexual function and marital interaction. *J. Sex Marital Ther.* **5**, 169–224.

18. Teal, J. C. and Athelstan, G. T. (1975) Sexuality and spinal cord injury. Some psychosocial considerations. *Arch. Phys. Med. Rehabil.* **56**, 264–268.

19. Wagner, G. (1981) Methods for differential diagnosis of psychogenic and organic erectile failure, in *Impotence: Physiological, Psychological, Surgical Diagnosis and Treatment*, pp. 89–130. (Plenum, New York).

10

Desire Dysfunctions

Beverly Hotchner

Introduction

Upon first regaining consciousness or a clear understanding of the extent to which a spinal cord trauma has damaged the body, the injured are full of queries about three basic areas of their lives: physical survival and limitation; economic capability; and sexual functioning. The sexual concern centers on several important questions:

1. "Can I still satisfy my partner?"
2. "Can *I* be satisfied sexually?"
3. "Will I still be desirable?"

The fact that sexual capability is so prominent in the minds of the disabled indicates the centrality of sex in the lives of people. It also highlights the degree to which sexual interest and functioning is a deep and pervasive aspect of personality, and one that is essential to an integrated self and to a sense of general well-being. Human beings are social animals. Recent clinical data (Leyson) (*18*) have shown that there are four phases of human psychosocial sexual response:

1. Transition (the psychosocial urge to arrange or go out on a date and sexual encounter)
2. Preliminary desire (libido)
3. Sexual arousal/excitement and
4. Orgasmic-resolution phase.

When sexual functioning is called into question or is feared to be irretrievable, a lack of interest in sex can become a protective mask for an overwhelmed ego. Furthermore, sexual interest can be affected by the enormous psychosocial ramifications of the spinal cord injury.

Sexual Rehabilitation of the Spinal-Cord-Injured Patient
Edited by J.F. Leyson, © 1990 The Humana Press, Inc.

Whatever the case, inhibited sexual desire (ISD), the clinical term for lack of sexual interest, strikes at the very foundation of what is important to people: to be normal, to be adequate, to love, and to be loved.

Since most Americans place an inordinately high premium on sex, they feel distressingly deviant when they find themselves feeling asexual and disinterested in America's favorite sport. Because desire was once so automatic and unquestioned, its arcane disappearance is easily (but often mistakenly) attributed to the spinal cord injury. This can lead to a sustained and untreated dysfunction that can ravage self-esteem, and inordinately stress or rupture a marriage or long-term relationship. These sequelae make it clear: abstinence does not make the heart grow fonder.

The spinal cord injured can easily conjure up fantasies of an entire world satisfyingly engaged in frequent and fantastic sex. They believe that the sexual revolution, Masters and Johnson, *The Joy of Sex*, and the Grafenberg spot have made it possible for intact Americans to have entered into sexual nirvana. Nothing is further from the truth. Although largely unrecognized, the lack of sexual desire in marriage is extensive. Edwards (*1*) calls it "commonplace." Deckert (*2*) indicates that "the lack of sexual desire in marriage is almost universal sometime in the natural history of almost any marriage."

That the "*bacterius asexualis*" is widespread is testified to by data from clinics and private practitioners of sex therapy across the country. Kaplan (*3*) indicates that ISD "is probably the most prevalent of the sexual dysfunctions" and reports information from the Marriage Council in Philadelphia showing that about 40% of patients applying there for help were suffering from low libidinal states. Lo Piccolo (*4*) reports that, of 39 consecutively treated cases at New York's Stony Brook Sex Therapy Center, 69% included a diagnosis of low sexual desire in at least one spouse.

There are indications that men experience ISD in approximately equal ratio to women. Renshaw (*5*) reports that, over an 8-y period at the Loyola University Sexual Dysfunction Clinic, they treated 24% of their male patients compared to 30% of the women for sexual disinterest. In my own practice, I see 1.4 women to 1 man with hypoactive disorders.

The extent of sexual disinterest in the spinal-cord-injured patient is difficult to assess since various studies report different findings. Bors and Comarr (*6*) indicate no change in desire; Hohmann (*7*) and Weiss and Diamond (*8*) show a slight decrease. Jochheim and Wohle (*9*) report a marked decrease (in intercourse only), and the Weiss and Diamond (*8*) data reflect an increase in interest in women. Keeping in mind that sexual interest and the criteria by which it is measured are poorly defined and difficult to assess, overall the data, according to Higgins (*10*), show that, although the spinal cord injured experience sexual arousal in a different manner, a large number of them continue to be active and enjoy sex in some way.

This kind of data helps to put the SCI patient's feelings about the diminution of desire in a somewhat different perspective. The recognition that they are not alone in feeling a lack of sexual interest, that ISD might have struck them even if they had not experienced a damaging blow to their bodies, and that significant numbers of them do ultimately work out some kind of an enjoyable sex life is heartening.

Diagnosis and Assessment

Establishing a diagnosis of ISD has also been difficult because of the lack of objective diagnostic criteria for this sexual dysfunction. Even the American Psychiatric Association's *Diagnostic and Statistical Manual of Mental Disorders* (DMS-III) (*11*), which for the first time in 1980 included ISD as a psychosocial sexual dysfunction, did not define the term. Fortunately, the opacity of the picture is being rendered clearer with the help of an instrument like the Multi-Axial Problem-Oriented Diagnostic System for the Sexual Dysfunctions developed by Schover et al. (*12*). This system offers a behavioral description of ISD with some objective, measurable assessment criteria. Among these are: (a) Low frequency of sexual activity (i.e., less than one per 2-wk period excepting greater frequency resulting from acquiescence to spousal pressure), and (b) a subjective lack of sexual interest manifest in an absence of erotic dreams, fantasies, and desires for erotic materials, and a lack of wishes for sexual activity or frustration because of its absence.

Diagnosis is also made earlier by the current recognition that ISD falls along a continuum from normal lack of interest in sex to more intense disinterest, to phobic aversion (*see* Table 1). At the low end of the continuum, there are normal dips in desire that tend to parallel the passages of marital development. These tend to come, according to Hotchner (*13*), in the first year of marriage after the hormonal highs of courtship wane; during pregnancy when fatigue and other body discomforts, and anxiety about responsibilities depress interest; during the rearing and careering years when other priorities and a broadening of the affectional network make sex less urgent or important; at middleage when boredom, body image concerns, or the malaise and depression common to the mid-life crisis take a sexual toll; and in old age as the myths, misunderstood physiological changes of sexual functioning, and

Table 1
Lack of Sexual Desire Continuum*

Type of low libido level	Intensity level	Therapeutic intervention
Normal developmental dip in desire	1	Demythification; information; permission to be nonsexual (let time pass); reduction of marital conflict; stress management
Inhibited sexual desire	3	All of the above plus insight; reduction of anxiety; sensory awareness and amplification; cognitive restructuring; behavior changes
Aversion	5	All of the above plus tricyclic medications, behavior desensitization or hypnosis; very small behavioral steps spread over a longer than usual time frame

*Based on a five-point Likert-type scale.

depression attached to becoming a valueless person in our society erode interest.

Professionals are urged to be aware of these sexual crisis points in the lives of their spinal-cord-injured clients since the disabled will confront these stressful times just as their ambulatory cohorts do. This means establishing whether or not ISD is related to the injury, a developmental stage, the psychosocial disruptions created by the injury, or some combination of these.

There are those with intense fears that make sex so dangerous or threatening that they are unable to involve themselves in physical encounters. These kinds of fears will find the affected experiencing a diminution in desire at a more serious point on the continuum than that of a developmental dip. If a partner reacts to such a sexual withdrawal with inordinate fear, anger, frustration, hurt, pressure, or castigation of the low interest person, the dysfunction can be exacerbated. Hotchner (*13*) has developed the diagnostic Checklist for a Sexually Disinterested Person and its companion Checklist for the Partner of a Sexually Disinterested Person to help each person in a relationship see his or her contribution to the sexual disinterest and to serve as a starting point for therapeutic intervention.

The most severe point on the continuum is that of aversion to sex. This might be an aversion to intercourse, to the genitals, or to touch of any kind. The fear that underlies this recoil from sex is of phobic proportions and engenders panic states in the troubled individual. The aversive client might even become phobic about getting undressed or going out to dinner for fear these acts might set in motion a desire for sex in the partner.

Diagnostic evaluation demands that the primary and secondary nature of the ISD, in addition to its point on the continuum, be determined. Primary ISD occurs in all situations, with all partners, at all times, and for any kind of sexual activity (including masturbation and fantasy). Secondary ISD means the dysfunctional state is situational (e.g., occurring monthly just before and during one's menstrual period or each time mother comes to visit).

There are several important diagnostic questions to ask a spinal-cord-injured person about his or her sexual interest and functioning. One is: "Who is it that says your are uninterested in sex?" If it is the mate who believes the client's sexual desires are "abnormal," and who has convinced him or her of a sexual deficiency, you might be dealing with a desire discrepancy that is not necessarily a true state of ISD. Some individuals' aggressive personality structures or low self-esteem states are such that they demand daily or even more frequent sex. For such individuals, a partner who enjoys sex once every week or two weeks seems to lack normal libido.

A second important diagnostic question to ask is: "What was your preinjury pattern of sexual interest and activity?" Often spinal-cord-injury clients will become aware that things were not functioning very satisfyingly sexually even before the traumatic events of their injury, hospitalization, and reentry to homelife. This may have been related to their age, general health, marital health, alcohol, or drug consumption. They might have ignored, denied, or rationalized that sexually troubled period, and have continued to do so postinjury as it now seems blissful by comparison with their current state. If there was little interest of activity or another dysfunction before the spinal cord injury, there will be little or no sex afterwards. The professional must take this into account and work through the preinjury difficulties as well as the trauma and its aftermath.

An accurate diagnosis is the *sine qua non* of success in therapy with sexually dysfunctional clients. In fact, Kaplan (*14*) established the desire phase of her triphasic response cycle by examining the failures in sex therapy at the Cornell University Medical Center. She attributed the negative outcomes to misdiagnoses, which led to inappropriate treatment plans. Accurate diagnosis is particularly critical for ISD clients since the majority of them will not respond to the brief behavioral methods widely and successfully used in the amelioration of other sexual dysfunctions.

The diagnosis cannot be made during the period of "spinal shock," lasting from a few weeks to several months, during which Coxe and Grubb (*15*) report an absence of deep and superficial reflexes, an atonic paralysis of the bladder and rectal sphincters, and sensory loss. Assessment of sexual potential during this period will not necessarily reflect the long-term capabilities of the paralyzed. After the shock subsides, there is a period of stabilization when identification of testosterone levels, sensory and motor levels of the lesion, its completeness, the presence or absence of reflex or psychogenic activity, depression, anxiety states, and marital conflict will reflect the nature and extent of the sexual dysfunction.

Etiologic Factors

Androgens

Androgens have been long thought to be responsible for low libidinal states. Until recently, findings regarding the production of testosterone in spinal-cord-injured men have been contradictory. Recent data by Claus-Walker (*16*) and by Kikuche et al. (*17*) indicate that testicular and pituitary function remains remarkably normal or returns to normal by 9–18 mo postinjury. According to Leyson and his colleagues (*18*) testosterone production was found to be normal even in the spinal shock period, except in 1% of the cases. Reasons for the impaired libido, therefore, must be sought elsewhere, unless testosterone (the hormone responsible for desire in both men and women) is low because of age, stress, pituitary disorders (LHRH—gonadotrophic releasing hormone deficiencies), or other physical dysfunctions.

Anxiety

Anxiety is at the base of almost all sexual dysfunction, but nowhere is it more intense than in desire-phase problems (*see* Table 2). In the spinal cord injured, this profound anxiety is primarily related to extreme performance fears. Their adequacy concerns are often associated with reality factors: the inability to get reflex, stimulative, or psychogenic erections, to ejaculate, or to reach orgasm. Often, they find it preferable

Table 2
The Role of Anxiety in Sexual Dysfunction

Time of anxiety	Intensity of anxiety	Primary causes	Sexual dysfunction
Anxiety develops late at peak of arousal, just before orgasm or ejaculation	Mild	Relatively mild performance fears; overconcern for partner; unrealistic expectations; control issues	Ejaculation disorders; anorgasmia
Anxiety occurs earlier in response cycle at point of erection, lubrication, or penetration	Moderate	Moderately intense fears of failure or success; fears of intimacy (rejection or entrapment)	Erectile and lubrication problems
Anxiety occurs very early in response cycle when desire begins	Profound	Very intense fears of failure/success; childhood or adult trauma; low self-esteem; intense fears of pregnancy or bodily harm; strong religious/parental interdicts against sex; very strong fears of control, absorption or rejection	Inhibited sexual desire

to be disinterested in sex rather to try and to fail. Renshaw (*19*) believes that, if you "scratch a desire disorder, you will find a dysfunction underneath." Psychogenic dysfunction cannot be ruled out, since the desire to please the partner may be particularly intense in the injured. This could lead to spectatoring and acute performance anxiety.

Anxiety can also be related to fears of success as well as of failure. A spinal-cord-injured person can be consciously or unconsciously saying: "If I succeed at sex, then you will expect me to succeed in other areas of my life where I am even more threatened." Fears of success can also be related to guilt, especially if the disabled person feels responsible for the injury. The dysfunction is then often presumed to be a punishment for misdeeds, and pleasure of any kind, including sexual pleasure, is not deserved. The possible inability to work or to be independent can also induce guilt that makes the spinal cord injured feel undeserving of sexual success.

Fears of failure and success are often intensified by fears of pregnancy, fears about the inability to conceive or to impregnate, and fears of bodily harm. The male can produce children only if he continues to produce sperm and ejaculate [90% lose ejaculatory capacity, according to Bors and Comarr (*6*)]. Those who continue to ejaculate often do so in a retrograde fashion (*20*), and recovery of semen for purposes of artificial insemination has met with little success (*21*). The spinal-cord-injured woman's ability to conceive is not impeded if she continues to menstruate, although she is somewhat more vulnerable to complications of pregnancy (e.g., premature delivery, especially if the lesion is above T_{10}) according to Eisenberg and Rustad (*22*).

Rational fears about pregnancy are usually related to the added responsibilities of supporting or caring for a child; the irrational fears are related to dying in childbirth and to having a malformed child, a possibility no more likely than in the population at large (*22*). Anxiety centered on bodily harm is more often related to Foley catheters and drainages than to pregnancy or delivery. Information about managing these during sex (*see* Information) can help to preclude this kind of anxiety.

Low Self-Esteem

Low self-esteem is another major etiologic factor in ISD. In our culture, sex has been associated with orgasm and ejaculation; femaleness with attractiveness; and maleness with an erect penis, the ability to play sports, and to be a successful wage earner. The inability (or perceived inability) to fulfill these stereotypic expectations strikes the spinal cord injured at the meridian of their identity and stability. Lifeless limbs, wheelchairs, catheters, muscle spasms, and bladder or bowel incontinence egregiously violate the well-entrenched media-fostered ideal of desirability, and often lead to intense self-consciousness and embarrassment that erode self-esteem. Even if a person's self-esteem was good prior to the injury, he or she will probably need some time to successfully integrate body and lifestyle changes into the self-concept. During the period between disintegration and positive reintegration, the injured will typically engage in self-negations with irrational statements, such as: "I am undesirable now; therefore, I am worthless"; "Nobody could love me or my inert body"; "My spouse will leave me, and I will never find anyone to love or to love me again."

Because of functional limitations of all kinds, the spinal cord injured can readily back away from sexual intimacy and anticipated hurt, loneliness, or feelings of undesirability. They find it preferable to remain safe, even if bored and alone. Fears of intimacy can also be related to sexual merging and feelings of entrapment that threaten to erase the fragile boundaries of the self. The injury *per se* may precipitate this fear. Overprotective, controlling parents, or spouses (past or present) may also cause the injured to be so fiercely protective of their independence that they must completely avoid sexual closeness.

Anger

Anger and the control issues related to it, although often out of awareness, irrational, and unexpressed, are other large contributors to ISD. The spinal-cord-injured person might feel angry about blame for being the agent of destruction, about overprotection and feelings of dependency, about pity, about distance or rejection (imagined or real), about affairs (imagined or real), or about criticism of any kind. The anger, if not expressed directly, can be communicated in the silent language of sexual disinterest. In addition, a partner who represses or volatilely expresses anger about the injury, the resulting economic deprivations, his or her increased burdens, or the changes in sexual functioning will often seem reproachful and, thus, unapproachable. Behind the log-jammed libido often lies the fragile personality or disordered communications of a spouse and/or lover.

Depression

Depression is a major etiologic consideration is ISD since the spinal cord injured are at high risk to develop this condition. Powerlessness, worthlessness, and feelings of entrapment in an irreversible paralysis commonly engender a sense of futility and despair that spirals downward into depression. The sleeplessness, ennui, irritability, and tearfulness of the depressive state are not conducive to erotic feelings. Furthermore, there is little energy or desire for any kind of activity or interpersonal contact, much less for sex. The will is as paralyzed as the body.

Relationship Monotony/Fatigue

Marital Monotony from sex with a long-term partner can be attributed to a declining "excitement or novelty factor." Marriage boredom coupled with post-traumatic depression can precipitate sexual desire and arousal problems. Similar but somewhat different from marital ennui, psychophysical fatigue can also inhibit sexual desire (ISD) and decrease transition-phase energy. Fatigue can become an enemy of sexual desire as a result of depression or from struggling with the physical limitations and psychological stresses of the cord injury. Since there is no Red Cross to come to the aid of SCI persons, they must draw on their own energies to cope with the flood of new adjustments the chronic condition demands: accepting physical and sexual limitations, finding new or adjusted ways to make a living, dealing with relative dependency and boredom as well as with the insecurities and fears of their partners, to mention only the more obvious of a long list. These accommodations can deplete the energy storehouse and leave little personal strength to fuel the libido. Anxiety, depression, pain, stress, fatigue, and boredom can lead one to drink or to other drugs to assuage the assaults on the body and spirit.

Alcohol and Drug Use/Abuse

Alcohol, often sought as a palliative, depresses the central nervous system and can, unfortunately, suppress the sexual system as well. Marijuana, sometimes used by cord patients to cope with severe muscle spasm and pain, has "limited effectiveness," according to sparse clinical data (*18*). Furthermore, Leyson (*18*) has demonstrated that chronic marijuana users present with hypotestosteronemia with ISD. Valium and other psychotropic drugs, in large doses, may also diminish desire. The psychological benefits of these in the overall adjustment picture, however, must be weighed against the loss of libido. The spinal-cord-injured patient may also take prescribed drugs for other illnesses that develop alongside the paralysis, such as hypertension, which may also be implicated in the ISD diagnosis.

Absence of Genital Sensation

Absence of genital sensations can also obviate sexual desire, since arousal is commonly heavily dependent on sensory input in these erogenous zones. Fears, myths, and rigidities in the personalities of the spinal cord injured or their partners may make experimentation with new kinds of sensations, or new ways to produce them, threatening or impossible. *Mental anesthesia* perceived as an absence or decrease of erotic dreams may occur in patients with primary or secondary hypogonadism and may contribute to impaired libido or ISD.

Sexually Dysfunctional Partner

A sexually dysfunctional partner may also be the major factor in ISD. A spinal-cord-injured person can experience a lack of desire in sex as a way to protect a dysfunctional partner. As one client said: "If you can't have it, you might as well learn not to want it. It's less painful that way."

The Therapeutic Regimen

Treatment for ISD requires interventions supplemental to the typical behavioral approach used in sex therapy, as has been pointed out by Kaplan (*14*) and by Lo Piccolo (*4*). Some combination of the following modalities is usually ameliorative.

Demythification

Debunking the sexual myths pervasive in the culture that we are all heir to might be necessary. Zilbergeld's (*23*) list of male myths, the most pernicious of which is that a man needs to have a stiff penis to be a good lover, and the SAR guide (*24*) list of myths that victimize women, the most invasive of which is that a woman needs to be attractive to achieve sexual fulfillment, provide a starting point for awareness and disavowal. In addition, the myths that Anderson and Cole (*20*) outline as particularly destructive to the sexuality of the spinal-cord-injured must be challenged. These truths include: (1) that the loss of genital function does not mean the end of sexuality; (2) that the loss of sensation does not mean the loss of feelings; and (3) that the lack of ability to move does not mean the lack of ability to please and be pleased sexually.

Information

The spinal-cord-injured need special information about urinary and bowel concerns. They should, for example, be instructed to avoid drinking fluids for a few hours prior to sexual celebration and to empty the bladder just beforehand. To avoid embarrassing accidents, the bowel should also be evacuated.

Information about catheters and drainages is very important in reducing sexual anxiety. Foley (indwelling) catheters as well as suprapubic and ilealoop drainages can be left intact and taped to the penis or abdomen for short periods of time without interference with bodily functions or sexual activity, although Eisenberg and Rustad (*22*) believe it is wisest to counsel patients to void before sex, to remove the catheter, and to know they will be safe for up to 4 h. The SCI patient will also find that sex is possible, easier, and more desirable if they have information about artificial lubrication, the stuffing technique, the use of vibrators, and alternative modes of pleasuring.

Pain Control

Pain associated with muscle spasm may need medical treatment, although some combination of muscle relaxation therapy, physical therapy, phenol injection, and/or percutaneous rhizotomy may help. Pain control should be established on an individual basis related to etiology. A reduction in the amount of sedative and analgesics, plus dorsal column stimulation, transcutaneous nerve stimulation, biofeedback, comprehensive pain management, and some surgical ablative procedure may be necessary to treat chronic pain (*28*). Complex pain (psychological and physical) should be managed with comprehensive pain clinic/program therapy.

Insight

Awareness of why the spinal-cord-injured patient and/or spouse has little or no sexual desire is often an important component of therapy. Talk, introspection, and readings about past or present thoughts, fears, inhibitions, values, wants, and behaviors will help the couple to see how these factors interact to create patterns of tension and conflict that criss-cross like a cat's cradle, binding sexual interest. The exploration and resolution of hidden relationship problems should be inaugurated by the therapist.

Sensory Awareness and Amplification

The spinal-cord-injured will generally experience an impoverishment of external sensory-body cues to respond to. They might also have a paucity of or absence of internal arousal cues if they were heavily or totally dependent on physical stimulation as preinjury triggers of sexual arousal. In addition, they may have little to no awareness of the sensual qualities of their environment.

Therapy should involve the development of enhanced sensory awareness. This will typically involve experimentation with scents, tastes, sounds, and sights that elevate the erotic consciousness. Caresses of each pore and orifice with a variety of touches (with *water-soluble oils*, powders, and vibrators to see what stirs and delights the senses), especially above the area of the lesion, which has been reported by Bors and Comarr (*6*) and Hohmann (*7*) to become an inordinately erogenous area, are important so that the spinal cord injured and his or/her mate can learn: that touching is a good in and of itself, that primary responsibility for turn-ons, pleasure, and orgasms is one's own, and that a sharp focus on one's own body and pleasure is facilitative of these.

Sensory amplification can also be enhanced by the assignment of tasks that will help a couple to create a sensual ambience through experimentation with candles, incense, mood music, costumes, poetry, erotic magazines, shared fantasies, shared feelings, or their own creative embellishments.

Cognitive Restructuring

This portion of therapy involves the mind, which is as important as the body and the environment in shaping desire. The cognitive work might involve Wolpe's (*25*) thought-stopping procedure or Burn's (*26*) method of challenging and converting such cognitive distortions as the all-or-nothing statement, "My wife will leave me if I cannot get an erection," to such logical, rational statements as "There is a lot more for her to love than my penis." Cognitive restructuring might also involve examination of expectations, the castles in the head, to see if they are unrealistic Normal Rockwell idylls of marriage, Hugh Hefner visions of ideal body-type, Harold Robbins views of megasex, or popular notions of sex via magic buttons. Some of the most self-defeating expectations that people cling to and that need to be challenged are those pertaining to partners: (a) "If my partner loved me, he or she would know what I like or want"; and (b) "If I have to ask for what I want, I will be begging, and it will not feel good if I get it." When these beliefs operate, the individual relinquishes responsibility for his or her needs, and trusts to luck, faith, or x-ray vision when a partner is neither a wizard, nor a god, nor a superman or superwoman.

In addition to challenging negative thoughts, cognitive distortions and unrealistic expectations, sexual scripts (overt and covert) that are laid down in childhood and that pertain to sex and gender roles, deviant conduct, lifestyle commitments, and bodily attitudes, however rarified, should be clarified. Those that commonly need modification are the traditional, dog-eared ones that have become leitmotifs in one's life: men are genital and women are romantic; men initiate and women ingratiate.

Fantasy is another cognitive process that should be addressed, as this can become an important enabler or enhancer of sexual interest. What individuals include in their phantasmagorical life can be a key to unlocking desire. If fantasy is a sexually impoverished desert, blocked by religious or parental interdicts, permission and suggestion through films, readings, and discussion can be facilitative. The spinal-cord-injured should know that Mooney et al. (*27*) report that, through fantasy and concentration on physical stimuli, they can amplify the sensations in their minds and experience "mental orgasm."

Behavior Change

People can learn how to get to a particular destination, but they must first get in their cars and drive to arrive there. Similarly, sex therapy necessitates that people have homework assignments that will involve risk-taking and trying out new behaviors. These might include: acting as if they were a very sexy Clark Gable or Marilyn Monroe; practicing communication skills to assert themselves and ask for what they want with a spouse or a doctor (e.g., to change or reduce the dosage of medications that impede sexual functioning), expressing anger appropriately; fighting fear; expressing fears and concerns about the injury or other aspects of living; giving and accepting criticism or compliments; negotiating differences with a spouse; controlling stress levels; or taking steps to seek a surgical operation for a sexual prosthesis. If the latter is contraindicated for medical or psychological reasons, the client should be asked to challenge the belief that intercourse *per se* is essential to happiness.

In learning new behaviors or skills, clients need to know that they will not move from an inhibited position to one of grace overnight or in a steady, linear progression. The therapist's role is to help the spinal-cord-injured strike out into new territory by finding an artful balance between risk and security. Moreover, therapists should not attempt to fit all of the disabled into standardized behavioral molds, but should individualize the tasks to suit particular needs, values, and abilities to endure anxiety.

Conclusions

Inhibited sexual desire is the most common and severe of all the psychosocial sexual dysfunctions, yet diagnosis has been difficult because of a lack of clear definition and criteria for assessment. Libidinal or arousal sexual dysfunctions are generally caused by some combination of a developmental life passage, fear, anger, low self-esteem, fatigue, depression, absence of genital sensation, or a dysfunctional partner. Brief (12–15 sessions) behavioral treatment methods used for the other dysfunctions will not remediate low libido states. Some combination of demythification, information, insight, sensory awareness and amplification, cognitive restructuring, pain control, and behavior changes in small steps over a long period of time is ameliorative. Love, understanding, and support from family members and friends are the best ingredients for SCI patients with post-traumatic psychosexual alterations to recapture their sense of self-worth, and regain their sexual desire and sensual sensitivities.

References

1. Edwards, J. N. (1981) How prevalent is lack of sexual desire in marriage? *Med. Asp. Human Sex.* **15**, 73–82.
2. Deckert, G. (1981) How prevalent is lack of sexual desire in marriage. *Med. Asp. Human Sex.* **15** 73–82.
3. Kaplan, H. S. (1979) Inhibited sexual desire. *Med. Asp. Human Sex* **13**, 26–47.
4. Lo Piccolo, J. (1982) Treatment effectiveness for dysfunctions of sexual desire. *J. Sex & Mar. Therapy* **8**, 179–197.
5. Renshaw, D. (1981) Roundtable: Sexual apathy. *Med. Asp. Human Sex.* **15**, 68B–68S.
6. Bors, E. and Comarr, A. E. (1960) Neurological disturbances of sexual function with special reference to 529 patients with spinal cord injury. *Urol. Survey* **10**, 191–222.
7. Hohmann, G. W. (1966) Some effects of spinal cord lesions on experienced emotional feelings. *Psychophys.* **3**, 143–156.
8. Weiss, A. and Diamond, D. (1966) Sexual adjustment, identification and attitudes of patients with myelopathy. *Arch. Phys. Med. & Rehab.* **47**, 245–250.
9. Jochheim, K. A. and Wahle, H. (1970) A study on sexual function in 56 male patients with complete irreversible lesions of the spinal cord and cauda equina. *Paraplegia* **8**, 166–172.
10. Higgins, G. E. Jr. (1978) Aspects of sexual response in adults with spinal-cord injury: a review of the literature, in *The New Sex Therapy* (Lo Piccolo and Lo Piccolo, eds.) pp. 387–410, Plenum, New York.
11. American Psychiatric Association (1980) Diagnostic and statistical manual of mental disorders. 3rd ed. (Washington, DC).
12. Schover, L. R., Friedman, J., Weiler, S. M., Heiman, J. R., and Lo Piccolo, J. (1981)The multi-axial problem-oriented diagnostic system for

the sexual dysfunctions: an alternative to DSM-111. *Arch. Gen. Psychiat.* **39**, 614–619.

13. Hotchner, B. (1982) Not tonight, I have a headache dear: a guide to understanding and overcoming lack of interest in sex. Unpublished manuscript, St. Louis.

14. Kaplan, H. S. (1979) *Disorders of Sexual Desire*, Plenum, New York.

15. Coxe, W. S. and Grubb, R. L. (1974) Central nervous system trauma: spinal, in *Neurological Pathophysiology* (Eliasson, Prensky, and Hardin, eds.) pp. 284–292, Oxford University Press, New York.

16. Claus-Walker, J., Scurry, M., Carter, R. E., and Campos, R. J. (1977) Steady state hormonal secretion in traumatic quadriplegia. *J. Clin. Endocrin. Metab.* **44**, 530–535.

17. Kikuchi, T. A., Skowsky, W. R., El-Toraei, I., and Swerdloff, R. (1976) The pituitary-gonadal axis in spinal cord injury. *Fert. and Ster.* **27**, 1142–1145.

18. Leyson, J. F. J. (1982) Personal communication. Veteran's Administration Medical Center: East Orange, N.J.

19. Renshaw, D. (1979) Sexual boredom. *Med. Asp. Human Sex.* **13**, 16–25.

20. Anderson, T. P. and Cole, T. M. (1975) Sexual counseling of the physically disabled. *Postgrad. Med.* **58**, 117-123.

21. Kolodny, R. C., Masters, W. H., and Johnson, V. E. (1979) *Textbook of Human Sexuality for Nurses*, Little, Brown, New York, pp. 258–263.

22. Eisenberg, M. G. and Rustad, L. C. (1974) Sex and the spinal cord injured: some questions and answers; 2nd ed., US Government Printing Office, Washington, D.C.

23. Zilbergeld, B. (1978) *Male Sexuality*, Little, Brown, Boston.

24. Staff of National Sex Forum (1975) *SAR Guide for a Better Sex Life*, National Sex Forum, San Francisco.

25. Wolpe, J. (1958) *Psychotherapy by Reciprocal Inhibition*. Stanford University Press, Stanford, California.

26. Burns, D. (1980) *Feeling Good.* Morrow, New York.

27. Mooney, T. O., Cole, T. M., and Chilgren, R. A. (1975) *Sexual Options for Paraplegics and Quadriplegics*. Little, Brown, Boston.

28. Leyson, J. F. J. (1988) Sex Odyssey 2001. Presented at the Annual Meeting of the Association of Philippine Physicians in America., July 26-31, Long Beach, CA.

11

Diagnosis of Sexual Dysfunction in Spinal-Cord-Injured Women

Dorothea D. Glass

Introduction

Spinal cord trauma impacts on an injured woman's sexuality in a variety of ways, depending not only on how, how much, and where in the spinal cord the damage occurred, but also on the soma and psyche that she had developed preinjury and that will determine her responses postinjury. Much remains to be learned about both the somatic and the psychological aspects. Research and reliable reporting about spinal-cord-injured women has been scant. It is important to keep in mind that there is great variation from one individual to another and, even in the same individual, from one time to another. The goal of sexual activity is satisfaction for the particular individual within the limits possible, not reaching for a standard and probably impossible ideal of function and feeling (*1*,*2*).

Changes in Sexuality Post-SCI

Many aspects of the spinal-cord-injured woman's sexuality may be affected after her injury, including libido or sexual desire, arousal,

Sexual Rehabilitation of the Spinal-Cord-Injured Patient
Edited by J.F. Leyson, © 1990 The Humana Press, Inc.

response, and specific sexual behaviors. Changes in desire and arousal may result from the impact of the changes in her physical status on her perception of herself, from role changes that may occur as a result of the injury, and/or from the anger and depression that usually accompany grieving for the losses she has sustained. Changes in physical responses and specific sexual behaviors follow the effects of the spinal cord lesion on the various parts of the sexual response system. All of these changes are interwoven, and can make the diagnosis of sexual dysfunction and remaining sexual potential difficult and inexact (*3*). However, it is important to make this diagnosis as early and as accurately as possible, because many of the postinjury changes are preventable or treatable. Proper diagnosis and prompt institution of appropriate therapy can save the patient much suffering, or rescue her from a future of sexual denial and frustration.The purpose of evaluation is to include/exclude treatable medical disease or impairment that may influence sexual function, and to diagnose organic and psychosocial causes for sexual problems that, even though not treatable, must be understood to facilitate the patient's adjustment and proceed with rehabilitation planning (*4*).

Factors in Sexual Dysfunction

Many factors other than the injury may cause sexual dysfunction to occur; these are discussed fully elsewhere in this volume, so I will just touch on them. Since sexual desire and arousal are so intimately linked with the woman's affective status, the emotional reactions postinjury that may negatively influence this—grief, anxiety, fear, anger, and loss of self-love—need to be explored. There may be changes in sexual response because of damage to the neurological centers supplying the genitalia. These will vary depending on the site and extent of the spinal cord lesion, and the type of injury. Allowance must be made for the period of neurological inactivity or spinal shock immediately following the injury, which may last only hours or days or, less frequently, may persist for weeks or months. Physical impairments that are present for six months or more are likely to be permanent. Since the autonomic nervous system is the main neurologic conduit for sexual response, the amount of damage to this system can be assessed by its effects on other autonomically innervated functions such as bowel and bladder, vasomotor responses, and so on. In addition, the autonomic system is very sensitive to emotional influences and may show changes

Table 1
Female Sexual Responses

	Able-bodied	SCI
Wall of vagina	Moistens	±
Clitoris	Swells	±
Labia	Swells and opens	±
Uterus	Contracts	±
Inner ⅔ of vagina	Expands	±
Outer ⅓ of vagina	Contracts	±
Muscles	Tense, spasms	Tense, spasms
Nipples	Erect	Erect/no response?
Breasts	Swell	Swell/no response?
Breathing	Increases	Increases
Pulse	Increases	Increases
Blood pressure	Increases	Increases/hypertensive
Skin, neck, face	Sex flush	Sex flush
Skin of trunk	Sex flush	(Paras) sex flush (Quads) equivocal

(Adapted from Cole, T. M. (1975), Sexuality and the Spinal Cord Injured in Human Sexuality, (Green, R., ed.), Williams (Wilkins Co., Baltimore, p. 164(8)).

resulting from these rather than from any direct physical damage. We must first appraise those losses caused by physical damage, but not forget that either may mask the other (*4–6*).

Psychosocial influences causing dysfunction may be just as disabling as the physical injury. Often dysfunction is attributed to the physical impairment, and psychological components are overlooked. For instance, painful intercourse resulting from vaginismus may be attributed to spasticity from a high cord lesion, whereas the basic cause may be anxiety, which can greatly increase spasticity. Dysfunction is usually the result of a combination of organic and psychological factors, but some patients, unwilling to accept adjustment problems as the basis for the dysfunction, prefer a medical problem viewed as beyond their control.

It is important to keep in mind the multiple body systems that work together to produce sexual response in the human being, and that SCI sexual dysfunction may result from damage to any of these systems and the emergence of compensatory mechanisms (Fig. 1). There are also, therefore, many alternate ways for a human being to respond sexually even if the nerve supply to the genitals has been impaired. Many of the extragenital areas of sexual stimulation and response remain intact (Table 1).

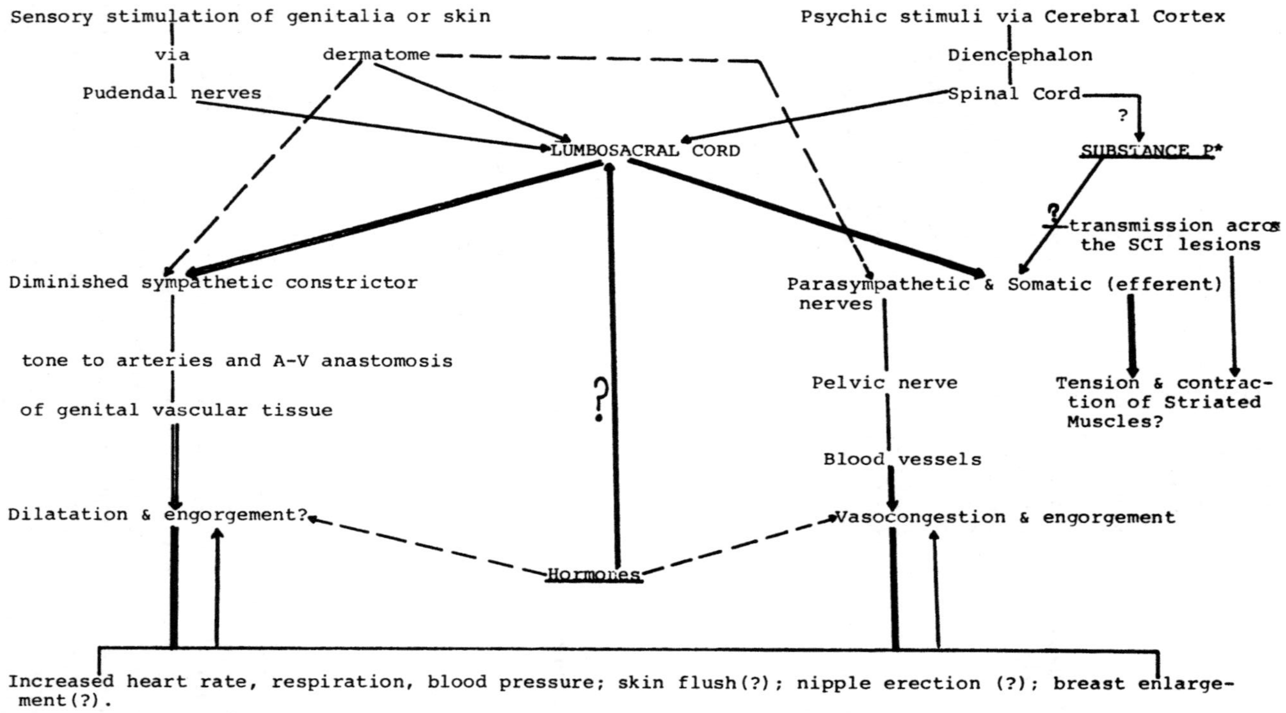

Fig. 1. Multiple body systems involved in sexual response of SCI patients (modified from Downey, J. A. and Darling, R. C. (1971) *Physiological Basis of Rehabilitation Medicine*. WB Saunders, Philadelphia). Substance P is believed to carry neuronal impulses beyond the damaged area, which may facilitate urinary bladder (*30*) and sexual recovery or function (*31*).

Too little reliable research has been done with spinal-cord-injured women to know exactly the effects of spinal cord trauma at different levels on women's genital responses. Much of the information available has been arrived at only by analogy with male counterpart functions. Many spinal-cord-injured people who should not be able to respond, do. Again, the multiplicity of the body systems involved, interactions and overlapping of the nerve supply, and other compensatory mechanisms probably account for this. The neurophysiologic effects of injury, which are discussed in other chapters, also need to be assessed carefully as we attempt to delineate sexual losses and potential.

Rarely is the cord totally severed into two separate parts; the usual injury is a fracture-dislocation, causing compression or shearing of the cord, and resulting in hemorrhage and necrosis at various levels of varying extent (*2,10*). With greater disability, there is usually an increased incidence and severity of sexual problems (*8*). No permanent hormonal changes have been described that might cause loss of libido or arousal, but a significant decrease in sexual interest, activity, and orgasm has been noted by many authors. Also noted to occur are cognitional or fantasied orgasms, paraorgasms, or orgasms following stimulation of nongenital areas (*2,9,11*). Changes may be the result of aging, or other illness unrelated to the injury.

Lack of control of the bladder and/or bowel, as well as fear of incontinence, can have serious antiarousal effects. There may also be difficulty with intercourse because of loss of vaginal lubrication, adductor spasticity, and motor and sensory impairment. Depression, adaptations in sexual activities, devaluing of self-image, performance fears, anxieties concerning a partner's reactions, and frightening experiences with autonomic dysreflexia may lead to secondary inhibition of sexual desire (*12*). This may account for some of the decrease in sexual interest and activity reported postinjury. The woman's own attitudes as well as the attitudes of her partner or other significant people in her life toward her disability and her sexuality influence her sexual expression. Women who have been brought up in an atmosphere of strict religious, family and social taboos appear to be the most vulnerable. Certainly, the decreased opportunities for socialization and intimacy often imposed by the disability, especially for women, are a significant factor.

Many medications used in the treatment of the spinal patient may also alter sexual desire, arousal, or response—psychotherapeutics, autonomic nervous system blockers and enhancers, antihypertensives, sedatives and hypnotics, analgesics, stimulants, recreational drugs—

the list grows ever longer (*13*). It is, therefore, important to know what drugs are being used or have been used, and what their possible effects on sexuality may be.

All of these potential factors must be carefully considered in any evaluation process. Because of the complexity and variability of the interaction of physiologic and psychological elements in the human sexual response, tracking down the precise mix of physical–psychosocial components that are the sources of any dysfunction can be a laborious process requiring special expertise. Identification of sexual problems often reflects the diagnoser's initiative in seeking sexual information and ease in discussing sexual material. What is left unsaid, undone, or avoided may be as important as what is said and done (*2,9,14,15*).

Evaluation—When, Who, How

When in the course of the treatment program to first evaluate the spinal-cord-injured person's sexuality has been a matter of some controversy. It may vary greatly because of the variability of the patients and the many factors involved. Duration of the disability has been shown to be important in the patients' awareness of sexual dysfunction and concerns. Cole and Cole (*4*) found that, among recently hospitalized spinal-cord-injured patients, about 50% felt their sexual adjustment was good and 9% that it was poor at the time of discharge. One to two years later, the number who reported poor sexual adjustment had risen to 38%. This suggests an early lack of awareness of the overall effect of the disability on sexual activity.

Some feel that investigation during the immediate posttrauma hospitalization is too early; that the recently disabled patient needs a period of physical and psychological adjustment to the impact of the disability; that changing physical, psychological and social circumstances may lead to unforeseen outcomes; that discussion of sexuality at this time is not likely to be productive; and that the professional should therefore respond only to the patient's expressed needs (*2*). Others have found that it is unwise to wait for the patient to initiate questions, since many patients are so overwhelmed or fearful that they will not initiate and seem to need permission to ask; that the professional must anticipate need, and offer the patient an avenue toward intimacy in order to prevent the sense of isolation that many feel; and that it is important to total rehabilitation to open the door to intimate discussion as early as possible (*4*). Since sexuality has a broader and deeper meaning than genitality and the sex act, making sexuality part of the rehabilitation program from the beginning and placing it within the context of continuing discussion of all the problems related to the spinal-cord-injured person's rehabilitation is important.

There has been much discussion about who should participate in the evaluation. This varies depending on the therapeutic setting, the knowledge and experience of the professionals involved, and the relationship of the patient with these professionals. It is important that a physician knowledgeable about spinal cord injury and the the medical causes of sexual dysfunction participate in the evaluation and specific diagnosis, as well as in the interpretation of the relationship of the injury to the degree and type of sexual response (*3,14,16*). The team member who has the best insights into the patient's problems and has established the closest relationship with the patient and family often assumes the role of primary counselor. Expertise concerning both the physical and psychosocial aspects of the sexuality of the SCI woman is necessary to make a working diagnosis. Each professional must decide the level at which she/he wishes to be involved, according to her/his training, knowledge, skills, comfort, and interest (*2,3,15,16*).

The evaluator must have learned to be comfortable with the sexual rehabilitation of SCI patients and with him/herself as a sexual person. He/she must take care to keep personal ethical and moral values out of the picture, so as to serve as a nonjudgmental resource. Until recently, most professionals have not been prepared to deal with sexual problems. Many feel incompetent or embarrassed with the subject, and are fearful of doing harm. This can block communication and investigation, leading to a devastating effect on the patient and reinforcing her belief that there is nothing to be done to help her with her sexual problems (*8,14,16*).

The language used should be explicit, express interest and intent clearly, and should be understandable and comfortable to both patient and professional. It is important to be familiar with the variety of idiomatic vocabularies used to discuss sexuality by patients from different ethnic and socioeconomic backgrounds. Euphemisms are to be avoided as much as possible, as are careless or flippant language or professional jargon (*2,15*).

A complete and careful evaluation gives respectability and importance to the subject of sexuality for the person with a disability. Good communication, openness and frankness about intimacy and sexual specifics are essential to validate the reasonable concerns the patient has. This not only delineates what exactly is functioning and not functioning, but also tells the patient that it is acceptable to be sexual. Unnecessary confrontation of the patient and/or her partner is to be avoided.

Evaluation as precise as possible is needed because accurate knowledge of the patient's functional losses is necessary to determine treatment and potential (*2,4,8,16,17*).

The evaluation procedure should be carried out systematically in order to provide a reliable and accurate analysis of present and potential sexual problems. Every problem need not originate from the physical limitations of the injury. Attendant psychosocial stresses may precipitate problems that are not organic, though they may at first seem so. Physical difficulties are often amplified by guilt, anxiety, depression, and poor self-esteem (*18*).

Contributory Factors

Sexual problems also develop from ineffective interpersonal communication, rigid sex role stereotypes, and goal-oriented sexual values. Patients may lack knowledge that allows sexual satisfaction within the boundaries of the person's physical limitations. We must differentiate between those who have limited their sexual options because of ignorance, misinformation, fear, and guilt, and those who reject sexual activity on moral and/or esthetic grounds.

Sexual dysfunctions that persist despite counseling about alternatives and options are often rooted in dysfunctional sexual attitudes, restrictive childhood family environment, behavioral problems, interpersonal relationships, and early traumatic sexual experiences. Any of the sexual dysfunctions may occur in spinal-cord-injured women whether induced by injury or not. The professional therefore needs to know and consider the ordinary sexual dysfunctions, as well as the ways in which sexual function may be changed by other physical disease. It may take years to adjust sexually after the onset of severe disability. It is also necessary to recognize that homosexual and bisexual orientations occur among the disabled; there is no place for value judgments about this when evaluating a patient (*4*).

History

All of the above factors must be assessed and recorded during evaluation, including information on:

1. Background—age, education, work history, marital status
2. Origins of the dysfunction—physical, mental, and/or family–social

3. Time of onset in the patient's sexual development—before/after puberty, established dating patterns, social skills, sexual experience, aging
4. Limitations associated with the injury—motor, sensory, pain, coordination, limiting mobility; tolerance for activity; cognitive, emotional, educational-vocational restrictions; availability of a suitable and cooperative partner; access to privacy
5. Adjustment to the disability—coping abilities, acceptance, self-esteem, motivation for rehabilitation, denial, compensation, other defense mechanisms
6. Relevant sexual history—pre- and postinjury sexual patterns; specific sexual behaviors including preparation and foreplay; knowledge of techniques for bowel and bladder control, positioning, erotic facilitation, assistive devices; difficulties and dysfunctions; sexual trauma; sexual orientation; sexual satisfaction; variety of extragenital responses to stimulation such as warm sensation, increased spasticity, headaches, which may not be recognized as sexual; range of sexual behaviors; sexual attitudes and values; current relationship(s); current and future expectations; worries and problems about sexuality, reproduction and relationships
7. Relevant medical and family history with a detailed review of the patient's medical records—past and current illnesses, medications, recreational drugs (alcohol), medical procedures, reproductive history; awareness of autonomic dysreflexic symptoms that may occur with sexual activity
8. Social and vocational resources—family support; marital or partner relationship(s); friends and social activities; religious, educational-vocational, community agencies (*2,9,19,29*)

Reassurance concerning normality and acceptability should be given as often as seems desirable. The patient must know that any information or question she offers is acceptable. The interviewer must be readily approachable, so that the patient feels safe in bringing up any concerns or questions not mentioned. Maintenance of confidentiality is essential to trust. Interviewing should be done in private and discussion limited to those professionals who are working directly with the patient.

Input from the husband/partner must always be included if at all possible. We must know not only how the patient feels about herself as a sexual person, but also how she relates to others sexually. Consideration of the interpersonal aspects and the effect of the disability on the partner is critical. Sequelae of injury often call for role changes for both. The dependency needs of the patient may put the partner into a nurse–lover relationship with attending difficulties sexually. Partner's feelings of anxiety about possible injury during sexual activities, aversion, and attendant guilt must be explored. Sometimes the disability offers one or both a welcome escape from sexual activity that was always undesired.

Methodologies should be flexibly applied in accordance with individual characteristics and variations among patients and examiners. There are almost as many outlines, forms, and suggested routines as there are writers on the subject. The professional needs to select those that suit her/his interest, knowledge, time allotment, and patient accessibility. History-taking may be done in relatively brief (half hour) interviews over a period of time, perhaps with a form to be completed by the patient with assistance if needed, or in one or two closely spaced in-depth interviews (*2,3,9,10*). What is learned during the interview serves as the basis for the physical examination, laboratory investigation, and possible consultations that follow.

Sexological Examination

A relevant and thorough physical examination, which is an essential part of every evaluation, beginning with examination of the total body, offers clues to possible difficulties for further exploration. In addition, the examination offers the opportunity to explore further the patient's sexual attitudes, fears, and myths, and to develop confidence and trust in the patient. It can set the tone for the pelvic–genital examination, which is often frightening to the patient. The possibility of a conjoint physical and sexological examination with the partner present and participating may be suggested and discussed. This can give significant insight into the patient's and partner's sexual knowledge, attitudes, self-image, mutual support and concern, and willingness to explore and experiment (*14,20*).

The manner in which the physical examination is conducted is extremely important. Every effort should be made to keep the situation as nonthreatening as possible, with a running explanation of what the examiner is doing and what is to come, so that the patient knows what is going on and why. The examination should progress from the more routine and least sensitive portions such as blood pressure, temperature, weight, pulse and respiratory rate, to examination of body parts, leaving the genital–pelvic–rectal examination for last. The examination should be detailed and recorded to delineate any physical changes that might be affecting the patient's sexual functioning. General alertness, cooperation, responsiveness are significant. Decline in general health, pain, anemia manifested by changes in color of skin and mucus membranes, skin breakdown, infection, cardiopulmonary abnormalities can contribute to malaise and low energy level with loss of libido. Care must be taken to note clues to possible contributory endocrine or vascular problems, such as hair growth and distribution, local temperature changes, peripheral circulation and pulses, skin response, breasts, and nipples. Spasms of extremities and contractures may not only be uncomfortable, but may also interfere with positioning for sexual activities.

A complete neurological examination—from peripheral nerves to spinal cord to cerebrum—is necessary to establish as accurately as possible the level and completeness of the injury and delineate areas of change related to sexual function. This should include evaluation of cognition and perception, muscular impairments, weakness, reflex activity, and abnormal reflexes. Any of these may affect sexual mobility, response, and positioning. The neurologic examination serves also to assess sensory and motor segmental levels by presence or absence of reflex activity, muscle strength of trunk and limbs, sitting balance, and sensory awareness to touch, pain, temperature, position, and vibration. Diagnosis of the completeness or incompleteness of a lesion must often rely on inference from the functional examination rather than definite observable physical evidence (*19*).

A detailed genital–pelvic–rectal examination is performed in order to disclose abnormalities and losses bearing directly on genital functions. It also provides the examiner with a further opportunity to discuss and explore the range of the patient's sexual fears about such subjects as normality, deficiencies in size, color, odors, shape of the genitalia, and patient's degree of ease with her own body parts. It should always include a bimanual vaginal–rectal examination of the uterus. If a conjoint sexological examination has been decided on, the partner can be asked to participate by standing behind the examiner to adjust the light, pass instruments, cotton swabs and so on. Elevation of the patient's head, and a mirror placed so that the patient can observe the examination is desirable. The manner of doing the genital examination is critical. The examiner must be aware of the possibility of some physical discomfort and the psychologic impact of exposing intensely private areas about which the woman herself may be ignorant or which may have past associations of mystery, shame, embarrassment, and "do not touch." It is especially important to continue the explanation of what the examiner is doing and why, what is to come, possible discomfort, and also to elicit questions about the patient's feelings or concerns about her body. The mirror can be used to point out the various body parts of which many women are surprisingly ignorant, since they have been brought up not to look or touch. Most women have been conditioned to regard their anal–genital areas as intensely private, yet here they are expected to surrender themselves in a helpless position to invasion of their most secret body orifices by someone who is at best a friendly stranger. There may also be a subconscious fear that some sexual response may occur. If this does happen, the examiner should recognize it and explain to the patient that these are normal responses that are positive since they indicate intactness of the nerve reflexes supplying these parts. This should never be exploited by the examiner for personal reasons. This is less likely to be a problem with the patient's partner or a neutral observer present (*14,15,21*).

Gentleness is essential. Any limitation of accessibility to the perineal area because of increased spasticity or contracture should be measured. Note should be taken of impairment of local sensation to pinprick, light touch, and pressure of the thigh, groin, perineum and buttock areas, which share similar innervation. Degree and nature of sensory loss in the saddle area can be discussed with patient and partner in relation to possible erotic zones and potential gratifying alternatives for arousal and orgasm (*16*). The labia, vagina, clitoris and introitus should be examined: appearance, adhesions, inflammation, lesions, abrasions, fissures, pain, color, vaginismus, discharge, abnormal dryness or bleeding. The bulbocavernosus reflex may be checked, though its significance is controversial. If sensation is absent, considerable inflammation or trauma may be present, without the patient being aware of it. With severe adductor spasticity and difficulty with perineal hygiene, bacterial or fungal infection may occur. It is important to be alert regarding signs of arousal, including changes in mucous membranes, vasocongestion, enlargement of labia and clitoris and vaginal lubrication, which indicate an intact reflex arc (*14,20,21*).

The urethral meatus is identified, pointing out, if sensation is present, its extreme sensitivity to touch and pain, and the importance of proper toilet hygiene in this area. The clitoris should be identified using the mirror and noting its position relative to the labia, its increase in size, exquisite sensitivity and retraction with arousal, and its role in sexual arousal and intercourse.

The entrance to the vagina is now examined for sensation and voluntary contraction to test for muscle tone, flaccidity or spasticity, and weakness. If voluntary contraction is present, it may be discussed as a possible exercise for vaginal muscle laxity of urinary incontinence, and as a technique for increasing sexual enjoyment for the patient and her partner. A Kegel perineometer may be used for baseline measurements and to demonstrate muscle action (*16*).

The speculum examination should be explained to the patient, and she should be instructed to open her mouth and breathe slowly to help prevent contractions of the muscles around the introitus. If severe spasticity, vaginismus or dyspareunia is present, the speculum examination should be deferred until after treatment. A warmed speculum should be inserted gently to examine the vagina and cervix. The examiner can use this opportunity to point out to the patient and partner the delicate, strong, intricate and usually hidden internal genitalia, the vaginal wall, and its automatic probable lubrication response. This is also a good time to discuss contraceptive measures, and the couple's feelings and fears about them.

The bimanual abdominal–rectal–vaginal examination for assessment of the uterus and rectal sphincter follow, with frequent reassurances about the threat or discomfort it may represent. The tone and presence or absence of volitional control of the external rectal sphincter should be noted. The presence of pain or discomfort greater than the amount expected from the examination itself should be marked for further investigation.

Genital sexual potential may be determined, based on the presence or absence of sensation in the genital and saddle areas bilaterally, volitional control of the introitus and external rectal sphincter, as well as increase, decrease or absence of rectal sphincter tone. Depending on the correlation with other findings such as reflex activity, the level and completeness of the cord injury may be inferred. (*3*). This is discussed fully in other chapters.

This examination can be a valuable bonding experience between the examiner and patient if both are comfortable with the experience. When the partner participates, it enables the patient and partner to share an intimate sexual education. For the sexually ignorant or misinformed, this can be very therapeutic and may be enough to correct sexual misconceptions, so that the couple can begin to work out a satisfactory sexual adjustment on their own. For the physician, it can give useful insights on how each relates to this new sexual experience. The examination should always end with a request for any questions, and an "open door statement" that they may come back or call back at any time with further questions (*21*).

Other Evaluation

To complete the evaluation, routine laboratory studies including blood and urine analyses, serology, X-rays or tomograms of the chest, MRI of the spine, and urinary tract, and other studies suggested by the history and physical examination should be done unless already available. Significant hormonal changes have not been usual, but if indicated, measurements of the patient's level of relevant hormonal activity can be performed (*3*). Other specialized testing, not generally included in the routine examination, may be done if it is clinically indicated. When specific endocrinological problems are suspected, gonadal and related hormones, thyroid assays, and vaginal cytology are indicated (*3*). Researchers have isolated sex attractant pheromones from human vaginal secretions and smear (*13*) that may be useful in the future to measure female sexual arousal status. SCI lesions may influence the secretion of these sex scents. Assessment of local vascular and neurological responses is discussed later as "Special Procedures."

Psychiatric Examination

The multitude of physical (somatic) dysfunctions following cord trauma can also place a tremendous strain on the psyche. Most sexologists believe that psychic inhibitory mechanism(s) can dampen the compromised post-SCI sexual functions. Thus, the psychological and psychiatric evaluations are vital to the diagnosis of this multifaceted sexual dysfunction. Psychological testing may include MMPI, state-trait anxiety inventory, profile of mood status, body image test, fundamental interpersonal relations orientation and Derogatis sexual functioning. Additional specialized psychometrics are detailed under the specific chapter. The purposes of the psychological evaluations are to detect psychopathology, cognitive impairment, and hetero-homosexual disturbances, and to delineate current moods, interpersonal expectations, and body boundaries. Psychiatric evaluations are reserved for those patients with abnormal psychometric results. This examination will provide an independent opinion regarding the etiology of sexual problems and measure the degree of maladjustment to a new but distorted soma or body image.

Special Procedures

In order to delineate minute but possibly significant spinal-cord lesions, evoked potential testing and/or electromyographic (EMG) studies of nerves subserving the external genitalia may be useful (*23*). In addition, urodynamic studies are used to document possible urinary bladder recovery and predict sexual potentials (*22*).

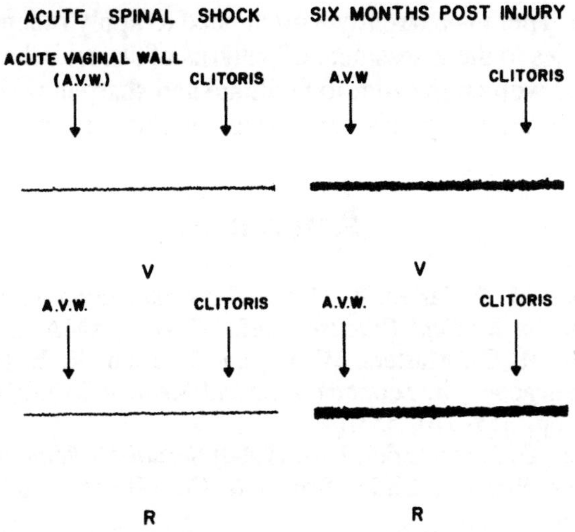

Fig. 2. EMG tracings of both vagina (V) and rectum (R) demonstrating no electrical spike response with anterior (acute) vaginal wall and clitoral stimulations, even up to 6 months postcord trauma.

Hormonal and vascular assessment has been mostly noncontributory, impractical, cumbersome and questionably reliable (*31*). More research is needed. In order to predict the degree of vaginal lubrication or vasocongestion in SCI women, intravaginal temperature and pressure has been recorded by a number of investigators during erotic stimulations (*24–28,31*). Leyson has advocated the use of an electromyographic (EMG) urodynamic anal probe (Fig. 2) to predict vaginal contraction response during sexual activity postinjury (*29,30*). The most commonly used assessment of local genital response is with a vaginal photoplethysmograph transducer, which measures vaginal contraction pressure, blood volumes and volume pulse (*24–27*).

Conclusions

Exact diagnosis of sexual dysfunction may be difficult because of the unfortunate paucity of reliable data on specific physiological genital and extragenital responses in spinal-cord-injured women. Most investigations indicate that, although the nature of sexual excitation and response is often somewhat changed, sexual activity persists and is enjoyed by a large percentage of spinal-cord-injured women (*19*). Careful and competent evaluation of each patient's physical and psychological factors is essential. There is currently a great need to apply recently developed methodologies to the assessment of patterns of sexual behavior in spinal-cord-injured women in order to facilitate and sharpen precise diagnosis and improve the prognosis for sexual satisfaction and fulfillment.

References

1. Diamond, M. & Karlen, A. (1981) *The sexual response cycle*, in *Sexual Problems in Medical Practise* (Lief, H., ed.), AMA, pp. 37–51.
2. Kolodny, R. C., Masters, W. H., and Johnson, V. E. (1979) Sex and the handicapped, in *Textbook of Sexual Medicine*, Little Brown & Co., Boston pp. 353–370, 533ff.
3. Munjack, D. J. and Oziel, L. J. (1980) *Sexual Medicine and Counseling in Office Practise*. Little, Brown & Co., Boston, pp. 3–24, 43–70, 143–159.
4. Cole, T. and Cole, S. (1981) Sexual health and physical disease, in *Sexual Problems in Medical Practise*, (Lief, H., ed.), AMA, pp. 191–198.
5. Shabanah, E. H. (1964) Role of the autonomic nervous system in uterine contractility I & II, *Am. J. of Obstet. Gynecol.* **89**, 841ff.
6. Kaplan, H. S. (1974) *The New Sex Therapy*. Brunner/Mazel Inc., New York.
7. Downey, J. A. and Darling, R. C. (1971) *Physiological Basis of Rehabilitation Medicine*, W. B. Saunders, Philadelphia, 1971.
8. Cole, T. M. (1975) Sexuality and the spinal cord injured, in *Human Sexuality*, (Green, R., ed.), Williams and Wilkins Co., Baltimore, pp. 147–170.
9. Cole, T. M. (1976) Sexual Problems of Paraplegic women, *Med. Aspects Human Sex.* **10(6)**, 105.
10. Stewart, W. F. R. (1979) *The Sexual Side of Handicap*. Woodhead-Faulkner, Cambridge, England.
11. Money, J. (1960) *Phantom Orgasm in the Dreams of Paraplegic Men and Women*, Archives of General Psychiatry, **3**, 373–382.
12. Glass, D. D. Sexual arousal responses and disability, in *Sexual Arousal: New Concepts in Basic Sciences, Diagnosis and Treatment* (Fisher, M., Fishkin, R., and Jacobs, J., eds.) Chelsea Thomas Publishers, Springfield, Illinois (in press).
13. Buffum, J., Smith, D. E., Moser, C., et al. (1981) Drugs and sexual function, in *Sexual Problems in Medical Practise* (Lief, H., ed.) pp. 211–243.
14. AASECT (1978) *The Physical Examination in Sex Counseling and Therapy*, American Association of Sex Educators, Counselors and Therapists, Washington, D.C.
15. Labby, D. H. (1981) Disturbances in the physician-patient relationship: Effects of sexual functioning, in *Sexual Problems in Medical Practise*, (Lief, H., ed.) AMA, Monroe, WI., pp. 113–119.

16. Evans, Halar, DeFreece, Larsen, (1976) Multidisciplinary approach to sex education of spinal cord injured patients, *Phys. Ther.* **56(5)**, pp.541-544.
17. Lief, H. J. and Berman, E. M. (1981) Sexual interviewing, in *Sexual Problems in Medical Practise*, (Lief, H., ed.), AMA, pp. 119–129.
18. Burgoyne, D. (1982) How self-esteem affects sexual behavior, *Med. Aspects Human Sex.* **16(12)**, pp. 70D–70H.
19. Higgins, G. E. (1979) Sexual response in spinal cord injured adults: A review of the literature, *Arch. Sex. Behav.*, **8(2)**, pp. 173–196.
20. Leyson, J. F. J. and Powell, R. B. (1979) *Counseling the female spinal cord injured patient, Med. Aspects Human Sex.* pp. 59–60.
21. Renshaw, D. C. and Lief, H. L. (1981) The sexological examination, in *Sexual Problems in Medical Practise* (Lief, H., ed.), AMA, pp.341-344.
22. Khanna, O. P. (1978) *Practical Urodynamics*, Proceedings of Symposium of Practical Urodynamics, Hahnemann Medical College & Hospital, Philadelphia.
23. Sridhara, C. R. (1983) Personal Communication, Albert Einstein Medical Center, Dept. of Physical Medicine and Rehabilitation.
24. Geer, J. H. (1975) Direct measurement of genital responding, *Am. Psychol.*, pp. 415–418.
25. Geer, J. H., Morohoff, P., and Greenwood, P. Sexual arousal in women: the development of a measurement device for vaginal blood volume, *Arch. Sex. Behav.* **3(6)**, pp. 599–564.
26. Geer, J. H. (1983) Personal Communication, State University of New York at Stony Brook, Dept. of Psychology.
27. Cohen, H. D. and Shapiro, A. (1970) A method for measuring sexual arousal in the female, *Psychophysiology* **8**, 251 (abstract).
28. Leyson, J. F. J. (1982) Intravaginal temperature recording as an adjunctive tool in the diagnosis of sexual dysfunctions in female spinal cord injured patients. Paper presented at American Asso. of Sex Educators, Counselors and Therapists, New York City. March 13–15.
29. Leyson, J. F. J., Stefaniwsky, L., and Martin, B. F. (1979) Effects of transcutaneous nerve stimulation on the vesicourethral function in spinal cord injury patients. *J. Urol.* **121**, 635-639.
30. Leyson, J. F. J. (1983) Electromyographic (EMG) urodynamic anal probe as a diagnostic tool in the management of sexual dysfunctions in female spinal cord injured patients. *J. Am. Paraplegia Soc.* **6**, 79–80.
31. Schover, L. R. and Soren, B. J. (1988) *Sexuality and Chronic Illness* (The Guilford Press, New York), pp. 146–149.

12

Management of Sexual Dysfunction in Spinally Injured Women

Domeena C. Renshaw

Introduction

In health care, a basic dictum is "first things first"—i.e., survival and crisis care of the patient take priority. Sexual problems and sexual well-being, therefore, will ordinarily not receive attention from the professional until after the acute phase of any injury or the most serious aspect of an illness had been dealt with. Too often the physician delays talking about sexuality until the patient asks about it. However, today rehabilitation professionals are receiving more training and practice in sexual medicine so that the rehabilitation phase, with its relatively relaxed pace of care, has become the time to discuss sexual issues.

For a man or woman who has newly sustained a spinal cord lesion—limb pain, isolated paralysis of a limb muscle group, paraplegia, or quadriplegia—immediate (not delayed) and recurring questions may be: Will I still be attractive (sexy)? Will I be sexually disabled? Will I be sexually helpless? These are expectable and quite normal concerns. For most persons, sex means closeness and love. For some persons, sex is synonomous with intercourse, a pleasurable release of tension. Whatever value the spinal-cord-injured (SCI) woman has attached to her sexuality, the thought of losing some or all of it will be there and must be dealt with. This awareness strongly suggests that, early on, a clinician should say something of the order of: "As soon as you stabilize, we will talk about your bowel, bladder, and sexual functions."

Sexual Rehabilitation of the Spinal-Cord-Injured Patient
Edited by J.F. Leyson, © 1990 The Humana Press, Inc.

This is both open and optimistic, and sets the stage for effective rehabilitative management.

For the health professional who manages any medical condition, the standard approach is:

1. Define the problem
2. Establish its cause(s)
3. Evaluate how much of the problem is the result of *physical* causes and how much arises from an emotional "overlay" or "underlay."

This same basic approach is also optimal for the sexual dysfunctions of SCI persons who will have mixed pathology: a human psychosomatic tangle to be unraveled in the course of diagnosis and treatment. How much of the sexual problem results from the cord lesion? How much from worry about self-image, attractiveness, dependency, rejection, and further damage?

Management of the sex problems of the SCI woman begins the very first time that sexual issues are avoided, dismissed, or discussed, which may occur early in the postacute phase or later, but which always should be dealt with openly before discharge.

The sex therapy approach for an SCI woman with sex problems must include:

1. An explicit, individual, personal medical and sexual history-taking from her childhood up to actual time of her interview: fantasies and facts.
2. A personal, medical, and explicit sexual history-taking from her partner
3. A physical examination that must include (a) a careful neurologic examination to establish the sensory-motor sparing, as well as the deficits and (b) a thorough educative sexologic genital examination with a mirror to teach the SCI woman about her own sexual self.

If she is married, her spouse, with her consent, is asked to be present during her sexologic examination, as she is for his. If she has a committed partner whom she wishes included in sex therapy, she will have to indicate consent for each visit, as he will have to do for her presence in his sexologic exam. Permission is required for medicolegal reasons whenever partners have no legal bond.

Why this special emphasis on a therapeutic sexologic examination? Because every medical problem lies somewhere along a continuum between psychological and somatic:

Somato-psychic ⟷ Psycho-somatic

A first important step in the treatment of any disorder is to find where, along this continuum, the problem lies, because no spinal cord lesion occurs in an emotional vacuum. The Sexological Examination is special because:

1. It follows a principle of sound conservative medical practice (*14,19*)
2. It gives the individual an awareness of her/his own body and how it works
3. It is a bonding experience: (a) for a couple committed to their relationship and (b) between the couple and the physician
4. It can be a valuable source of information about the couple and how they interact and relate under the stress of the new experience of the combined examination
5. It utilizes the partner as chaperone, although some physicians may still include a nurse chaperone. For a solo patient, however, because of the sensitivity of sexual dialog and to avoid accusations of sexual exploitation, an assistant or nurse chaperone is essential.

Specialization dictates "body" doctors and "soul" doctors. Good physician sex therapists are "both"! Since so much of sex therapy is sex education, frontline sex therapists for the SCI woman may be a sensitive and sexually educated neurologist, urologist, gynecologist, internist, physiatrist, psychiatrist, or family physician (*3,4,7,10,11,11A, 15,18*).

How does sexual dysfunction in an able-bodied woman come to the attention of a health professional? In much the same way as for an SCI woman: too often only by direct complaint during a search for information and help. Better medical management for all patients would incorporate a protocol for a thorough personal history-taking, which includes at least this one routine question: What part has sex played in your life up to now? If this gentle question meets with a negative response, simply say, "This is a routine question. I respect your privacy. However, if you ever want to discuss sexual issues, be sure to ask."

Should the response to this question be that it was vital and there are fears in the SCI woman that she now will lose her sexuality, it may be best to simply say: "We will have to ask you more questions if we are to help you remain as sexual a person as is humanly possible for you." Then begin formal sex therapy by continuing the sex history:

1. Do you have sexual desires/dreams/fantasies?
2. Did you express yourself regularly sexually before your spinal injury or problem? (Details)
3. Were you orgasmic before the spinal problem? (Details)
4. How did you attain this before (reading, movies, masturbation, fantasy only, foreplay, kissing, breast play, partner's hand/mouth on the clitoris, intercourse, or other)?
5. Have you attained orgasm since the spinal problem? How? (Details)
6. Do you have sleep (dream) orgasms? (Details) (*2*)
7. What was the frequency prelesion of (a) loveplay (b) intercourse per month?
8. How did your partner attain satisfaction?
9. Did you/partner have any sexual problems?
10. What type of sexual problem: Anorgasmia (primary/secondary). Dyspareunia? Vaginismus? Sexual aversion? Unconsummated marriage? Impotence? Premature or delayed ejaculation for your partner?
11. Were there sexual desire differences?
12. Can you/partner discuss sex and your feelings frankly?
13. Does your partner love you as a person as well as sexually?
14. What position(s) did you and partner use?
15. To what extent pre-SCI had you experimented with sexual positions?
16. Do you or partner have intercourse to please the other although not in the mood yourself?
17. Have either of you used contraceptives? Details?
18. Have you had individual/marital/sexual counseling?
19. Are you satisfied with your current sex education/knowledge?
20. Have you experienced any troubling sexual event: rape, incest, child molestation, other? (*17*) (Details)
21. Do you have any troubling sexual questions or thoughts? (Details)
22. Are you attracted to women? Have you expressed these feelings? (*10,13*)
23. What are your feelings about your sexual attractiveness now?
24. Would you like to hear how other SCI women are coping sexually?

If some or any of these questions trigger patient discomfort and avoidance, the sensitive clinician may say, "Sex is not an easy topic to talk about. Most of us have not learned how. Feel free to bring it up again when you are ready.'' This leaves an open-door option for her. Usually the comfort of the professional determines the comfort of the patient. Initially for the professional, the experience of taking an explicit sexual history violates the taboo of sexual privacy, plus possibly also that of man–woman explicit sexual dialog (if the professional is a man), and then another even more difficult taboo—sex and the disabled, who are often disenfranchised and mistakenly considered asexual. After taking three or so explicit clinical sexual histories, the professional will be amazed and gratified by the patient's responses and relief. Consequently, the expectable ''entry anxiety'' into the initially unfamiliar field of sex therapy is reduced.

What if the SCI woman is hurt and offended by a sexual history? Then the professional may simply state that sexuality is part of every normal person's life, just as are the menses and bowel function, so that at least one routine sexual question is a part of any history protocol. Her right to privacy on this topic will be respected.

What if these questions trigger a flood of tears from the SCI woman? Let them flow. Just as tears protect the eyes from grit and other noxious factors, so tears protect the emotions and allow overflow of hurt, anger, and grief at the possible loss of her sexual function, her mobility, and her opportunities to interact sexually. It is quite normal and relieving to cry, although many, even professionals, feel personally uncomfortable with tears. Be silent for a few minutes. Stay with her. Offer kleenex. Ask, ''What are the tears about?'' Just listen, and then say how important it is to have some release of her normal feelings related to the disability. Tell her it is fine to talk again, with or without tears. This is reassuring, but also does not set up a ''condition'' that attention and time will only be provided for being very upset and tearful.

What are female sexual dysfunctions specific to spinal cord injuries? No single answer is possible. Many personal variables are involved.

1. Her age at the time of the spinal lesion
2. Her previous sexual self-esteem, attitudes, desires, fantasies, and functioning
3. The degree of motor disability (legs/arms)
4. The degree of loss of reflexes (bladder, bowel, and genitals)
5. The availability of a loving, accepting sexual partner in the past and now
6. Her own willingness to discuss and experiment with her own thoughts and body to establish the limits of her current sexual capacity
7. Her moral values about the latter (7)

8. Her general health prior to and after the spinal lesion
9. Associated physical complications: general illness; vaginal, bowel and bladder infections; vasomotor changes, and so on.
10. Associated psychological complications: her attitude to the disability and her changed self-image; *sustained* emotional withdrawal/anger/depression/dependency/anxiety beyond expected normal grieving, distress, confusion, and anger.

There are no reliable statistics for the overall prevalence of SCI persons in the US or a breakdown of the male/female ratio of ages. One non-US statistic has a 9/1 male/female SCI ratio with a dominant etiology of stab wounds. No age range was given. A 1971 US epidemiology SCI overall statistic mentions that traffic (car and motorcycle) accidents caused 50%, mountain falls 25%, and all other causes (recreation: diving and other sports; firearms; polio; tumor; congenital diseases, and so on) the remaining 25%. The 1985 prevalence of SCI women may, therefore, be anything between 200 and 20,000 persons. It is not a well-documented group, to say the least. Thus, the specific sexual dysfunctions to be expected from the spinal lesion are not predictable because of paucity of data and the many prelesion variables (*5*).

On the surface, the situation might seem very different sexually for an institutionalized paraplegic teen with congenital SCI and presumed nondevelopment of a sexual relationship when she is contrasted with a healthy 30-year-old married woman with SCI after a fall from a cliff (presumed to have a good sexual relationship). However, the married mountaineer may be sexually restricted, may even not have consummated her marriage because of severe vaginismus, or she may be anorgasmic, whereas the teen may have romanced with another able or disabled person of either sex, or awakened and developed her own sexual feelings and function by very aware experimentation with her own body and reacting with others in her environment, by contact, reading, watching the soap operas, by daydreaming or night dreaming, and thus, found gratifying sexual responses and releases. Assumptions on the part of the professional may usurp the SCI patient's right to a sexual history and, later, to needed sex education and sex therapy.

For the mountaineer, the SCI may actually be a "silver-lining," because her pubococcygeus muscle will be partially paralyzed, as also her lower limbs if the injury is above S_2. The symptom of vaginismus may disappear. Random muscle spasms in the pubococcygeus may certainly occur, but theoretically these should be neither sustained nor anxiety-related and, therefore, should not prevent penetration. In such a case, careful reproductive education for the couple must then be part of sex education given by the responsible health professional. Both husband and wife must be told and explicitly asked about their current desire to resume attempts at intercourse. Raise questions about pregnancy, so that they may think and talk it through. The patient's periods will resume, and she may well remain fertile although disabled.

Step one, therefore, for formal sex therapy with SCI women is a good explicit sex and medical history based on trust. Then step two: personal sex education through a sexologic examination, as mentioned earlier. Step three might be didactic sex education: talking, reading, diagrams, slides, films, lecture, and group discussions (*4,19*). The steps need not be in sequence, and may be individualized to meet each SCI woman's needs and pace.

Sex Education for SCI Women

This aspect of sex therapy is a major and essential feature for the reversal of sexual ignorance and sexual inhibition in able-bodied women. It is also true for the disabled woman, because sexual illiteracy still remains the heritage of most women today. In most families there is sexual silence, interpreted by a child as: "We cannot talk about sex here. It upsets Mom and Dad." Few schools have the heroism to teach explicit human sexuality. They may offer menstrual and childbirth information for girls and VD details for both sexes. However, there is a critical gap—the vital one—of how the child can understand and handle the rich flood of natural and normal sexual feelings. Masturbation, although a natural and normal release, is thought and taught to be unnatural, damaging, and depraved (*15*). Most girls grow to womanhood treating their genitals as a "nonpart" of themselves because of the many negatives learned: "Don't touch! It's dirty—wash your hands. It's bad/sinful and don't get pregnant!" Needless guilts result, and often there may be suppression of the developmental sexual self-learning needed by many women until 20–60 yrs. later.

Where then do able-bodied girls learn about sex if not at home or school? From peers and from books mainly. What about SCI women? Probably in the same way before the spinal lesion. Lack of mobility and independence may restrict access both to peers and to sexual materials for the girl with a congenital spinal problem and for the post-SCI teen or woman, until mastery and assisted movement is attained so that sexual dialog, reading, video, or movie viewing as well as mating or dating opportunities may be experienced.

What about sex education in a rehabilitation setting? Is it appropriate? Who should provide it? How should sex education be offered to SCI women? (*4,13,20*) Yes, sex education is highly appropriate, since sexuality is a vital function of every individual, able-bodied or disabled. It is perhaps best offered as an elective program, so that the right of any SCI woman to refuse is respected if she feels she is not interested or not yet ready (because she is still grieving, angry, or uncertain) to confront this aspect of herself.

The two main qualifications of the SCI sex education (as with any educator) are *competence* and *comfort. Competence* includes knowledge of female and male sexual responses, dysfunctions, and treatment; physical changes of spinal lesions; compensatory sexual pleasuring; the capacity to encourage the patient to experiment and to enjoy (*3,5,7, 10,17-22*). Competence also includes the capacity to say, "I don't know" when the educator does not and to follow with, "I certainly will try to find out for you." Physicians, rehabilitation therapists, social workers, nurses, psychologists, and counsellors with "sex therapy training" plus some special education about the expectable changes of spinal lesions could make good sex educators and therapists for SCI women.

Comfort will come from knowledge and practice (clinical application of knowledge), which will then allow skill to be attained by the professional. Skill provides comfort and reassurance in the clinician. Expectably, there will be "entry anxiety" for the educator or therapist when the new teaching or clinical situation is first encountered. After the third lecture or discussion experience, however, matters will generally prove easier, and by the tenth time, the initial nervousness will barely be recalled.

Sex education has two elements: (a) distant or cognitive: listening, reading, watching, e.g., movie, slides, illustrations, people, and so on, (b) personal application: from the two-dimensional page or screen to the three dimensions of "me" physically by the SCI woman. Then there are her internal emotions and reactions during the prelude to sexual exchange and afterwards. These may be warm, positive, and pleasurable. For some person, they may be controlled and "neutral." For other, they may be empty, negative, and even painful., dramatizing that sex and love are not necessarily synonymous.

For the SCI woman, the same range of responses may have been experienced prespinal lesion and may remain or change afterwards—for better or for worse, depending on her reaction to her lesion and that of her partner to her. Ideally experienced sexuality in humans involves both the "soul" (total essence or inner person) and the body. Although the SCI woman has sustained physical damage, her personhood may remain unchanged, she may mature and grow, or she may become embittered and withdraw sexually and socially. This is reflected in her facial expression—the most vital accessory worn by any person—young, old, man, or woman. Facial friendliness, openness, and interest in others is highly attractive, whereas hostility, tension, and frowning are repellant, in or out of a wheelchair. Grooming—cosmetics, perfume, and clothing—are all important for her own good feelings as well as responses from friends and family. Since sexual exchange is an interaction, eye contact is an essential preliminary encounter then to be followed by words and touch: affectionate touch first, then intimate sexual touch. These factors must all be incorporated into the sex education phase of sex therapy.

Expectably, quite normally, the *internal self-image* and *sexual self-esteem* will suffer after a spinal lesion for a man or a woman of any age. Do they ever recover? That depends on each SCI person. If an SCI woman accepts the residual "me" as real, and worthy of respect and care, this allows others to do the same when relatives and health professionals show their regard, respect, and care for her (*19*). Specific sexual problems in SCI women may include: sexual aversion, inhibited sexual desire, dyspareunia, or inhibited orgasm.

Sexual Aversion in an SCI Woman

This state may be fully conscious and relate to sexual trauma, such as rape or conflicts around incest or molestation or to strong negative learning resulting from religious beliefs. Sometimes the aversion is so strong that it resembles a phobic-anxiety state quite isolated from other daily function. It is the SCI patient's human right to avoid sexual discussion and contact if avoidance alone relieves her aversion, and this avoidance defense must be respected if revealed upon inquiry. It should not be assumed or imposed by the professional.

However, if she is married, sex avoidance may have caused marital problems. The SCI woman may perhaps now lessen her partner's pressure for sex. If he is loving and altruistic, he may stay in the marriage even though his last hopes for her sexual response and enjoyment seem shattered by the spinal lesion. Divorce may be another choice for him. For the SCI patient, being in bed gives time to request sex education and to explore questions more fully. Some sex therapy may in fact now help avert separation, promote closeness, and bring new sexual joy to both the SCI woman and her partner, perhaps for the first time.

How does the rehabilitation professional begin? Does one just ask whether the aversive SCI woman wishes to change? Whether she will read? Whether she will discuss her sexual feelings with the professional, and/or her religious advisor, or with a sex therapist in a women's group? Whether she will agree to individual or couple sex therapy? Assistance with referral can then be given (*6*). Does sexual ignorance cause sexual aversion? Does misinterpretation of sexual dogma cause sexual aversion or inhibiton? Yes. That is why a religious consultation can be most relieving after years of distress. Although highly controversial, SCI women without partners may be referred by some therapists to sexual surrogates for treatment, but other professionals have strong medical (STD or AIDS), ethical, and legal reservations about this practice (*9,17*). Celibacy by free choice is a normal sexual alternative, and may be differentiated from sexual aversion by the adequate general adjustment of the person, and awareness of the redirection of sexual drives or the absence of sexual distress.

Sexual Arousal Disorders in SCI Women

Until some additional laboratory studies are done on SCI women during masturbation (*9*) and coitus that are analogous to those done on able-bodied women by Masters and Johnson (*11*), it will only be speculative whether the patient's brain–autonomic nervous system–genital connections have been spared. Therefore, the DSM III-R definition of sexual arousal: "the persistent or recurrent partial or complete failure to attain and/or maintain the lubrication–swelling response until the completion of the sexual act" may be inappropriate for SCI women. Even if present, these reactions may not be consciously felt by her as sensations because of the injury if her linkage "circuit" has been interrupted (*5*).

For her (as also for able-bodied women), questions about desire must include inquiry about sexual fantasies. Does she have them/suppress them/enjoy them? Is she upset or negative about her sex fantasies? Does she long for and enjoy affectionate touch? Does she long for sexual contact? How long has this been so? If she is not interested and does not want to be interested, preinjury and presently, then this negative sexual state is her normal right, and needs to be acknowledged and respected. If her inhibition of sexual desire predates the SCI and she wishes to explore her inhibitions, then sex education may proceed, and psychosexual therapy may be considered as a possible way of modifying her negative attitudes and allowing her natural; positive sexual feelings to surface for enjoyment. Dealing with the possibly negative antecedent sexual experiences that may have started the problem will be an essential part of the psychosexual therapy she needs (*6*). Permission, support, and the suggestion that she exercise and explore her sexual fantasies is a necessary preliminary to exploring her body when she is alone or when with her partner. This way, she may get in touch very literally with her sexual self. If she has selective inhibition of sexual desire related to her partner (conflicts/doubts/mistrust) or to a clinical depression in herself, then these must be appropriately addressed by psychosexual treatment of the couple (*10*).

Demoralization (which includes desperation, feeling "down," crying, irritability, some sleep difficulty) is to be expected for up to 24 wks after a spinal disability occurs. It persists until adjustments are made. Demoralization is not necessarily a clinical depression, but a normal way of "regrouping" the patient's coping mechanisms. Persistent nihilism, insomnia, anorexia, and preoccupation with death and suicide indicate that a clinical depression has set in, and may be altering all of her appetites: for food, for sleep, for sex, and for life. Whenever this occurs—one day or one year later—it is a life crisis in need of psychotherapy, with or without antidepressant medication. Effective therapy will usually (in about 4–6 wks) restore sleep, zest for eating, and desire for sex. If the patient's sexual disinterest is thought to be related to a clinical depression, but remains after the depression clears, and if the patient wishes to address the issue, then the sex therapy approach described above is indicated: fantasy, self-exploration, and guided partner exploration of his and her sexuality (*6*).

Dyspareunia in an SCI Woman

Depending on the level of the spinal lesion, pain in and around the vagina is not to be expected when the spinal lesion is above S_2 because sensory fibers will have been affected. However, each SCI woman is unique and must be very carefully examined neurologically for her perineal responses to light touch and pinprick sensation. The therapist should watch her facial expression and reflex movements when this, as well as manual and speculum pelvic examinations, are done. The vaginal walls must be examined to note their thickness and moisture. If there is dryness or a mechanical problem, the couple should be advised to use a lubricant (KY jelly) and a more comfortable position for intercourse. On the other hand, hyperhidrosis may be treated with phenoxybenzamine: 10 mg orally or 3 times daily (alpha-adrenergic blocker). However, prolonged and excessive use of the drug (dibenzyline) may compromise orgasm (*9*).

A positive bulbocavernosus and the presence of external anal reflexes indicate *reflexic* bladder, bowel, and sex functions. The "mental dyspareunia" (if there is actual or real loss of a sphincter) may be a big factor for a previously meticulous SCI woman. She may fear partner upset and rejection because of an accident from possible reflex loss of bowel or bladder control during intercourse or orgasm, and be mortified and shamed if it does occur. This is an appropriate response. Talk about the possibility openly with both partners. Suggest they use old towels plus a big open Pamper (paper diaper) as a top layer under her hips to cope with such a possible accident. For her, careful preliminary (pre-loveplay) evacuation of her bladder and bowel can also be helpful. Large doses of humor in the bedroom can accompany preventive precoital preparations and reduce their tensions. Routine female hygiene is also a must to prevent unpleasant vaginal/urinary odors. Relaxation techniques include bathing together to promote bonding and enhance pleasure.

Intercourse may set off, for the SCI woman, a headache, facial sweating, and raised blood pressure, if the spinal lesion is above T_6. This "dysreflexia" may be triggered by a noxious stimulus (usually not consciously felt by the SCI person) in the urethra, vagina, or perineal area or by a full bladder/bowel. The first experience of this "dysreflexia" response may be anxiety-provoking, but once she and her partner know what it is and that it will pass in a few hours, dysreflexia becomes less of a problem (*2*). Avoiding the cause by emptying any full viscera or removing irritating stimuli is the best approach. The Foley catheter can be taped to the abdomen or removed prior to sex, but its waterbulb should be emptied to prevent mechanical injury to the sphincter. Embarrassing flatus (passage of gas from the vagina, bowel, or ostomy barrel) can be avoided by gentle penile thrusting, coital positioning, and by reducing gas-forming foods in the diet. Pain and muscle spasms should be treated or controlled with medications or surgical ablative procedures, keeping in mind the preservation of sensor/motor sensual circuitry (*9*). Frozen hips or joints that may interfere with coital positioning must be surgically released. Biofeedback is ideal therapy for incomplete lesions that cause pain and muscle spasms.

Sex therapy follows the same format: careful history, careful physical/neurological examination, sexological examination, sex education, and then suggestions for sensual touch on the face and body. This is a good opportunity for an SCI woman to explore (and tell her partner about) those areas that give her good sexual feelings, which may include a new and compensatory erotic area, such as a 1-inch transverse band

---

Ed note: Sexual incontinence can be minimized by emptying the bladder or oral "Ditropan" 5 mg an hour before sexual celebration.

below the level of the spinal lesion (*2*) or earlobes or lips that have become more eroticized. They should explore and enjoy one another, and then proceed to intercourse after a few weeks (*11,11A,12*). SCI women complaining of lax vaginal introitus may strengthen their "sex muscles" by performing Kegel's perineal exercises monitored by an electronic perinometer.* Comfortable alternative coital positions can be discussed using flexible pipecleaner dolls or cutout paper dolls to illustrate these positions three dimensionally. Week by week followup of their sexual progress by the sex counselor/therapist is important and supportive in sex therapy.

Inhibited Orgasm in SCI Women

Primary anorgasmia (namely, that never ever in any way has the patient experienced a sexual climax) may be newly discovered only after an explicit post-SCI sexual history reveals it. Depending on her age, primary anorgasmia is usually pre-SCI. If she is a teenager, it may represent nonlearning about her sexual self (*22*). Are there able-bodied women who do not know that they have not had an orgasm? Yes. With sexual ignorance, some women expect little except the good feelings of closeness and compliance in meeting the sexual needs of their partners. SCI women with primary anorgasmia may be helped by both psychosexual therapy and couple therapy: both partners should be counseled, and mention should be made that the SCI injury can cause orgasmic delay or nonresponse. Thus, SCI women may require long hours of sex play before they experience mini-orgasms or even just a feeling of exhilaration (*9*). They and their partners need patience, love, and humor.

Is the treatment of primary anorgasmia different from that of secondary anorgasmia? In principle, no. In practice, yes. A woman (able-bodied or SCI) who has not gotten in touch with her own sexuality needs much larger doses of permission from a respected professional authority to do so (*1,13,21,22*). Very few women, even contemporary teens, explore themselves sexually. Many expect their partner "to give me an orgasm," while they remain passive and receptive. An able-bodied or SCI woman needs to recognize her own sexual responsibility to explore and *find* her special pleasure centers, and then guide and encourage partner exploration in their lovemaking (*11*). Accepting and then enjoying her own sexuality is an important task of maturity for every woman. It is a giant emancipatory step from negatives and sexual illiteracy to positives and sexual knowledge. It is a personal odyssey for every

* Farrall Instruments, Inc., PO Box 1037, Grand Island, Nebraska 68802.

woman—disabled or able-bodied (*13*). An SCI woman with primary anorgasmia needs guidance and direction from a professional who can describe what she will experience: "After some period of sexual thoughts and fantasizing, your general response will be slightly increased mouth breathing, increased heart rate, and increased temperature. Your nipples will erect if the lesion is below T_5, and there will be increased tension in every functioning body muscle. For you, this will be in your face, neck, shoulders, arms, and so on (depending on her spinal lesion level). Then there will be a few contractions in those same muscles, followed by complete relaxation and perhaps some general sweating." Control of the environment by adjusting the room thermostat to the individual's comfort may help prevent sympathetic dysreflexia (*9*).

For the SCI woman with good arm and finger movement, suggestions from the therapist should include that, at home in *private*, she try exploring rubbing her earlobes (these contain erectile tissue), her lips (using fingers, scarf, cotton, powder brush, feather, and so on) and do the same on the face, neck, breasts, nipples, torso, clitoris, and wherever she can reach and feel. She is always the best sensual and sexual expert on herself. Self-exploration is enjoyable, vital, and health-affirming. It is also a developmental step towards mutual sexual exchange later (*1,22*).

Talking one-to-one about her sexual feelings to another SCI woman or in a small group of SCI women with a sensitive rehabilitation counselor or physician can be additionally relieving and helpful. Each woman will go at her own pace and in the framework of her own belief system. Sex therapists must recognize that no person can go further or faster than he or she is ready for. Some will take longer to integrate new sexual knowledge and feelings before they are ready to express and enjoy them. Their pace must be respected.

Secondary anorgasmia describes a woman who was able, in some way, to attain sexual release (orgasm) after arousal—at least once. She then knows what the experience is, so that it may be somewhat easier for her than for a primary anorgasmic SCI woman. If this happened before the SCI, she now must try to see how much of her previous responses she will enjoy again. It is also possible that an SCI woman only became orgasmic after her injury and enjoyed the experiences, but has now lost that former capacity to climax, perhaps because of social, marital, or interpartner conflicts. A recent sexual embarrassment, anxiety unrelated to sex but nonetheless intruding into the bedroom, family problems, a death, job or financial worries, and so on, may all need to be unraveled first with a sensitive sex therapist.

There may also be physical and/or chemical factors to check out: changes in her medical condition that may be causative or about which she is anxious, for example, bladder infections, muscle spasms, and others. What about needed medications that may have sexual side effect (*3,7,10*)? How much alcohol is being consumed? Are over-the-counter or street drugs being used? Even in hospital corridors, the contraband of "recreational chemicals" continues. Also, substance abuse and chronic illness are closely associated. The alert clinician must gently, routinely, and repeatedly check these out as sex therapy proceeds. Basic suggestions from the therapist should be: At home, relax, bathe, and be good to yourself; use lots of sexual fantasy, perfume, and lotion if you want to. Explore your whole self. Take your time. Read your favorite sexy book or novel, and so on. These are identical to the recommendations offered for the primary anorgasmic SCI woman. The goal, not to be lost sight of, is to obtain the most sexual enjoyment possible for her and her partner.

Counseling the partner of the SCI woman is an important part of sex therapy, if that partner is committed. His personal, medical, and sexual histories can help the sex therapist and his SCI partner understand him better. His sexual and social fantasies, experiences, and expectations are as important as those of the SCI woman in their post-SCI adjustment. Both will need good medical information (updated repeatedly if complications in her condition arise) so that physical problems are taken care of when necessary, rather than being considered resistances to sexual contacts—which they sometimes may be.

Sex education, therefore, must include information about a man's sexual responses, too, so that an SCI woman can also "get by giving." Recommended readings, with an opportunity to ask questions or to discuss what she has read, are also of help (*1,2,6,11–13,21,22*). Sexual discussion may be done individually, in a group of SCI women, or mixed with able-bodied women. Each situation will dictate what sex therapy options there are available.

The male's reactions to her spinal lesion's effect on her body, her activity, and her emotions will be as varied as the personality of each partner. A husband who vowed "in sickness and in health" may simply break down and cry, as one 31-year-old man did in individual history-taking: "I prayed she would die, and I feel terrible about that. How can I look after a cripple? I hate the word, but it came into my head. I was so proud of her looks and figure. I still have trouble staying near her wheelchair in public. It's like I'm ashamed to be her husband. I'm so messed up. It's like I love her and hate the wheelchair. . . ."

Is he brutal and unfeeling? Not at all. He has normal intense and honestly expressed confused and negative feeling about a severe crisis in their lives that neither anticipated. Could this interfere with their sex lives? Unless they are able to "avoid avoidance" in dealing with these feelings, it may. How can they be dealt with? On the part of the therapist, by nurturant confrontation: "How are you feeling right now—John/Mary? Let's talk about it. That's a natural response. Feelings *feel*; they don't think. We think and behave afterwards. It's important that you're honest. Both of you are grieving the loss of Mary's independence and her good-looking legs. She still has a great face, a bright mind, lots of love, and warmth. She also has sexual feelings, as do you. Can you accept the challenge of caring and sharing the exploration of your sexual selves for new, different, compensatory, and even possibly more enjoyable alternatives?" The partner of the SCI woman must not be allowed to suffer benign neglect in the management of the SCI woman's sexual adjustment. He/she can continue to be, or newly become, a full 50% of her sexual pleasure.

Conclusions

Management of the sexual problems of the SCI woman necessarily entails truly caring for the well-being of the whole person—soul and body. For the sensitive clinician, adding sexual help in rehabilitation is a "close encounter" of the best and most human kind!

References

1. Basbach, L. (1975) *For Yourself*, Doubleday, New York.
2. (1978) Becker, E. F. *Female Sexuality Following Spinal Cord Injury*, Accent Special Inc. Bloomington, Illinois.
3. Boller, F. and Frank, E. (1982) *Sexual Dysfunction in Neurological Disorders*, Rave, New York.
4. Cole, R. M. and Cole, S. S. (1982) Sexuality and Disability, in Krusen, F. H., Kottke, F. J. and Elwood, P. M. *Handbook of Physical Medicine and Rehabilitation*, 3rd Ed. (Krusen, F. H., Kottke, F. J., and Elwood, P. M.).
5. Griffith, E. R. and Treischmann, R. B. (1975) Sexual functioning in women with spinal injury, *Arch. Phys. Med. Rehabil.* **56**, 19–21.
6. Kaplan, H. S. (1979) *Disorders of Sexual Desires*, Simon & Schuster, New York.

7. Kolodny, R. C., Masters, W. H. and Johnson, W. E. (1979) *Textbook of Sexual Medicine*, Little Brown, Boston.
8. Leyson, J. F. J. (1983) Sexual surrogate—A new sex therapy alternative, *J. of Mult. Sclerosis Quarterly*. Summer, 3-7.
9. Leyson, J. F. J. and Powell, R. (1979) Counseling the female spinal cord injured patient, *Med. Asp. Human Ses.* **13**, 59-60.
10. Lief, H. (ed.) (1981) *Sexual Problems in Medical Practice*, AMA, Monroe, WI.
11. Masters, W. H. and Johnson, V. E. (1970) *Human Sexual Inadequacy*, Little, Brown, Boston.
11A. Masters, W. H., Johnson, V. E., and Kolodny, R. C. (1986) *Sex and Human Loving*, Little, Brown, Boston.
12. Mooney, T. D., Cole, T. M., and Chilgren, R. N. (1979) *Sexual Options for Paraplegics*, Little, Brown, Boston.
13. *Our Bodies Ourselves*: a book by and for women, (1975) Simon & Schuster, New York.
14. Poma, P., "The Sexological Examination" *The Female Patient*, **4:8**, p. 40–42.
15. Renshaw, D. C. (1973) Sex education for educators, *J. School Health*, **XLVI/10**, pp. 645-650.
16. Renshaw, D. C. (1982) Sexual surrogates, *Sexual Medicine Today* **2(7)**, 39.
17. Renshaw, D. C. (1982) *Incest: Understanding and Treatment*, Little Brown, Boston.
18. Rosensweig, N. and Pearsall, P. (ed.s) (1978) *Sex Education for the Health Professional.* Grune and Stratton, New York.
19. Semmens, J. (1979) The sexological examination. *Medical News*, 11-14.
20. Shaked, A. (ed.) (1981) *Human Sexuality and Rehabilitation Medicine.* Williams and Wilkins, Baltimore.
21. Simon, S. (1976) *Caring, Feeling, Touching.* Argus Communications, Illinois.
22. Yates, A. (1978) *Sex Without Shame.* Morrow, New York.

13

Holistic Massage

Rachel J. Harris

Introduction

The holistic approach to massage is more an attitude than a set of techniques. Holistic Massage considers the unity of the body, psyche, and spirit, and recognizes that intervention at any of these levels affects the whole system of the person. Furthermore, the whole person is more than the sum of body, psyche, and spirit (*24*), and needs to be perceived as such. Thus, holistic massage practitioners are distinguished more by their special perceptions than by techniques.

Traditional massage offers a multitude of techniques for reducing pain, increasing circulation, channeling energy flow, relaxing or stimulating muscles, balancing the structure, increasing range of movement at joints, improving posture, experiencing pleasure, and many other benefits. Holistic massage may use none or all of this wide variety of techniques. The qualitative difference is that the individual technique is used within the context of a greater goal, that is, for the optimum well-being of the whole person.

Practitioners of holistic massage respect the capacity of the recipient to be responsible for his or her own well-being. This responsibility begins with a interaction unfolds, the whole person evolves. Any barriers to well-being are considered to be both a misfortune and an opportunity for discovery (*12*) leading to further evolution. Holistic massage seeks to stimulate, facilitate, and support progress along this path.

Thus, holistic massage is not symptom oriented. Although symptoms may be acknowledged and even explored, they are not considered simply a challenge to be relieved. Rather, many such complaints are viewed as a message from the body containing important feedback regarding balance, daily life habits, and stress. It is the conscious awareness

Sexual Rehabilitation of the Spinal-Cord-Injured Patient
Edited by J.F. Leyson, © 1990 The Humana Press, Inc.

of everyday habits at all levels of physical functioning, psychological patterns, and spiritual perception that provides the personal learning necessary for growth and evolution (*2*).

Another distinguishing characteristic of holistic massage is the relationship between the giver of the massage and the receiver. Both are active participants in the experience of the massage. Both enter into an altered state of consciousness through the use of relaxation and meditation techniques that will be explained later. This meditative approach increases the sensitivity and empathic receptiveness of both people, and allows for an almost mystical communication to occur via the massage. People often report profound feelings of oneness with their massage partner, regardless of whether they are giving or receiving the massage.

In summary, holistic massage perceives the unity of the body, psyche, and spirit; respects the right and capacity of the recipient to be responsible for his or her own well-being and evolution; emphasizes the process of awareness rather than utilizing goal-oriented techniques; and uses a meditative relationship between the giver and receiver of the massage. Holistic massage depends upon the awareness, intention, and communication between both participants of the massage. In this way, both the giver and receiver are enhanced by the experience of the holistic massage.

Body Image

One of the major goals for holistic massage is to provide the opportunity for the receiver to experience the whole body as a unit. This is appropriate for the spinal-cord-injured person, because the body can be experienced in many different modes of perception other than neurologically. The wholeness of the body can be perceived visually, remembered in kinesthetic imagery, held as a concept in the mind, or sensed as an energy field. The perception of the whole body can include the physical body, the inner space of the body, or the space surrounding the body. Holistic massage seeks to facilitate these and other perceptions of the whole body through the use of touch, energy channeling in both the giver and receiver, imagery, and cognition.

The psychological concept of body image is useful in understanding the importance of experiencing the whole body. Fisher (*7*) described this term to mean the attitudinal framework that defines the long-term concept of the body and also influences body perception. It is through the body image that the feelings and experiences emanating from the body are integrated. The importance of body image in the development and maintenance of the sense of self can be inferred from this definition. However, Burton (*1*) stated this connection more directly: "The psychological concept of self is so minutely bound up with our conception of our organs and body that it is difficult to conceive of a holistic or balanced psychic self with an incomplete body self." Even more profound is Freud's original statement that the ego is, first and foremost, a body ego (*9*). Thus, the importance of body image to the sense of self can be readily acknowledged.

Holistic massage reinforces the body image by reminding the receiver that he or she is a whole body at whatever level the receiver is capable of perceiving that wholeness. This sense of wholeness is also reinforcing to the person's sense of self. It may even help the spinal-cord-injured person reconnect with a sense of self before the trauma and discover some helpful psychic resources and strengths.

It should be noted that some dimensions of body image reflect psychological material (*10,18,23*), whereas other aspects of body image relate to actual physiologic functioning of the body (*5,6,8*). It is not possible either conceptually or practically to isolate "which dimensions of body image are linked to the actual state of the body and which are projections on to the body of basic personality attitudes which do not fluctuate with variations in bodily conditions" (*4*). In the case of the spinal-cord-injured person, the physical and psychological dimensions of body image are minutely intertwined. It should therefore be recognized that, when one touches the physical body, one is also touching the psyche.

Holistic massage for the spinal-cord-injured person provides an opportunity to gradually explore and experience those parts of the body that are considered less attractive. Therapeutically, this means becoming conscious of the physical parts of the body that are usually kept to the unconscious by a variety of defense mechanisms. Furthermore, it means exposing those very same parts to an intimate partner. This can feel threatening to the sense of self, as well as to the relationship.

One recommendation is to concentrate first during the massage in those parts of the body that are considered most attractive. Then slowly the less attractive parts can be incorporated into the massage until the whole body is covered (*25*). In this way, the acceptance of the whole body, including the disability, by both the spinal-cord-injured person and the partner will enhance self-esteem and affirm sexuality.

Psychological Meaning of Touch

The need to be touched and to touch, perchance to heal at whatever level, may be one of the oldest known needs of humankind. Yerkes

(*26*) even speculated that our need to touch is an evolutionary expression of the primates' grooming behavior. Later Yerkes (*27*) observed that such grooming in primates serves a healing as well as a cosmetic purpose. It is possible that this same need to be touched and to touch is expressed in all the different forms of massage.

Certainly it is well known that the newborn infant's need to be touched is as basic as the need for food and shelter (*20*). The role of touching in the establishment of the original mother–infant bond has been documented by Kennall and Klaus (*16,17*). They found that babies who were touched by their mothers immediately after birth were distinguishable from infants who were removed from their mothers at birth by the speech patterns of the mother–child interaction at two years of age (*22*). Holistic massage can stimulate preverbal memories from the early months of life and release feelings stemming from the original mother–infant relationship. Awareness of early feelings of dependency and deprivation can become confused with more current emotions for the spinal-cord-injured person. Partners using holistic massage need to be aware of this dynamic and be able to discuss whatever feelings arise.

The need to be held is related to touch in the sense that body contact is being sought in both cases. Research regarding the need to be held found it to be related to depression, anxiety, sexual behavior, and orality (*14*). Hollender (*13*) even described the need to be held as a "major determinant of a particular characterologic pattern of life." People vary tremendously in their need to be held, and their willingness to experience and acknowledge it (*11*). Some people can be quite defensive and uncomfortable with nurturant touching and holding, often because of the intense feelings that arise. Others are starved for this type of contact and blossom when their need is met. That the need for physical contact is so great may be the result of at least two factors. First, the nurturing aspect of such touching is reminiscent of the early mother–infant relationship. Secondly, such touching reinforces the receiver's experience of the body and that, in turn, affirms the sense of self. The touching involved in holistic massage is extremely nurturing and affirming at these levels.

Holistic Massage as a Sexual Alternative

When holistic massage is used between intimate partners, the touching involved can also be sexually stimulating. For spinal-cord-injured persons, the massage can be used to develop heightened sensations in areas of the body unaffected by the disability. People report extremely sensual experiences in various areas of the body, including the neck, ears, armpits, and so on. Since such a response is uniquely individual, it is recommended that a massage be given with an open, exploratory approach. Variations in speed, rhythm, pressure, and technique of massage can also affect the response. The more relaxed the partners can be about such exploration, the more discoveries will emerge.

During such shared exploring the ability to communicate what is and is not pleasurable is crucial. Such feedback needs to be given and received neutrally, without blame of defensiveness. Often problems of communication that are linked with intimate sexual behavior emerge during a holistic massage and can be identified by a therapeutic person. Alternative communication modes can then sought that may also prove helpful in discussing the private experience of intercourse. Such improvements in communication serve to increase emotional trust and bonding between partners.

Positive memories of sexual experience before the spinal cord injury can be cognitively and kinesthetically stimulated to enrich current sensation (*25*). The spinal-cord-injured person can intentionally use his or her memory, imagery, and fantasy to enhance current feelings of sensuality. The body itself also records previous experience, and this can be stimulated by touching and reintegrated into the present capacity for sensual pleasure.

In many ways, holistic massage between intimate partners shares some similarities with Sensate Focus. Expectations regarding orgasm are eliminated, so that failure is impossible. This establishes ideal conditions for the extinction of sexual anxiety (*15*). The goal is merely to discover what gives pleasure. McCary (*19*) defined sensate focus as a "therapeutic technique which emphasizes the sense of touch in which body surfaces are gently, manually explored by self or partner to reestablish the sexual reactions of childhood." The emphasis of sensate focus is similar to that of holistic massage, in that it is a means of physical awareness not intended specifically or solely for sexual pleasure. The emphasis is on touching as a personal sensual experience that consists of exploring textures, contours, temperature, and contrasts.

Preparation

Equipment for a holistic massage is minimal. Ideally, it is nice to have a massage table, mostly for the giver's comfort and channeling of energy. Often there is an undiscovered massage table in people's homes, although it is usually thought of as a dining room table, desk, or bureau. Simply by placing some blankets or a sleeping bag over the top and then covering with a sheet, many such pieces of furniture can be transformed into massage tables. If this is not possible, two sawhorses can be linked by a sturdy piece of wood, such as a door, which can then be padded and covered to serve as a massage table (this arrangement may be a little unsteady and care should be taken). It would also be possible to give a holistic massage with the spinal-cord-injured person in a wheelchair, although techniques would need to be adapted to the new position.

Using a regular bed to perform massage can be debilitating to the giver. The height of the bed is likely to create back problems, and the softness of the bed seriously drains energy. Any physical pressure the giver applies to the receiver is usually transferred to the soft mattress, and the massage giver becomes depleted without realizing what happened.

The best height for a massage table is approximately at the level of the wrist of the giver when standing. If the table is higher, the masseur will develop tension in the shoulder girdle. If the table is lower, that person will stress the lower back as a result of bending over. Thus, the height of the massage table mostly benefits the giver. However, *holistic massage is a systemic event, meaning that whatever increases the giver's energy is also of benefit to the receiver.* The effect of many of the massage strokes depends upon the giver being balanced, aligned, and able to channel his of her own energy from the feet all the way up through the body and out through the hands.

Since holistic massage entails the delivery of many smooth strokes, a water-soluble lubricant is recommended. This lubricant can also be oil, lotion, or even baby powder. Any of the vegetable oils may be used, either alone or with a few drops of a scented oil, such as lemon, wintergreen, eucalyptus, sandlewood, and so on, depending upon personal preference. Any oil used on the body should be edible, since it soaks into the skin. This eliminates mineral oil, which is often the base for baby oil.

The best preparation for holistic massage is for both the giver and receiver to enter into a state of meditation. There are many forms of meditation (*21*) and any can be used, especially ones that have actually been practiced by either person. One basic form of meditation is simply to be aware of the process of breathing. Just notice your breath. Thoughts and feelings will interrupt this process. When you notice that you have drifted away from being aware of your breath, you can gently guide your awareness back to its focus. Simply notice, without praise or blame, whatever thoughts of feelings arise. This is not an easy task. Perhaps the image of sitting by a river watching without judgment whatever floats by will enrich the instructions. Then, whether you see a flower float by, a canoe full of children, or a beer can, there is still no praise and no blame.

Thus, the holistic massage is literally a meditation in itself, and both the giver and receiver are following the same instructions for their state of consciousness. This allows many levels of communication to develop between the partners. Talking, especially about everyday kinds of things, is highly discouraged, since that will interfere with other levels of communication. During the massage, there will often be a moment of oneness between the giver and receiver. This is a special time, and needs to be recognized and appreciated. There are no words to describe such connection. This level of touching can occur at any time during the massage, whether it is an elbow, finger, or knee being touched. Just be alert to the possibility.

Before beginning the massage, the giver needs to become centered and connected with the energy flow in his or her own body. The giver can imagine breathing a stream of golden light upwards from the feet, and then that it streams through the body and extends out through the hands. By placing his or her hands about two to four inches apart, the giver can actually experience a feeling of energy flow or magnetism between the hands. This feeling can be explored by altering the distance between the palms, closing the eyes, or breathing more deeply. Energy can be felt even without direct body contact, and this needs to be remembered throughout the massage.

The giver can sensitize his or her hands to feel the partner even before the actual physical touch. This can be practiced by placing the hands about two to four inches over the partner's body, and being open and receptive to whatever is sensed through the hands. At first, the partner's body warmth may be felt, and then another level of feeling that is more elusive may develop. It may feel similar to what was experienced between one's own hands. This sensitivity to subtle energy within one's own and one's partner's, body is central to the experience of the holistic massage.

The massage giver is more likely to develop this level of sensitivity to energy flow if his or her own body is used in an aligned, balanced way. Basically, this means keeping the back straight, bending using the knees, keeping the shoulders relaxed, and using the whole body for leverage.* Figure 1 shows an incorrect (left) and a correct (right)

---

*For more information on body alignment and balance, consult *Structural Awareness*, self-study program consisting of three 60-minute tapes and three illustrated booklets available from the author.

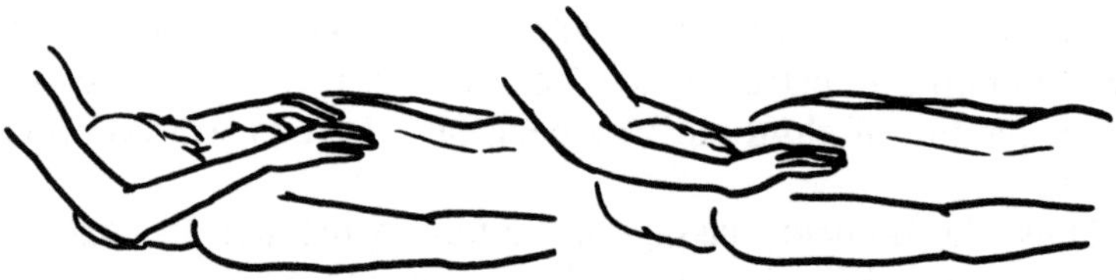

Fig. 1. Incorrect (left) and correct (right) use of body in giving a holistic massage.

use of the arms in giving a holistic massage. Ideally, the giver too should feel revitalized after the massage, rather than simply depleted.

The massage giver is also more likely to experience and learn how to channel subtle energy if the hands are used in a relaxed manner. Practice placing your hands anywhere on your own body, and allow them to melt into the contours of your body. The shape of your hands can be determined by the body part you are touching. This means allowing your fingers and palm to relax, and even to merge with what you are touching. Think of touching beneath the surface of the skin. Downing (*3*) described additional suggestions for learning how to use your hands in massage.

Anticipating the massage, the receiver may have concerns regarding nudity, touch, and sexuality, as well as the disability. However, once the receiver adjusts to being massaged, a deeper issue arises. The receiver asks, "Do I really deserve to feel this much pleasure?" Resistance to such pleasure comes in the form of guilt, worrying about the partner, not taking time for the massage, mundane talking, or feeling badly about not reciprocating. Some people can learn how to accept and enjoy this much nourishing attention; others, however, may need therapeutic help to feel worthy of such an expression of personal caring.

Technique

The most basic stroke of the holistic massage is what is commonly known as effleurage. This is the approach used to spread the oil over the body as well as to warm up the muscles. This stroke also allows the giver to begin to stimulate the receiver's energy flow. Effleurage is a smooth stroke that follows the contour of the body. Allow your hands to be molded to and shaped by the body.

As you use this long, smooth stroke, imagine that your hands are giving an energy message to your partner's body. Examples of positive messages to communicate are: let go of tension and feel relaxed; allow your neck to be long and free; fill this part of your body with awareness and light; allow the energy to flow through your arm (leg) and out your hand (foot); feel the space above the crown of your head; you deserve to feel pleasure; this is your whole body; this is you; you are okay just the way you are. These messages can be communicated directly from your touch into your partner's body. Holistic massage contends that the giver's intention is extremely important in conveying these messages. So be conscious about your intention as you touch your partner.

Figure 2 shows the basic outline of holistic massage using effleurage. These movements provide a guide for covering the whole body. The order of what body part is done first can be completely left to the giver's intuition. For the torso, arms, and neck, stand at the head of the massage table with your partner lying on his or her back. Begin by placing your hands on your partner's sternum, over the heart center. Just let your hands rest there a moment in the manner of laying on of hands rather than massage. Allow yourself to feel into your partner's heart space underneath your hands. Then gently glide your hands toward your partner's shoulder. Press firmly as you slide across the shoulder and down the arms. Circle back with your hands by sliding gently up the front of your partner's body and return to the heart. Repeat this large, circular movement a number of times, altering the speed and amount of pressure for variety and specific purposes. For instance, press downward toward the feet when at the shoulders in order to relieve chronic tension.

Begin again from the sternum to the shoulders, and then gently trace up the sides and back of the neck. As your hands leave the head, give a gentle sense of traction to the neck by pulling directly toward you from your partner's occiput. Only lift the head enough for your hands to slide underneath. Repeat the effleurage movement, and add the variation of turning the head to one side. Trace the side of the neck from the ear to the shoulder. Think of erasing or lifting out any accumulated tension and stress. Repeat on both sides of the neck and shoulder.

For specific areas of tightness, such as the trapezius muscle, you can knead deeply into the muscle. Be sensitive to any discomfort this may cause your partner, and use only as much pressure as feels good to the partner. With firm pressure, you can trace the bony structure of the body. For example, outline the clavicles during some of the broader effleurage movements. With gentle pressure, you can outline the bony landmarks of the face. Allow plenty of time to do a laying on of hands on the forehead and the crown of the head.

Walk around to the side of the table, and use an effleurage movement from the stomach and heart center outward to one shoulder and

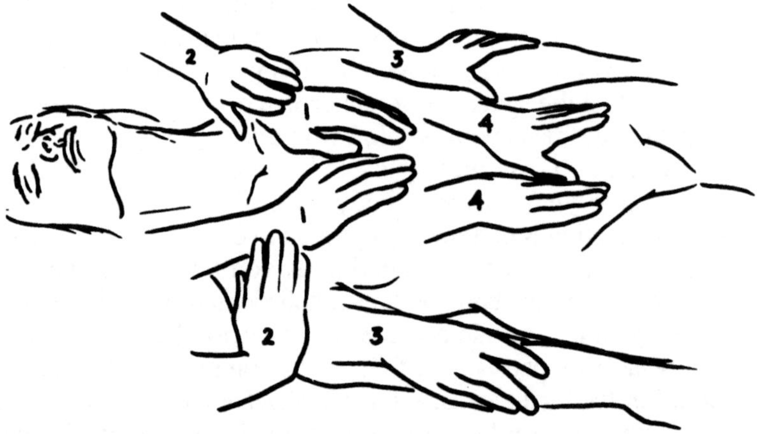

Fig. 2. Manual techniques of effleurage.

down the arm to the hand. Work with pressure into the palm of the hand and along each of the fingers. Then with varying degrees of pressure and speed, use petrissage along the whole length of the arm and shoulder. Petrissage is a firm circular stroking, alternating hands in rhythm. Use petrissage as you work your way up and down the arm. Complete the arm by repeating the basic effleurage stroke. Repeat this whole sequence on the other arm and hand.

Move footward along the side of the table to about the knee. Again, use effleurage from the stomach down one leg to the foot. Repeat this long stroking a few times, using pressure as you go upward on the leg. Figure 3 shows how the movement back to the foot slides along the inner and outer side of the leg. Imagine you can remove any tenseness in the leg with this movement. Concentrate on the foot, specifically each of the toes, the sole, and the ankle, outlining the bony structure with your fingertips. Then return to the leg using petrissage and kneading on the large muscles of the thigh. Again, end with effleurage of the entire leg and foot. Repeat this whole sequence on the other leg and foot.

Gently help your partner to roll over onto the back. Repeat the same movements to the back of the leg that you used on the front. This time, include the buttocks. Use petrissage and deep kneading to work into the muscles of the buttocks. Stand just at the side of the hip for best leverage. Figure 4 shown the circular movements for the buttocks. Allow plenty of time for deep kneading of the calf and back of the thigh muscles. Complete the leg and buttocks with long, smooth effleurage movements. Repeat this sequence on the other leg.

For the back, almost any technique feels wonderful. Use a combination of effleurage and kneading especially of the trapezius, around

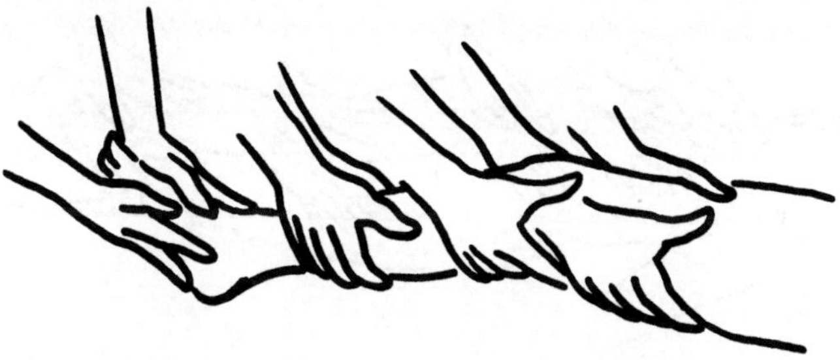

Fig. 3. Schematic illustration of arm and hand motions during petrissage.

the scapula, and the pelvis. Remember to include the sides of the body as you petrissage the back. Use the most pressure of the whole massage to trace the long back muscles on either side of the spine from the neck all the way down to the pelvis. Complete with a walking effleurage movement from the shoulders, down the back, over the buttocks, down the legs, and off the feet (Fig. 5). This long, total body stroke ends the massage with a feeling of wholeness.

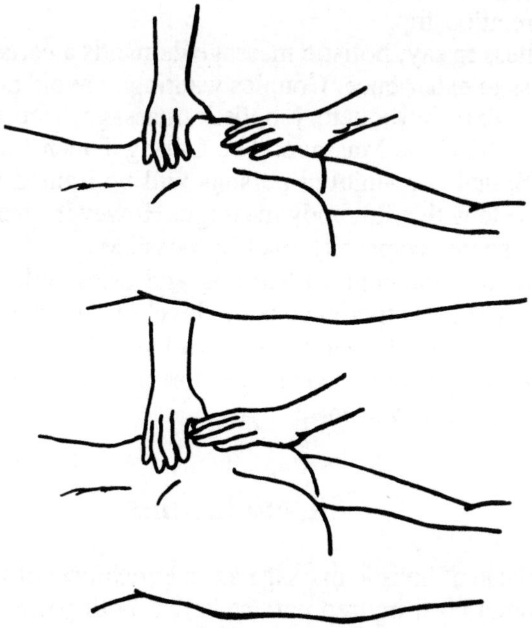

Fig. 4. Massaging motion of both hands over the gluteal areas.

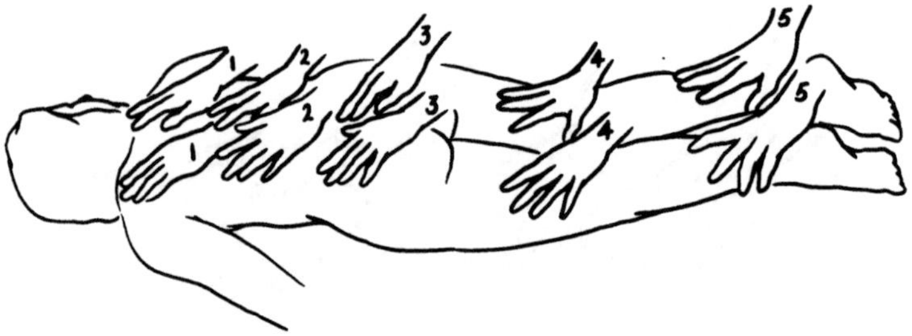

Fig. 5. Hand-sliding movements from the thigh along the inner and outer sides of the leg, toward the foot.

Limitations

Holistic massage is usually taught in an intensive experiential workshop. An important element in the workshop is that the massage is done with both giver and receiver nude. Participants become more comfortable with their own and with other's bodies as they adjust to the nudity. The suggestion is made that couples learn the techniques of holistic massage on someone other than their partners. In this way, they develop confidence in a new skill that they can then bring into their intimate relationship.

Needless to say, holistic massage demands a certain openness and willingness to experience. Couples wanting to avoid public nudity may be able to learn introductory holistic massage from the instructional videotape, "Holistic Massage: The Caring Touch" developed by the author.* Spinal-cord-injured persons will be limited in their capacity to reciprocate with a full body massage. However, depending upon the disability, some reciprocity may be possible.

The major challenge to learning and using holistic massage as a sexually enriching experience is the level of communication. Couples may need to be taught clear communication skills and monitored as they practice nonjudgmental feedback, reporting what feels pleasurable and asking for what they want.

Conclusions

The value of holistic massage as an enrichment of sexual experience for the spinal-cord-injured patient is that both partners become more

*Available from Broadcast Quality, 7800 SW 57th Ave., Suite 219, South Miami, FL 33143.

comfortable with their own and each other's bodies. Increased comfort can then expand into learning how to give and receive pleasure as the couple becomes more proficient in holistic massage. As each partner achieves increased comfort with his or her own body, self-concept improves and the sense of self as a lovable person is reinforced. For some people, the experience of energy during the holistic massage may open up or enrich an inner spiritual life (*28*). Thus, the holistic massage involves and benefits the whole person at all levels of body, psyche, and spirit.

References

1. Burton, A. and Adkins, J. (1961) Perceived size of self-image body parts in schizophrenia. *Arch. Gen. Psychiatry.* **5**, 39–48.

2. Deikman, A. J. (1982) *The Observing Self* (Beacon Press, Boston).

3. Downing, G. (1972) *The Massage Book* (Random House, New York).

4. Fisher, S. (1959) Body image boundary and the aged. *J. Psychiatry* **48**, 315–318.

5. Fisher, S. (1960) Head-body differentiations in body image and skin resistance. *J. Abnorm. Soc. Psychol.* **60**, 286–285.

6. Fisher, S. (1967) Organ awareness and organ sensitivity. *Psychosom. Med.* **29**, 643–647.

7. Fisher, S. (1970) *Body Experience in Fantasy and Behavior* (Appleton-Century-Crofts, New York).

8. Fisher, S. and Cleveland, S. E. (1957) An approach to physiological reactivity in terms of body image schema. *Psychol. Rev.* **64**, 26–27.

9. Freud, S. (1927) *The Ego and the Id* (Hogarth Press, London).

10. Greene, L. R. (1976) Body image boundaries and small group seating arrangements. *J. Consult. Clin. Psychol.* **44**, 244–249.

11. Harris, R. and Linn, M. W. (1980) Differential response of the need to be held. *Br. J. Med. Psychiatry* **53**, 243–248.

12. Hastings, A. C., Fadiman, J., and Gordon, J. S. (1980) *Health for the Whole Person* (Westview Press, Boulder, CO).

13. Hollender, M. H., Luborsky, L., and Harvey, R. R. (1970) Correlates of the desire to be held in women. *J. Psychosom. Res.* **14**, 387–390.

14. Hollender, M. H., Luborsky, L., and Scaramella, T. J. (1969) Body contact and sexual enticement. *Arch. Gen. Psychiatry* **20**, 188–191.

15. Kaplan, H. S. (1975) *The Illustrated Manual of Sex Therapy* (NY Times Book Co., New York).

16. Klaus, M. H., Jerauld, R., Kreger, N. C., McAlpine, W., Steffa, M., and Kennell, J. H. (1972) Maternal attachment. *N. Engl. J. Med.* **286**, 480–484.

17. Klaus, M. H., Kennell, J. H., Plumb, N., and Zuehike, S. (1970) Human maternal behavior at the first contact with her young. *Pediatrics 46*, 187–191.
18. Kolb, L. C. (1959) Disturbance of body image, in *American Handbook of Psychiatry* (Ariet, S., ed.) (Basic Books, New York).
19. McCary, J. L. (1978) McCary's human sexuality; Vol. 3 (Van Nostrand, New York).
20. Montague, A. (1971) Touching: *The Human Significance of the Skin* (Harper and Row, New York).
21. Naranjo, C. and Ornstein, R. E. (1971) *On the Psychology of Meditation* (Viking, New York).
22. Ringler, N. M., Kennell, J. H., Jarvella, R., Navojosky, B. J., and Klaus, M. H. (1983) Mother to child speech at two years: Effects of early postnatal contact. *Behav. Pediatr.* **86**, 141–150.
23. Secord, R. F. and Jourard, S. M. (1953) The appraisal of body cathexis: Body-cathexis and the self. *J. Consult. Clin. Psychol.* **17**, 343–347.
24. Smuts, J. C. (1926) *Holism and Evolution* (MacMillian, New York).
25. Task Force on Concerns of Physically Disabled Women (1978) *Toward Intimacy* (Human Sciences Press, New York).
26. Yerkes, R. M. (1933) Genetic aspects of grooming: A socially important primate behavior pattern. *J. Soc. Psychol.* **4**, 3–11.
27. Yerkes, R. M. (1943) *Chimpanzees* (Yale University Press, New Haven).
28. Leyson, J. R. (1988) Updates in Sexual Medicine. Presented at the annual winter meeting, Association of Physicians (Phil.) in America, Philippine Convention Center, Dec. 14–17, 1988 Manila, Philippines.

14

Reproductive Aspects of Spinal Cord Injury in Females

Shirley McCluer

Introduction

Although a great deal of attention has been paid to the effect of spinal cord injury (SCI) on sexuality and fertility in males, very little has been reported about the effect on females. This is partly because of the lower incidence of SCI in females (only 18% of all SCI patients) (*29*), and partly because the effects are subtler in women than in men. This chapter deals with the effect of SCI on reproduction, rather than on sexuality of psychosocial effects.

In order to understand the changes that are caused by SCI, normal female reproductive anatomy, physiology, and endocrinology will be reviewed. Reproductive anatomy consists of the vagina, uterus, fallopian tubes, and ovaries. When a female is born, each of her ovaries contains about one million oocytes (ova), which decrease to about one half million by puberty. No new ova are produced, and only about 450 of these will proceed to ovulation during a woman's reproductive lifetime. Each ovum is located within a capsule called a graafian follicle, which is surrounded by connective tissue cells called theca cells (Fig. 1) (*19,27*).

The physiologic changes that comprise the menstrual cycle occur primarily within the ovary and uterus. The cycle begins with the gradual enlargement of several follicles, which continue to grow for about 14 d. Only one of these follicles is preselected (by a process not yet

Sexual Rehabilitation of the Spinal-Cord-Injured Patient
Edited by J.F. Leyson, © 1990 The Humana Press, Inc.

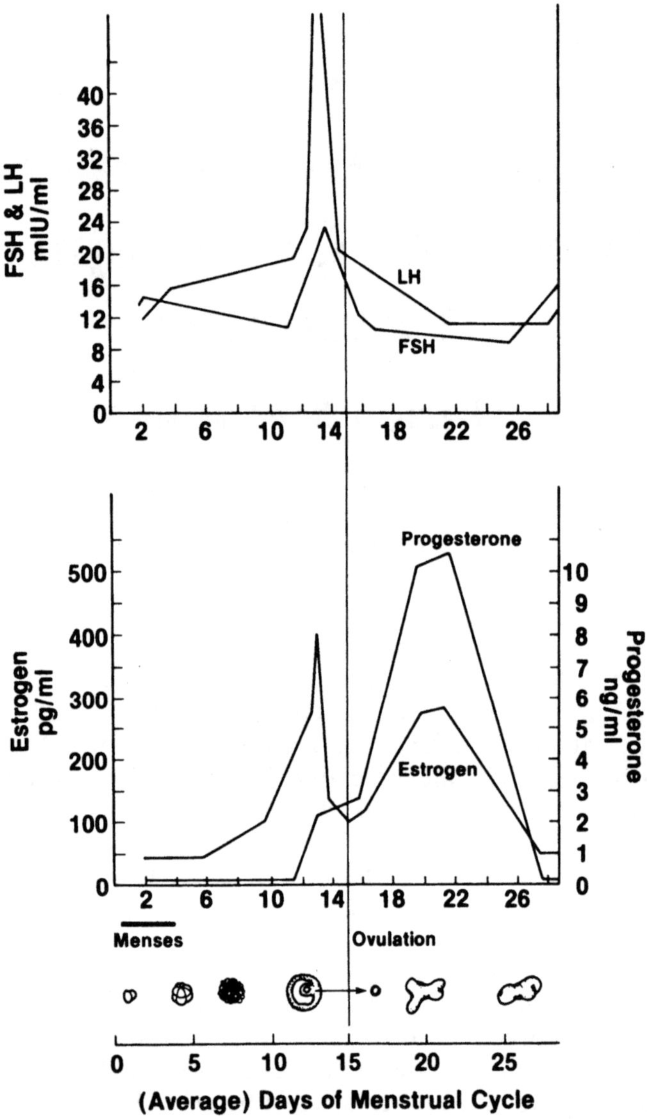

Fig. 1. The sequence of events occurring each month within the ovary.

understood) to grow more rapidly than the others, until it ruptures and expels its ovum into the fallopian tube. The ruptured follicle then undergoes a degenerative change, with production by its granulosa cells of a yellowish pigment called lutein; thus the term corpus luteum. The follicles that become enlarged, but are not selected for ovulation, will

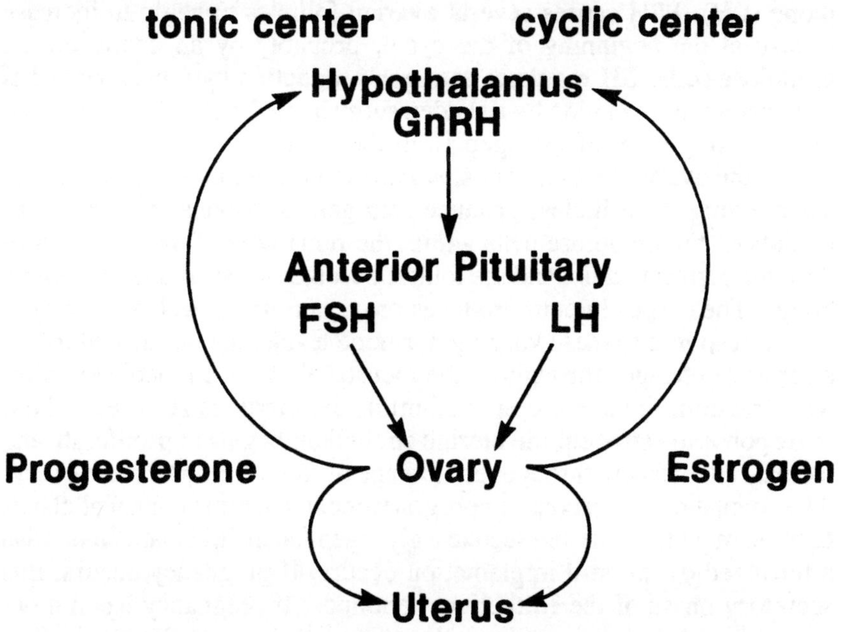

Fig. 2. Organs involved in hormone regulation of the menstrual cycle.

atrophy and deteriorate. If pregnancy does not occur, the corpus luteum begins to degenerate after the 8th d, and 14 d after ovulation, menstruation repeats itself.

The average menstrual cycle is about 28 d in duration, but the normal range is from 23 to 35 d (*19*). The time from ovulation to menstruation is fairly constant at 14 d, and any variability in the cycle length occurs because of the time required for follicle growth and maturation prior to ovulation.

This sequence of events in the ovary is influenced by the complex interaction of numerous hormones, many of which are not yet understood. The primary organs involved are the hypothalamus, anterior pituitary, ovary, and uterus (Fig. 2). The hypothalamus contains a tonic and a cyclic center for the secretion of a gonadotropin-releasing hormone (GnRH). The tonic center maintains a constant baseline level of gonadotropins and responds to the negative feedback effect of the ovarian steroid levels (estrogen and progesterone). The cyclic center is responsible for the mid-cycle surge of gonadotropins (LH and FSH) that results in ovulation and is responsive to the positive feedback of estrogen. This cyclic center is probably inhibited by androgens.

The anterior pituitary responds to GnRH by the production of two hormones, a Follicle Stimulating Hormone (FSH) and a Luteinizing Hormone (LH). FSH causes several ovarian follicles to begin to increase in size at the beginning of the cycle, probably by an action on the granulosa cells. LH regulates estrogen production by the ovary and is responsible for ovulation by a sudden surge in the level of LH stimulated by the rising level of estrogen from the ovary.

In the ovary, the theca cells, which are part of the connective tissue surrounding the follicles, produce estrogen in response to LH. After ovulation, the granulosa cells within the remainder of the follicle produce the pigment lutein, and the follicle becomes a corpus luteum (yellow body). The corpus luteum produces progesterone, as well as estrogen.

In response to these varying hormone levels, the uterus undergoes a series of changes throughout the menstrual cycle. Immediately after menstruation, the surface epithelium of the uterus is repaired. Then, in response to estrogen, the uterine epithelium begins to proliferate and increase in thickness throughout the stage of follicle growth in the ovary. After ovulation, in response to progesterone, the uterine epithelial glands become more tortuous and secrete a glycogen-laden fluid that will nourish a fertilized ovum until implantation occurs. If pregnancy occurs, this secretory phase of the epithelium continues. If pregnancy has not occurred by 14 d after ovulation, the epithelial lining is sloughed off in a menstrual period that usually lasts 4–7 d, and the cycle then repeats.

Figure 3 is a summary of all of the events occurring simultaneously to illustrate the complicated interactions involved in a 28-d menstrual cycle. It is perhaps easier to understand if all of the events are considered in relationship to estrogen levels.

1. A decrease in estrogen level (d 25) is necessary to initiate the rise in FSH (d 28), which stimulates the growth of the ovarian follicles.
2. Continued estrogen production is necessary to maintain sensitivity of the ovarian follicles to FSH.
3. An increase in estrogen level (d 10–14) is necessary to stimulate the surge of LH (d 13–14) for ovulation (d 14) to occur.
4. Decreased estrogen may be the trigger for the regression of the corpus luteum (d 24).

High levels of progesterone can exert a profound negative feedback on the hypothalamus and block the mid-cycle surge of LH that triggers ovulation. The negative feedback effect of progesterone will only occur, however, in the presence of estrogen. This effect of the combination of progesterone and estrogen is utilized in the birth control pill to inhibit ovulation.

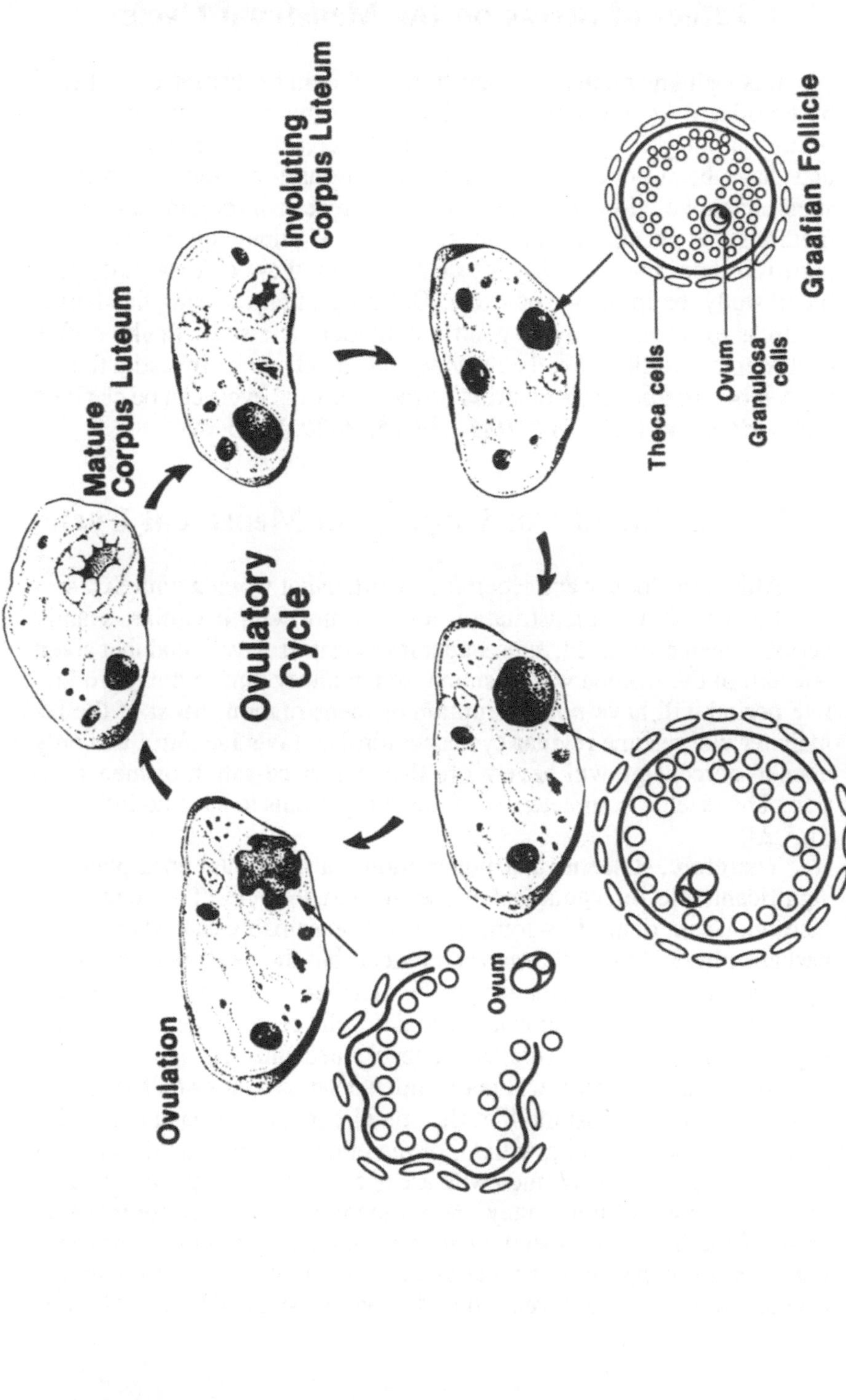

Fig. 3. Relationship of hormone levels to events occurring in the ovary during the menstrual cycle.

Effect of Stress on the Menstrual Cycle

It is well known that the menstrual cycle can be disrupted or altered by emotional or physical stress, but the mechanism(s) by which this occurs is not yet understood. Most of the investigations published to date have been done to determine the reasons for infertility in long-standing anovulation (*12,16,25*). Until the recent development of assay methods that permit accurate measurement of minute quantities of the numerous hormones that may affect the menstrual cycle, it was not possible to study the influence of stress. Defining and measuring the degree of stress experienced by a specific individual is also difficult. A few preliminary studies have been done, but much more investigation is needed before the effects of stress on the menstrual cycle can be clarified and understood (*1,2,7,8,9,10,11,14,15,16,20,22,26,30*).

Effect of Spinal Cord Injury on Menstrual Cycle

Although Cooper and Hoen (*6*) reported that women with SCI suffered a cessation of menstruation for 3–6 mo, with irregular, scantly periods when it resumed, subsequent investigators have found that about one half of the women who sustain a spinal injury during the reproductive period will have no interruption of menstruation. Most of the remainder will resume regular cycles within 1 yr (average 5 m), and only a small percentage will have more than a 1-yr cessation of menstruation. The level of completeness of the injury seems to have no influence (*3,5,23*).

Therefore, it seems that innervation via the spinal cord plays no significant role in regulation of the menstrual cycle. The temporary disruption experienced by some women is presumably caused by stress, perhaps physical as well as psychological, but the exact mechanism(s) by which this occurs remain(s) to be clarified. It has been suggested that stress affects the hypothalamic tonic/cyclic centers, thereby disrupting the normal neurohormonal feedback mechanisms.

Many times, women will not mention delayed menses to their physician, because they assume that the spinal cord injury has altered this part of their bodies along with all of the other changes and they do not expect to menstruate. Women who are not interested in having children may be very grateful that they are not menstruating, because management of the hygienic aspects of menstruation is one more annoyance that they are happy to postpone as long as possible. When menstruation is known to be delayed, should it be investigated? Yes. There is evidence that continued anovulation with its attendant abnormal hormone levels could have some harmful effects, in addition to the obvious one of infertility. These include hirsutism, excessive menstrual bleeding (anovulation), and increased risk of cancer of the endometrium and breast (*27*). Therefore, it is suggested that any woman who has missed at least three menstrual periods should have an evaluation. One simple procedure to evaluate amenorrhea is to give progesterone (Provera 10 mg, daily p.o. × 5 d or progesterone in oil, 200 mg, i.m.) and watch for withdrawal bleeding 2–7 d after discontinuing the progesterone. Positive withdrawal bleeding confirms at least minimal function of the ovary, pituitary, and central nervous system, and suggests an integration problem causing the anovulation. Normal cycles will sometimes resume following the test with no other treatment needed.

Hygienic Aspects of Menstruation

When women do resume menstruation, how do they deal with this as a self-care function? This question was addressed in a questionnaire survey in 1978, in which SCI women were asked whether they used tampons or external pads, and whether they were able to manage this function independently (McCluer, unpublished). Seventy-three quadriplegics and 147 paraplegics responded. Over 79% in both categories preferred tampons. In the paraplegic group, 108 (73%) used tampons and 39 (27%) used some type of external padding, either napkins with belts, beltless pads, Pampers, or other types of padding devices. Eighty-seven percent indicated that they were able to manage this independently; 4% indicated that they were independent with some type of assistive device; and 9% required assistance. In the quadriplegic group, 52 (71%) used tampons and 21 (29%) used some type of external padding. Of the group using tampons, 62% required assistance by another person, and 38% were independent. Of the group using external padding, 57% required assistance from another person, and 43% were independent. Women who reported that they used tampons plus pads were counted in the tampon group. The following individual comments from the questionnaire give further insight into some of the complications or difficulties experienced in relation to menstrual hygiene:

1. Unable to change tampons while sitting in the wheelchair, requiring transfer into bed (mentioned frequently)
2. Tampon worn all day because of difficulty changing it
3. Two tampons worn at the same time because of heavy flow or difficulty changing it

4. Some women reported that the "stick-type" tampon was easiest to insert
5. Others preferred tampons without applicators when fingers were impaired (quadriplegia)
6. Difficulty with tampons falling out during transfers of crutch walking
7. Perineal pressure sores from use of napkins
8. Insertion of the tampon into the urethra when urethra was dilated
9. Tampon becoming "lost," necessitating removal at a hospital.

The results of this survey suggest that rehabilitation personnel should pay more attention to the hygienic aspects of menstruation as part of self-care training for disabled women.

Premenstrual syndrome (PMS) may affect women with SCI, as it does nondisabled women. Symptoms such as depression, headache, fluid retention, joint pains, or paresthesias should be evaluated for a relationship to the menstrual cycle. The etiology and treatment of PMS remain controversial, although many treatments have been proposed, including progesterone, vitamin B complex, diet modifications, diuretics, bromocryptine, and counseling (*24*) with "bright light" therapy.

Contraception in Spinal Cord Injury

Since normal menstrual cycles and ovulation are expected in a woman with spinal cord injury, with the resulting potential for pregnancy, the issue of contraception must be considered. What is the best method of contraception? What are the potential complications? Are they any different from those experienced by able-bodied women? The present status of contraception for able-bodied women will be reviewed before attempting to answer these questions.

The ideal contraceptive should be 100% effective and safe, as well as esthetically acceptable to both partners, with minimal interference with spontaneous sexual activity. It should also be inexpensive, readily available, easy to use, foolproof, and reversible. Unfortunately, such an ideal does not exist at the present time, although research is continuing to pursue this goal. Contraceptive methods currently in use can be considered in the following categories:

(1) Reversible—temporary:
   (a) Barrier—any method designed to mechanically prevent sperm from reaching the uterus for fertilization—condom, spermicidal jelly, diaphragm, cervical cap

   (b) Hormonal—preventing ovulation by artificially manipulating hormone levels
   (c) Natural—includes methods such as coitus interruptus and avoiding intercourse during fertile periods (rhythm method)
   (d) Preventing implantation—IUD
   (e) Abortion.
(2) Nonreversible—permanent:
   (a) Tubal ligation
   (b) Hysterectomy
   (c) Vasectomy of partner.

Each method has a potential for complications or failure that varies considerably depending upon how carefully the recommended procedure is followed. However, the risks of the method of contraception should be considered in relation to the risks of pregnancy. Ory et al. (*18*) showed that, in nondisabled women of all age groups except 40–44, the risk of fatality was greater with pregnancy than with birth control pills, IUD, or abortion. Therefore, each woman, together with her physician and her partner(s), must carefully review her reasons for preventing pregnancy, her lifestyle, her personal preferences, and the relative risk of complications before deciding which contraceptive method to choose.

Unfortunately, little is known about the relative risks of pregnancy and contraception in women with spinal cord injury. The concerns that have been expressed involve primarily the use of birth control pills and the IUD. Birth control pills have been associated with an increase in thrombotic phenomena, and it is but whether or not this actually happens is not known.

With the use of an IUD, the potentially serious complications, such as perforation of the uterus or infection, would be recognized in normal women initially by a complaint of pain. Would a woman with loss of sensation in the pelvic area be able to recognize symptoms of such acute complications early? Unfortunately, the answers are not available. Late complications, such as acute inflammatory disease or peritonitis, may precipitate a sympathetic crisis (autonomic dysreflexia) or increased spasticity as a presenting symptom.

Medical literature does not provide much help for a woman or her physician in choosing an appropriate method of contraception with a clear understanding of the relative risks involved. Therefore, in 1978, a questionnaire survey of spinal-cord-injured women was conducted by mail to determine what their experiences had been with complications from contraceptive methods (McCluer, unpublished). Two hundred twenty-seven women responded, of which 74 (33%) were quadriplegics and 153 (67%) were paraplegics. Of these, 76% of the paraplegics and 56% of the quadriplegics reported that they had been sexually active since their injury.

Four of 70 women who reported use of birth control pills had an episode of thrombophlebitis. This greatly exceeds the estimated frequency of 1/1000/year in the able-bodies population. However, it must be kept in mind that there are many causes for thrombophlebitis, and the birth control pill may or may not have contributed to this frequency. Thirty-four women reported the use of an IUD, 21 of them for longer than one year. Complications included one ectopic pregnancy and two infections. However, the complication rate is high among the general population, and the numbers were too small to draw any definite conclusions.

In summary, there is still inadequate information available about the risks of various methods of contraception in women with spinal cord injury, but there seems to be a greater chance of thromboembolic complications from using birth control pills. As with any woman, the choice of contraceptive method for a woman with spinal cord injury must be carefully considered on an individual basis. Factors such as frequency of intercourse, number of partners, medical contraindications to pregnancy, age, whether or not children may be desired in the future, and degree of physical disability can influence the final decision. The risks must be understood as well as the advantages and disadvantages of individual methods.

Pregnancy and Spinal Cord Injury

Women with SCI who desire to have children also have difficulty obtaining reliable advice about the medical risks involved. Physicians who are unfamiliar with spinal injury will sometimes overemphasize the dangers of pregnancy and delivery. Very little information is available in the literature to assist a physician who is genuinely interested in giving correct advice. The cases reported in the medical literature tend to emphasize the complications, rather than normal uneventful pregnancy and delivery.

The following general guidelines, based on verbal reports from patients and general knowledge of spinal injury, are presented for consideration.

(1) Before pregnancy:

(a) Medications—Because the potential for causing birth defects is unknown for most medications, it is suggested that each drug being used by the SCI patient be reviewed carefully, and that as many as possible be discontinued whenever a woman is trying to become pregnant. The greatest risk for birth defects occurs during the first three months of pregnancy; therefore, a woman cannot wait until she knows she is pregnant to discontinue drugs.

(b) X-rays—Routine kidney and bladder evaluations usually involve X-rays, which also have potential for causing birth defects. Therefore, when possible, ultrasonography and/or a complete urologic evaluation should be done prior to a planned pregnancy. SCI women who do not use a catheter, or those with a history of frequent urinary complications, should have detailed discussions with their urologists, about the effects pregnancy may have on their urinary care. Temporary alternatives, such as the use of a catheter, may be advisable.

(c) Scoliosis—Many women with SCI, especially those with onset at an early age, have a scoliosis or other skeletal deformity that may either interfere with their ability to carry a pregnancy to term, because of inadequate space in the abdomen, or with delivery, because the pelvic outlet is small. These possibilities should be discussed with an obstetrician prior to becoming pregnant.

(2) During pregnancy:

(a) Keep all medications to a minimum.

(b) Activities of daily living—As the fetus gets larger (primarily during the last 3 mo), this will probably have a significant effect on balance, transfers, mobility, and especially on ambulation for SCI women who are ambulatory. For a paraplegic, a "reacher" may be useful to help her maintain access to objects that would otherwise be inaccessible. Even able-bodied women vary greatly in how much of a problem reaching becomes during pregnancy, but women who are otherwise completely independent should not be surprised if they require some assistance during the last few weeks. On the other hand, at least one T5 paraplegic reported that she continued to be completely independent until delivery, with some awkwardness during the last 2 wk.

(c) Urinary management—In all women, the increasing size of the uterus causes pressure on the bladder and decreases bladder capacity. The mechanism of bladder emptying should be carefully evaluated and any potential problems during pregnancy discussed with a *urologist familiar with SCI.* An indwelling catheter will probably cause little or no difficulty, but a woman with a balanced bladder or one who uses intermittent catheterization will probably have to modify the program during the last few weeks of pregnancy. If there has been a previous history of hydronephrosis or frequent bladder infections, more careful attention must be paid to ensuring good bladder drainage, especially during the last trimester. Women who have an ileal loop should discuss this with their urologist. Much will depend on the surgical technique that was used and how well the loop drains, but it should not be a contraindication to pregnancy if it is working well.

(d) Nutrition—It is customary to give supplementary vitamins with iron during pregnancy. The iron may disrupt an otherwise regulated bowel program. This should be discussed with the obstetrician and the dosage regulated so that such effects are negligible. Iron can be obtained by eating foods high in iron rather than with supplements. Calcium—Many patients with SCI have been cautioned to restrict their calcium intake to prevent stone formation. However, calcium supplements are routinely given during pregnancy. This should be discussed with the obstetrician (perhaps in cooperation with the urologist) and an effort made to find a level of calcium supplementations, that will meet the mother's increased need for calcium without causing urinary stones. Constipation—This is a common problem in pregnancy because of the increasing size of the uterus and pressure on the colon. with careful attention to a high-fiber diet, this should be controllable without recourse to laxatives.

(e) Skin care—As the body's center of gravity changes because of the increasing size of the uterus, the weight-bearing surfaces may change, and extra care must be taken to prevent pressure sores. Special attention should be given to hygiene and frequent weight shifting.

(f) Edema of legs—This is a common problem in the later stages of pregnancy because of the pressure of the uterus on the pelvic veins. This pressure is even worse in someone who cannot stand or walk. When edema occurs, frequent periods of lying down with the feet elevated are essential to relieve the swelling. Elastic stockings may also be helpful.

(g) Thrombophlibitis with pulmonary embolism is a greater risk because of the impaired venous circulation.

(3) Delivery:

(a) Cesarean section—Many women have been told that a Cesarean section will be necessary just because they are paralyzed. However, this is not true. The uterus is under hormonal (not neurologic) control and will begin to contract reflexly at the appropriate time, even when a woman has complete motor and sensory loss. Therefore, the indications for a Cesarean section in an SCI woman would be essentially the same as for any other woman.

(b) Early labor—When the uterus begins to contract (labor pains), a woman with a sensory level below the level of the umbilicus will probably feel sensations normally. However, complete loss of sensation above the umbilicus will mean an inability to feel the contraction. Therefore, a woman may not recognize when she is in labor and may deliver before she can get to the hospital. For this reason, some obstetricians advise hospitalization during the last 2 w of pregnancy. Labor pains will probably feel similar to bladder spasms, so women who have experienced these will know what to watch for.

(c) Late labor—A woman who has no voluntary control over her abdominal muscles will be unable to assist in the last stage of delivery by "bearing down." Therefore, if the uterine contractions are not sufficient, it may be necessary to use forceps to assist more often than with able-bodied women. However, when there is no perineal sensation, no pain medication is necessary, and there should be minimal discomfort with the delivery. Labor is often shorter than normal, and SCI women should therefore advised to get to the hospital promptly.

(d) Premature labor—From the limited number of cases reported, there is a suggestion that premature onset of labor is more frequent among SCI patients than normals, for reasons that are not clear. Therefore, women should pay careful attention to the possible onset of uterine contractions after the 7th m. Verduyn reported that premature labor could be stopped by Brethine (Terbutaline) (*28*).

(e) Autonomic dysreflexia—This is a syndrome that occurs frequently with injuries above the level of T6 (*28*). It is usually caused by the contraction of a hollow organ—most commonly the bladder—but can also be caused by uterine contractions. It is characterized by profuse sweating and flushing of the skin above the level of injury, pale skin below, headache, and marked elevation of the blood pressure. Very few physicians are familiar with this phenomenon, and obstetricians frequently confuse it with toxemia of pregnancy, which would require entirely different management. Any patient with a lesion at or above T6 should be sure that both she and her doctor are familiar with the symptoms and the treatment of autonomic dysreflexia before labor begins (*13*). In severe cases, if untreated, the blood pressure can reach extremely dangerous levels and cause seizures or a stroke. Verduyn suggested treatment of autonomic dysreflexia with amyl nitrite, calcium channel blocker and Arfonad or nitroprusside. For uncontrollable intrapartum dysreflexia, a C-section may be necessary (*28*).

(4) Post delivery:

(a) Heat lamp to perineum—This is a common practice in obstetrical units, but when there is loss of sensation, the benefits of the heat do not outweigh the danger of burns. Thus, heat should not be used.

(b) Thrombophlibitis—At the time of delivery, changes occur in the mother's blood that make her more susceptible to blood clots. This was once a common complication with childbirth, but it has been almost completely eliminated by having women get up and walk around frequently after delivery. For a woman whose activity is restricted by paralysis, special care should be taken to prevent this complication. This could include elevation of the foot of the bed when lying down to promote venous drainage, elastic stockings when sitting, and frequent passive range of motion (ROM) of the legs.

(c) Nursing—There is no reason to believe the spinal injury will interfere with milk production, so any woman who desires to nurse her baby should plan to do so.

(d) Orthostatic hypotension—For women who have no control over the abdominal muscles, there will probably be a tendency to faint when sitting up for several d after delivery. This can be minimized by the use of a tight abdominal binder and elastic stockings.

(e) Episiotomy—It has been suggested that wound healing below the neurological injury is impaired (*4*). Thus, careful surgical technique with minimal tissue trauma is advisable.

(5) For additional suggestions by Verduyn, please refer to Chapter 15, Reference no. 28 and literature listed below.

Conclusions

A spinal cord injury alone is not a contraindication to pregnancy for any women who desires to have children. There are a number of special factors to be considered, and most of them have been discussed here. One of the principal problems reported by pregnant SCI women is simply finding a physician who understands her problems or is willing to learn about them.

References

1. Adashi, E. Y., Rebar, R. W., Ehara, Y., Naftolin, F., and Yen, S. S. C. (1980) Impact of acute surgical stress on anterior pituitary function in female subjects. *Am. J. Obstet. Gynecol.* **138**, 609–614.
2. Aono, T., Kurachi, K., Miyata, M., Nakasima, A., Koshiyama, K., Uozumi, T., and Matsumoto, K. (1976) Influence of surgical stress under general anesthesia on serum gonadotropin levels in male and female patients. *J. Clin. Endocrinol. Metab.* **42**, 144–148.
3. Axel, S. J. (Sept–Oct 1982) Spinal Cord injured women's concerns: menstruation and pregnancy *Rehabil. Nurs.* **7**, 10–15.
4. Basson, M. D. and Burney, R. E. (1982) Defective wound healing in patients with paraplegia and quadriplegia *Surg. Gynecol. Obstet.* **155**, 9–12.
5. Comarr, A. E. (1966) Interesting observations on females with spinal cord injury. *Med. Serv. J. Can.* **22**, 651–661.
6. Cooper, I. S., and Hoen, T. I. (1952) Metabolic disorders in paraplegics. *Neurology* **2**, 332–340.
7. Cutler, W. B. and Garcia, C. R. (1980) The psychoneuroendocrinology of the ovulatory cycle of woman: a review. *Psychoneuroendocrinology.* **5**, 89–111.
8. De Marchi, W. G. (1976) Psychophysiological aspects of the menstrual cycle. *J. Psychosom. Res.* **20**, 279–287.
9. Dimsdale, J. E. and Moss, J. (1980) Plasma catecholamines in stress and exercise. *J.A.M.A.* **243**, 340–342.
10. Du Ruisseau, P., Tache', Y., Brazeau, P., and Collu, R. (1979) Effects of chronic immobilization stress on pituitary hormone secretion, on hypothalamic factor levels, and on pituitary responsiveness to LHRH and TRH in female rats. *Neuroendocrinology.* **29**, 90–99.
11. Groll, M. (1978) Gonadotropic patterns in psychogenic amenorrhea. *Int. J. Gynaecol. Obstet.* **16**, 53–553.

12. Karahasanoglu, A., Barglow, P., and Growe, G. (1972) Psychological aspects of infertility. *J. Reprod. Med.* **9**, 241–247.
13. Kewalramani, L. S. and Orth, M. S. (1980) Autonomic dysreflexia in traumatic myelopathy. *Am. J. Phys. Med.* **59**, 1–21.
14. Lachelin, G. C. L. and Yen, S. S. C. (1978) Hypothalamic chronic anovulation. *Am. J. Obstet. Gynecol.* **130**, 825–831.
15. Legros, J. J., Demoulin, A., and Franchimont, P. (1975) Influence of chlorpromazine on the positive and negative feed-back mechanism of oestrogens in man. *Psychoneuroendocrinology.* **1**, 185–198.
16. Mc Donough, P. G. (1978) Amenorrhea—etiological approach to diagnosis. *Fertil. Steril.* **30**, 1–15.
17. Marinari, K. T., Leshner, A. I., and Doyle, M. P. (1976) Menstrual cycle status and adrenocortical reactivity to psychological stress. *Psychoneuroendocrinology.* **1**, 213–218.
18. Ory, H. W., Rosenfield, A., and Landman, L. C. (1980) The pill at 20: an assessment. *Fam. Plann. Perspect.* **12**, 278–283.
19. Page, E. W., Villee, C. A., and Villee, D. B. (1981) *Human Reprodiction: Essentials of Reproductive and Perinatal Medicine.* (W. B. Saunders, Philadelphia).
20. Persky, H. (1975) Adrenocortical function and anxiety. *Psychoneuroendocrinology.* **1**, 37–44.
21. Peyser, M. R., Ayalon, D., Harell, A., Toaff, R., and Cordova, T. (1973) Stress induced delay of ovulation. *Obstet. Gynecol.* **42**, 667–671.
22. Quigley, M. E., Sheehan, K. L., Casper, R. F., and Yen, S. S. C. (1980) Evidence for increased dopaminergic and opioid activity in patients with hypothalamic hypogonadotropic amenorrhea. *J. Clin. Endocrinol. Metab.* **50**, 949–954.
23. Reame, N. (April 1982) Menstrual Cycle Function and Hygiene Practices of Women after Traumatic Spinal Cord Injury. Paper presented at Sixth Midwest Nursing Research Society Conference.
24. Reid, R. L. and Yen, S. S. C. (1981) Premenstrual syndrome. *Am. J. Obstet. Gynecol.* **139**, 85–104.
25. Seibel, M. M. and Taymor, M. L. (1982) Emotional aspects of infertility. *Fertil. Steril.* **37**, 137–145.
26. Singh, K. B. (1981) Menstrual disorders in college students. *Am. J. Obstet. Gynecol.* **104**, 299–302.
27. Speroff, L., Glass, R. H., and Kase, N. G. (1978) *Clinical Gynecologic Endocrinology and Infertility*. 2nd ed. (Williams and Wilkins, Baltimore).
28. Verduyn, W. H. (Nov 22–26 1982) Pregnancy and Delivery of SCI Women with Tetraplegia: A Patient Survey and Literature Review. Read at the Third Far East and South Pacific Spinal Cord Injury Conference, Melbourne, Australia.
29. Young, J. S., Burns, P. E., Bowen, A. M., and McCutchen, R. (1982) Spinal Cord Statistics. Good Samaritan Medical Center, Phoenix, AZ.
30. Zacur, H. A., Chapanis, N. G., Lake, C. R., Ziegler, M., and Tyson, J. E. (1976) Galactorrhea-amenorrhea: psychological interaction with neuroendocrine function. *Am. J. Obstet. Gynecol.* **125**, 859–862.

15

Spinal-Cord-Injured Women

Pregnancy, Delivery, and Sexual Behaviors

W. H. Verduyn

Introduction

Women, whether married or single, physically sound or disabled, believe that having a child completes the family unit. With the improvement of acute care and effective post-cord-trauma rehabilitation, pregnancy and delivery in spinal-cord-injured women will occur more frequently. Our staff from the Spinal Cord Injury (SCI) Rehabilitation Unit felt fortunate when we had two tetraplegic patients who were pregnant. Staff members were involved in both the prenatal and the postnatal care of these women. This chapter presents our personal experiences, along with mail and literature survey results, on pregnancy, delivery, and sexual behaviors during the pre- and post-partum stages.

There were 33 women (20 patient survey, 13 literature review) studied. Twenty-one were T6 and above; 12 were below T6. There were a total of 50 deliveries (one intrauterine death, two sets of twins).

Cause of paralysis			
Arachnoiditis	1	Gunshot (*7*)	1
Car accident (*5,11*)	15	Unknown trauma	4
Motorcycle accident	1	Baseball bat	1
Horse accident (*6*)	2	Rock slide	1
Tumor and surgery	1	Airplane crash	1
Scoliosis surgery (2)	1	Fall off garage roof	1
Transverse myelitis	2	Cord hematoma	1

Sexual Rehabilitation of the Spinal-Cord-Injured Patient
Edited by J.F. Leyson, © 1990 The Humana Press, Inc.

Four women were pregnant at the time their paralysis developed.

Circumstances of Pregnancies		
Tumor and surgery	22 wk	Normal baby
Car accident	14 wk	Normal baby
Car accident	21 wk	Normal baby
Gunshot (*7*)	14 wk	Intrauterine death, induced at 20 wks

The spinal-cord lesions were divided into two categories:

A. *T6 and above:* 21 women; 27 deliveries (one intrauterine death, one set of twins).
  13 vaginal and forceps
  7 vaginal (one breech)
  7 C-sections (*5*)

During 22 of these deliveries, hyperreflexia was experienced. (One patient developed intraventricular bleed with coma) (*5,6,7,11*).

B. *Below T6:* 12 women; 23 deliveries (one set of twins).
  3 vaginal forceps
  8 vaginal
  12 C-sections (1 pt. 4; 1 pt. 2; 5 pts. 1) (one set of twins).

Indication: One fear of bladder damage; one ruptured membrane; one premature twins with presenting cord.

Physicians managing pregnancy and delivery			
SCI specialist	2	Family practice plus obstetrician	1
Obstetrician	38	Obstetrician plus SCI specialist	4
Family practice/general practice	4	Father	1

Problems Related to Pregnancy and Delivery		
Pedal edema	1	
Increased seizures	1	
Overweight with difficulty of transfer	3	Patients in 6 pregnancies
Thrombophlebitis	1	Treated with Heparin
Premature labor 7 wk treated with bedrest/Terbutaline	1	Delivery at 39 wk
Premature labor 6 wk treated with bedrest/Isoxsuprine	1	Delivery after induction at 35 wk
Premature labor 8 wk; Twins presenting cord	1	C-section

Urinary tract infections (*11,13*)	8	Although patients reported taking antibiotics during an additional 14 pregnancies for bladder infection
Pyelonephritis	2	
TIA-like episode	1	
"Sick all the time"	1	
Anemia	4	
Decubitus ulcers	5	
Treatment of Hyperreflexia		
Epidural (*5,11*)	6	
Anesthesia	1	Patient reported physician stated she had hypertension
5 C-sections (3 in C5-6 tetraplegic, 2 in C6 tetraplegic)	2	
Amyl nitrate	1	
Ditropan triple anesthesia, guanethidine	1	
Arfonad	1	
Sodium nitroprusside	1	
Magnesium sulfate and demerol	1	Physician thought she had pre-eclampsia
Apresoline	1	Only one dose after pt. went in coma
Diazepam plus diphenhydramine (*13*)	2	
Hydralazine + diphenhydramine (*13*)	1	
Hydralazine + diphenhydramine and promethazine (*13*)	1	

Age of respondents in 1982/83 varies from 26 to 66. (The 66-year-old was 21 when injured and had five children, the last one at age 44). Age of injury varied from age five to age 39. (Five-year-old is a C5-6 quadriplegic; 50 at the time of survey had three children all by C-section).

Age	*Age at Injury Number*	
5	1	
9	1	
12	4	
14	1	
15	2	
16	2	11

(Continued)

Age at Injury

Age	Number	
18	4	
19	2	
20	1	
21	3	
22	2	
24	2	
26	3	
27	1	
28	1	19
33	1	
34	1	
39	1	3

Previous Pregnancies

4 women had 1 previous pregnancy
1 woman had 2 previous pregnancies (1 miscarriage, 1 child)
1 woman had 3 previous pregnancies (2 miscarriages, 1 child)
1 women had 5 previous pregnancies (3 children, 2 miscarriages)
1 woman had 6 previous pregnancies

Prematurity

Above T6		Below T6	
3	2 wk	2	2 wk
5	4 wk	4	3 wk
1	5 wk (induced)	2	4 wk
2	6½ wk	1	8 wk (twins, C-section)

Post Maturity

Above T6		Below T6	
1	1½ wk	1	3 wk
		1	4 wk

Congenital Abnormalities

Persistent ductus arteriosus	1	
Down's syndrome	1	(5th child, mother age 44 at time of birth, other four children normal)

Death of Babies

10 mo, electrolyte imbalance resulting from GI infection	1
6 months, anoxia, brain damage at birth	1

Medications Taken During Pregnancy			
Vitamins	28	Ditropan	5
Iron	25	Gantrisin	6
Dilantin/Mysoline	1	Probanthine	4
Dantrium	1	Macrodantin	5
Darvon	1	Antibiotics (Ampicillin, Keflex, penicillin, nalodixic acid)	9
Thyroid	1		
Heparin	1		
Monostat	1	Uroqid	3
Brethine (Terbutaline)	1	Gentamycin	1
Mandelamine	1	Tobramycin	1
Lioresal	1	Sulfa	1
Valium	3	Septra	1
Daricon	4		

Bladder Management		
Ileal conduit	1	
Controlled voiding, 19 below T6, 1 incomplete C5-6	20	(8 were catheterized a short time after delivery)
Foley catheter	19	
Intermittent catheterization	5	
Suprapubic catheter	2	
Not reported	3	

Induction		
Pitocin/oxytocin (*5,11*)	2	
Laminaria plus oxytocin (*7*)	1	
Pitocin	2	(Intraventricular bleed, 1)

Professions			
PhD Psychology	2	Engineer	1
MD	1	Master's degree	2
Cytotechnologist	1	Key punch operator	1
Owner service station and bulk plant	1	Two years college	1

Birth Control			
Unknown	9	Diaphragm	1
Condom	1	Foam	1
Pills	4	Pills—IUD	3
Pills—IUD—foam	1	Pills—condom	1
Rhythm	1	(T-10, 5 pregnancies)	
No birth control	7		
Pregnant at time of paralysis	4		
Artificial insemination	1	(Twins)	

Birthweight

Variation from 1361 to 4848 g. One patient delivered 2098-g baby and also a 4621-g baby. The babies of T6 and above varied from 1361 g to 3941 g.

Anesthesia

General	12	No anesthesia	31
Epidural	6	Pudendal	1

Delivery and Postpartum Complications

Bleeding, post-C-section	1	(2000 mL transfusion)
Large cervical laceration and bleeding	1	(2000 mL transfusion)
Retained part of placenta plus bleeding	1	(850 mL blood loss)
Bleeding and infection	1	
Prolapsed cord	2	
Decubitus ulcer	5	
Dehisence of episiotomy (*6*)	2	
Thrombophlebitis plus pulmonary emboli (*6*)	1	
Peritonitis (post-C-section)	1	
UTI	1	

Problems in Child After Delivery

Anoxia, brain damage (one of twins)	1
Valium withdrawal	1
Possible Valium withdrawal	1

The separation of the women into two groups, those with a neurological level of T6 and above, and those with a level below T6, was made primarily to isolate those women that were likely to suffer hyperreflexia. Of the 27 deliveries in the category T6 and above, 22 reported hyperreflexia. Seven had Cesarean sections (one patient reported hyperreflexia as an indication for Cesarean section. Of the total of 50 deliveries, there were 19 C-sections, certainly a high incidence. These were confined to only 11 patients, with 1 patient having four C-sections, one having three C-sections, three patients having two C-sections, and six patients each having one. The indications were as follow: hyperreflexia, ruptured membranes, fear of bladder damage. The incident of forceps use was 15, which seems fairly high. There was one breech delivery.

Prematurity

Actually there were only four: one at 5 wk, two at 6½ wk, and one pair of twins at 8 wk. One was treated with terbutaline successfully and delivered on her due date. Another was treated with Isoxuprine for 1 wk and induced 5 wk early. One pair of twins, was born at 8 wk, post-C-section, because of presenting cord. There were some deliveries from 2 to 4 wk prior to the expected due dates, but not really premature. Postmaturity did not seem to be a real problem. The time varied from 1½ wk to 4 wk.

In regard to birth control, pills were used by nine women, either alone or in combination with an IUD, condoms, and foam. The rhythm method was used by one individual who had five pregnancies. One women reported artificial insemination.

Birth Weight

There were nine babies under 2500 g (1361, 1531, 1616, 1701, 1871, 2013, 2098, 2296, and 2325 g).

Anesthesia

Most of these babies were delivered without anesthesia. Some of the Cesarean sections were done under general anesthesia, and epidural anesthesia was used for six deliveries because of hyperreflexia.

Delivery complications were minor, except for hyperreflexia. One patient, while induced with Pitocin, sustained intraventricular bleeding and went into a coma. There were two patients with prolapsed cords and one patient with ruptured membranes. Postpartum complications: I feel the dehiscence of the episiotomy in two patients probably is significant for spinal-cord-injured women. Thrombophlebitis plus pulmonary emboli should also be considered a risk of pregnancy for these women. The problems occurring during pregnancy and delivery included a significant number of women with urinary tract infections. Very likely, this was related to the large number of women that had Foley catheters in place. Two women reported bladder stones, and five women had decubitus ulcers. It was interesting to note that two women indicated they had difficulties with their transfers towards the end of their pregnancies because of weight gain.

The treatment of hyperreflexia showed significant variation from epidural anesthesia to general anesthesia to the use of drugs, varying from amyl nitrate to magnesium sulfate and Demerol. Some of this seemed to reflect the preferences of the individual physicians managing these deliveries. It was noted that only two deliveries were managed by a spinal-cord-injury specialist. In four deliveries, the spinal-cord-injury specialist was a consultant. The great majority (38) of the deliveries were done by obstetricians and only four by family practitioners/general practitioners. One delivery was done by the father, on the ranch, because they had barely made it to the hospital the first time.

The congenital abnormality rate does not reflect the presence of any specific types of abnormality among the offspring of these spinal-cord-injured women. I am sure the sample is too small to have any definite impressions (*4*).

Postnatal problems found in the child after delivery were: 1 anoxia, 1 Valium withdrawal, 1 possible Valium withdrawal. It was noted that four women were pregnant at the time of their paralysis, and three of them delivered normal babies (*3,4*). The fourth one suffered an intrauterine death with induction at 20 wk.

Bladder management showed use of a wide variety of techniques, from ileal conduit to intermittent catheterization. There was controlled voiding in women whose injuries were categorized as occurring below T6. One was an incomplete quad at C5-6. Many of the controlled-voiding women apparently needed a catheter for a short time after delivery.

There were five inductions in this group. One was for intrauterine death; two were for recurring hyperreflexia; two were done on the due date. In one of these, the induction was directly responsible for hyperreflexia, intraventricular bleeding, and coma. Only three blood pressures were taken over a 4-h period: 124/80, 140/90, 210/100, prenatal: 106/60, 98/60, 110/64.

Comments by the women included: "Problems with labor and delivery room staff" and "I knew more than the doc." One woman reported she called a nurse from the neighboring spinal-cord-injury hospital to come and manage her hyperreflexia. Several of the women felt they were either overtreated or were not believed about what they felt was necessary for their care.

One individual was severely overtreated. At the time of delivery, she had an arterial line, CVP line, epidural catheter, intrauterine catheter, fetal scalp electrode, and a Foley catheter. She delivered a 2013-g baby approximately five weeks prior to due date. It was delivered vaginally by outlet forceps, after amniotomy and oxytocin. Indication for induction was hyperreflexia. Fortunately, this patient did not have any iatrogenic complications after her delivery.

Pre- and Postpartum Care

1. Most spinal-cord-injured women know their disability well. Listen to the patient. Ask questions about skin care, bowel reflexia) during orgasm, it is prudent to advise their sexual partners to reduce the force and depth of penile thrusting after the second trimester of pregnancy. Furthermore, during this period vaginal sex should be limited to once every two weeks for women with lesions above T6 and once a week for those with T6 and below.
2. At the onset of the third trimester, because of the high incidence of premature labor, women with lesions above T6 should avoid the frontal or missionary sexual position. It is also advised that the male partner should approach the woman from behind or from a kneeling position. This posterior (rear) approach would reduce the incidence of the glans penis reaching the cervical os, thus preventing the orgasmic contraction response. Vaginal sex should be performed only once every three weeks (*14*). Anal sex is still not advisable, for it may precipitate sympathetic crisis. The urinary bladder must be emptied before and after sexual intercourse.
3. At the seventh month of pregnancy, vaginal intercourse is ill-advised, for it can precipitate premature labor. Nonvaginal sexuality offers such other options as: male masturbation either by manual, intrainguinal (in between the thighs), intramammary (in between the squeezed breasts), or oral sex. For women, possible substitutes for sex are passionate kissing, hugging and petting. Female masturbation may trigger sympathetic crisis and premature labor during the orgasmic response after the seventh or eighth month of pregnancy.

Conclusions

In reviewing the figures, I feel very strongly that those of us dealing with spinal-cord-injured patients should take the initiative to be involved with pregnancies and deliveries of spinal-cord-injured women, perhaps not actually doing the deliveries, but certainly maintaining close communication with the obstetricians so that these patients will be managed properly. Autonomic hyperreflexia or dysreflexia is a severe threat to the SCI women whose injuries are at T6 and above.

I also feel it is essential for the staff of the spinal-cord-injury center to be involved in the postpartum care of these women, particularly to teach the quadriplegic women how best to care for their babies during the immediate postpartum period. I feel that additional hospitalization to assure completion of that training is certainly worthwhile.

References

1. Daw, E. (1972) Pregnancy problems in a paraplegic patient with an ileal conduit bladder, *Practitioner,* **211.**
2. Dickinson, F. T. (1977) Paraplegia in pregnancy and labor: Report of case and review of literature, *J. Am. Osteopath. Assoc.* **76.**
3. Goller, H. and Paeslack, V. (1980) Our experiences about pregnancy and delivery of the paraplegic women, *Paraplegia,* **8.**
4. Goller H. and Paeslack, V. (1972) Pregnancy damage and birth complications in the children of paraplegic women, *Paraplegia,* **10.**
5. Nath, M., Vivian, J., Cherny, W. (1979) Autonomic hyperreflexia in pregnancy and labor: A case report, *Am. J. Obstet. Gynecol.* **134.**
6. Oppenheimer, W., (1971) Pregnancy in paraplegic patients: Two case reports, *Am. J. Obstet. Gynecol.* **110.**
7. Ravindran, R. S., Cummins, D. F., and Smith, I. E. (1981) Experience with the use of nitroprusside and subsequent epidural analgesia in a pregnant quadriplegic patient, *Anesth. Analg.* **60, No. 1.**
8. Rossier, A., Ruffieux, M., and Ziegler, W. (1970) Faits cliniques, *Gynecologie et Obstetrique,* **69.**
9. Rossier, A., Ruffieux, M., and Ziegler, W. (1969) Pregnancy and labour in high traumatic spinal cord lesions, *Paraplegia,* **7.**
10. Spector, R. (1983) Intravenous nitroglycin: New uses for an old drug. *J. Iowa Med. Soc.* **73 (3),** 96.
11. Tabsh, K. M. A., Brinkman, C. R., Reff, R. A. (1982) Autonomic dysreflexia in pregnancy, *Obstet. Gynecol.* **60, No. 1.**
12. Watson, D. W. and Downey, J. O. (1980) Epidural anesthesia for labor and delivery of twins of a paraplegic mother, *Anesthesiology* **V 52 (3).**
13. Young, R. K., Katz, M., and Klein, S. A. (1983) Pregnancy after spinal cord injuries: Altered maternal and fetal response to labor, *Obstet. Gynecol.* **62 (1).**
14. Leyson, J. (1988) Sex Odyssey 2001. Association of Phil. Physicians in America Meeting. July 26–31, Long Beach, CA.

15A

Recommendations for Sexual Precautions During and After Pregnancy

J. F. Leyson

Intrapartum Sexual Activity/Behaviors

1. Although there is no recent published datum on the exact percentage of SCI women experiencing sympathetic crisis (hyperreflexia) during orgasm, it is prudent to advise their sexual partners to reduce the force and depth of penile thrusting after the second trimester of pregnancy. Furthermore, during this period vaginal sex should be limited to once every two weeks for women with lesions above T6 and once a week for those with T6 and below.
2. At the onset of the third trimester, because of the high incidence of premature labor, women with lesions above T6 should avoid the frontal or missionary sexual position. It is also advised that the male partner should approach the woman from behind or from a kneeling position. This posterior (rear) approach would reduce the incidence of the glans penis reaching the cervical os, thus preventing the orgasmic contraction response. Vaginal sex should be performed only once every three weeks (*1*). Anal sex is still not advisable, for it may precipitate sympathetic crisis. The urinary bladder must be emptied before and after sexual intercourse.
3. At the seventh month of pregnancy, vaginal intercourse is ill-advised, for it can precipitate premature labor. Nonvaginal sex-

Sexual Rehabilitation of the Spinal-Cord-Injured Patient
Edited by J.F. Leyson, © 1990 The Humana Press, Inc.

uality offers such other options as: male masturbation either by manual, intrainguinal (in between the thighs), intramammary (in between the squeezed breasts), or oral sex. For women, possible substitutes for sex are passionate kissing, hugging and petting. Female masturbation may trigger sympathetic crisis and premature labor during the orgasmic response after the seventh or eighth month of pregnancy.

Postpartum Phase

1. In women who have no sensation below the level of injury, vaginal sex can be resumed according to their sexual appetites 3–4 wk after delivery. For those women with associated perineal or rectal diseases, it is advisable to wait a week longer after the above pathology has been corrected (*1*).
2. In women who have had an episiotomy, love-making can be resumed only after 5–6 wk because of delayed tissue healing from spinal-cord-injury. Urinary tract infections should be treated before sex is allowed postpartum. Vaginal sex is appropriate 4–5 wk after Cesarean section.
3. For women who have incomplete lesions, with sensory recovery, premature (early) resumption of vaginal sex may precipitate pain. This condition may occur in older, multiparous women because of a low-lying uterine cervix from loose uterine and round ligaments.

References

1. Leyson, J. (1988) Sex Odyssey 2001. Association of Phil. Physicians in America Meeting. July 26–31, Long Beach, CA.

16

Diagnosis of Erectile Dysfunction

Ananias C. Diokno
and
Jay B. Hollander

Introduction

Spinal-cord injury (SCI) is usually associated with multiple-organ injuries, all of which must immediately be attended to upon institution of medical care. Total rehabilitation of the spinal-cord-injured patient is begun as soon as the acute process is stabilized. As part of any such program, sexual functionality must be explored to determine, among other things, whether erectile ability has been preserved. During the investigation, one should be aware that erectile function may be evolving just as would any other function that depends upon the integrity of the spinal cord. Significant recovery of erectile function may be observed within the first 12 mo and occasionally several months thereafter. In addition, since erection is in itself a multifactorial process, numerous factors besides the neurogenic component should be considered. A thorough knowledge of the various etiologies of impotency is necessary if one is to be accurate in pinpointing the exact mechanism of this dysfunction.

Impotency, the inability to initiate or sustain erection to complete the act of coitus, is traditionally classified as organic or psychogenic, depending upon the etiology of the process. However, a combination of causes is not unusual; an impotency that is obviously an organic-type may be associated with a functional or psychogenic etiology as well. The scope of this chapter will deal mainly with the diagnosis of

Sexual Rehabilitation of the Spinal-Cord-Injured Patient
Edited by J.F. Leyson, © 1990 The Humana Press, Inc.

organic impotency. In general, the organic etiology of impotency is divided into vascular, neurogenic, and hormonal causalities, each of which may relate alone or in combination. Although the etiology of impotency in most of our SCI patients is most likely neurogenic in origin, the other causes should always be considered as well.

Any total evaluation of erectile dysfunction should start with a medical history taking, followed by a thorough physical examination. When further studies are needed, numerous tests are available and should be utilized according to the problem being addressed. Generally, the initial step is to establish whether erection is absent, partial, or complete. This can be done by the use of a nocturnal penile tumescence monitor. Once erectile dysfunction is established, the next step is to determine the etiology of impotency. In a patient with complete conus or cauda equina lesion, impotency is generally the rule. Once established, no further test is necessary. When the lesion is incomplete or lies above the sacral segments, impotency is unusual. Comarr (*3*), in his long experience with SCI patients, has observed the reflexogenic reflex in over 90% of those with upper motor neuron lesions. When loss of erection is observed in this group, further evaluation is needed to find the cause, which may be neurologic, vascular, hormonal, psychogenic, or a combination of these.

Medical and Sexual History

The history is important to establish both the presence and the nature of any impotency. Some patients are confused about the terminology, and they should be asked to define the problem in their own words. Occasionally, a patient suffering from retrograde ejaculation misuses the word "impotency" as his chief complaint.

The specific characteristics of the SCI patient's erectile dysfunction should be clarified. Thus, the degree of erection loss should be evaluated to determine whether it is complete or partial. If erection can be achieved, the degree of residual tumescence should be ascertained in terms of percent. The duration of erection as well as the frequency of episodes should be assessed. The presence and degree of erections at night or upon awakening in the morning should be determined, since their presence may indicate psychogenic dysfunction.

Another area of sexual history that needs to be probed is the intensity of sexual drive (libido), episodes of ejaculation, and orgasm. On occasion, problems of ejaculatory dysfunction (retrograde or absent) and depression causing loss of sexual desire or lack of orgasm are the main problems rather than a true erectile impotency.

Once the characteristics of the patient's erectile dysfunction has been determined, the medical history should be explored to determine whether there are causes besides the presumed neurologic etiology. Medications (antihypertensives, psychotropics, and antisecretory drugs) that can suppress or reduce erection should be inquired about. The patient's vascular history may point to a preexisting vascular lesion or to risk factors for vascular disease that can be involved in impotence. Endocrinologic and metabolic disturbances may also be present and should be identified; foremost in this group are diabetes, adrenal dysfunction, hypogonadism, renal failure, and so on. Concomitant pelvic injury, with extensive vascular and urologic complications, should always make one suspect vascular problems in the differential diagnosis of impotency. The patient's sexual value system, marital status, education, and economic level should be noted. The frequency of intercourse per week and the percentage of failure to complete intercourse should be evaluated.

Sexologic–Physical Examination

The objective of this examination is to identify not only the possible causes of impotency, but the level or types of SCI lesions that can affect therapy. In this examination, the genitalia must be evaluated thoroughly. In an uncircumcised patient, the prepuce should be examined for phimosis or tight foreskin. The glans penis and shaft should be inspected for ulcerations, plaques, deformities, and so on. Congenital anomalies such as hypospadias, micropenis, and chordee should be identified. The scrotum should be evaluated for the presence of hydrocele or other mass, and the testes palpated to rule out congenital and acquired abnormalities. Testicular tumors as well as inflammatory lesions of the testis and epididymis should be identified during testicular palpation.

The perineal space should be inspected to identify lesions such as ulcers and deformity. Perineal sensation should be tested to determine whether there has been any sensory sparing of this area in the SCI patient. Anal sphincter tone should be evaluated, as well as the presence or absence of the bulbocavernosus reflex. As a rule, the presence of this reflex is highly correlated with reflexogenic impotency.

Examination of the abdomen should include identification of any stoma or other lesions that might interfere with surgical treatment. The neck should be palpated to check for thyroid masses. The cranial nerves and cerebral functions should be tested to rule out brain pathology. These latter diagnostic approaches may uncover the 10% or so of SCI patients whose recovering or incomplete cerebral lesions account for their impotency. Thyroid abnormalities and anosmia with hypogonadism (Kallman's syndrome) may point to an endocrine deficiency syndrome that will impair the erectile capacities of patients recovering from spinal-cord injury (SCI).

Psychological and Psychiatric Examinations

Some spinal-cord-injured patients may have psychological difficulties that either antedate their injury or arose as a result of the injury. The Derogatis Sexual Inventory Test, the Minnesota Multiphasic Personality Inventory (MMPI), and the Male Impotence and Body Image tests can be valuable in the early detection of personality dysfunctions and their response to postoperative penile prostheses implantation. However, the validity of using the MMPI test as the sole diagnostic evaluation procedure in the differential diagnosis of impotence has recently been questioned and is believed to be inadequate (*14*). A psychiatric evaluation to rule out psychosis and to determine intellectual and cognitive functions is also essential. This, along with a psychological evaluation, will eliminate unsuitable candidates from elaborate physiologic testings (*14*). The details of these psychological and psychiatric examinations and treatments are discussed in the appropriate chapters elsewhere in this volume.

Laboratory and Urologic Workup

A complete blood count and biochemical testing, including routine liver and renal function testing, should be used as a screening test for generalized organ systems. It must be stressed that chronic alcoholism and preinjury renal dysfunctions can compromise the full recovery of erectile dysfunction in these patients. Urinary drug screening should also be routine in patient populations with drug abuse tendencies. Urinalysis and urine culture should be done to rule out severe or acute genitourinary (GU) disease. The detailed GU workup, including lower urinary tract dynamics, is discussed in the chapter on sexuality and urology.

Endocrine Evaluation

From the endocrinologic standpoint, diabetes mellitus should always be ruled out. Generally, a fasting blood glucose can suffice for screening, with glucose tolerance testing being reserved for uncertainties, or for those with a family history of diabetes. Blood levels of testosterone and prolactin, and thyroid function tests should be evaluated when abnormalities are suspected. If the patient's libido appears normal, it is unusual to find hormonal abnormalities that are the source of impotence. When hormonal evaluation does reveal abnormalities, they should be pursued. Hyperprolactinemia can occur in older patients, present as either impotency or a benign pituitary tumor. Low testosterone levels can represent either primary hypogonadism (a testicular problem) or secondary hypogonadism (a pituitary or hypothalamic problem). To differentiate between the two, serum LH and FSH determinations are necessary. Reversal of abnormal thyroid states can improve sexual function.

Special Diagnostic Tests

Vascular Evaluation

Vasculogenic causes for impotence are now well recognized and can result from lesions anywhere—from the major pelvic arteries to the penile arterioles and penile erectile tissues (*11*). In addition, penile venous abnormalities may be involved.

The evaluation of vasculogenic impotence has changed markedly in the last five years. Testing is best performed by a specialist, and ranges from simple penile blood pressure testing (*1,5,9*) to complex physiological testing during artificial erection using intrapenile pressure monitors and contrast with fluoroscopic monitoring (*16,17*). These studies, referred to as penile cavernosometry and cavernosography, are still developing. In addition, ultrasonic pulse doppler (Fig. 1) evaluation of the penile vasculature can give information on the adequacy of penile blood flow during erections that are pharmacologically induced (*15*). Use of newer vasoactive drugs injected into the penis (i.e., papaverine and phentolamine) can be useful in differentiating vasculogenic and neurogenic impotence.

A simple penile pressure measurement can be done using the Doppler probe (Fig. 1). The penile brachial index is calculated from the formula: dorsal penile artery pressure divided by brachial artery doppler pressure. Penile vascular integrity is usually assured if the index is 0.8 or greater. Another way of measuring penile pressure is to record penile volume by placing the pulse volume recorder around the penis at its base and inflating to the mean brachial diastolic artery blood pressure plus one-third the pulse pressure. The pulse volume is recorded in an EKG machine, and a permanent record is obtained. When a

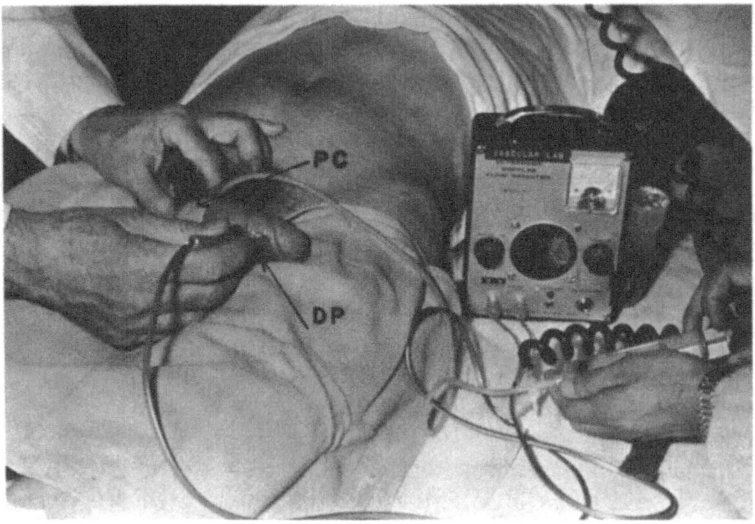

Fig. 1. Penile pressure (Doppler) studies are done with a doppler probe (DP) placed over a deep dorsal artery. The penile cuff (PC) is inflated until the arterial sounds are muffled, and a reading of the sphygmomanometer is taken as penile dorsal artery pressure as the sound starts to disappear.

vascular block is suspected, pelvic and selected internal pudendal arteriography can be performed to search for the blockage.

Jevtich has demonstrated that the penile urethral temperature correlates well with penile doppler blood flow studies (*7*). In his experience, patients having more than 3 °F difference between sublingual and internal penile temperature are most likely to have significant penile arterial obstruction. This premise was extended by Leyson, who studied the same parameters among spinal-injured men. His data revealed that most of the 105 men studied had normal values, suggesting a nonvasculogenic etiology of impotency in this group of patients (*13*) (Fig. 2). The pharmacocavernosography, detailed vasculogenic, vibratory audiovisual, neurogenic-somatosensory evoked potential tests, and responses are addressed in the last chapter.

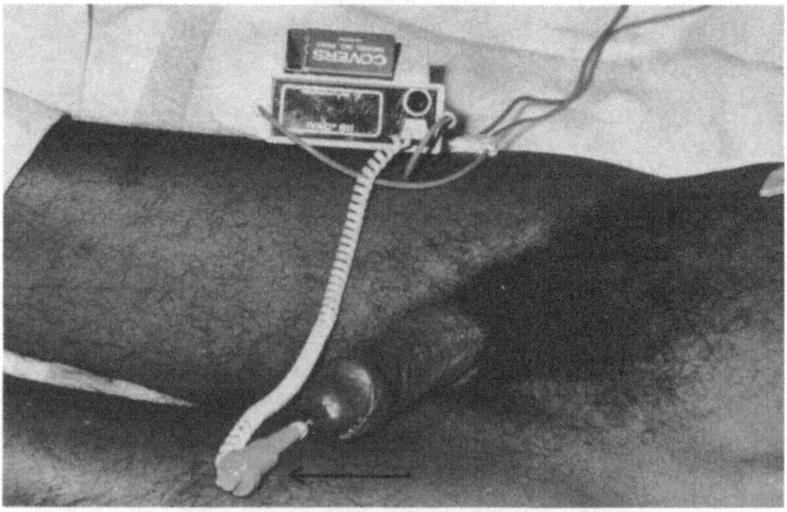

Fig. 2. Determination of intraurethral (internal penile) temperature by means of an electronic thermometer (arrow).

Nocturnal Penile Tumescence Study

Noctural penile tumescence (NPT) is generally found in normal males during sleep (*6*). Karacan et al. (*8*) have demonstrated that these nocturnal erections occur in direct association with rapid eye movement (REM) sleep. In Karacan's sleep laboratory, it was demonstrated that all normal young adult volunteers (20–26 yr old) exhibited this nocturnal penile tumescence. The average number of episodes of tumescence in young adults was observed to be 3.33 times per night. In this group, 66% of the episodes were associated with REM sleep, and each tumescence lasted an average of 37 min. In a series of 12 patients whose ages ranged from 30 to 39 yr, the average frequency of nocturnal tumescence was 3.7 times per night (*4*). In this same group, the average duration of each episode was 32.98 min.

The observations have been the basis for the introduction of nocturnal penile tumescence monitoring in clinical practice. Although the sleep laboratory is the ideal place to monitor NPT and EEG, it is obviously very impractical and expensive. As a result, several portable NPT/rigidity apparatuses have been introduced and are now in use. Each uses a mercury ring gage transducer and a strip-chart recorder. The penis is monitored at two levels, the base and the corona (Fig. 3), to observe

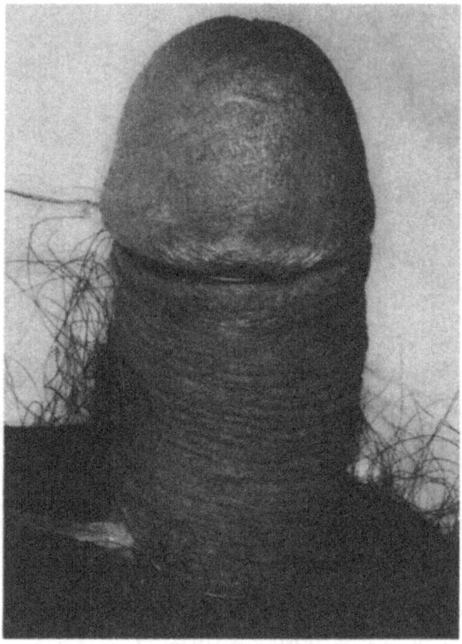

Fig. 3. NPT strain gauge (ring transducer) placed around the coronal sulcus and at the penile base.

any discrepancy between tumescence at the proximal and the distal halves of the penis. Among paraplegics using a condom collecting device, the ring transducer should be placed under the condom sheath. The monitoring can be done either in the comfort of the home environment or in the hospital. Although there appears to be no difference between the frequency of tumescence between the first and second night, monitoring for 2–3 d is recommended to reduce false negative readings. The apparatus is returned the day after monitoring completes, the graph is analyzed, and the patient is informed of the findings. Although the degree and duration of tumescence that will be satisfactory to the patient and his partner is unknown and variable, our unit considers an 80% tumescence lasting at least 20 min to be within normal range (Figs. 4,5).

The portable NPT apparatus is not without problems. The patient must be taught to use the device, which on occasion malfunctions, leading to patient frustration. Lastly, there is always a question of the validity of the findings. To further simplify documentation of the presence or absence of erection, the postage-stamp test was introduced by Barry (*2*). It involves wrapping a strip of postage stamps around the penis, moistening the overlapping stamp to provide a one-half to one stamp overlapping seal. The stamps are placed before retiring for the night

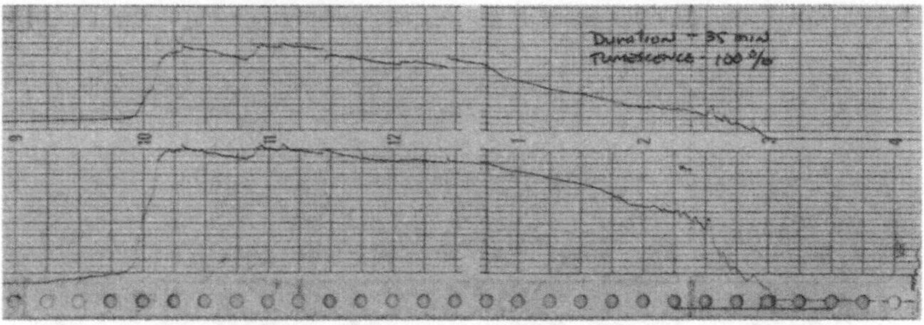

Fig. 4. Sample of a normal nocturnal penile tumescence (NPT) tracing showing abruptly ascending and smoothly descending wave patterns.

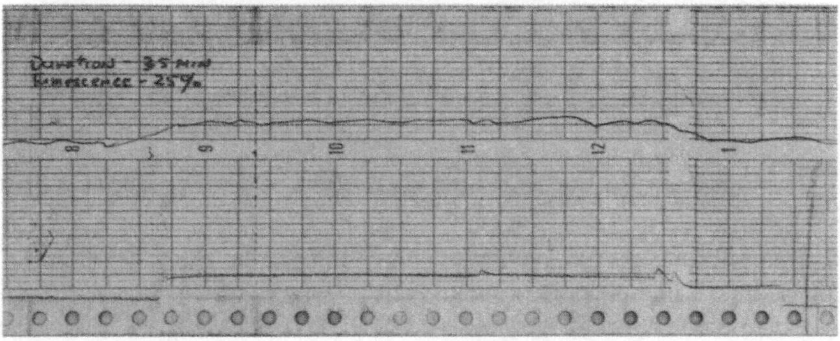

Fig. 5. Sample of an abnormal (weak) NPT recording denoting a poor erection wave pattern.

and inspected in the morning. Patients with normal tumescence are expected to break the stamps along the perforations. Intact postage stamps suggest the absence of or weak nocturnal erections. The major disadvantage of this test is that it does not measure either the duration or degree of the erection. Its use is further limited among paraplegics with incontinence and those wearing external collecting devices. Leyson, in a study of 105 men with SCI, compared the value of penile stamp tumescence with that of the strain gage is far superior to the stamp tests in evaluating erectile dysfunction in SCI patients (*12*), because the stamps can roll inside the condom urinary appliance.

Also useful in the measurement of nocturnal penile tumescence (*4*) is the Snap Gauge™ introduced by Ek and Bradley (Fig. 6). The gage consists of three bands that snap at different forces, depending upon the degree of penile expansion. As in the postage-stamp test, it is worn around the penile shaft during sleep. Limited clinical studies have verified

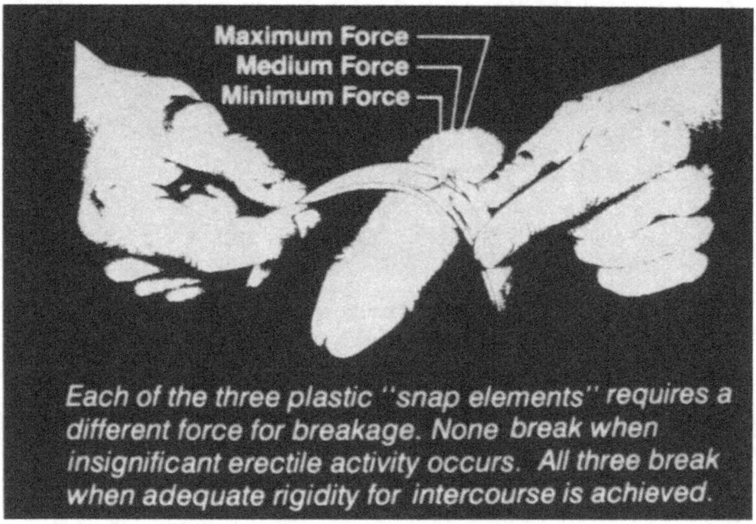

Fig. 6. Snap gauge showing three (strips) bands that break at different degrees of tumescence (erection). Snap Gauge™ photo courtesy of the DacoMed Corp.

the reliability of the Snap Gauge when compared to the NPT monitoring device. The major drawback, as in the stamp test, is that the duration of erection cannot be measured. The erectiometer (Fig. 7) is a device that is applied around the penis to measure penile expansion with the stamp test or Snap Gauge, duration of erections is not measured.

Newer nocturnal erection monitoring devices have recently been developed. The Rigiscan®, also manufactured by the DacoMed Company, is a device placed and worn in a manner similar to other NPTR devices. It measures both girth changes (tumescence) and firmness (rigidity) with its monitoring loops worn on the proximal and distal penile shaft overnight.

Neurologic Evaluation

Whenever the neurologic etiology of impotency is in question, a thorough examination—including direct electromyography of the perineal and extremity musculature, as well as cortical/sacral evoked-potential studies—should be carried out. Direct perineal electromyography can be done using needle electrodes to sample the anal, bulbocavernosus, and external urinary sphincter muscles. The presence of denervation potentials tends to further reinforce the likely presence of lower motor neuron dysfunction.

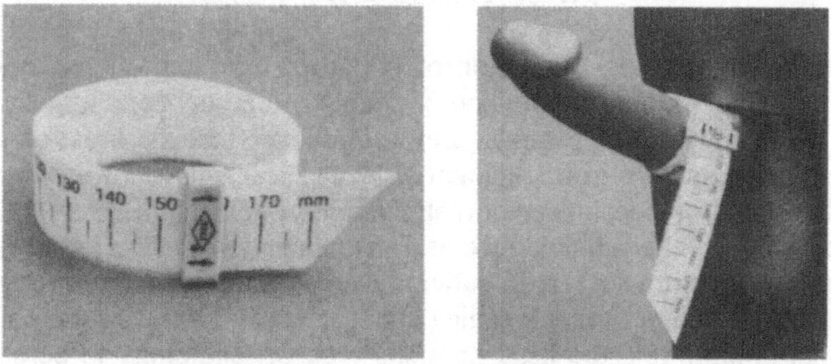

Fig. 7. A calibrated band (tape) with a sliding collar, which determines the penile shaft expansion circumference during erection.

Evaluation of sacral evoked potentials can be carried out using an EMG apparatus with a signal averager. Platinum or tin plate surface electrodes applied to each side of the phallus can be used as stimulating electrodes. A monopolar or concentric electrode can be used to monitor the bulbocavernosus muscle response to the stimulus. Square wave stimuli with a frequency of 1/s and a duration of 0.5–1 ms are generally used to stimulate the penis. Stimulation is usually started with 0 V and gradually increased until sensory and reflex thresholds, as well as the minimum latency, are determined. Usually, several stimulations are applied and the responses are averaged. In a normal subject, the reflex is usually evoked with a 100 V or smaller stimulus, with a latency time of 30–40 ms. These studies, although not a direct measure of the nature of impotency, provide fairly good incriminating evidence of its cause. Krane and Siroky reported their experience with the electrically evoked bulbocavernosus reflex in a series of patients with sacral and suprasacral lesions (*10*). The latency of the bulbocavernosus reflex was generally lower in the suprasacral group, and increased in the conus and cauda equina group. The mean latency time in the suprasacral group was 32.7 ms and, in the sacral group, 58.1 ms. This special neurologic evaluation is vital in detecting occult or minimal spinal-cord lesion(s).

There is no good way to directly evaluate the efferent nerves responsible for erection (pelvic parasympathetics primarily). However, abnormalities in EMG and/or cortical/sacral evoked potentials may suggest occult or minimal spinal-cord or peripheral-nerve lesions when they are not otherwise obvious. A vibratory sense-testing device—the biothesiometer—provides a noninvasive means to test penile afferent sensory status and may be helpful if sensory deficits are not otherwise obvious.

Other Diagnostic Tests

Quantitative determination of the adrenergic corpora cavernosal receptor population in able-bodied diabetes mellitus patients may not be useful in the SCI patients. Leyson believes that the impotent SCI population suffers from regional neuronal transmission impairment, rather than from local receptor malfunctions or deficiency (*13,14*). Thermography has been abandoned as a diagnostic aid in the evaluation of impotency, more so in SCI patients in whom the primary etiology is neurologic and not vasculogenic (*13*). The use of CAT scanning of the spinal column and the head may show occult pathology to be a collorary factor to erectile dysfunction. However, nuclear magnetic resonance (NMR) procedures may be 10% more accurate than the CAT scan in the detection of spinal cord/brain diseases.

Penile Buckling and Indenter Devices

These devices measure or calibrate penile rigidity during erection. However, most erections in SCI patients are reflexogenic/stimulative, and thus are usually fleeting. It is therefore difficult to utilize these diagnostic aids. Leyson and Powell believe that the nocturnal penile tumescence (NPT) monitor tracings can approximate penile rigidity if the erections last for at least 25 min (*14*). NPT monitoring can prognosticate the return of erectile function by periodic recording of the patient's nocturnal penile tumescence for at least 1 yr posttrauma (*12*). The multisystems diagnostic flow diagram is discussed in the last chapter.

Conclusions

The tests discussed in this chapter are not intended for use on all patients complaining of impotency. Rather, they should be utilized in a fashion tailored to the specific patient. Lower-cord-injured patients with a history of impotence and related findings (such as neurogenic bowel and bladder injury) may need no more workup other than a simple snap gage or postage stamp-test. Likewise, routine hormonal studies in young spinal-cord-injured males with normal libido may be of little value. On the other hand, depending on the initial evaluation, a large and continuously evolving armamentarium of instruments and techniques are available to the spinal-cord injured for diagnosing and determining the etiology of impotence. Regardless of how simple or sophisticated our evaluation may be, knowing the patient and understanding his sexual history is imperative to the determination of appropriate therapy.

References

1. Abelson, D. (1975) Diagnostic value of the penile pulse and blood pressure: a doppler study of impotence in diabetes. *J. Urol.* **113**, 636–639.
2. Barry, J. M., Blank, B., and Boileau, M. (1980) Nocturnal penile tumescence monitoring with stamps. *Urology* **15**, 171–172.
3. Comarr, A. E. (1971) Sexual concepts in traumatic cord and cauda equina lesions. *J. Urol.* **106**, 375–378.
4. Ek, A. and Bradley, W. (1982) A new concept in the measurement of penile rigidity. Proc. Amer. Urol. Assoc., Kansas City, Kansas, May 17–21.
5. Engel, G., Burham, S. J., and Carter, M. D. (1978) Penile blood pressure in the evaluation of erectile impotence. *Fertil. Steril.* **30**, 687–692.
6. Hursch, C. J., Karacan, I., and Williams R. L. (1972) Some characteristics of nocturnal penile tumescence in early middle-aged males. *Comp. Psychiat.* **13**, 539–548.
7. Jevtich, M. J. (1981) Penile body temperature as screening test for penile arterial obstruction in impotence. *Urology* **17**, 132–135.
8. Karacan, I., Hursch, C. J., Williams, R. L., and Thornby, J. I. (1972) Some characteristics of nocturnal penile tumescence in young adults. *Arch. Gen. Psychiat.* **26**, 351–356.
9. Kempczinski, R. F. (1979) Role of the vascular diagnostic laboratory in the evaluation of male impotence. *Am. J. Surg.* **138**, 278–282.
10. Krane, R. J. and Siroky, M. D. (1980) Studies on sacral-evoked potentials *J. Urol.* **124**, 872–876.
11. Lerich, R. and Morel, A. (1948) The syndrome of thrombotic obliteration of the aortic bifurcation. *Ann. Surg.* **127**, 193–206.
12. Leyson, J. F. (1982) Comparative study between stamp and strain gauge nocturnal penile tumescence monitoring in the diagnosis of impotence in spinal cord injured men. Proc. Amer. Spinal Injury Assoc., New York, April 18–20.
13. Leyson, J. F. (1983) Penile temperature recording in the diagnosis of impotence in spinal cord injured men. F. C. Valentine Urology Contest. AUA New York Section, New York City, April 6.
14. Leyson, J. F. and Powell, R. (1982) Comparative study of two nocturnal penile tumescence monitor. *J. Med. Society of NJ* **79**, 647–650.
15. Lue, T. F., Aricale H., Marich, K. W., and Tanaglio, E. A. (1985) Vasculogenic impotence evaluated by light resolution ultrasonography and pulsed doppler spectrum analysis. *Radiology* **155**, 777.
16. Lue, T. F., Aricale H., Schmidt, R. A., and Tanaglio, E. A. (1986) Functional evaluation of penile veins by cavernosography of papaverine-induced erection. *J. Urol.* **135**, 479.
17. Shabsigle, R., Fishman, I., and Scott, F. B. (1988) Evaluation of erectile impotence, *Urol.* **Vol. 32 #2**, 83.

17

Neuroendocrine Evaluation and Management of Erectile Dysfunction

W. Ronald Skowsky

Introduction

Generally, medical therapy of erectile disturbances in patients with spinal-cord injury (SCI) is fraught with failure and appears to be limited to a very selected subgroup of patients with documented hypogonadism. This is not to understate the importance of male erectile failure in SCI, which varies in incidence and magnitude according to the level and completeness of the lesion. Although the physiology and neural regulation of penile erection has been discussed in detail elsewhere in this volume, a brief discussion here is needed to emphasize certain aspects germane to the present topic.

Physiology

The change in penile size that occurs when passing from flaccidity to tumescence to full erection can be anatomically and physiologically related to the following processes:

1. Arterial dilatation—passive and/or active dilation of the arterial vasculature to the intracavernous sinuses
2. Venous constriction—active narrowing of the arteriovenous shunts preventing drainage from the arterial system
3. Sinusoidal relaxation—active relaxation of the smooth muscle within penile erectile tissue corpora cavernosa and corpus spongiosum (*1–4*).

Sexual Rehabilitation of the Spinal-Cord-Injured Patient
Edited by J.F. Leyson, © 1990 The Humana Press, Inc.

Neural control of involuntary or reflex penile erection is regulated via at least two distinct mechanisms. Psychogenic erections (in response to centrally perceived erotic stimuli of an auditory, visual, olfactory, tactile, and/or imaginative nature) arise in supraspinal centers and have their efferent pathways in either the thoracolumbar (T12-L3) or the sacral (S2-S4) autonomic trunk (*5*). On the other hand, reflexostimulative erections—arising by direct tactile stimulation of the afferent sensory terminals of the pudendal nerve on the male external genitalia—are mediated through the spinal cord via the sacral reflex center with the efferent limb in the sacral parasympathetic nerves.

Pathophysiology

Because there are reflex erection centers within the spinal cord, patients with a spinal cord lesion above T12 may still undergo reflexogenic/stimulative erections, although psychogenic erections are abolished. Conversely, patients with lower spinal-cord lesions involving the sacral segments, with lesions of the cauda equina, or with pelvic parasympathetic plexus injuries are unable to exhibit reflexogenic erection, although psychogenic erections may still occur via the sympathetic presacral innervation to the penis (*6,7*).

During the immediate "spinal shock" period following acute SCI, the effect of cord lesioning on sexual functioning is variable and unpredictable (*8*). In subjects with complete cervical-cord transection studied several months after the initial spinal-shock period, 100% of patients retained reflexogenic erection patterns (*6*), but only 7% (*9*) to 27% (*6*) of patients with lower motor-neuron lesions reported psychogenic erections. Likewise, in another large series, 95% of patients with complete upper motor-neuron lesions had spontaneous reflex erections, although this occurred in only 12% of complete lower motor-neuron lesions (*10*). In the latter study, preservation of pinprick sensation, more than light touch, seemed to be prognostically important for the retention of penile erection.

Neuropharmacology

Intimately associated with the neuronal control of physiologically normal erection is the functional role of neurotransmitters in controlling erectile patterns. It was first proposed that the parasympathetic nerves from the sacral plexus to the Ebner pads and cavernous tissue were the only pathway required for vasodilation (*11,12*), although other studies documented neural pathways through the sympathetic hypogastric nerve (*13*). It is still uncertain whether penile vasodilation is mediated exclusively through cholinergic nerves, although in humans erection can be produced by electrical stimulation of the sacral nerve roots S2, S3, or S4 (*14*). Recent electron microscopic studies of the nerve endings within the corpus cavernosum describe vesicles that are suggestive of peptidergic, cholinergic, as well as adrenergic neurotransmitter content (*15*).

Several pharmacologic studies of the neural regulation of penile function have been undertaken in the rabbit, in which two sets of vasodilatory pelvic nerves can be demonstrated: one containing noncholinergic postganglionic parasympathetic fibers and the other containing cholinergic postganglionic sympathetic (hypogastric) fibers (*16*). The latter are believed to suppress adrenergic vasoconstrictor tone and transform a flaccid penis to an erect one. Other animal studies have also suggested cholinergic control of penile erection since atropine will partially inhibit, and anticholinesterases will augment, erections elicited by autonomic nerve stimulation (*13*). However, atropine infusion in normal, young human volunteers failed to inhibit the ability to produce a rapid and complete erection, elicited by both visual stimulation or local vibration (*17*).

Since atropine fails to completely abolish electrically stimulated or spontaneous penile erection, some investigators have suggested the concept of noncholinergic vasodilation (*18,19*), i.e., sympathetic vasoconstriction in which blood is shunted to the cavernous sinuses (*20*). However, animal studies suggest that tonic sympathetic vasoconstrictor tone may have an inhibitory effect since alpha-adrenergic pharmacologic blockers will produce penile erection (*2,12,21*). Human male volunteers receiving an alpha-adrenergic blocking agent, phenoxybenzamine, or a beta-adrenergic blocking agent, propranolol, had no impairment of the speed or completeness of penile erection nor of its stiffness (*4*). Thus, current knowledge does not support the concept of either cholinergic or adrenergic dominance in penile erection, nor recommend cholinergic-adrenergic pharmacologic manipulation alone as therapy for erectile dysfunction in SCI males. However, the muscular contractions that occur during the process of semen emission do definitely appear to be regulated by norepinephrine receptors (*22,23*) and possibly modulated by cholinergic activity (*24*).

The immunocytochemical presence of vasoactive intestinal polypeptide (VIP) in the corpora cavernosa of the cat has been documented (*25*). Pharmacologic administration of VIP produces smooth muscle relaxation. Preliminary work has suggested the presence of this peptide in human erectile tissue (*4*), but its role as a putative neurotransmitter is still speculative.

Hormonal Control Mechanisms

Since the development of secondary sexual characteristics is dependent on functioning gonads, much speculation has centered upon the possible role of androgens in penile erectile function. Although gonadal androgen secretion is important in adolescent penile growth, there is little to support any role in erectile ability in normal adult males. A few well-publicized studies have gained public support, since the results have claimed improvement in sexual function following testosterone administration (*26,27*), but these reports cannot be scientifically evaluated, since they lack descriptions of any controls, of any patient medical evaluations, or of any placebo group. One double-blind clinical study (*28*) claiming increases in erection and organisms following testosterone therapy failed to distinguish between psychogenic and organic cause of impotence, and lacked careful patient evaluation. Another double-blind crossover study included behaviorial evaluations and hormonal blood sampling (testosterone, free testosterone, sex-hormone-binding globulin, luteinizing hormone, and prolactin) before and during testosterone administation to 29 males without clinical or biochemical evidence of androgen deficiency (*29*). This study emphasizes the importance of a placebo in a double-blind study, since nearly 60% of the subjects claimed significant clinical improvement whether they received placebo or hormone.

Although there is no rationale for androgen therapy of erectile dysfunction in eugondal males without evidence of sex steroid deficiency, testosterone is clearly beneficial to hypogonadal subjects, improving the incidence of total erections, nocturnal erections, sexual desire, and coital frequency (*30,31*). In addition, preliminary reports suggest a beneficial effect of luteinizing hormone releasing hormone (LHRH) on increasing penile erectile function and libido in hypogonadal men (*32,33*). There also appears to be an effect of this hypothalamic peptide in eugonadal, sexually active, normal adult males who received a single dose of LHRH and experienced greater sexual arousal following erotic visual stimuli; they were observed to have climaxed faster following masturbation with a greater degree of tumescence, as compared to placebo administation (*34*). No studies have been undertaken with LHRH therapy in psychogenic erectile failure. In addition, prolonged chronic therapy with LHRH agonists (for infertility studies) have demonstrated degenerative effects on testicular function via downregulation of the pituitary and testicular receptors or by a direct effect on the Leydig cells (*35*), which may limit its therapeutic usefulness in the pharmacologic therapy of erectile dysfunction.

The effects of hyperprolactinemia are now appreciated as an important factor in the pathologic state associated with male and female reproductive dysfunction. Over 90% of males with elevated prolactin secretion have evidence of sexual and/or reproductive abnormalities at the time of diagnosis, with varying degrees of hypogonadism. Presenting symptoms in the adult male include impotence, impairment of libido, loss of morning erections, and a decrease in seminal volume (*36,37*). Elevated levels of prolactin appear to have an inhibitory effect on both the hypothalamic/pituitary release of LHRH and gonadotropins as well as on the gonadal secretion of testosterone (*38,39*), producing a net decrease in circulating androgens. Also, a recent report (*40*) suggests that a hypothalamic prolactin-inhibiting peptide resides within the LHRH precursor molecule, implying a close inverse relationship between prolactin and gonadotropin secretion.

Elevation of serum prolactin levels can result from a variety of causes, the most common etiology being a pituitary adenoma, which may be radiographically undetectable; other types of hypothalmic disease, including hypophyseal stalk disruption, also may elevate prolactin secretion. Additional etiologies of the hyperprolactinemic state include primary hypothyroidism, chronic renal insufficiency, and a variety of drugs including antipsychotic dopamine-receptor-blocking agents and antihypertensive catecholamine-depleting agents. Treatment is aimed at the removal of the causal process—either surgical tumor removal, therapy of the underlying disease, or removal of the offending drug. In addition, medical therapy with dopamine agonist drugs, including the semisynthetic ergot alkaloid bromocriptine, will significally lower and normalize prolactin serum concentration in many of the abovementioned pathologic states. Chronic therapy with this pharmacologic agent to normalize prolactin levels in selected hyperprolactinemic males will reverse the hypogonadal state, improve the libido, restore erectile penile function, and increase serum testosterone levels and sperm counts (*36–38,40–42*).

Endocrine Evaluation

In view of the preceding emphasis on hypogonadism, it is important to determine whether changes in gonadal function truly exist in SCI males. Early studies suggested seminiferous tubular atrophy, and normal or hyperplastic Leydig cells in the testes of paraplegic males (*43*). Serum hormonal quantitation documented elevated concentrations of follicle-stimulating hormone and luteinizing hormone, normal prolactin, and borderline low testosterone in 30–50% of SCI males (*44–48*). Subsequently, it became apparent that the hormonal changes in circulating androgens depended upon the time elapsed since the spinal-cord trauma, suggesting that the hypothalamic–pituitary–testis axis is disturbed for the first 4–8 mo after initial SCI (*47–49*). Eventually, plasma testosterone returns to normal values (*47–49*) as the clinical status of the cord-injured patient stabilizes.

Selection of candidates for medical therapy of erectile penile dysfunction in SCI males is not an unduly difficult task. Although there is a small subgroup of hypogonadal males who can benefit from endocrine therapy, in the absence of documented testicular deficiency, any beneficial effect of androgen treatment for erectile disturbances appears to be only a placebo response. In view of the possibility of seminiferous tubular hyalinization or hepatic damage with chronic testosterone administration, there is little rationale for unwarranted use of this agent.

Detailed workup for erectile dysfunction in SCI males should probably be delayed until more than 6 mo from the time of initial trauma to avoid the transient disturbances observed in the hypothalamic–pituitary–gonadal axis. At that time, the physician should search for signs of diminished gonadal size, or persistent alterations in libido and secondary sexual characteristics (frequency of facial shaving, body skin and hair distribution, texture, and so on). Development of a bilateral decrease in testicular size in a previously normal adult male generally implies germinal tubular atrophy, which may be either primary or secondary to diminished pituitary secretion of follicle-stimulating hormone. Loss of secondary sexual characteristics implies diminished Leydig cell secretion of testosterone, which may be either primary or secondary to diminished pituitary secretion of luteinizing hormone.

As a result of negative gonadal feedback to the hypothalamic–pituitary axis, a decrease in Leydig cell secretion of testosterone would be expected to produce a reciprocal increase in pituitary luteinizing hormone release, although a decrease in normal seminiferous tubular function would produce an increase in pituitary release of follicle-stimulating hormone; thus, primary gonadal failure is associated with a hypergonadotrophic hypogonadal state. If the hypogonadal state results from hypothalamic–pituitary pathology and failure of gonadotropin secretion, this produces a hypogonadotrophic hypogonadal state. Such conditions can usually be ascertained by serum measurement of testosterone and gonadotropins. All hypogonadotrophic hypogonadal patients should be further examined for the possibility of associated anterior and/or posterior pituitary deficiencies with appropriate serum measurement of thyroid hormones, cortisol, prolactin, and osmolality. If basal levels of these parameters are normal, it may be necessary to undergo pertubation studies with thyrotropin-releasing hormone (TRH), luteinizing-hormone releasing hormone (LRH), insulin hypoglycemia (to evaluate the hypothalamic–pituitary–adrenal axis), and fluid deprivation (to evaluate vasopressin reserve). Radiographic investigation with computerized axial tomography (CAT) may also be warranted, depending upon the medical examination and endocrinologic workup.

Hyperprolactinemic states can easily be diagnosed by serum measurement of this peptide. If observed, a careful search for an underlying pituitary adenoma is mandatory. Mild to moderate elevations of serum prolactin may be drug related, and the offending agent should be discontinued. The elevated prolactin of chronic renal insufficiency is usually not suppressed with regular hemodialysis, but can be therapeutically lowered with bromocriptine administration with a marked improvement in clinical symptoms.

It behooves any physician evaluating erectile dysfunction in male SCI patients to attempt to distinguish psychogenic from organic causative factors. This may present a diagnostic dilemma at times, one that has been addressed elsewhere in this volume. Additional medical disorders associated with erectile disturbances in both SCI and non-SCI patients include diabetes mellitus, atherosclerotic vascular disease, chronic renal disease, alcoholism, epilepsy, and postabdominal surgery (perineal prostatectomy, abdominal perineal colostomy, and so on). Further discussion of these disease states as well as of the multitude of pharmacologic agents affecting erectile function is beyond the scope of this chapter.

Hormonal Therapy

Appropriate therapy is directed toward the basic pathology. There is no convincing evidence that therapy with cholinergic agonists or adrenergic antagonists has any proven therapeutic value in the penile erectile dysfunction associated with SCI. Documented gonadal deficiency is the only justification for testosterone treatment as therapy for erectile failure. The androgen is generally administered intramuscularly as an ester of testosterone* in a dose of 200–300 mg every 2–3 wk. If

---

*Transdermal testosterone (10–15 mg) can be worn as a patch on the scrotum for 22 h/d.

the hypogonadal state is associated with elevated serum levels of gonadotropins, a subsequent decrease in serum gonadotropin values, along with improvement in body hair and muscle growth, indicates pharmacologic adequacy of dosage upon the hypothalamic–pituitary axis and peripheral androgen receptors.

Erectile dysfunction associated with hyperprolactinemic states should include therapy directed toward the underlying pathologic causation. If it is elected to undertake medical treatment with bromocriptine (as primary or ancillary therapy), gradually increasing doses of 2.5 mg given one to three times a day will lower and usually normalize serum prolactin, depending upon the underlying etiology, and may improve clinical symptoms of sexual dysfunction.

Erection Mineralogy and Other Vital Elements

The complex process of erection involves a multitude of neurohormonal transmitters and still undefined "electrochemical" reactions. Zinc as a testosterone cofactor is indirectly involved in erection. The zinc levels of SCI patients with normal renal functions, complaining of erectile dysfunction are usually normal. On the other hand, oral replacement therapy for documented zinc deficiency-induced impotence in SCI patients on hemodialysis has been claimed to be effective. There has been no correlation between impotence and serum magnesium deficiency. Copper has been implicated in some infertility problems in non-SCI patients, but has not been thoroughly investigated in spinal-cord injury cases. Vitamin deficiency in SCI patients has no clearly defined effect on erectile function. Furthermore, clinical observations have failed to demonstrate improved tumescence and duration of reflexostimulative erections following massive doses of vitamins.

Conclusions

Although much remains to be learned about the interaction of various minerals, vitamins, and neurotransmitters and how they modulate sexuality, certain diagnostic and therapeutic guidelines can be adopted in evaluating erectile dysfunction in the SCI patient. Sophisticated methods of assessing neuroendocrine function should be able to identify the small, but present, treatable subgroup.

References

1. Degroat, W. C. and Booth, A. M. (1980) Physiology of male sexual function. *Ann. Intern. Med.* **92(Part 2)**, 329–331.
2. Weiss, H. D. (1972) The physiology of human penile erection. *Ann. Intern. Med.* **76**, 793–799.
3. Newman, H. F., Northup, J. D. and Devlin, J. (1964) Mechanism of human penile erection. *Invest. Urol.* **1**, 350–353.
4. Wagner, G. (1981) Erection, physiology and endocrinology, in *Impotence. Physiological, Psychological, Surgical. Diagnosis and Treatment.* (Wagner, G. and Green, R., eds.) Plenum, New York, pp. 25–36.
5. Root, W. S. and Bard, P. (1947) The mediation of feline erection through sympathetic pathways with some remarks on sexual behavior after deafferentiation of the genitalia. *Am. J. Physiol.* **151**, 288–290.
6. Bors, E. and Comarr, A. E. (1960) Neurological disturbances of sexual function with special reference to 529 patients with spinal cord injury. *Urol. Survey* **10**, 191–222.
7. Furlow, W. L. (1979) Diagnosis and treatment of male erectile failure. *Diabetes Care* **2**, 18–25.
8. Cole, T. (1979) Sexuality and the spinal cord injured, in *Human Sexuality: A Health Practioners Text (2nd ed)* (Green, R. ed.) Williams and Wilkins, Baltimore.
9. Cibeira, J. B. (1970) Some conclusions on a study of 365 patients with spinal cord lesions. *Paraplegia* **7**, 249–254.
10. Comaar, A. E. (1970) Sexual functions among patients with spinal cord injury. *Urol. Int.* **25**, 134–168.
11. Langley, J. N. and Andersen, K. H. (1896) The innervation of the pelvic and adjoining viscera. Part VI. *J. Physiol.* **20**, 372–406.
12. Semans, J. H. and Langworthy, O. R. (1938) Observations on the neurophysiology of sexual function in the male cat. *J. Urol.* **40**, 836–846.
13. Bacq, F. M. (1935) Recherches sur la physiologie et la pharmacologie du systeme nerveux autonome. *Arch. Internat. de Physiol.* **40**, 311–321.
14. Habib, H. N. (1967) Experimental and recent contributions in sacral nerve stimulation for voiding in both man and animal. *Brit. J. Urol.* **39**, 73–83.
15. McConnell, J. A. (1979) EM analysis of the adrenergic and possible peptidergic innervation of the human vas deferers and corpus cavernosum. *The Anat. Record* **193**, 168.
16. Sjöstrand, N. O. and Klinge, E. (1979) Principle mechanisms controlling penile retraction and protrusion in rabbits. *Acta. Physiol. Scand.* **106**, 199–214.
17. Wagner, G. and Brindley, G. S. (1978) Effects of atropine on erection (abstract). First Internation Conference on Vasculogenic Impotence, New York.

18. Henderson, V. E. and Roepke, M. H. (1933) On the mechanism of erection. *Am. J. Physiol.* **106**, 441–448.
19. Dorr, L. D. and Brody, M. J. (1967) Hemodynamic mechanisms of erection in the canine penis. *Am. J. Physiol.* **213**, 1526–1531.
20. Newman, H. F., Northup, J. D., and Devlin, J. (1964) Mechanism of human penile erection. *Invest. Urol.* **1**, 350–353.
21. Domer, F. R., Wessler, G., Brown, R. L., and Charles, H. C. (1978) Involvement of the sympathetic nervous system in the urinary bladder internal sphincter and in penile erection in the anesthetized cat. *Invest. Urol.* **15**, 404–407.
22. Kedia, K. and Markland, C. (1975) The effect of pharmacologic agents on ejaculation. *J. Urol.* **114**, 569–573.
23. Anton, P. G. and McGrath, J. C. (1977) Further evidence for adrenergic transmission in the human vas deferens. *J. Physiol.* **273**, 45–55.
24. Sjöstrand, N. O. and Kinge, E. (1977) What function have cholinergic nerves in the smooth muscle of the male genital tract? *Acta. Physiol. Scand.* (Suppl) **452**, 89–91.
25. Larsson, L. I., Fahrekrug, J., and Schaffalityzky De Muckadell, O. B. (1977) Occurrence of nerves containing vasoactive intestinal polypeptide immunoreactivity in the male genital tract. *Life Sci.* **21**, 503–508.
26. Margolis, R. and Lesley, C. (1966) Review of studies of a mixture of nux vomica, yohimbine and methyl testosterone in the treatment of impotence. *Curr. Therap. Res.* **8**, 280–284.
27. Margolis, R., Sangree, H., Prieto, P., Stein, L., and Chinn, S. (1967) Clinical studies on the use of Afrodex in the treatment of impotence: Statistical summary of 4000 cases. *Curr. Therap. Res.* **9**, 213–219.
28. Sobataka, J. (1969) An evaluation of Afrodex in the management of male impotence: A double-blind crossover study. *Curr. Therap. Res.* **11**, 87–94.
29. Benkert, O., Witt, W., Adam, W., and Leitz, A. (1979) Effects of testosterone undeconate on sexual potency and the hypothalamic pituitary gonadal axis of impotent males. *Arch. Sexual Behav.* **8**, 471–480.
30. Davidson, J., Camargo, C., and Smith, E. (1979) Effects of androgens on sexual behavior in hypogonadal men. *J. Clin. Endocrinol. Metab.* **48**, 955–958.
31. Skakkebaek, N., Bancroft, J., Davidson, D., and Warner, P. (1981) Androgen replacement with oral testosterone undeconate in hypogonadal men: A double blind controlled study. *Clin. Endocrinol.* **14**, 49–61.
32. Mortimer, C., McNeilly, A., Fisher, R., Murray, M., and Besser, G. (1974) Gonadotrophin-releasing hormone therapy in hypogonadal males with hypothalamic or pituitary dysfunction. *Brit. Med. J.* **4**, 617–621.
33. Davies, T., Mountjoy, C., Gomes-Pan, A., Watson, M., Hanker, J., Resser, G., and Hall, R. (1976) A double-blind crossover trial of gonadotrophin releasing hormone (LHRH) in sexually impotent men. *Clin. Endocrinol.* **5**, 601–607.
34. Evans, I. and Distriller, L. (1979) Effects of luteinizing hormone releasing hormone on sexual arousal in normal men. *Arch. Sexual Behav.* **8**, 385–395.

35. Bergquist, C., Nillius, S. J., Bergh, T., Skarin, G., and Wide, L. (1979) Inhibitory effects on gonadotropin secretion and gonadal function in men during chronic treatment with a potent stimulating LHRH analogue. *Acta. Endocrinol.* **91**, 601–608.
36. Thorner, M. O., Martin, W. H., Rogol, A. D., Morris, J. L., Perryman, R. L., Conway, B. P., Howards, S. S., Wolfman, M. G., and Macleod, R. M. (1980) Rapid regression of pituitary prolactinomas during bromocriptine treatment. *J. Clin. Endocrinol. Metab.* **51**, 438–445.
37. Perryman, R. L. and Thorner, M. O. (1981) The effects of hyperprolactinemia on sexual and reproductive function in men. *J. Androl.* **2**, 233–242.
38. Ben-David, M., Danon, A., and Sulman, F. G. (1971) Evidence on antagonism between prolactin and gonadotropin secretion. *J. Endocrinol.* **51**, 719–725.
39. Bex, F. J. and Bartke, A. (1977) Testicular LH binding in the hamster: modification by photoperiod and prolactin. *Endocrinology* **100**, 1223–1226.
40. Nikolics, K., Mason, A. J., Szony, E., Ramachandran, J., and Seeburg, P. H. (1985) A prolactin-inhibiting factor within the precursor for human gonadotropin releasing hormones. *Nature* **316**, 511–517.
41. Bommer, J., Del Pozo, E., Ritz, E., and Bommer, G. (1979) Improved sexual function in male hemodialysis patients on bromocriptine. *Lancet* **ii**, 946–947.
42. Vircburger, M. I., Prelevic, G. M., Peric, L. A., Knezevic, J., and Djukanovic, L. (1985) Testosterone levels after bromocriptine treatment in patients undergoing long-term hemodialysis. *J. Androl.* **6**, 113–116.
43. Stemmerman, G. N., Weiss, L., Ansbach, O., and Friedman, M. (1950) A study of the germinal epithelium in male paraplegics. *Am. J. Clin. Pathol.* **20**, 24–34.
44. Morley, J. D., Distiller, L. A., Lissoos, I., Lipschitz, R., Kay, G., Searle, D. L., and Katz, M. (1979) Testicular function in patients with spinal cord damage. *Horm. Metab. Res.* **11**, 679–682.
45. Hayes, P. L., Krishnan, K. R., Diver, M. J., Hipkin, L. H., and Davis, J. C. (1979) Testicular endocrine function in paraplegic men. *Clin. Endocrinol.* **11**, 549–552.
46. Mizutani, S., Sonoda, T., Matsumoto, K., and Iwasa, K. (1972) Plasma testosterone concentration in paraplegic men. *J. Endocrinol.* **54**, 362–364.
47. Cortes-Gallegos, V., Castaneda, G., Alonso, R., Arellano, H., Cervantes, C., and Parra, A. (1981) Pituitary—Testis relationship in paraplegic men. *J. Androl.* **2**, 326–330.
48. Claus-Walker, J., Scurry, M., Carter, R. E., and Campos, R. J. (1977) Steady state hormonal secretion in traumatic quadriplegia. *J. Clin. Endocrinol. Metab.* **44**, 530–535.
49. Kikuchi, T. A., Skowsky, W. R., El-Toraei, I., and Swerdloff, R. (1976) The pituitary gonadal axis in spinal cord injury. *Fertil. Steril.* **27**, 1142–1144.

18
Sexual Harmony Despite Impotence

Roberta B. Trieschmann

Introduction

The focus of this chapter is the variety of issues and approaches that need to be considered when one member of a partnership, the man, acquires a spinal-cord injury that results in an altered ability to obtain and maintain an erection. Other chapters have introduced and discussed the importance of cultural and religious influences on sexual functioning, psychological considerations, and marital status, and these chapters should thus be considered to complement the discussion herein.

A Definition of the Problem

Three Components of Sexual Functioning

Any discussion of sexual functioning following a severe disability, such as spinal-cord injury, should include a differentiation among sex drives, sex acts, and sexuality in order to conceptualize the nature of the problem and plan appropriate interventions (*9,10*).

Sex drive is the primary drive that results in copulation and propagation of the species. In males, there is a specific physical urge that seeks release in the form of ejaculation and orgasm. In lower organisms, this drive is instigated by subcortical regions of the brain and controlled by the presence or absence of a partner. In humans, this drive is instigated subcortically, but is controlled by the neocortex, which is the seat of social learning. Therefore, the issues of love, relationship, and satisfaction of a partner become components of the sex drive in humans.

Sexual Rehabilitation of the Spinal-Cord-Injured Patient
Edited by J.F. Leyson, © 1990 The Humana Press, Inc.

Sex acts are the variety of ways in which individuals have learned to express caring and love, and to provide pleasure to one another. A continuum of actions from casual to intimate would include kissing, casual caressing, intimate caressing, direct stimulation of the erogenous zones, and sexual intercourse. Frequently, discussions of sexual functioning tend to suggest that there is only one sex act, penile–vaginal intercourse, but we need to expand our focus as professionals in order to provide assistance to persons with physical disabilities. The subcortical sex drive tends to seek penile–vaginal intercourse as its primary focus. The neocortex, however, as the seat of social learning, may include a variety of learned sex acts, such as manual and oral stimulation, as part of the repertoire of activities that can lead to sexual pleasure and that can express caring and love. However, in each individual, social learning will profoundly influence which sex acts are considered to be acceptable and which are unacceptable.

Sexuality is the self-image of the individual that encompasses the sense of maleness or femaleness and the learned behavior patterns associated with these statuses. Sexuality is inherently tied to a sense of self in all of its dimensions, and is highly influenced by what society in general and one's particular culture or ethnic group defines as appropriate male or female roles, patterns of functioning, and specific behaviors.

Following the onset of spinal-cord injury in males, the physical release aspects of the sex drive become less important since the physical sensation of ejaculation and orgasm is no longer present. Thus, the initiation of a sexual interaction for the physical release it entails will decline (*6*). However, the neocortical parameters of the sex drive remain active, and the person will initiate a sexual interaction with a partner with whom he has a relationship in order to express loving and caring within the context of that relationship. In the absence of a partner, many men with spinal injury (and many of those without spinal injuries) can become acclimated to a celibate life without extreme difficulty.

Depending upon the level and completeness of the injury, some sex acts may be available to the individual and some may not. Kissing, fondling, and caressing of the female partner remain available to *all* men with spinal injury through use of the hands, lips, and tongue. Persons with high levels of quadriplegia may not use their hands functionally, but they can still be lovers with their lips and tongue. The degree to which sexual intercourse is possible depends upon the erectile capability of the male (the firmness and *duration* of the erection). If erectile capacity is impaired, intercourse will remain a component in the sexual repertoire of the partners, depending upon the needs and frustration tolerances of the individuals concerned. Thus, some sex acts, but not all, may be altered by the onset of spinal injury, and the personal preferences of the partners will be a crucial feature in postinjury sexual adjustment. The role of cultural, ethnic, and religious proscriptions of certain sex acts may complicate the situation, and the professional must be sensitive to these issues (*7*).

The sexuality of the individual with spinal injury will be significantly influenced by the onset of the disability, at least initially (*9,10*). The physical disability challenges one's definition of self, and this altered definition is confirmed by the reactions of family, friends, and strangers. *Ideally*, family and friends will perceive the essential sameness of the person and not allow the physical changes to alter the relationship, though this may take some time depending upon the individuals involved. However, a major component in the process of adjustment to disability is the devaluation of the disabled person by society. Every day the person will receive subtle and not so subtle messages from people in his environment that he is not "as good as" men who can walk. Furthermore, these are the very feelings that he has about himself: he is not the man he used to be. Thoughts and feelings along these lines do not enhance self-confidence and well-being, and thus most of his relationships will be influenced by these issues until he comes to terms with the fact that he is a worthwhile and lovable person. His ability to express and receive love will relate to the status of his self-image and will influence the outcome of any efforts aimed at sexual rehabilitation.

Consequently, the sexuality of the man with spinal injury will be influenced by the onset of the disability. Any approach to sexual rehabilitation, then, should view *sexuality* as the context within which the *sex drive* may be expressed through a variety of *sex acts*, depending upon the capability and preferences of the persons involved. All three components of sexual functioning—sex drive, sex acts, and sexuality—will be influenced by the spinal injury, though in different ways. Thus, this conceptualization should be kept in mind as we consider primary and secondary sexual dysfunctions.

Primary and Secondary Sexual Dysfunctions

Primary sexual dysfunctions are those in which the dysfunction has an organic etiological basis, whereas secondary sexual dysfunctions are those in which attitudes, emotions, and behavioral factors interfere with sexual satisfaction. Most persons with spinal injury will experience both types of dysfunction, at least initially, and the distinction between the two should be remembered, since the types of interventions will differ.

The primary sexual dysfunctions that may accompany a spinal injury include the loss of psychogenic erections, the impairment in sensation, and the impairment of ejaculation. These dysfunctions will often become the major focus for intervention during the initial phases of rehabilitation. Specific suggestions may be given to manage these conditions or surgical intervention may be considered. However, most persons with spinal injury would agree that the physical parameters of the sexual dysfunction are not the whole problem. Rather, the challenge to self-image influences one's sexuality in profound ways. Thus, secondary sexual dysfunctions arise from changes in the nature of the relationship, attitudes toward disability, attitudes toward changes in sexual functioning, and the various emotions that can influence postinjury adjustment (*10*).

Treatment for primary and secondary dysfunctions will differ. In the former, surgical and pharmacologic approaches are frequently used interventions; whereas, with secondary dysfunctions, the interventions will include counseling and behavior therapy. Treatments aimed at the primary dysfunction usually propose to change "what is" (the physical aspects of the problem). Interventions aimed at the secondary dysfunction focus on helping the person to live with "what is" and to find satisfaction in the relationship by focusing on "what can be." Unfortunately, all too often, the interventions focus only on the primary problem, and the secondary dysfunctions are ignored. Thus, persons with disabilities have occasionally referred rather dismissively to the many professional articles on sexuality and disability as "Electricians' Guides to Sexual Ecstasy." It is therefore important for professionals who propose to participate in sexual rehabilitation programs to realize that treatment of the primary problem, without interventions aimed at the sexuality issues (secondary dysfunctions), will have limited success. As all able-bodied men realize, a fully functional set of genital equipment does not guarantee adequate sexual performance or sexual satisfaction. Fluctuations in stress, emotions, and self-image influence sexual performance and satisfaction in able-bodied and spinal-injured men alike. Consequently, attention to the secondary sexual dysfunctions becomes an essential component of all sexual treatment programs for those with severe physical disabilities, such as spinal injury.

An Integrated Approach to Sexual Dysfunctions

The three components of sexual functioning (sex drive, sex acts, and sexuality) should be evaluated in terms of the primary and secondary dysfunctions present (Table 1). The primary dysfunctions will be

Table 1
Primary and Secondary Sexual Dysfunction Following Spinal-Cord Injury

Components of sexual function	Primary dysfunction	Secondary dysfunction
Sex drive	Physical urge may be reduced	Emotional attitudes in the relationship can interfere with satisfaction
Sex acts	Erection and ejaculation may be impaired Sensation may be impaired Intercourse may be unsatisfactory to both partners	Attitudes toward sex acts other than intercourse may influence satisfaction. Cultural, religious, and established patterns of behavior may create anxiety and guilt
Sexuality	Not applicable	Self-image as a male will be challenged initially, and issues of self worth may interfere with sexual performance and satisfaction

associated with the sex drive and sex acts (particularly intercourse), and sexuality will not be directly affected. However, all three (sex drive, sex acts, and sexuality) are highly vulnerable to secondary sexual dysfunctions. Thus, if surgical or pharmacologic interventions are planned, they should be only one component of a sexual-therapy program that views sexual functioning as a relationship between two people who have individual perceptions of the disability, of the proper roles for males and females, and of the acceptability of various sex acts. Thus, the impact of the disability itself on the lives of the partners will create an emotional atmosphere that can inhibit sexual function and satisfaction well beyond the influence of the primary dysfunction. Consequently, when planning a sexual-therapy program for persons with spinal injury, the secondary aspects *should always be treated* and the primary aspects *may be treated.*

The Sexual Relationship

Very few males with complete spinal injuries masturbate as a source of sexual satisfaction following onset of the disability. Initially, masturbation may be utilized to determine erectile capability, but usually, when sensation and ejaculation are impaired, masturbation does not continue because it is not intrinsically rewarding. Thus, when the urgency of physical release is no longer an important factor in the initiation of sex acts with a partner, the expression of love and caring within a relationship serves as a major impetus for continued sexual activity. The relationship, then, of the spinal-injured male and his partner should become the focus of the sexual rehabilitation program, so that attention can be given to all three components of sexual functioning and to both the primary and secondary dysfunctions that may be present.

When the emphasis in a sexual rehabilitation program is placed on the relationship in this manner, a thorough sexual history from both the spinal-injured male and partner is essential. If the relationship existed prior to the injury, it will be important to determine sexual likes and dislikes, preferences and aversions, expectations of oneself and one's partner, cultural and religious proscriptions regarding the variety of sex acts available, and sex-role expectations for oneself and one's partner.

When a relationship was initiated preinjury, it is very important to elicit attitudes toward the disability. How has the disability affected the relationship? What changes in expectations for each other have occurred? How does the man with spinal injury view himself as a person, a man, and a lover? Often the man has quite a negative self-image arising from the onset of the disability, whereas the female partner does not view him in the same negative light. Women, in general, are less put off by the onset of a disability than men are, and therefore, a very important feature of the postinjury adjustment phase is the reaffirmation of love by the woman for the man. Such a reaffirmation can provide the context for the man to begin to love himself again. This does not mean, however, that there are not disappointments and adjustments to be made by both parties in the relationship. Nevertheless, attempts to open the lines of communication are a helpful first step in adjustment. Just lying in bed together and hugging without any further sexual advances is a very important form of communication and loving.

The role of the partner needs to be emphasized in sexual rehabilitation programs. Most professional articles describe the importance of including the partner in the rehabilitation process, but there has been little information in the literature about the reactions of partners of males with spinal injury. However, a recent study by Coffman (*1*) provides information on the sexual attitudes and behaviors of female partners of men with spinal injury. Interviews were conducted with 25 women to gain information on:

1. Acquisition of sex-related information about the disability
2. Attitudes about the importance of sex
3. Predisability and postdisability sexual behavior

4. Attitudes about the physical limitations of the spinal injured partner
5. Levels of sexual satisfaction attained with this partner
6. The spinal-injured male's adjustment to the disability and its effect on the couple's sexual activity.

Group averages indicated that these women were 31 yr old, in the relationship for 4 yr, and the man had been disabled 5 yr. Fourteen were married to the man, and 11 were unmarried. All levels of spinal injury were involved and all religious backgrounds were represented, but the women did not, on the average, describe themselves as deeply religious.

Most of the women obtained sex-related information regarding the implications of the disability from the man with spinal injury. Only four obtained such information from professionals trained in the area of spinal-cord-injury sexuality. Almost one-half of the women sought such information actively and, as a result, received a fair amount of input. Of the women who did not actively pursue information regarding sexuality and disability, most were given little or no information by others. Thus, women need to seek input aggressively in order to be knowledgeable in this area. The rehabilitation system does not regularly provide it. Twenty-one of the women reported that sex was important to them, and this was also true even if there were physical limitations that affected the execution of certain sexual activities. Over one-half of the women disclaimed the notion of being involved in sex only for their partner's satisfaction.

The sexual behaviors of the partners changed from predisability to postdisability by emphasizing male hands and mouth on female breast, female hands and mouth on male breast, and male mouth on female genitals. Manual stimulation and oral genital contacts increased in cases in which the man had erectile problems. The major petting technique that declined significantly postdisability was female mouth on male genitals. Many women reported that managing a catheter or ostomy appliance can have a disruptive effect on the spontaneity of sexual activities.

For those who engaged in intercourse, the female superior position predominated. The women reported that they did not masturbate to achieve sexual satisfaction in the relationship. Rather, they reported a high rate of orgasm through petting with their partner. Most of the women said that their spinal-injured partner was a more attentive and satisfying lover than most able-bodied men they had known, because the spinal-injured men were truly interested in doing what pleased the female partner.

Pre- and postdisability statistical analyses revealed that masturbation decreased, petting increased, and intercourse decreased in frequency. Most of the women's orgasms were achieved during petting, not during intercourse. Interestingly, only 28% of the males were diagnosed as having erectile dysfunctions. Nevertheless, ten of the women complained that their partner experienced erectile dysfunction during intercourse. In these cases, the erection was not sustained long enough for her to achieve satisfaction. Thus, we obviously need to clarify the definition of erectile dysfunction. The fact that a man *can* have an erection is not very meaningful functionally if its duration is limited so that intercourse for the woman becomes more frustrating than fulfilling. In addition to erectile problems, eight of the women reported that spasticity interfered with sexual activities to a significant degree, as did the catheter and urinary appliances.

Level of sexual satisfaction for the women was assessed for various sexual activities. Most of the women were very satisfied with their sex lives. A majority reported that they attained high or medium levels of satisfaction by using a variety of sexual activities rather than relying on any one sex act alone. However, only two reported high levels of satisfaction from intercourse, and seven reported medium levels of satisfaction; 19 rated their petting activities as satisfying. Most of the women reported that their satisfaction in their sex lives derived from the use of sex acts to express emotional tenderness and communication in bed, so that there would be physical closeness. Wheelchair sex was not rewarding. They felt that the spinal-injured partner understood their physical needs and desires better than any previous male partner, and this generally made their sex lives better.

One-half of the women reported that the men with spinal injury experienced emotional reactions that interfered with the overall relationship and, thus with the sexual relationship. Anger by the male toward the disability was reported by seven, withdrawal and depression were reported by four, and three reported overcompensatory behavior by the man as disruptive to the relationship. Generally, during these emotional phases, there was a reduction in the frequency of sexual overtures by both parties as part of the disruption of communication within the relationship itself.

Coffman's study provides a great deal of valuable information regarding sexual relationships following spinal injury. The women found that their sex lives with their spinal-injured partners were more fulfilling than with able-bodied men, because the men with spinal injury showed more care for their partner's satisfaction. There was little concern for the mechanics of individual sex acts. Rather, there was a focus

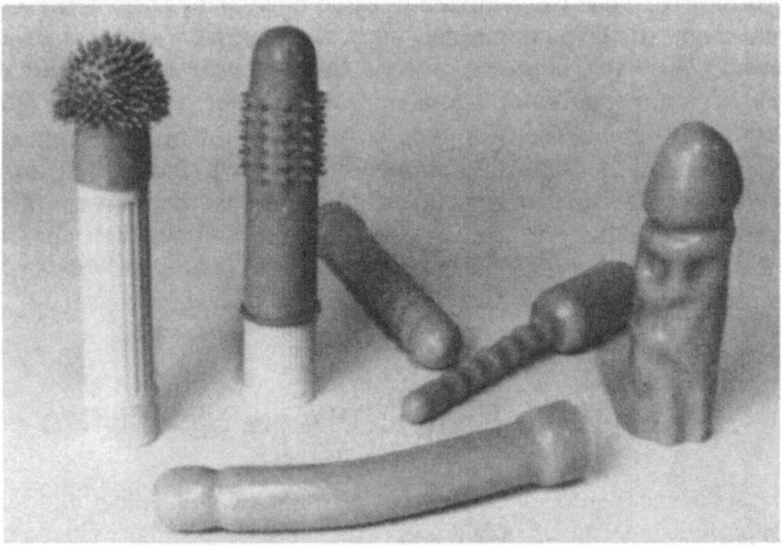

Fig. 1. Multiple types of hetero–homosexual stimulators: from battery powered vibrators and dildoes. SCI men who dislike penile prostheses may use the hollow dildoes (intercourse-assistive devices), which can be strapped around the pelvis and simulate an erect penis.

on the expression of the sex drive through a combination of pleasurable activities to express love and tenderness. The women were not concerned, in general, with erectile problems, unless the erection was lost during intercourse. Thus, a little bit of a penis is not necessarily better than no penis at all in the opinion of a large percentage of women. Sexual satisfaction can be obtained through a variety of sex acts and need not include intercourse. Yet, a great deal of the professional literature focuses on intercourse as the primary sex act. When the erection is lost during intercourse, this can damage the self-image of the man and prove to be a frustrating experience for both parties involved. Consequently, clear communication between partners as to preferences becomes crucial in successful relationships. It should also be noted that a loving woman will, of course, attempt intercourse if this would please the man. Also, an equally loving man will, of course, stimulate his partner in a variety of ways that are satisfying to her (Fig. 1).

The issue, then, is one of love between two people, and sex acts are just one way of expressing this love. If, however, we isolate sex acts from the context of the relationship, we are treating sexual functioning in a very mechanical fashion; we are dealing only with the subcortical drives; and we are treating sexual functioning as not much more than an animalistic mating ritual. *What distinguishes humans from most animals, however, is the neocortical, learned aspect to sexuality that focuses on the relationship between two people who care for each other.* Therefore, the essense of a good sexual rehabilitation program is to help the partners establish a communication style that allows for the free expression of love, and sex acts become just one feature of this communication pattern. Consequently, this requires a holistic approach to the patient and partner during evaluation and treatment, with special attention being given to the secondary sexual dysfunctions.

Strategies to Enhance Sexual Satisfaction

After the therapists have evaluated the male with spinal injury and his partner in terms of sexual and personal history and provided an atmosphere that opens communication between the partners, guidance may be given regarding the specifics of various sex acts that are acceptable to both partners. First of all, in any sexual therapy program, the professionals should present the basic information of sexual functioning—the anatomy and physiology of male and female sexual activities. Many people have misconceptions about the basics of sexual functioning and often major gaps in their information about normal sexuality. Following the presentation and absorption of this information (using nonmedical, layman terms), the variations in sexual function imposed by the disability can be presented with ample opportunity for the partners to ask questions. It is especially important that the female partner be involved rather than having a discussion with the man alone, as unfortunately happens all too often. This type of discussion can be presented to the couple alone or in groups. Group discussion, followed by individual counseling, can be an important facet of any sexual rehabilitation program. Furthermore, Sexual Attitude Readjustment (SAR) workshops can help to desensationalize the issue of sexuality, so that the spinal-injured person and his/her partner can examine their attitudes toward various aspects of sexual function. However, it should be noted that didactic sessions, group sessions, and sexual attitude readjustment workshops may not be sufficient to lead to behavior change in the area of sexual function (*10*). Thus a more behaviorally oriented approach is often warranted. Furthermore, sexual functioning after spinal injury evolves over time; therefore, a combination of the previously mentioned approaches may be appropriate at different points in the adjustment process.

Because of the complexity of the adjustment process, the team approach of physician (sexologist) and psychologist or other individual skilled in the behavioral sciences is recommended for sexual therapy programs. However, all members of the rehabilitation team should be knowledgeable about human sexuality and disability, and should provide an atmosphere in which the person with spinal injury feels comfortable discussing the issue of sexuality.

During the inpatient rehabilitation phase, a private hospital room may prove to be a major resource to the man and partner (*3,4*). This room is helpful as a place for intimate conversation and practice of many of the behaviors associated with sexuality and intimacy. Initially, the man may use the room to explore his body, and to determine methods and sites of sensual pleasure and arousal. Fantasy, transposition of stimuli from a sensate area to insensate erogenous zones, sensory amplification, music, pictures, aromas, variations of tactile stimuli (light touch, massage, pinch, tickle, scratch, hair pulling, catheter manipulation, vibration, and so on), and exposure to cool or warm air should all be explored as possible sources of pleasure, arousal, or penile erection (*2,5*). Attempts to create a pleasurable reaction and erection (Fig. 2) should include stimuli to the mouth, ears, neck, and skin segments just proximal to the line of sensory demarcation, nipples, penis, scrotum, adjacent perineum, anus, inner thighs, or any other body site that seems appropriate. Scratching the leg or foot may result in a mass withdrawal reflex accompanied by erection. The man may benefit from the opportunity to explore his body alone initially in order to determine changes in function since onset of the disability.

If therapy is begun soon after the onset of disability, the couple should initially relax together, caress, and reestablish communication. As with the management of functional sexual disorders, performance should not be stressed. Preliminary sessions should focus on communication, nongenital contact, review of preparatory activities, exchange of information about pleasurable sensations, and mutual body exploration, which can gradually proceed to more explicit sex acts. When erection is a high priority for either or both partners, the most effective methods of inducing and maintaining it should be sought. Any of the methods that had worked during the solitary trials can be attempted. If acceptable to the partners involved, cunnilingus can be tried and the option of fellatio presented. As Coffman (*1*) found, however, fellatio is not usually part of the sexual repertoire of couples following spinal injury, because it is not particularly rewarding to either party when the male has impaired sensation in the genital region. Depending upon the male's ability to fantasize, he may be able to experience a phantom orgasm,

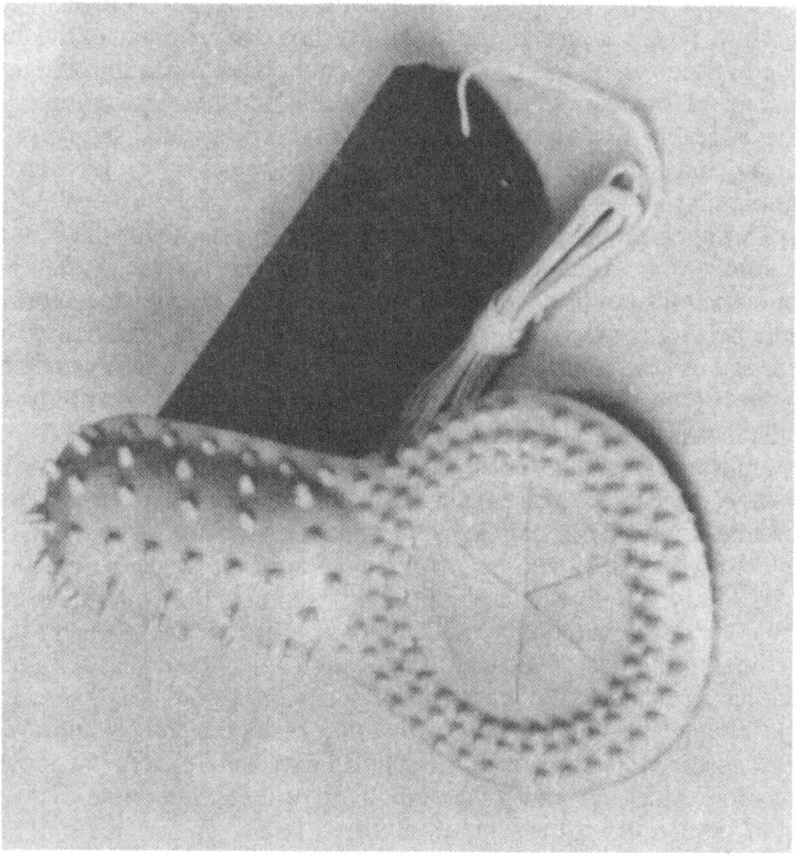

Fig. 2. The half erect penis is inserted through the aperture of the Equalizer (Erotems Inc., San Francisco, CA) to enhance the erection, while the erotic bristles directly stimulate the clitoris.

an orgasm-like reaction achieved by stimulating highly sensitive body areas while recalling and imaging previous orgasm experiences.

As a resource, the book by Mooney et al. (*8*) describes and presents pictorially the sexual options available to persons with spinal injury. These authors present the wheelchair as a site for sexual activity, and this can be considered by the couples when spontaneity and transfer problems are an issue (Fig. 3). However, Coffman's (*1*) interviewees reported that they much preferred to relate to their partners in bed, where there was the opportunity for closeness, relaxation, and physical contact in a comfortable position. Most wheelchairs are not built for two.

Preparations for sexual activities will have to be worked out by the couple to maintain some degree of spontaneity and to prevent the

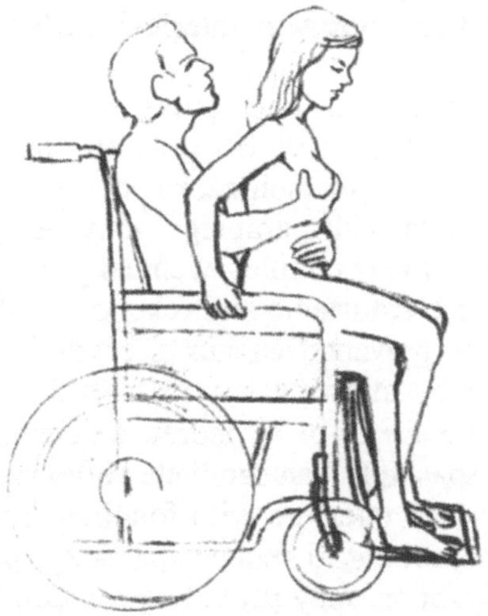

Fig. 3. Wheelchair sex is possible for the low paraplegics who are liberated. In high paraplegics (T4 lesion and above), this position may trigger unpleasant spastic episodes. Most prefer sexual activity out of the wheelchair.

preparations themselves from becoming such a chore that all of the fun disappears from the interaction. Bowel and bladder preparation need to be given special thought, since this was a major area of nuisance for Coffman's informants. If the person with spinal injury needs assistance with such matters, it can be a decided disadvantage to have the female partner assist with such procedures, because this changes the nature of the relationship in subtle, but potentially significant ways. The assistance of a third party is ideal when possible. Ordinarily, the bladder and bowel should be emptied before intercourse. However, if intercourse is not part of the couple's repertoire of sexual activities, this may not be necessary. An indwelling catheter may be doubled back on the penis and covered by a condom. This prevents traction on the catheter during thrusting and, thus, avoids bladder or urethral trauma. Collection bags and tubing should be positioned so that they are not obstructed by kinking or pressure, and so that reflux of urine into the bladder does not occur. Thus, the receptacle should be placed in a dependent position.

Men on intermittent catheterization programs should empty the bladder immediately before sexual activity. External drainage systems can be temporarily replaced by a condom, and a towel can be placed nearby in case of an accident. Men with a urinary diversion should position themselves so that the collection bag is not subject to pressure or shearing. As with all of these procedures, careful attention to cleanliness will reduce the chance that odor will interfere with the pleasure of the moment.

A variety of positions for intercourse may be tried by the couple to determine which technique works best. Persons with quadriplegia often find it preferable to lie on their back with the women in the superior position. Some persons with paraplegia may be able to assume the superior position, but many couples eventually find that the female on top may be the most comfortable and relaxing to all concerned. Caution should be taken to prevent decubitus ulcers during prolonged periods of relaxing together by allowing for occasional position changes.

Spasticity can be a help or a hindrance during sexual activity. A certain amount of spasticity can facilitate reflexogenic erections, but too much spasticity can interfere with fondling, caressing, and intercourse. Careful positioning to reduce spasticity, plus wise timing of antispasticity medications, may provide a solution to these problems. However, these medications have the potential to reduce reflexogenic erections; thus, a balance can be achieved through experience over time. Autonomic dysreflexia is a potential problem for individuals with spinal injuries at or above T4–6. Sudden diastolic hypertension; slowed heart rate, flushed, warm, moist skin of the face and upper torso; pale, cool dry skin on the remainder of the body; throbbing headaches; pupillary constriction; nasal congestion; and goose flesh may be noted. When this occurs, all activity should cease, and the head should be elevated. If symptoms persist, a full bladder or rectum may be the cause, and emptying should be accomplished as soon as possible. Medical advice should be sought if the symptoms continue or if they occur repeatedly (*2,4*).

When the male partner has a partial erection, the couple needs to determine what their individual needs are. If intromission is important to the man, the stuffing technique may be helpful in simulating the experience of intercourse for him. Few women, however, will find this to be a source of sexual satisfaction in and of itself, but usually will be happy to please the partner. Reciprocity will require the man to also be willing to engage in a variety of stimulating activities that will provide her with the opportunity to have an orgasm.

Sexual adjustment following a spinal injury may be a long-term process, and the timing of the specific activities described in this chapter will depend upon the person involved. Some will be very receptive during the initial rehabilitation program, and others may need to face the various accommodations that the disability requires over a longer period of time. Thus, the issue of timing will require skill and judgment by the therapeutic team. In any event, the issue of sexuality should be introduced during the initial inpatient rehabilitation program, and the person should be given the opportunity to become involved to the degree that he is capable at that particular time. If the couple has received sexual training while he is an inpatient, outpatient followup sessions should be scheduled to monitor progress in this area and other areas of psychosocial functioning. If the couple did not avail themselves of the opportunity to receive such training while in the hospital, the option of participating in such a program on an outpatient basis should be available.

If the man does not have a partner at the time of his contact with a sexual rehabilitation program, he should be given information regarding his disability, its impact on his sexuality, and the opportunity to become familiar with his body and its new means of functioning. The opportunity to explore his attitudes toward sexuality, his role as a man in a relationship with a woman, and his attitude toward a variety of alternative sex acts can still be available to him through the therapeutic team, so that he will serve as an educated informant to a future partner. Furthermore, it is helpful to provide the opportunity for future partners to meet with the therapeutic team to discuss any specific questions or concerns that she may have.

Conclusions

In order to implement a complete sexual rehabilitation program, the three components of sexual functioning need to be evaluated, so that the proper treatment strategies can be planned. Sex drives, sex acts, and sexuality may each be influenced by the onset of spinal-cord injury, and thus, each should be considered separately during the initial evaluation. Each of these three components of sexual functioning should be considered in terms of the primary and secondary dysfunctions that may occur—primary dysfunctions having an organic etiology and secondary dysfunctions arising from emotional, attitudinal, and learned reactions to sexual functioning. Both primary and secondary dysfunctions tend to occur initially. The primary dysfunctions may be treated; the secondary dysfunctions should always be treated. However, the essence of all treatment programs is the encouragement of a healthy, communicative, and giving relationship between two people that will provide the context for sex acts as one type of expression of love. To remove sex acts from the context of human relationships is to reduce them to subcortical expressions of drives, and to deny the neocortical components of loving, sharing, and relating.

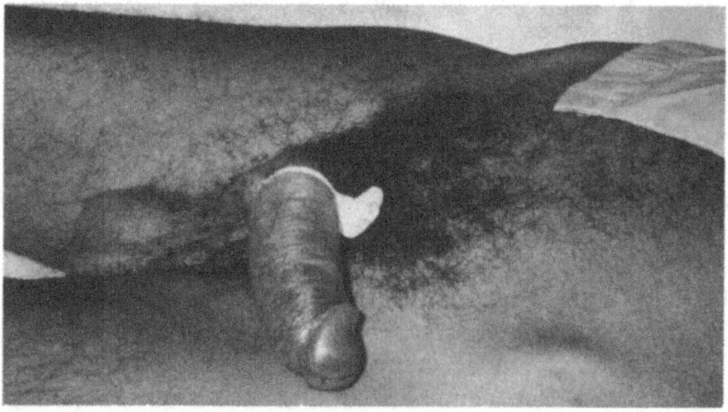

Fig. 4. Erection band: a shortened elastic leg bag strap wrapped around a half-erect penis to enhance tumescence. Commercial types are available.

Inclusion of the female partner is essential to success when a partner is available. Female partners of males with spinal injury report that they are very satisfied with their sex lives, because the male is a more attentive and responsive lover than most able-bodied men they have known. Intercourse is not the primary focus of the sexual interaction, particularly in instances in which the male has impaired erectile capacity. It should be noted that erectile capability should be defined to include ability to *obtain* and *maintain* an erection (Fig. 4) of sufficient hardness for the female partner to achieve an orgasm. Because of impairment in the duration of the erection, many couples include a variety of petting activities that produce an orgasm in the woman within the context of loving, caring communication in bed.

When a partner is not available during therapeutic contacts with the male, he should be given the opportunity to explore all dimensions of his sexuality and be given sufficient information that he can serve as an educated effective informant for his future partner. Ideally, the therapeutic team will make itself available to the future partner on an outpatient basis to help her resolve any issues that influence her relationship with the male with spinal injury.

References

1. Coffman, R. (1981) "Sexual Attitudes and Behaviors of Female Partners of Spinal Cord Injured Males." Unpublished Doctoral Dissertation, United States International University, San Diego, California.
2. Griffith, E. and Trieschmann, R. (1976) Sexual functioning in patients

with physical disorders, in *Clinical Management of Sexual Disorders* (Meyer, J., ed.) Williams and Wilkins, Baltimore.

3. Griffith, E. and Trieschmann, R. (1977) Sexual function restoration in the physically disabled: Use of a private hospital room. *Arch. Phys. Med. Rehabil.* **58**, 368-369.
4. Griffith, E. and Trieschmann, R. (1978) Use of a private hospital room in restoring sexual function to the physically disabled. *Sex. Disabil.* **1**, 179–183.
5. Griffith, E. and Trieschmann, R. (1981) Sexual training of the spinal cord injured male and his partner, in *Human Sexuality and Rehabilitation Medicine: Sexual Functioning Following Spinal Cord Injury* (Sha'Ked, ed.) Williams and Wilkins, Baltimore.
6. Hohmann, G. (1966) Some effects of spinal cord lesions on experienced emotional feelings. *Psychophysiology* **3**, 143–156.
7. Hohmann, G. (1972) Considerations in management of psychosexual re-adjustment in the cord injured male. *Rehabil. Psychol.* **19**, 50–58.
8. Mooney, T., Cole, T., and Chilgren, R. (1975) *Sexual Options for Paraplegics and Quadriplegics.* Little, Brown, and Company, Boston.
9. Trieschmann, R. (1987) *Aging with a Disability.* Demos Publications, New York.
10. Trieschmann, R. (1988) *Spinal Cord Injuries: Psychological, Social, and Vocational Rehabilitation* (Second Edition), Demos Publications, New York.

19

Surgical Treatment of Impotence

Prostheses for Sexual Enhancement

Jose Florante J. Leyson

Introduction

The loss of sensory and motor functions below the level of a spinal cord injury is both life-threatening and depressing to the patient. As he realizes, natural body functions may never or only partially return, and the psyche may then feel the true impact of the extent of physical and psychological trauma. Loss of sexual function is devastating to the "macho" image of the sexually active male and, at times, may affect his total postinjury rehabilitation (*6*). Those who may luckily have sustained only incomplete lesions or who have recovered fully probably need only sex counseling or therapy for their erectile impotence. However, for those patients, with stable relationships who have unfortunately sustained complete lesions and who have ineffective (i.e., less rigid, quick and random) reflexostimulative erections and who want penile–vaginal intercourse, penile prosthesis implantation can be suggested. However, before a penile prosthesis—either a solid or inflatable one—can be implanted, the patient must be given a comprehensive presurgical examination and evaluation.

Selection of Candidates

The detailed evaluation of candidates for surgery has been discussed previously. However, the patient's sexual partner must agree, in prin-

Sexual Rehabilitation of the Spinal-Cord-Injured Patient
Edited by J.F. Leyson, © 1990 The Humana Press, Inc.

ciple, to the surgery, too. The patient's decision to undergo the surgery surely should not conflict with his religious and sexual values; some Jewish men, for instance, are not permitted to have artificial devices or sex prostheses implanted in their bodies. The selection of candidates for surgical penile prosthesis implantation frequently requires a team approach that involves many medical specialities, including sexologists, urologists, psychologists, and psychiatrists (*2*).

History and Physical–Sexological Evaluation: General Medical and Sexual History

It is vital to elicit a premorbid and surgical history (*6*). Are there associated pre-SCI diseases, the presence or absence of hypertension, diabetes mellitus, cardiovascular problems, arthritis, malignancy, or immune deficiency syndromes? The use of antihypertensive agents or of some cardiac and psychiatric medications can put a damper on already recovering sexual functions. Uncontrolled diabetes mellitus is known to aggravate neurologically impaired posttraumatic erectile impotence. Any extensive vascular preinjury as well as cancer surgery and myelographic (spinal) diagnostic procedures, may add more neurovascular insult to the already compromised compensatory system of the SCI patient. Drug addiction and alcoholism prior to injury (sometimes continued post-SCI) are also detrimental to full or even partial sexual recovery.

The patient's sexual history must include his personal marital status and sexual values (*2,6*). If he is comfortable with oral sex, sex therapy usually is sufficient and a sex (penile) prosthesis is only a last resort. The patient's interpersonal relationships must also be evaluated. It has been suggested that patients who want a penile prosthesis should have a steady (stable) sexual partner. A sexological examination consists of a neurological examination of the sex organ's comparative oral–intraurethral temperature. This offers a significant collaborative index to duplex doppler vascular examination in determining penile blood flow in men with suspected vascular insufficiency (*7*). A more invasive method entails penile injection of papaverine, with ultrasonographic (doppler) vascular evaluation. Penile and perineal sensations, as well as rectal and bulbocavernosus reflexes, must be known in order to delineate the level of SCI lesions; thus, the type of erectile and bladder dysfunctions can be determined.

Urologic Evaluation

The urologist plays a crucial role in the evaluation of prospective surgical candidates, interviewing the patient, performing the indicated physical examinations, and conducting any special examination the patient's history suggests may be needed. Patients with SCI have special problems that may influence the outcome of the surgery. Since the incidence of renal deterioration in SCI patients is well known, both the upper and lower urinary tracts of these patients must be evaluated prior to surgery. As noted in the later discussion of the inflatable penile prosthesis, the method of urinary drainage employed is also important. Patients on a program of successful intermittent self-catheterization do not require an extensive lower urinary tract evaluation because the device is compatible with this form of bladder drainage. If an external type of condom (catheter) is used, urodynamic evaluation is important to exclude significant bladder outlet obstruction, the most common type of which is detrusor-sphincter dyssynergia. This voiding dysfunction must be corrected before any type of penile prosthesis is implanted (in pairs), because incoordination between the urinary bladder and urethral sphincters causes significantly high residual urines. Prolonged use of an indwelling urethral catheter may also cause urethral erosion as a result of pressure necrosis. The presence of a chronic (permanent) indwelling urethral catheter, even for as long as 10 yr, is regarded as a "relative" contraindication to the surgery because of the high risk of infection, whereas a vesicostomy or suprapubic tube puts the patient at an even higher risk of infection because of the associated chronic bacteriuria. It must be stressed that any urinary outlet obstruction (anatomic or neuropathic) should be corrected before implant surgery is contemplated.

The infrapubic, penoscrotal or perineal approaches are ideal for these situations. Prior to surgery, like any other genitourinary prosthesis, the patient's urine must be sterile, and since bacteriuria is common among these patients, urinary cultures are required for antibiotic sensitivity studies and treatment. Antibiotic treatments are started on an outpatient basis, if possible, but it may sometimes be necessary to admit the patient to the hospital a few days before surgery to administer antimicrobial agents intravenously in order to be certain of sterile urine, and to carry out final preoperative sexo-urological evaluations.

The urologist also checks the patient's dexterity to ensure that he will be able to manipulate the solid (Jonas) malleable or uninflatable (Omniphase) (Fig. 1F) penile prosthesis. If the patient is unable to per-

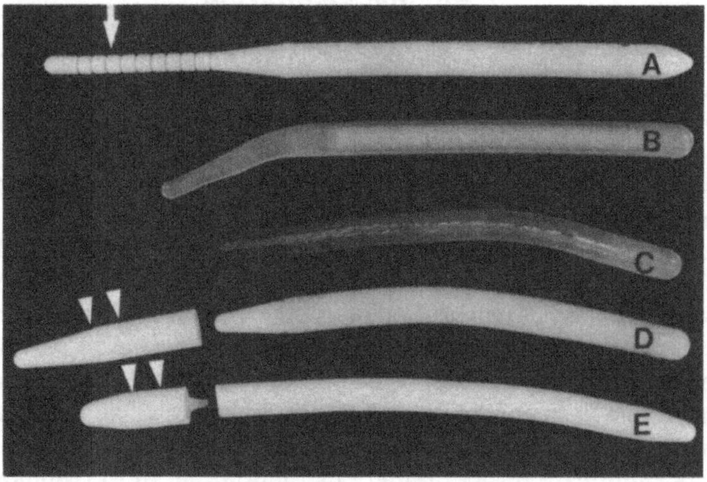

Fig. 1. Five different types of solid penile prostheses. (A) Flexirod—has calibrated grid (arrow) so that it can be trimmed to a perfect fit; (B) Small-Carrion (semirigid); (C) Jonas; (D) AMS-600; and (E) Mentor, which have rear tip extenders (arrows) for an intraoperative length fitting.

form the necessary tasks, his spouse or partner will need to learn the techniques; this has in fact been necessary in some of our cases.

The patient's expectations relative to the penile prosthesis are also discussed with him. Since most patients have some residual degree of tumescence, they must be made to realize that, after the operation, significant natural erection may no longer be possible. In addition, the inflatable, but not the solid, prostheses (a pair) will inflate only the shaft of the penis, and not the glans. However, the surgery will not significantly interfere with tumescence of the glans, if it were present preoperatively. It is possible that some degree of insignificant "natural tumescence" may occur postoperatively, once the device is in place.

The solid prosthesis and the surgery used to implant it will in no way add to the neurological lesion already present. Penile skin, in particular, is not altered by the operation and neither is bladder sensation. However, the glans penis may lose its sensation of warmth, especially with solid prostheses. As in the case of the inflatable type, the ability to achieve orgasm and ejaculation is related primarily to the underlying neurologic lesion and will not be influenced by the presence of a solid prosthesis. In patients with poor penile sensation, the infrapubic approach should be avoided, for this incision may injure the dorsal penile sensory nerves. Penile anesthesia post-op can be improved by oral dopamine (Levodopa) at 1.5–2 Gm/d for 3–4 wk, with a rest period every two months for up to 10 months (*11*).

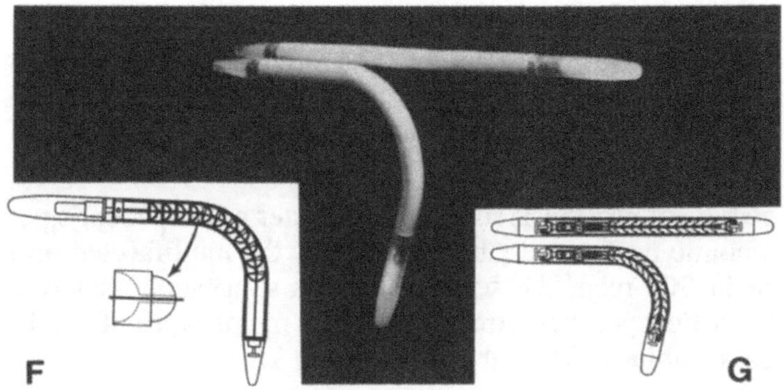

Fig. 1F,G. Omniphase (center picture) The straight prosthesis is in a rigid state, and once bent; the other (below) is in a flaccid natural position. The inset (left) shows the cross-section, which reveals articulated joints (a series of cup-like mechanisms) that temporarily lock when bent, and can maintain such a state until it is bent again to change its position or state. The inset (right) is the cross-section of the Duraphase [same external appearance as the Omniphase (F)] with a series of spring-like mechanisms for bending to switch from one position to another (G).

Psycho-Psychiatric Evalautions

The urologist will request psychological and psychiatric testings if he or she finds them necessary, as prescribed in the section on inflatable penile prostheses (*3*). If a relevant relationship or marital problem is detected, it should be communicated to the implant surgeon for sex or marital discussion and counseling. No patient with an absolute psychiatric contraindication to the operation should be accepted for penile prosthesis implantation (*2,3*).

Special Diagnostic Tests

Because it has been shown that most impotence in SCI men is neurogenic in etiology (*5*), duplex doppler penile examinations are reserved only for those with suspected vascular problems. Spinal evoked potentials and electromyographic examinations may have a place in the evaluation of patients with incomplete or new occult cord lesions. Nocturnal penile tumescence and rigidity monitoring have been accepted as diagnostic aids in differentiating between the organic and psychogenic causes of impotence. Patients with SCI, especially those with minimal lesions, are not immune to depression with its concomitant interference in penile tumescence/rigidity. The papaverine (chemoerection) test, accompanied by cavernosography and cavernosometry to rule out venous leaks, is discussed elsewhere.

Solid Penile (Sex) Prosthesis

The type of prosthesis selected is a matter of the patient's personal and economic preferences, but because of the multifaceted problems inherent in SCI men, the sexo-urologist's suggestion usually counts heavily. In Europe, there are two or three major types of solid penile prostheses, while in USA there are seven kinds:

- (A) Flexible (Fig. 1 A & B) (hinged or semirigid)
  - (1) Small—Carrion, which is the least flexible
  - (2) Finney (Flexirod I and II) which are more flexible
- (B) Malleable (Fig. 1 C-G)
  - (1) Jonas
  - (2) American Medical Systems—AMS 600
  - (3) Mentor
  - (4) Duraphase (positional)
  - (5) Omniphase* (mechanically activated)

All prostheses are made of silicone (elastomer), which is an inert (nonreactive) material to human tissue. Both the Small-Carrion and the Finney prostheses are pure elastomer and cost up to $1200 a pair. On the other hand, the malleable types contain: a center core of memory silver wire (Jonas and Mentor); stainless steel in AMS 600; a series of springs in the Duraphase; and (Omniphase) interlocking cups mechanisms that enable the patients to bend their prostheses in different directions. These types cost up to $1800. The malleable prostheses provide excellent rigidity and a flaccid appearance. The Duraphase and Omniphase sex prostheses adjust or revert from the flaccid to the rigid state through a unique "on/off switch" technique. The patient's functional hands or partner simply bends the prostheses until a click is felt. Bend once, and

*Photos courtesy of: Small-Carrion prosthesis—Am. Med. Systems, Minnetonka, MN 55343; Flexi-rod—Surgitek, Racine, Wisconsin 53404; Jonas—Dacomed, Minn., MN 55420; AMS-600—American Med. Systems, Minnetonka, MN 55345, Mentor—Mentor Corp., Goleta, CA 93117; Omniphase—Dacomed, Minn., MN, and Duraphase (Dacomed).

the device is rigid. Bend again, and the prostheses relax into an extremely natural flaccid position. This Duraphase remarkable new biotechnology gives a result like that of a hydraulic-type prostheses with lower cost (less $1000) and a simpler surgical procedure. The inflatable prostheses with extra penile reservoir and pump usually cost up to $4200 per set and a high surgeon's fee, because it takes more than an hour to implant such an erection device. The utilization of a single solid penile prosthesis (instead of two) for sufficient vaginal penetration is an accidental episode, for the patient refused replacement of the extruded pair. However, in India and in some economically depressed countries, the use of single solid sex prosthesis for financial or austerity reasons has proven effective. The Dept. of Veterans Affairs Medical Centers rarely provide the inflatable type because of its cost, and only service-connected veterans are given the option to have a sex prosthesis implanted for organic impotence.

The purpose of penile prostheses is twofold: (a) treatment for organic impotence and (b) to lengthen the penile shaft so that an external urinary condom can be applied securely. Preoperative patient preparations include bowel care, perineal or genitalia scrubbing with Betadine, and sometimes application of antifungal solutions to the groin. As emphasized previously, urine must be sterile for at least 3 d prior to surgery and any urinary outlet obstruction corrected at least a month preoperatively. Lymphedema of the external genitalia (Fig. 2) should be surgically and cosmetically corrected before the prosthesis is implanted. It is also advised that sexual intercourse (celebration) be postponed for 6–8 wk postoperatively because of the need for compromised tissue to heal.

There are several surgical approaches to the implant procedure (Fig. 3). However, the author's clinical experience dictates that the subpubic (infrapubic) and perineal approaches are ideal. The suprapubic route is not suitable for SCI men, because of adhesions from previous trauma, surgery (cystotomy), and the chronic infections associated with urinary and bowel dysfunctions. Other surgical incisions are not advisable, especially in patients who wear an external urinary condom. Repeated condom applications and the use of adhesives to secure the condom irritate the postoperative scar, and can cause deep tissue infections or superficial bleeding. Also, if the penile prosthesis scar is constantly bathed with urine in the condom, the old scar may become infected and scar dehiscence may subsequently occur.

The paired penile prostheses are inserted into both corpora cavernosa (Fig. 4), with the tips situated about one-third beyond the coronal sulcus (groove) (Fig. 5A1). Other prostheses locations are not advised because they are fraught with complications (Fig. 5). Since the sub-

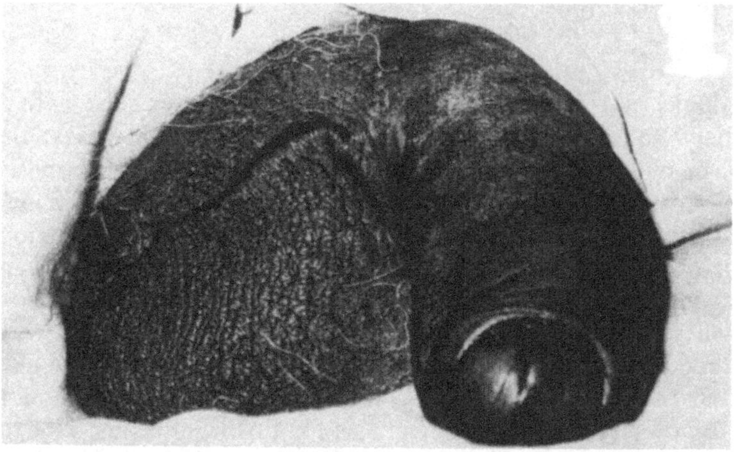

Fig. 2. A 56-yr-old diabetic, paraplegic male suffering post-irradiation swelling of the penis and scrotum from cancer of the prostate.

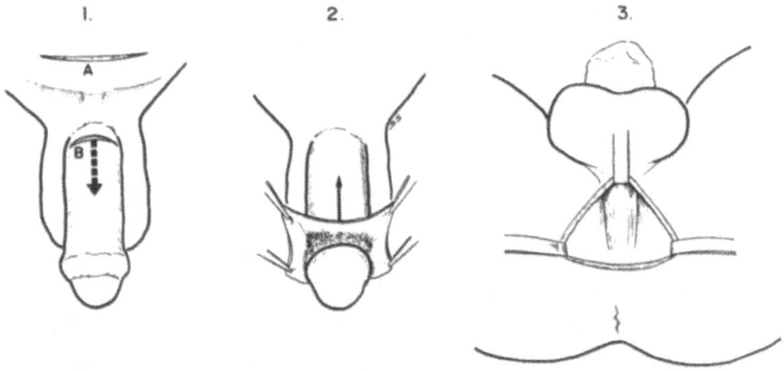

Fig. 3. Four different surgical incisions for penile prosthesis implantation. (1a) Suprapublic; (1b) penile; (2) coronal; (3) perineal. Not shown are the penoscrotal and infrapublic (subpubic) incisions, in which the latter is 2–2.5 fingerbreadths below the suprapubic approach.

pubic and perineal scars are away from the penile shaft, they are preferred. However, the SCI Health Team is aware that contamination of the perineal incision by feces postoperatively must be avoided for at least 2 wks. Consequently, an indwelling catheter must remain in place for at least 5–8 ds because postoperative edema sometimes impedes a good urethral flow, and application of a condom is difficult. The average hospital stay is 7–10 ds, and again it is advised that intercourse not be allowed for at least 6–8 wk postoperatively, because of poor tissue healing (5)*.

*Ed note: The risk factors that may lead the prostheses to erode into the bowel, bladder, and even groin are: prior radiation, neuropathic bladder and multiple operators, and associated metabolic diseases.

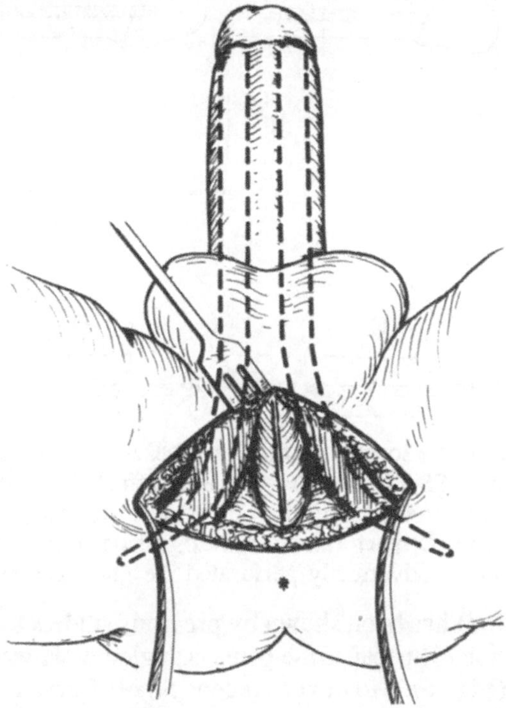

Fig. 4. Anatomical position of the penile prosthesis inside both corpora cavernosa (perineal insertion).

Results

One hundred and twenty SCI patients have undergone prostheses implantations. These patients range in age from 31 to 58 yr old, and 100 were paraplegic, whereas 20 were quadriplegic. Four of the 100 paraplegics have adult-onset diabetes, and one of the 20 quadriplegics had a repeat implantation. All patients have had their prostheses for the last 10–14 yrs.

Results are considered successful in 118 of these patients, meaning that sexual intercourse is satisfactory and partner acceptance is good. However, sexual partners who did not attend the postsurgery counseling sessions complained of dyspareunia (*5*). Both the Small-Carrion and the Finney prostheses were ideal for all patients, including those with no hand grasp, whether this condition was caused by either the cord injury itself or by associated arthritis. The malleable prostheses were well accepted and desired by young paraplegics who could play with them, bending them to desired angles or directions. The Finney pros-

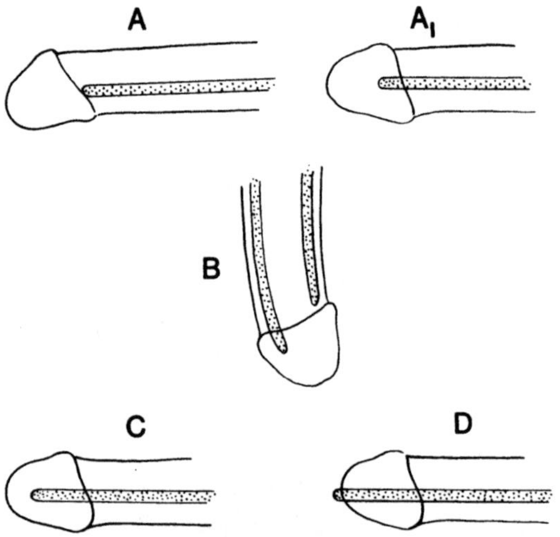

Fig. 5. Various tip locations of the prostheses. (A) Prosthesis length too short, producing an SST (concorde) "bending effect;" (A1) Proper tip location; (B) asymetrical prosthesis length, producing a lateral angulation; (C) prosthesis too long; and (D) perforated prosthesis (aside from being a long prosthesis, the surgeon inadvertently perforated the glans penis).

thesis (Flexi-Rod) has been shown by previous studies to be better than the Small-Carrion (*5*) because the penis is angled downward, facilitating urinary flow (Fig. 6). However, recent Small-Carrion modifications have made this prosthesis more flexible, and condom urinary drainage is almost similar to that of the Finney-type prosthesis or any of the malleable types. Overall success is 98% for sexual satisfaction and 90% for adequate condom application.

Two of the patients' wives complained that their husbands have become "sex maniacs" because they demand sex even at inappropriate moments. Two patients, one a paraplegic and the other a quadriplegic, have elected to insert an indwelling Foley catheter 6 mo postimplantation; their condom catheters kept slipping off because both patients are obese and have protruding abdomens*. The penis retracts even with an adequately implanted prosthesis. Repeated postoperative sex counseling resolved most of the above problems. Among the paraplegics studied, most preferred the inflatable prosthesis, but economic reasons and the fear of repeated surgery caused many of them to select the solid penile prosthesis. It must be stressed that a 12–18 mo postinjury waiting (adjustment) period with sex therapy is advisable before a prosthesis is implanted. Meanwhile, sex counseling/therapy should be tried in conjunction with other medical treatment options.

---

*Ed. note: In order to achieve extra penile length in patients with short penises, it is suggested to cut the penile ligament and partially detach the proximal crux of the penis from the pubic bone. A modified Z-plasty of the peno-scrotal skin may also help.

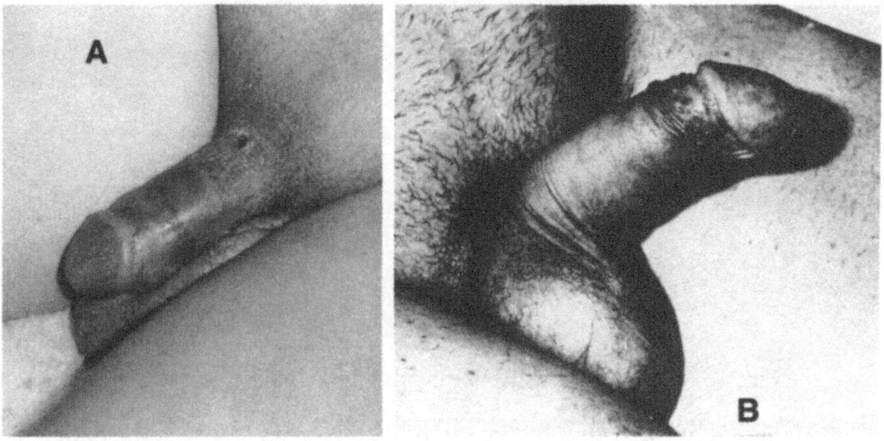

Fig. 6. (A) A quadriplegic male with a Finney (flexible) prosthesis. Note that the angle formed is less than 10 degrees and urine flows with ease. (B) Another SCI patient with a small-Carrion prosthesis whose angle is about 25 degrees and here urine must flow against gravity.

Intrapenile-Self Contained (Inflatable) Penile Prostheses

Self-contained (no extrapenile connections) sex prostheses are implanted in the whole corpora of the penis with pump-reservoir devices. The paraplegic or sexual partner can squeeze the proximal part (glans penis) of the prostheses to inflate the device. To deflate the prostheses, the operator should bend the whole device downward, by cradling the device with his/her hand. The two most popular types are the SurgiTek and AMS. There are reports that the SurgiTek devices can accidentally deflate with vigorous penile thrusting is done in a tight and dry vaginal introitus. However, the AMS (American Medical Systems) seem to withstand this bending or tort forces (see Chapter 20, Fig. 4).

Postoperative Complications

Of the 85 SCI men who have some sensory penile recovery, three complained that the warmth of the glans penis is gone. An empathetic

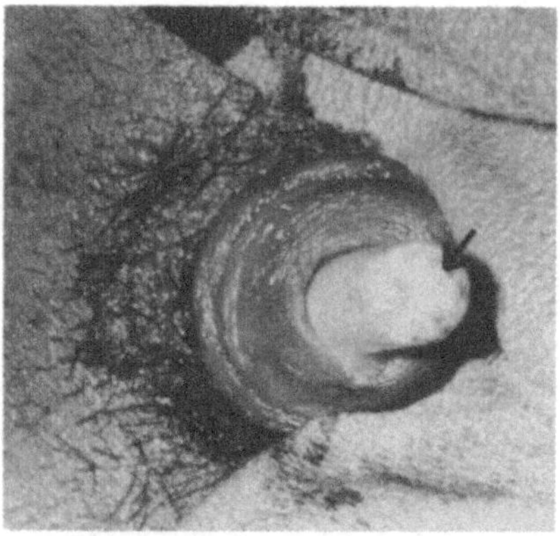

Fig. 7. A flexible prosthesis protruding through the glans penis.

explanation of the pathophysiology of the problem resolved the patients' sexual concerns and anxiety. One of the quadriplegic patients achieved "sexual celebration" less than 4 wks postop, which resulted in extrusion of one of his pair of prostheses (Fig. 7). Further evaluation showed that the diameter of the prosthesis was too large, and 3 mos later, reimplantation of a smaller caliber prosthesis resulted in complete success. With the malleable and Finney type prostheses it is not important to conceal the penis. However, the older type of Small-Carrion prosthesis presents minor problems, especially to those who experience spasms.

The infection rate in the above series was 4% while other surgeons reported up to 7% (*12*). The infections were mild, and a loss of six prostheses occurred. An additional 5 d of antibiotic therapy (total 15–20 d postop) eventually resolved the infection uneventfully. Although it is believed that a chronic indwelling catheter is a contraindication to penile prosthesis, data from the East Orange VA Medical Center in New Jersey showed that it is only a relative one (*5*). Five quadriplegics who had indwelling catheters for 10 yr were free of them after urinary rehabilitation and prostheses implantation. However, they have occasionally complained of penoscrotal discomfort and recurrent exacerbations of "abacteric" prostatitis. These patients responded to "Cipro" and Norfloxacin. Five of the patients—two high paraplegics and three quadriplegics—had repeat sphincterotomies for urinary bladder outlet obstructions. By gently pushing the prostheses toward the pelvis, TUR surgeries were no problem, even with a regular length resectoscope. The following protocol is suggested in managing infected penile prostheses:

(1) Remove the infected components thru the eroded site

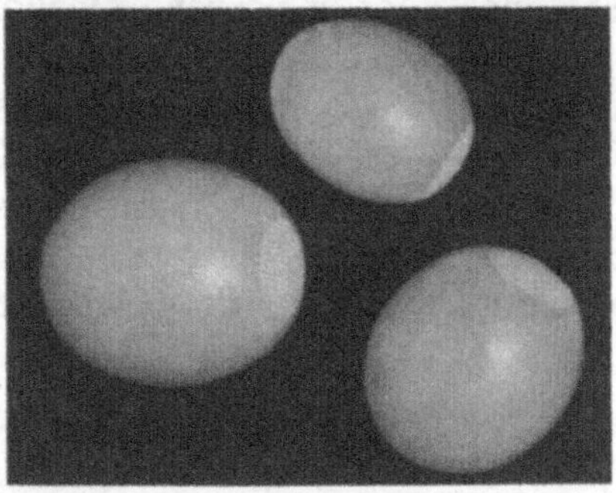

Fig. 8. Three different sizes of silicone testicular prostheses with reinforced (netted) tops so that the anchoring sutures will not inadvertently perforate the main body. Courtesy of Mentor Corp., Goleta, CA 93117.

(2) Divert the urine with an indwelling Foley catheter or suprapubic tube
(3) Consider placing drains (for deep infection) and irrigate wounds with antibiotics
(4) Appropriate antibiotics should be used for 2½ wk
(5) Reimplant in 3 months for superficial and 9–12 months for deep infections (use smaller caliber prostheses).

Testicular Prosthesis

In some cultures, the presence or absence of the testes (scrotum) determines one's virility. In four SCI paraplegic men who were found to have one testis, none noticed a preinjury sexual problem. In most cases, the absent testis had been removed surgically following chronic postinjury infection, whereas one patient had testicular atrophy and another had cryptorchid testis. All except two patients had a testicular prosthesis (Fig. 8) implanted for psychological and cosmetic reasons.* So far, no complications have been reported after 12 years followup.

Conclusion

There are several therapeutic options in the management of post-SCI sexual dysfunctions. However, if one is an ideal candidate for a penile (sexuality) prosthesis, it is advisable that a solid type should be

*Ed note: In patients with undeveloped or contracted scrotum, the use of tissue expanders can aid in enlarging the scrotal sac to accomodate a testicular prosthesis via a suprapubic approach.

implanted in patients with poor or no hand function at all. It is suggested that sexuality prostheses can be re-implanted in SCI men for up to 4 times in the absence of the following conditions: (1) metabolic or associated disabling cardio-respiratory diseases; (2) recurrent deep (cavernosal) infections; (3) severe cavernosal fibrosis and/or defects; (4) lower urological tract anomalies, obstructions, and/or diseases; and (5) psychiatric–marital disorders and drug dependency.

References

1. Divita, E. C. and Olsson, P. A. (1975) The use of sex therapy in a patient with a penile prosthesis. *J. Sex Marital Ther.* **1**, 305–311.
2. Butler, L. E., Karacan, K., and Ware, C. (1978) Psychological assessment of sexually impotent men, in *Sleep Disorders: Diagnoses and Treatment* Karacan, I. and Williams, R. L., eds.) Wiley, New York, pp. 383–394.
3. Byrd, G. (1978) Preoperative psychiatric evaluation, in *Sleep Disorders: Diagnosis and Treatment* (Karacan, I. and Williams, R. L., eds.) Wiley, New York, pp. 395–399.
4. Karacan, I., Scott, F. B., and Salis, P. J. (1977) Nocturnal erections, differential diagnosis of impotence and diabetes. *Biol. Psych.* **12**, 373–379.
5. Leyson, J. F. J. (1979) Solid penile prostheses and dyspareunia in spinal cord injury patients. Presented at 12th National Sex Institute, Wash., DC, April 4–8.
6. Leyson, J. F. J., and Powell, R. (1984) Evaluation of candidates for the surgical treatment of erectile dysfunction. *Sexual Med. Today* **18**, 12–16.
7. Leyson, J. F. J., and Scalera, J. (1983) Penile temperature recordings in the diagnosis of impotence in spinal cord injured men. Read at the F. C. Valentine Urology Contest, AUA New York Section, NY, April 6.
8. Light, J. F., and Scott, F. B. (1981) Management of neurogenic impotence with inflatable penile prosthesis. *Urol.* **17**, 341–345.
9. Scott, F. B., Light, J. K., and Fishman, I. J. (1982) Treatment of impotence caused by cancer therapy—the inflatable penile prosthesis. *Cancer Bulletin* **34**, 33–36.
10. Scott, F. B., Light, J. K., Fishman, I. J., and West, J. (1981) The artificial urinary sphincter. *Contemporary Surg.* **18**, 11–14, 16–25.
11. Leyson, J. F. J. (1988) Sex Odyssey 2001. Presented at the annual meeting of the Assoc. of Philippine physicians in America, Long Beach, CA, July 26–31.
12. Collins, K., and Hackler, R. (1988) Complications of penile prostheses in the spinal cord injury population. *J. Urology* **140**, 984–985.

Mentor testicular prostheses. Mentor Corp., Goleta, CA 93117.

20
Surgical Treatment of Impotence

Therapeutic Options and Prostheses for Sexo-Urological Comfort

Jeffrey L. Marks and J. Keith Light

Introduction

The personal and social implications of spinal cord injury are far reaching. The initial post-injury period frequently involves life-saving procedures because of the associated injuries. This is followed by a period of recovery that may last 18 months or longer. Once the full impact of the lesion is understood, numerous adjustments become necessary. Two important aspects that may have a significant effect on the rehabilitation of the patient are the sexual and bladder dysfunctions that invariably accompany this injury. Significant advances have been made during the last decade in treating problems of incontinence, impotence, and infertility. Pharmacological manipulation for both bladder and erectile dysfunction, together with mechanical improvements in the field of prosthetics, have demonstrated that urological intervention can play an important role in the rehabilitation of these patients.

Neuropathic Erectile Dysfunction

The degree of residual erectile dysfunction varies according to the level and completeness of the spinal cord lesion. Some patients may obtain sufficient recovery to be able to function normally. Others may

Sexual Rehabilitation of the Spinal-Cord-Injured Patient
Edited by J.F. Leyson, © 1990 The Humana Press, Inc.

respond to sex counseling for the erectile dysfunction. Generally speaking, most male patients experience some degree of erectile dysfunction consisting of either short duration of erection, poor rigidity, or both. These erections are usually reflex in character and often random. There is, therefore, a group of patients who will greatly benefit from urological intervention.

Evaluation

History and Physical

The urologist plays a crucial role in evaluating patients for the medical or surgical treatment of impotence. Patients with spinal-cord injuries have special problems that may influence the outcome of this treatment. The potential for renal deterioration is well known in these patients, and it is necessary to evaluate both the upper and lower urinary tracts in selected patients prior to surgery. The method of urinary drainage is important. The patient on successful intermittent self-catheterization does not require an extensive lower urinary tract evaluation since a penile prosthesis is compatible with this means of bladder drainage. If an external type of catheter is used, however, urodynamic evaluation is important to exclude any significant bladder outflow obstruction, the most common being detrusor-sphincter dyssynergia. This type of voiding dysfunction may require correction prior to implantation of a penile prosthesis as prolonged use of an indwelling urethral catheter following prosthetic surgery can produce urethral erosion from pressure necrosis. The presence of a permanent urethral catheter is regarded as a contraindication to the surgery because of the high risk of infection. A vesicostomy or a suprapubic tube places the patient at a higher risk for infection of any prosthesis because of the associated bacteriuria and potential contamination of the surgical field. Bacteriuria is common in this population group, and a urine culture is necessary to determine antibiotic selection for preoperative treatment.

The urologist also examines the dexterity of the patient in order to ensure that no problems will be experienced postoperatively in relation to manipulation of the penile prosthesis. Inflation of the device requires the ability to appose the thumb and forefinger while at the same time preventing displacement of the pump. If the patient is unable to perform this maneuver, his partner will have to learn the technique. This has been necessary with some patients, particularly those with cervical injuries.

The prosthesis or the surgery to insert the device will in no way add to the neurological lesion. In particular, penile skin and bladder sensation are not altered by the surgery. The ability to achieve orgasm and ejaculation is related primarily to the underlying neurological lesion and will not be influenced by the presence of the prosthesis.

Psychiatric Evaluation

Selected patients are referred for psychiatric evaluation (*1*). The interview is conducted in order to determine the patient's mental stability and his ability to adapt to a new form of treatment. If possible, the patient's sexual partner is also interviewed simultaneously. This is designed to detect relevant marital discord which, if present, is then communicated to the surgeon for further discussion with the couple. No patient with a psychiatric contraindication to the operation is accepted for surgery.

Psychological Testing

Though not commonly employed, this may be obtained by a urologist if deemed necessary (2). The commonest test is the MMPI, which is designed to disclose potential problems in four performance areas: (1) mental efficiency, (2) emotional stability, (3) interpersonal compatibility, and (4) susceptibility to performance anxiety. Ordinarily, the psychologist does not see the patient, but if this screening raises the possibility of serious problems, the patient may be referred for a more intense psychological evaluation at the surgeon's discretion.

Intracavernosal Injections of Vasoactive Drugs

A new method for the investigation and treatment of impotence was introduced in 1983. Brindley demonstrated that injection of vasoactive drugs into the corpus cavernosum produced a sustained erection (*3*). These drugs act directly on the smooth muscle of the erectile tissue, thus bypassing the normal cavernosal nerve stimulation required to initiate the vascular response.

The response to vasoactive drugs varies according to the etiology of the erectile dysfunction. Patients with spinal-cord injury generally have an excellent response (i.e., normal erection) to injection of vasoactive substances as they are young without significant vascular disease. Patients with vasculogenic impotence may have a varied response, depending on the severity of the vascular disease. A normal erection of short duration is suggestive of a venous leak. Patients with psychogenic erectile dysfunction generally have a good response with the development of a normal erection. Severe anxiety however may partially inhibit the response because the increased quantity of circulating catecholamines and the resultant stimulatory effect on the smooth muscle of the penile vasculature prevents vasodilation. The injection of a vasoactive substance may therefore aid in differentiating neurogenic from psychogenic impotence. A poor response requires further evaluation with cavernosometry, cavernosography, and Doppler studies of the penile arteries.

The most commonly used vasoactive substances in the US are papaverine hydrochloride, a smooth muscle relaxant, and phentolamine mesylate, an alpha-adrenergic blocking agent. These two drugs are frequently used in combination (*4*).

Since patients with neuropathic erectile dysfunction are extraordinarily sensitive to the drugs, low doses should initially be given to avoid a prolonged response.

The papaverine/phentolamine combination is prepared by mixing 5 mg of phentolamine in 10 mL of papaverine (30 mg/mL). This solution is stable for up to 40 d (*5*). The initial dose in these patients should not be greater than 0.25 mL. This is then gradually increased until a response of 1–2 h is obtained. Should priapism occur (persistent erection beyond 4 h), treatment with intracavernosal injections of ephedrine at a dose of 25 mg in 10 mL of normal saline becomes necessary.

As noted by Lue and Tanagho, there are currently six groups of medications that possess smooth-muscle-relaxation properties and are capable of inducing penile erections when injected intracorporeally (*6*). These include smooth muscle relaxants, alpha-blockers, calcium channel blockers, prostaglandins, beta-agonists, and antipsychotic agents such as thorazine.

Nocturnal Penile Tumescence

With the advent of intracavernosal injection of vasoactive drugs to assess erectile function, sleep tumescence studies are no longer routinely performed. In addition, patients with spinal-cord injury have a definite reason for erectile dysfunction (*7*). These patients, however, are not immune to depression with resultant erectile dysfunction. If there is any doubt that the erectile dysfunction is unrelated to the spinal-cord injury, sleep tumescence studies are obtained. These studies have evolved to the point where machines, such as the Rigiscan, can be used by the patient at home. The advantage of the Rigiscan is that both penile tumescence and rigidity are measured (*8*).

Treatment

Suction Erectile Devices

One option for the treatment of erectile dysfunction in the spinal cord injured patient is the vacuum device. There are currently several types available. The basic design is a cylinder that is placed over the penis to create a vacuum. This draws blood into the penis, which then becomes engorged. A constricting ring is placed around the base of the penis to maintain tumescence. The overall satisfaction with this device has been reported to be 80% (*9*). Prolonged compression at the base of the penis however may cause tissue necrosis if the constricting ring is left in place for a lengthy period. A detailed discussion of this device can be found in the last chapter.

Injection of Vasoactive Substances

The success rate with the long-term injection of vasoactive substances has been reported to be 84% (*10*). However, this method of treatment does have potential complications. The most important is cavernosal fibrosis, reported in 4% of patients treated by Zorgniotti and associates (*11*). Levine and associates found in a prospective study that 57% of patients developed palpable nodules at the site of injections after 12 mo. Forty percent of these patients had at least one abnormal liver function test (*12*). There is also the potential for patients to exceed the recommended dosage and frequency of the injections. The latter is 2–3 times/wk. Further, the long-term side effects of this medication are not yet fully recognized.

More recently, intracavernosal injection of prostaglandin E_1 has been used (*13*). Prostaglandin E_1 reacts directly on the smooth muscle of the corpus cavernosum, causing relaxation. Most of the drug is metabolized during a single passage through the lungs. No priapism occurred in a recent series of 135 patients treated with prostaglandin E_1 (*13*). A functional erection resulted in 95% of the patients with neurogenic impotence, but some non-neuropathic patients noted pain during the erection. For a complete discussion, please refer to the last chapter.

Penile Prosthesis (Inflatable Types—Extrapenile)

The introduction of the inflatable penile prosthesis in 1973 resulted in a surgical means of treating erectile dysfunction (*14*). The penile prosthesis creates an artificial erection and provides satisfactory cavernosal rigidity and good glandular support. The surgical technique has previously been described in detail (*15*).

There are several varieties of inflatable penile prosthesis in current use. It is beyond the scope of this chapter to discuss all of these. Only the AMS700 and the Mentor G.F.S. will be discussed. The reader is referred to the literature for details on some of the other devices (*16–18*).

Scott, Bradley, and Timm introduced the first three-piece inflatable prosthesis in 1973 (*14*). Since that time, numerous mechanial improvements have been made, resulting in the current device, the AMS700 (Fig. 1).

The annual revision rate for mechanical failure of the inflatable penile prosthesis was 75% in 1975, 15% in 1978, and 1–2% in 1985. The most significant improvements in the AMS700 inflatable penile prosthesis were introduced in 1983 with the introduction of the AMS700 CX cylinders. These cylinders provided controlled expansion, thereby eliminating the complication of aneurysmal dilatation of the corporeal bodies.

A total of 263 patients have had insertion of the AMS700 with CX cylinders by this author from July 1984 to the present. Only three patients have required revision for a cylinder leak to date. Survival time of the device, as computed from a life table analysis of this data yield a 4-yr survival rate of 98% for the device. No patient developed aneurysmal dilatation of the cylinder, thus eliminating a complication that was particularly common in patients with spinal-cord injury.

A two-piece inflatable penile prosthesis was introduced by the Mentor Corporation in 1986. The Mentor G.F.S. prosthesis was constructed from polyurethane, a biocompatible polymer that is reportedly more durable and less elastic than the silicone rubber which is utilized in the AMS700 penile prosthesis. The Mentor G.F.S. prosthesis utilizes a resipump, in which the pump and reservoir are both contained in a single unit which is implanted in the scrotum. This simplifies the surgical procedure by avoiding any retropubic placement of a reservoir.

The author has inserted a total of 20 Mentor G.F.S. penile prostheses. These include three Mark II penile prostheses, the second generation of the G.F.S. two-piece prosthesis in which the connectors have been eliminated (Fig. 2). The results have also been excellent to date using this device.

Adequate postoperative patient instruction is essential to ensure a good result. Failure to operate the device in the initial postoperative period may result in complications, especially with the AMS700 device. The formation of restrictive sheath around the cylinders or reservoir

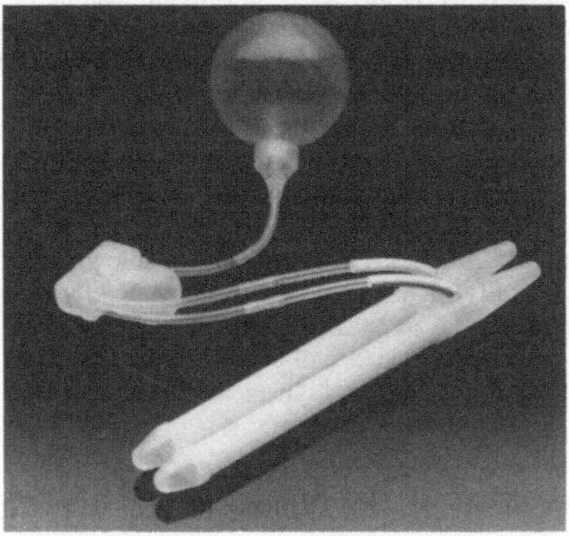

Fig. 1. The AMS700 inflatable penile prosthesis. Note the CX cylinders that provide for controlled expansion and the Teflon coating on the input tube to minimize friction against the cylinder. (Courtesy of American Medical Systems, Minnetonka, MN.)

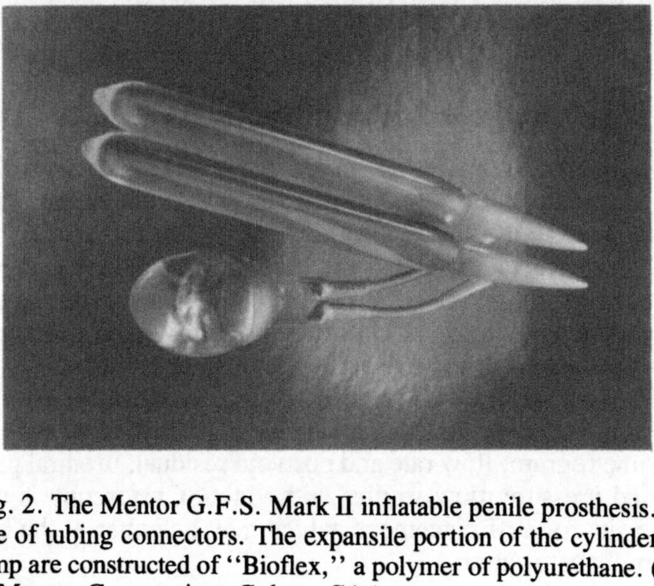

Fig. 2. The Mentor G.F.S. Mark II inflatable penile prosthesis. Note the absence of tubing connectors. The expansile portion of the cylinders and the resipump are constructed of "Bioflex," a polymer of polyurethane. (Courtesy of the Mentor Corporation, Goleta, CA.)

results from failure to cycle the device during the healing process. In the former instance, the restrictive sheath results in the development of chordee of varying degrees. The inability to empty the cylinders is usually indicative of a restrictive sheath around the reservoir or the resipump. The avoid these problems, the patients are instructed to manipulate the device as soon as the postoperative discomfort permits—usually 7–14 d. Once the sheath has formed, however, surgery is required to correct the deformity.

The incidence of infection of the inflatable penile prosthesis in this population is generally higher than that in patients with impotence of non-neurogenic etiology. This has been approximately 6% in the author's series (*19*). The increased incidence of infection in this population group is almost certainly related to the high incidence of bacteriuria.

Management of the Neuropathic Bladder

Neuropathic bladder dysfunction is a common problem among patients with spinal-cord injury. For a full discussion of this problem the reader is referred to various texts (*20–22*). A more thorough understanding of the neurourology has led to an improvement in the management of the bladder in spinal cord injury patients. These advances include the use of intermittent catheterization and the development of the artificial urinary sphincter.

The Artificial Urinary Sphincter (Fig. 3)

The surgery to implant the device has been previously described (*23*). In addition to the routine urological evaluation of patients with neuropathic bladder dysfunction, urodynamic testing is essential to document the type of bladder, assess the presence and severity of bladder outflow obstruction, and localize the anatomical site of the obstruction if present. This knowledge is important since it relates directly to the success of the artificial urinary sphincter, this being generally higher in patients with areflexic as opposed to hyperreflexic bladders. The urodynamic evaluation includes a varying combination of the following: cystometrogram, flow rate and postvoid residual, urethral pressure profile, and pressure–flow studies with video. Cystoscopy is used to assess the site for cuff placement, which may be either at the bladder neck or bulbous urethra.

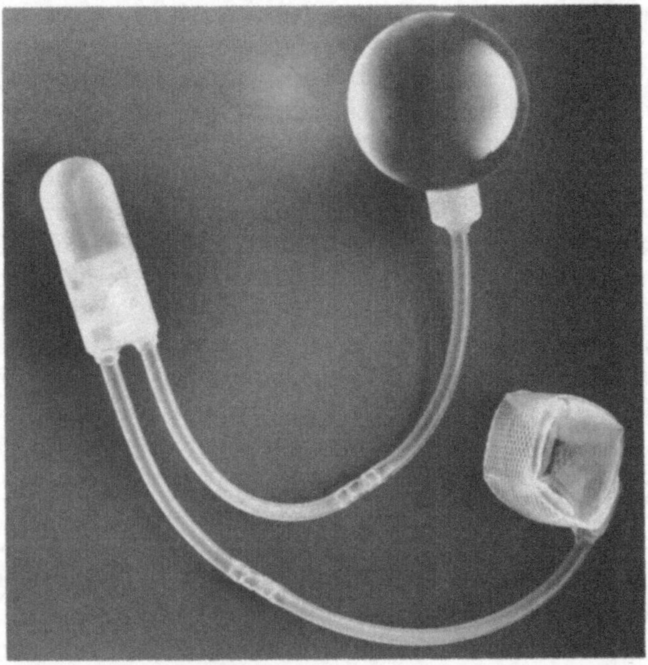

Fig. 3. The AS800 artificial urinary sphincter. (Courtesy of American Medical Systems, Minnetonka, MN.)

Bladder outflow obstruction requires relief prior to implantation of the sphincter. In the male, a transurethral sphincterotomy is required, with resection of the bladder neck being performed in selective cases. It should be noted that both suprasacral and sacral lesions will benefit from the sphincterotomy. Obstruction in the former is the result of active detrusor-sphincter dyssynergia and in the latter, from failure of relaxation of the paralyzed external urethral sphincter. Females require a bladder flap urethroplasty to ablate outflow obstruction. Males frequently require a sphincterotomy to decrease bladder pressure and preserve renal function as part of their general urological care. Females are usually totally incontinent following bladder flap urethroplasty, and this is important for a patient to understand, since the above procedure precludes return to successful intermittent catheterization should the artificial sphincter require removal.

Patients with hyperreflexia also require a trial of anticholinergic medication to ensure that an adequate volume of urine can be stored before detrusor contraction is initiated. The hyperreflexia will often improve with relief of outflow obstruction and control of urinary infection. Should pharmacological manipulation not be successful in controlling the hyperreflexia, augmentation cystoplasty can be performed to ensure a highly compliant, low-pressure storage system (*24*).

Seventy-nine patients with spinal cord injury have undergone implantation of the artificial urinary sphincter by this author. Success is related to the type of bladder found during urodynamic evaluation (*24*). Twenty patients with detrusor hyperreflexia secondary to spinal-cord injury underwent insertion of the artificial urinary sphincter. Satisfactory social continence without the necessity for protective clothing was achieved in 69% (*25*). These patients were all treated prior to the routine use of augmentation cystoplasty. More recently, the concomitant use of the artificial sphincter with augmentation cystoplasty has yielded a successful continence rate of 79% (*24*). Of the 50 patients with detrusor areflexia, 47 were totally continent for a success rate of 94%.

The incidence of infection requiring removal of the device is again higher than in the non-neurogenic patients because of the high incidence of bacteriuria. Successful reimplantation of the sphincter can be performed. Every effort should be made to ensure sterility in an effort to decrease the incidence of infected prostheses.

Electrical Stimulation

Electro-erection or the use of an erection pacemaker is addressed elsewhere in this volume. However, more recently, work has progressed on the use of electrical stimulation to aid in the management of the neurogenic bladder. Tanagho and Schmidt reported on treating 22 patients with neuropathic bladder dysfunction by implantation of sacral root electrodes (*26*). Seventy percent of the patients demonstrated improved reservoir function and obtained continence. The ability to obtain complete bladder evacuation while maintaining low bladder pressure was achieved in 50% of this group. This remains a promising treatment option in the restoration of bladder and sphincteric function.

The successful control of urinary incontinence is important in itself, and there is also a positive effect on the sexual rehabilitation of these patients. Their confidence is boosted with the removal of any type of collecting device together with the fear of involuntary urination. Special preparations for intercourse, such as emptying the bladder, are usually unnecessary.

Conclusions

Based on the above series, it is felt that either intracavernosal injection of vasoactive substances or the inflatable prosthesis is eminently

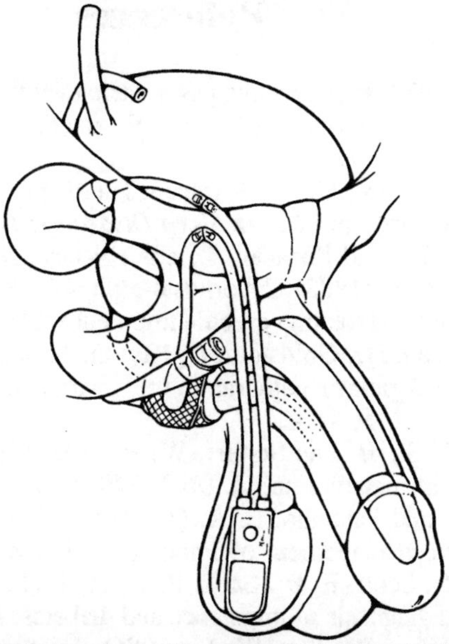

Fig. 4. Schematic presentation of implanted (both) "self-contained" inflatable penile prostheses and artificial urinary sphincter. (Courtesy of the American Medical Systems, Minnetonka, MN).

satisfactory in rehabilitating patients with sexual dysfunction following spinal cord injury. Most of the surgical complications associated with implantation of penile prostheses have been eliminated by device improvements and refinement of surgical techniques. The incidence of mechanical failure has decreased sharply over these past several years and is now uncommon with the current devices.

The artificial urinary sphincter results in attainment of total urinary continence in the vast majority of patients with spinal cord injury. This has certainly added further dimension to the total sexual rehabilitation of patients with spinal cord injury (Fig. 4).

Finally, is it no longer appropriate to assume that all spinal cord injury patients who desire sexual intercourse and fertility have a dismal prognosis because of the advent of several medical and surgical therapeutic options plus electrical and vibratory stimulation.

---

*Ed note: Simultaneous implantation of two (sex and urinary) prostheses is not advocated due to compromised tissue healing. A 4–6 wk interval between surgery is advised.

References

1. Byrd, G. (1978) Preoperative psychiatric evaluation. In *Sleep Disorders: Diagnosis and Treatment.* (William, R. and Karacan, I. eds.) Wiley, New York, pp. 395–399.
2. Beutler, L., Ware, C. and Karacan, I. (1978) Psychological assessment of sexually impotent men. In *Sleep Disorders: Diagnosis and Treatment.* (Williams, R., and Karacan, I., eds.) Wiley, New York, pp. 383–394.
3. Brindley, G. S. (1983) Cavernosal alpha-blockade: a new technique of investigating and treating erectile impotence. *Br. J. Psychiatry*, **143**, 332.
4. Padna-Nathan, H., Goldstein, I., Payton, T. and Krane, R. J. (1987) Intracavernosal pharmacotherapy: the pharmacologic erection program. *World J. Urol.* **5**, 160.
5. Benson, G. S., Jr. and Seifert, W. E. (1988) Is phentolamine stable in solution with papaverine. *J. Urol.* **140**, 970.
6. Lue, T. F. and Tanagho, E. A. (1987) Physiology of erection and pharmacological management of impotence. *J. Urol.* **137**, 829.
7. Karacan, I., Scott, F. B., Salis, P. J., et al. (1977). Nocturnal erection, differential diagnosis of impotence and diabetes. *Biol. Psychiatry* **12**, 373.
8. Kaneko, S. and Bradley, W. E. (1986). Evaluation of erectile dysfunction with continuous monitoring of penile rigidity. *J. Urol.* **136**, 1026.
9. Nadig, P. W., Ware, J. C. and Blumoff, R. (1986) Noninvasive device to produce and maintain an erection-like state. *Urology* **27**, 126.
10. Nelson, R. P. (1988). Nonoperative management of impotence. *J. Urol.* **139**, 2–5.
11. Zorgniotti, A. W. and Lefleur, R. S. (1985) Auto-injection of the corpus cavernosum with a vasoactive drug combination for vasculogenic impotence. *J. Urol.* **133**, 39.
12. Levine, S. B., Althof, S. E., Turner, L. A., et al. (1989). Side effects of self-administration of intracavernous papaverine and phentolamine for the treatment of impotence. *J. Urol.* **141**, 54.
13. Ishii, N., Watanabe, H., Irisawa, C., et al. (1989) Intracavernous injection of prostaglandin E_1 for the treatment of erectile impotence. *J. Urol.* **141**, 323.
14. Scott, F. B., Bradley, W. E. and Timm, G. W. (1973) Management of erectile impotence: Use of implantable inflatable prosthesis. *Urology* **2**, 80.
15. Light, J. K. and Scott, F. B. (1986) Penoscrotal approach for insertion of the Scott inflatable penile prosthesis. In *Modern Techniques in Surgery. Urologic Surgery.* (Ehrlich, R. M. ed.) Futura, New York, pp. 38–1.
16. Mulcahy, J. J. (1989) The hydroflex penile prosthesis. *Urol. Clin. North Am.* **16**, 33.
17. Brooks, M. B. (1988) 42 months of experience with the Mentor inflatable penile prosthesis. *J. Urol.* **139**, 48.
18. Stanisic, T. H. and Dean, J. C. (1989) The flexi-flate and flexi-flate II penile prosthesis. *Urol. Clin. North Am.* February, p. 39.

19. Light, J. K. and Scott, F. B. (1981) Management of neurogenic impotence with inflatable penile prosthesis. *Urology* **17**, 341.
20. Lapides, J., Diokno, A. C., Gould, F. R. and Lowe, B. S. (1976) Further observations on self-catheterization. *J. Urol.* **116**, 169.
21. Linder, A., Leach, G. E. and Raz, S. (1983) Augmentation cystoplasty in the treatment of neurogenic bladder dysfunction. *J. Urol.* **129**, 491.
22. Light, J. K. (1985) Restorative procedures for neuropathic bladder dysfunction: an overview. In *Recent Achievements in Restorative Neurology. I. Upper motor neuron functions and dysfunctions.* (Dimitrijevic, M. and Eccles, J. eds.) Karger, Basel, Switzerland, p. 128.
23. Light, J. K. (1988) The AS800 artificial urinary sphincter: surgical technique and troubleshooting. In *Controversies and Innovations in Urologic Surgery.* Edited by (Gingell, C. and Abrams, P. eds.) Springer-Verlag, New York, Chap. 20.
24. Light, J. K. and Engelmann, U. H. (1985) Reconstruction of the lower urinary tract: observations on bowel dynamics and the artificial urinary sphincter. *J. Urol.* **133**, 594.
25. Light, J. K. and Scott, F. B. (1983) Use of the artificial urinary sphincter in spinal cord injury patients. *J. Urol.* **130**, 1127.
26. Tanagho, E. A. and Schmidt, R. A. (1988) Electrical stimulation in the clinical management of the neurogenic bladder. *J. Urol.* **140**, 1331.

21
Ejaculatory Dysfunction

Jose Florante J. Leyson

Introduction

Most invertebrates are true hermaphrodites. Thus, transfer of sperm toward the egg does not require great propulsive power or ejaculation. In certain species of fish, breeding females can change into breeding males and by "redifferentiation," thus ensuring fertilization, even in the presence of probable ejaculatory dysfunction (*22*). As mammals evolved, their reproductive processes became specialized resulting in the use of an accessory reproductive apparatus, the penis, to deposit sperm into a fertilization recepticle. With the specialization of the penis, ejaculation in humans is coordinated with dual local (genital-reflexogenic) and central (cerebral-regionalized) controls. However, in primates, ejaculation is still genital (tactile) or reflexogenic (primitive) in nature. Thus, nature designs humans to be unique among all animals and to function as a coordinated unit, unlike the segmented function of invertebrates. Is it possible that, following spinal cord trauma, a man's ejaculatory power is lost because he reverts back to use of the primitive or reflexogenic unit and no longer uses the sophisticated centrally coordinated (corticospinal-somatic pathway) system? Is this nature's way of saying that only the fittest (ablest) and strongest should procreate?

Physiology of Ejaculation

Ejaculation, which is separate from erection and/or orgasm, is composed of two phases: (a) emission—the expulsion of prostatic fluid, semen, and sperm into the posterior urethra and (b) ejaculation proper—the rhythmic ejection of the ejaculate from the urethra (*18*). Although

Sexual Rehabilitation of the Spinal-Cord-Injured Patient
Edited by J.F. Leyson, © 1990 The Humana Press, Inc.

the exact neurophysiologic excitatory stimulus for ejaculation has not been clearly defined, the hypothalamus appears to play a central role in controlling the total ejaculatory phenomenon (*18*). It has been shown that the anterior hypothalamus facilitates ejaculation, whereas the serotonergic system seems to inhibit it (*16*). In the genital region, the penile dorsal nerves partly subserve the ejaculatory reflex (*28*). In monkeys, complete transsection of the afferent sensory dorsal nerves resulted in the absence of ejaculation. However, in man, destruction of these nerves does not always abolish ejaculation, but prolongs it. As long as the cortical stimulation is present, with a functional sympathetic chain and postganglionic fibers, ejaculation can still take place (*2,4*).

The efferent fibers subserving seminal emission originate from the cerebral cortex (thalamus) via the spinothalamic tract, and descend to the anterolateral columns to the thoracolumbar and sympathetic chain (T10-L3) (*28*). From these ganglia, postsynaptic adrenergic nerve fibers form the superior hypogastric plexus, descend downward, disperse to either side of the bladder and rectum, mingle with the parasympathetic branches of the sacral cord, and end in the bladder neck, vas deferens, seminal vesicles, epididymis, and prostate (*24,26*). Furthermore, short adrenergic fibers with a high norepinephrine content run throughout the vas deferens. The bulbocavernosus, ischiocavernosus muscles, and the urogenital diaphragm are innervated by the pudendal nerve, a somatic (mixed) sensory component of the ejaculatory afferent nervous circuitry (*28*).

Physiodynamics of Ejaculation

Marberger had proposed that there are actually three distinct rhythmic phases of ejaculation: (a) seminal emission, (b) formation of a pressure chamber, and (c) explusion of semen from the urethra. When a cerebral or genital emission stimulus occurs, it initiates the contraction of the sperm-rich part of the ampulla, vas deferens, and seminal vesicles, and subsequently the prostatic (smooth muscles) musculature (*18*). It is also believed that ampullar contractions appear to be dominant during this phase (*14,21*). The "pressure chamber" then forms between the vesical neck and the urogenital diaphragm. The above phenomenon occurs with emission. The ischiocavernosus, bulbocavernosus, and other pelvic floor muscles contract rhythmically against the gradient or closed bladder neck, while the urogenital diaphragm opens and the semen is propelled distally (*10*).

The closure of the vesical neck (mainly the ventral aspect) is the result of activation of the alpha-sympathetic-adrenergic receptors during the ejaculation phase. However, Stockamp and Schreiter have demonstrated that the vesical neck usually does not close completely; instead, the colliculus is pushed backward towards the bladder neck, plugging the anterior vesicourethral orifice (*27*). Furthermore, the external urethral sphincter, innervated by the somatic (mixed) efferent pudendal nerves originating from the sacral plexus, relaxes (opens) during ejaculation (*28*).

Pathophysiology of Ejaculatory Dysfunctions

Alterations in ejaculation post-SCI can arise from either of two main groups of etiologic factors: (a) ejaculatory dysfunction associated with pre-SCI disorders and (b) those with post-SCI diseases.

Prespinal-cord-injury problems (diseases) may include myopathic, neuropathic, metabolic, and iatrogenic causes. Myopathic caused diseases are usually those arising from transurethral resection of the prostate (TURP), sphincterotomy, prostatectomy, and Y-V urethrocystoplasties of the vesical neck (*28*). Neuropathic-factor diseases can be those caused by mechanical (surgery) and chemical (toxins) injury to the sympathetic chain, i.e., retroperitoneal lymph node dissection. Anterior resection of the rectum and abdominal–perineal surgery can result in 38–50% ejaculatory disturbances, respectively (*29*). Diabetes mellitus can cause retrograde ejaculation *per se* as a result of autonomic neuropathy (*13*). Various antihypertensive and other psychotrophic medications can produce drug-induced ejaculatory dysfunctions (*see* Table 1).

Diseases or conditions that may aggravate ejaculatory problems after cord trauma are similar to those causing pre-SCI problems. However, most of these factors rarely occur, except TUR prostate, sphincterotomies, saddle or pelvic trauma, and the use of various medications (Table 1).

Most ejaculatory dysfunctions following the SCI episode are either retrograde and/or total absence of ejaculation. The causes of retrograde ejaculation probably include paralysis (relaxation) of the vesical neck or neurogenic alterations in the closure mechanism of the bladder neck (internal urethral sphincter). A remote possibility is the so-called "blocked ejaculation." This phenomenon may occur where there is internal–external sphincter (ejaculation) dyssynergia—i.e., both internal and external urethral sphincters go into spasms during the phase of ejaculation proper. The above abnormality may be the result of a

Table 1
Drugs That May Adversely Affect Ejaculation[a]

Alcohol	Perphenazine
Amitriptyline	Pheneizine
Bethanidine	Phenoxybenzamine HCl
Chlorimipramine	Phentolamine
Guanethidine sulfate	Reserpine
Imipramine HCl	Trifluoperazine HCl
Methadone	Thioridazine
Naproxen	Diazepam (large doses)

[a]Modified from Thomas, A. J. (1983) Ejaculatory dysfunction. *Fertil Steril.* **39**, 445–453.

"minisympathetic crisis" (dysreflexia) during the ejaculatory and/or orgasmic phase of sexual activity.

The absence of ejaculation in those SCI men who suffer from it is probably the result of neurotransmitter disruption of the autonomic nervous system and/or direct injury to the sacral-cord reflex center. Thus, there is no contraction of the epididymis, vas deferens, seminal vesicles, prostate smooth-muscle fibers, and the bulboischiocavernosus muscles. Comarr and Gunderson reported that men with complete upper motor neuron (UMN) lesions rarely ejaculated, though 70% had adequate erections (*5*). Those with incomplete UMN lesions exhibited a somewhat greater frequency of ejaculation. Very few SCI men with complete lower motor neuron (LMN) lesions are likely to achieve ejaculation or erection. Half of the men studied with incomplete LMN lesions retained their ejaculatory capabilities. The majority of men with recovering lesions claimed normal ejaculation 6–12 mo postinjury. However, in our clinical experience, there are patients who have normal erections, but who continue to ooze semen after the ejaculatory experience.

The medical treatment of retrograde ejaculation without pre-SCI bladder neck incompetence consists mainly of the use of alpha-sympathomimetic medications (*see* Table 2) (*28*). However, these drugs are contraindicated in hypertension. One of the undesirable side effects with some of these agents is the development of tachyphylaxis as a result of the depletion of norepinephrine stores at the terminal nerve endings (*28*). To circumvent this problem, phenylpropanolamine (propadrine) can be tried, but our clinical experience has shown that this particular drug provides only minimal beneficial effects.

Hypertensive patients with retrograde ejaculation can be treated with beta-adrenergic blockers (i.e., propanolol) at 30 –60 mg/d, orally.

Table 2
Sympathomimetic Medications[a] Used to Treat Retrograde Ejaculation

Drug	Trade name	Dosage	Frequency of administration
Bromopheniramine maleate, phenylephrine hydrochloride plus phenylpropanolamine	Dimetapp Extentabs	One tablet	Every 12 hr
	Purebrom Compound Tabs	One tablet	Every 12 hr
Chlorpheniramine plus phenylpropanolamine	Ornade	One tablet	Every 12 hr
Ephedrine sulfate		25 mg, 50 mg	Every 6–8 hr
Pseudophedrine HCl	Sudafed	60 mg	Every 8 hr
Phenylpropanolamine	Propadrine	25 mg, 50 mg	Every 8 hr
	Phenylpropanolamine HCl	75 mg	Every 12 hr

[a]To be taken by the patient during the spouse's periovulatory interval (approximately 10 d during midcycle) and 3–5 d before the semen sample is obtained. In the author's clinical experience, only ephedrine sulfate is effective in up to 60%. However, sympathetic side effects may occur at doses of 250 mg/d.

Theoretically, by suppressing beta-adrenergic activity in the region of the bladder neck, alpha-adrenergic receptors may become dominant (indirect activation), thus causing vesical neck closure and preventing retrograde ejaculation.

Two major therapeutic approaches that can be used to induce ejaculation are: (a) intrathecal drug injection and (b) neuroelectrical stimulation. Guttman and Walsh injected neostigmine intrathecally to achieve both erection and ejaculation (*11*). Single or multiple ejaculations were noted in approximately 60% of 70 men with complete upper neuron (UMN) lesions and 75% of 29 men with incomplete UMN lesions. Two-thirds of those with complete LMN lesions failed to ejaculate (*11*). Intrathecal artificial ejaculation can induce complications similar to those following lumbar punctures—chemical (allergic) myelitis and autonomic (sympathetic) dysreflexia, which usually occur with high cervical lesions. These complications are treated symptomatically, whereas the hypertensive crisis (dysreflexia) is controlled with a fast, but short-acting, alpha-adrenergic blocker, i.e., nitroprusside (*28*).

Since the 1930s, electrical stimulation has been used to induce ejaculation in animals. Ten–15 yr later, electroejaculation was tried in just a few paraplegic men for fear of uncertain electrical or neurodermal complications. However, it was not until the late 1970s that Francois et al. (*7*) performed 116 electrostimulations, which resulted in 63 ejaculations that produced only one pregnancy. In the 1980s, Brindley modified Francois' technique and achieved 50 ejaculations (58%) in 84 patients (*3*). Amelar et al. later introduced a handheld vibrator that was found useful and safe, though studied in only a few patients (*1*). The vibrator is held against the glans penis or inserted rectally until ejaculation occurs.) Recent clinical trials and our own limited data with this battery-operated vibrator have shown that it is effective, especially in patients with recovering lesions and in chronic paraplegics whose sensations have returned and/or who have experienced orgasms.*

Techniques of Electroejaculation

We have tried three types of clinical neurodermal/rectal electroejaculation (Figs. 1B–D). Before the procedure, each patient should undergo proctosigmoidoscopy to assess the status of the rectal mucosa. The electroejaculation technique involves inserting short electromyographic needles (EMC) in the bulbocavernosus muscles (Fig. 1B), taking care not to perforate the urethra. Of the ten subjects (five quads and five paras with complete lesions) studied or stimulated, none ejaculated. Another method used to induce electroejaculation is the transcutaneous neurostimulation (TNS) pad (*17*). These pads are secured with tape over the bulbocavernosus region (Fig. 1C), and stimulation is applied until a tingling sensation was felt or a maximum rate of eight/impulse. Of the five subjects (one quad, three complete paras and one monoparetic L1-L2), only the monoparetic man experienced a weak ejaculation, even when the TNS dermal pads were placed in the lumbosacral areas. The third method is anal stimulation. Of the three electroejaculation techniques, only the anal (rectal) probe or plug (Fig. 1D) stimulator is effective, as demonstrated by Frankel and Mathias (*9*) and recently by Perkash et al (*24*). Mathias et al. suggested that vital signs should be monitored during electroejaculation (*20*). The above method consists of accessing blood pressure and heart rate via intraarterial catheters in the radial or dorsalis pedis artery, a separate intravenous open line, and an electrocardiogram (ECG). However, most physicians who perform electroejaculation prefer one intravenous line instead of two. Before the electrode (ejaculation-stimulator plug) is inserted, the rectum must be manually emptied. The stimulator or electrode is placed close to the seminal vesicles, and a rectal thermometer is inserted next to the electrode to insure that the intrarectal temperature does not rise

*Ed note: To minimize sexual dysreflexia, oral dose of 1–0.5 mg prasozin (Minipres) is advised 1–2 h before vibratory ejaculation.

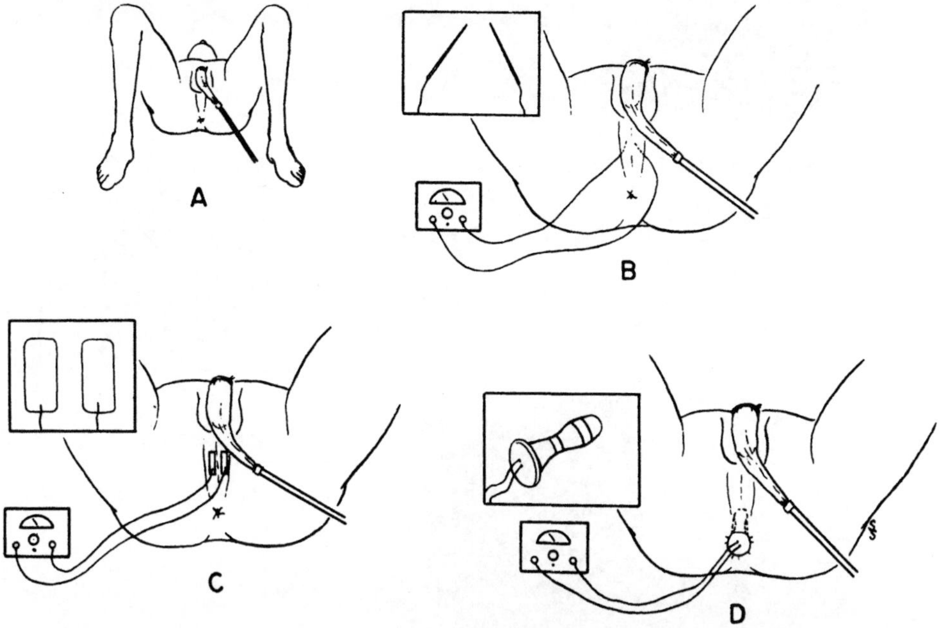

Fig. 1. The patient shown in the dorsal lithotomy position, exposing the perineal area for stimulation. A condom urinal can be placed with a semen collection bag. B, C, and D demonstrate the different techniques for possible electroejaculation. D—rectal probe electroejaculation. The bladder is initially irrigated with neomycin sulfate-polymycin B sulfate solution and drained. Before rectal probe stimulation, 150–200 mL of buffered lactated Ringer's solution is left in the bladder. The semen may be mixed with the bladder urine after the stimulation, and is then collected with a catheter flush in which various modifications have been done for better extraction.

above 99°F, which could cause local mucosal burns. Once the stimulator is positioned properly, a 20-Hz stimulus (with a current level between 0.70–0.35 $\mu A/\mu m^2$) is applied for 2 s intermittently, while vital signs are monitored (*9,25*). Electrostimulation is continued until ejaculation (Fig. 3 A,B,C). If ejaculation does not occur, even after five trials, a urologic workup, including vasoseminal and vesiculography, should be done to rule out congenital or obstructive pathology (*14*). In summary, ejaculation can be induced not only by masturbation/fellatio, but also by vibratory stimulation [Oster-75; Pifco and Ling 201] personal vibrators (Fig. 2) and by rectal probe electrostimulation.

Complications of Electroejaculation

The superiority of electroejaculation, compared to intrathecal neostigmine, in eliciting ejaculations is that it can provide a controlled

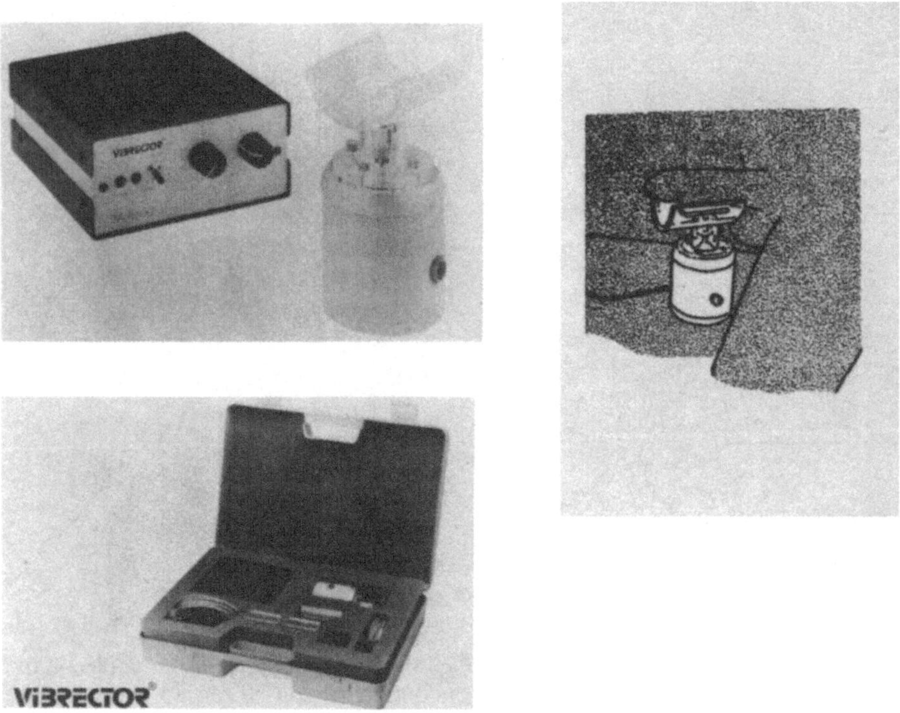

Fig. 2. In the absence of sensual human mechanical stimulation, another option for electroerection is by use of mechanical vibrations applied at 30–60 Hz. The Vibrector, can be used in combination with other stimulations including direct intrapenile vasoactive drug injections. Clinical studies reported 55% effective response in all types of SCI men.

stimulus for a short period of time. However, Frankel and Mathias have observed severe hypertension and bradycardia as a potential danger of electroejaculation in patients with cervical or high thoracic lesions (*9*). Headaches, flushing of the skin, and sweating over the face and neck were also noted as minimal problems during electrical stimulation (*8*). Frankel and Mathias believed that the profound cardiovascular changes are probably part of the syndrome of autonomic dysreflexia (crisis) secondary to visceral (rectal) stimulation, which results from uninhibited sympathetic nervous system activity via the distal part of the spinal cord (*9*). The presence of a functioning inhibitory pathway in the traumatized spinal cord is questionable. However, the presence of residually functioning Renshaw cells may be responsible for inhibiting or suppressing the severe cardiovascular changes in patients with incomplete or low thoracic (T7-T10) lesions.

Frankel and Mathias recently reported that severe hypertension occurred in patients with high cord lesions (C7 and above) during electroejaculation, which can be managed effectively with prostaglandin E_2 (PGE_2) (*9*). These investigators intravenously infused (Harvard Infusion Pump) prostaglandin E_2 (Prostin E_2, Upjohn) at a starting dose of 0.5 μg/min, increased to 1 μg/min after 5 min, and then titrated to between 3.5 and 8.5 μg/min to maintain a prestimulation (baseline) blood pressure during electroejaculation. Intravenous PGE_2 infusion can provide an advantage in that stronger electrical stimulation and electroejaculation can be used for a longer period of time (up to ten trials) with minimal rise in blood pressure (*9*). The precise mechanism by which PGE_2 reduces blood pressure is still unknown. However, Conway and Hatton had demonstrated in animal studies that PGE_2 produces vascular smooth muscle dilatation, thereby reducing the resistance and capacitance of blood vessels and causing low blood pressure (*6*). Hedqvist suggested that PGE_2 may exert a negative feedback over the sympathetic neural transmission (*12*). The latter mechanisms may impair the chance of successful ejaculation. However, in guinea pigs, PGE_2 enhances the contractile response of the vas deferens and seminal vesicle (*23*). Prostaglandin E_2 is a promising novel therapeutic approach to the management of electrocoagulation-induced hypertension but it seems to retard or impair ejaculation (*9*). However, other vasodilator drugs (prostacyclin) and/or vascular smooth-muscle slow-channel calcium blockers, which have no direct effect on the autonomic nervous, or ejaculatory smooth muscle, systems may be tried clinically as a possible adjunct in the management of electroejaculatory hypertensive crises. Frankel and Mathias suggested that, in addition to a cardiac arrest trolley, ganglionic and alpha-adrenergic blockers should be available for emergency use (*9*). Another drawback of electroejaculation is the low volume and recovery of sperm with less than 20% motility (*25*). The etiology of low sperm motility has not been elucidated. However, sperm motility may be improved by:

(a) Preventing or minimizing urinary tract infections
(b) Selecting an antibiotic for urinary tract infections or avoiding drugs that compromise sperm survival (i.e., mandelamine hippurate is directly toxic to sperm)
(c) Preventing sperm stagnation in the lower tract storage sites, perhaps by periodic sexual activity and/or use of rectal probe electrostimulation (*25*).

Furthermore, data by Ingerslev (*15*) has shown that the addition of 4.0 mL normal human serum to the 15–35 mL semen specimen significantly improved the motility of spermatozoa.

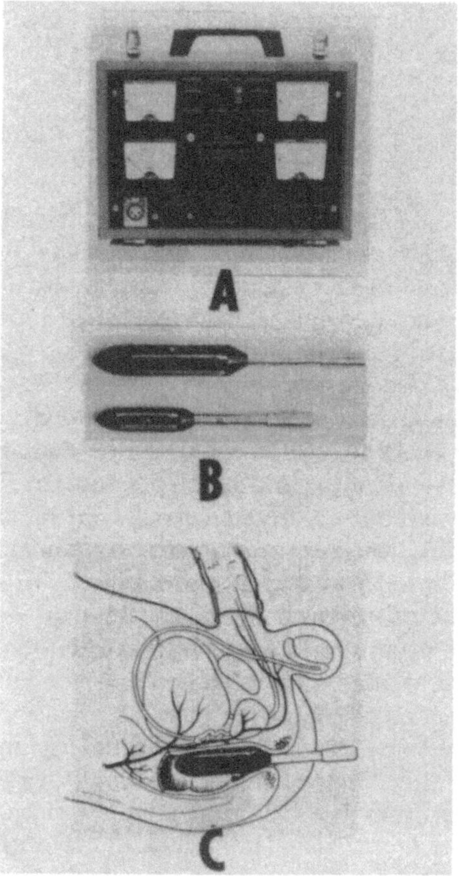

Fig. 3. A, Stimulator/generator for electroejaculation. B, Most commonly used rectal probes. C, Lateral view of the male pelvis with an inserted probe and an external condom for semen collection.

Electroejaculation, although fraught with hazards as a result of autonomic nervous system hyperstimulation, is a logical alternative for semen collection, either for fertility studies or for artificial insemination. In impotent patients with deficient penile tactile sensation only, vasoactive intestinal polypeptide (VIP) may be given or prostaglandin E_2 ointment used (when it becomes available commercially) to enhance the sensual or erotic penile sensory feedback needed to maintain erection, which may then result in ejaculation. It may also be logical to administer both the VIP and sympathomimetic-dopaminergic-like preparations to induce ejaculation medically, as well as to maintain erection. A futuristic approach is the direct stimulation of the sacral ejaculatory reflex center (?), or the thoracolumbar segment, with miniature electrodes selectively implanted in the ejaculatory stimulating fibers. Although 5–7% of SCI men ejaculate normally, several investigators have reached some conclusions:

(a) Thoracic level seems to be ideal and complete lesions ejaculate well with electrostimulations
(b) About 20% result in pregnancy, and
(c) Sperm penetration assay is not an accurate index for fertility (*5,7,15,25,30*).

Recent data have shown that the use of deoxyribonucleic acid (DNA) flow cytometry on testicular aspirates is a good predictor for fertility status in the outcome on SCI men requesting electroejaculation (*32*).

Sperm Allergy

In some cases, the wife is allergic to the spouse's ejaculate from the immunoglobulin E (IgE) of the seminal plasma protein. This form of sexual allergy is mainifested by vaginal irritative symptoms and even abacteric dysuria following sex. The treatment for sperm allergy consists of:

1. avoidance of semen contact with the vagina or skin
2. no fellatio and
3. use of condom during sexual activity until the allergy has been resolved (*31*).

The definitive therapy is immunotherapy. This desensitization consists of series of injections of a partially purified seminal plasma protein of the husband into the wife, until the symptoms have abated or the wife becomes asymptomatic following exposure to the ejaculate.

Fertilization by Intravaginal Voiding

A nonbionic (neuroelectroejaculation) alternative for fertilization is postejaculatory intravaginal voiding. Although it is an unorthodox method, this technique involves three phases of preparation:

(1) Alkalinization of the male urine (which has been sterilized by nonspermicidal drugs) 2–3 d prior to sexual celebration with 12–15 g of sodium bicarbonate orally
(2) Emptying the urinary bladder (either by voiding or catheterization) 2–3 h before sexual activity. Oral hydration with 750–800

mL water in order to fill the urinary bladder to prevoiding volume

(3) Finally after the postejaculatory or orgasmic sensations are felt, the male is instructed to void either voluntarily or reflexly into the vagina.

The woman is requested to keep her pelvis elevated with a pillow for at least an hour. This maneuver will, it is hoped, let the sperm gravitate into the cervix. After 60–90 min, the woman slowly gets up and lets the urine drip out of her. Prior to attempting the intravaginal voiding fertilization technique, the couple should be counseled by the sexologist that the technique is neither dirty or harmful, and though it sounds messy, it is neither humiliating nor insulting to the woman. When trying this method, the woman should be in her ovulatory (fertile) period, and must use an alkaline vaginal douche just prior to the fertilization attempt. So far, of the eight SCI patients studied (three complete paraplegics, two complete quadriplegics, and three incomplete quadriplegics), two paraplegics and one incomplete-central-cord-syndrome male have been successful in impregnating their wives. With recent advances in biotechnology, an infertile SCI couple may now have several better fertilization options.

Conclusions

Rectal probe electroejaculation in SCI men usually yields greater than 10 million sperm in a majority (71%) of cases (*30*). Most investigators report that there is a higher success rate in patients with complete and thoracic lesions. But sperm motility is better in those with incomplete lesions (*25,30*). Patient age and duration of injury had no effect. Patients on intermittent catheterization consistently did well. If sphincterotomy is indicated, a single 12 o'clock position should be done to avoid damage to the area around or opening of the ejaculatory ducts (*30,31*).

References

1. Amelar, R. D., Dubin, L., and Walsh, P. C. (1977) *Male Infertility*. Saunders, Philadelphia, p. 208.

2. Bors, E. and Comarr, A. E. (1960) Neurologic disturbances of sexual function. *Urol. Surv.* **10**, 191–195.

3. Brindley, G. S. (1981) Electro-ejaculation: its technique, neurological implications and uses. *J. Neurol. Neurosurg. Psychiatry.* **44**, 9–11.
4. Comarr, A. E. (1971) Sexual concepts in traumatic cord and cauda equina lesions. *J. Urol.* **106**, 375–379.
5. Comarr, A. E. and Gunderson, B. B. (1975) Sexual function in traumatic paraplegia and quadriplegia. *Am. J. Nurs.* **275**, 250–258.
6. Conway, J. and Hatton, R. (1975) Effects of prostaglandins E1, E2, Al and A2 on the resistance and capacitance vessels in the hind limb of the dog. *Cardiovas Res.* **9**, 229–235.
7. Francois, N., Maury, M., Jouannet, D., David, G., and Vacant, J. (1978) Electroejaculation of a complete paraplegic followed by pregnancy. *Paraplegia* **16**, 248–251.
8. Frankel, H. L., Mathias, C. J., and Walsh, J. J. (1979) Blood pressure plasma catecholamines and prostaglandins during artificial erection in a male tetraplegic. *Paraplegia* **12**, 205–211.
9. Frankel, H. L. and Mathias, C. J. (1980) Severe hypertension in patients with high spinal cord lesions undergoing electro-ejaculation management with prostaglandin E2. *Paraplegia* **18**, 293–299.
10. Gallizia, P. (1972) The smooth sphincter of the vesical neck, a genital organ. *Urol. Int.* **27**, 341–345.
11. Guttman, L. and Walsh, J. J. (1971) Prostigin assessment test of fertility in spinal man. *Paraplegia* **9**, 39–43.
12. Hedqvist, P. (1973) Autonomic neurotransmission, in *The Prostaglandins* (Randwell, P. W., ed.) pp. 101 Plenum, New York.
13. Hosking, D. J., Bennett, T., Hampton, J. R. (1978) Diabetic autonomic neuropathy. *Diabetes* **27**, 1043–1049.
14. Ichijo, S., Sigg, C., Ngasawa, M., Siraiwa, Y. (1981) Vasoseminal vesiculography before and after ejaculation. *Urol. Int.* **36**, 35–40.
15. Ingerslev, H. J., (1985) Can human serum improve motility of spermatozoa? *Lancet* **123**, 519–521.
16. Kimura, Y., Kisaki, N., Sakurada, S., Tadano, T. (1977) On the brain monoaminergic systems relating to ejaculation. II. Brain dopamine-serotonin and ejaculation. *Andrologia* **9**, 50–56.
17. Leyson, J. F. J. (1982) A treatise of human sexuality. Update in medicine. Cebu Institute of Medicine, Cebu City, Phil. June 10–12.
18. MacLean, P. P., Dua, S., Denniston, R. H. (1963) Cerebral localization for scratching and seminal discharge. *Arch. Neurol.* **9**, 485–494.
19. Marberger, H. (1979) The mechanisms of ejaculation. *Basic Life Sci.* (Part B) **4**, 99–103.
20. Mathias, C. J., Christensen, N. J., Corbett, J. L., Frankel, H. L., Goodwin, T. J., and Peart, W. S. (1975) Plasma catecholamines, plasma renin activity and plasma aldosterone in tetraplegic man, horizontal and tilted. *Clin. Sci. Molec. Med.* **49**, 291–299.
21. Mitsuya, H., Asai, J., Suyama, K., Ushida, T., Hosoe, K. (1960) Application of x-ray cinematography in urology. I. Mechanism of ejaculation. *J. Urol.* **83**, 86–90.

22. Money, J. (1984) Bisexuality and Homosexuality. *Sex. Med. Today* **8**, 24.
23. Naimzada, M. K. (1969) Effect of some naturally occurring prostaglandins (PGE, PGE2, PGA and PGFI) on the hypogastric nerve, vas deferens and seminal vesical preparations of the guinea pig. *Clin. Thera.* **4**, 34–42.
24. Owman, C. H. and Sjoberg, N. O. (1972) The importance of short adrenergic neurons in the seminal emission mechanism of rate, guinea pig and man. *J. Reprod. Fertil.* **28**, 379–383.
25. Perkash, I., Marin, D. E., Watner, H., Blank, M. S., Collins, D. C. (1985) Reproductive biology of paraplageics: Results of semen collections, testicular biopsy, and serum hormone evaluation. *J. Urol.* **134**, 284–288.
26. Sjostrand, N. O. (1965) The adrenergic innervation of the vas deferens and the accessory male genital gland. *Acta Physio. Scand.* **65**, 257–261.
27. Stockamp, K. and Schreiter, F. (1974) Function of the posterior urethra in ejaculation and its importance for urine control. *Urol. Int.* **29**, 226–230.
28. Thomas, A. J. (1983) Ejaculatory dysfunction. *Fertil. Steril.* **39**, 445–453.
29. Williams, M. H., Watson, P. C., Golligher, J. C., Riches, E. W., Gabriel, W. B., and Pyrah, L. N. (1951) Discussion on urological complications of excision of the rectum. *Proc. R. Soc. Med.* **44**, 819–822.
30. McGuire, E. (1988) Personal communications, June 1988.
31. Leyson, J. F. (1988) *Updates in Sexual Medicine.* Presented at the annual winter meeting, Asso. of Phil. Physicians in America, Philippine Convention Center, Manila, Philippines. Dec.
32. White, R. de., Stone, A., Hellstrom, W., and Deitch, A. (1989) The clinical application of aspiration DNA flow cytometry to neurologically impaired men entering an electroejaculation program. *J. Urol.* **142**, 309–312.

22

Infertility Evaluation and Management After Spinal-Cord Injury

Eli F. Lizza

Introduction

In the general population, approximately 15% of couples intending to have children are found to be infertile. In about 30–50% of these couples, the male partner is either totally or partially responsible for the infertility (22). From these satistics, it appears that between 5 and 7% of males intending to impregnate their spouses are infertile.

The etiology of infertility in the general male population varies widely. Greenberg et al. (*17*) found that the most common associated factor is a varicocele. This condition, representing dilated tortuous tributaries to the internal spermatic vein, was found in almost 40% of 425 men evaluated for infertility. Characteristically, a varicocele is found on the left side as a result of the difference in venous drainage between the left and right testes. The second largest diagnostic category, idiopathic infertility, was diagnosed in 25% of the patients studied. Other categories included primary testicular failure, obstruction, and cryptorchidism, each accounting for between 5% and 10%. Categories contributing less than 5% to the final diagnosis included ejaculatory failure, sexual dysfunction, and endocrine abnormalities, each of which accounted for 1–2%.

These statistics are important in treating the spinal-cord-injured (SCI) patient for infertility. In this population, the effect of the SCI augments the incidence of certain causes of infertility, such as the inability to achieve or maintain an erection, ejaculatory dysfunction, primary in-

Sexual Rehabilitation of the Spinal-Cord-Injured Patient
Edited by J.F. Leyson, © 1990 The Humana Press, Inc.

jury to the testes, acute or chronic infection with or without antibiotic therapy, and hormonal abnormalities. Although one must remain cognizant of other causes of infertility in the SCI male, collectively, they account for about 5% of the infertility in a group of patients for which the infertility rate has been estimated to be greater than 90% (*24*).

Advances in the care and rehabilitation of the SCI patients have markedly improved the duration and quality of life for these patients. As a result, many of them seek to live as normal a life as possible, both in employment and in raising a family. This chapter, therefore, concentrates on those causes of male infertility prevalent in SCI men and on their treatment. For a review of infertility in otherwise normal males, the reader is referred to the excellent text of Lipshultz and Howards, *Infertility in the Male* (*22*).

Diagnostic Evaluation

As with any medical problem, the importance of a thorough history and physical examination cannot be overemphasized. Consequently, when interviewing the SCI male, the history should include information concerning prior pregnancies, the ability to achieve and maintain erections, the methods used, and whether the erections maintained are satisfactory for vaginal penetration. One should also ascertain whether the patient can achieve an ejaculation and, if so, by what means. Also, is the ejaculation accompanied by seminal emission.

The initial evaluation should attempt to identify the level of SCI and whether the spinal-cord lesion is complete or partial, by associated symptoms. One should also determine how the patient empties his bladder, and whether or not he experiences incontinence with an ejaculation. As in any evaluation for infertility, the couple must be treated. Therefore, the patient's wife must be evaluated to ensure the presence of ovulation and the absence of obstruction. A history of previous pregnancies, offspring, infertility problems, and any prior infertility evaluations of either partner must be recorded. Information on prior surgery or hospitalizations should be included, since these may impact on the patient's infertility as would previous infections or inflammations of the testes or genital structures. The latter include acute or chronic urinary tract infections with a history of medication use. Any associated past or present toxic exposure, either through the environment or through the use of alcohol or tobacco, should not be overlooked.

During the physical examination, attempts should be made to assess the patient's general condition, as well as the level of his cord injury.

Examination of the genitalia proceeds with attempts to identify abnormalities or inflammation of the phallus; the testes are examined and measured to detect testicular atrophy. The author prefers to measure the testes in the superior inferior and medial lateral axes, the normal size being 4 × 2 cm or larger. The consistency of the testes is noted, and any irregularities or abnormalities are investigated further. The epididymides are palpated in their entirety for nodularity, and the vas deferens is palpated bilaterally. To detect a varicocele, the spermatic cord on each side is palpated while the patient performs the valsalva maneuver. Bilateral variococeles have been found in about 20% of the cases. The shape of the prostate gland, its consistency, and the presence of any nodularity as well as the tone of the external sphincter and the presence or absence of the bulbocavernous reflex are evaluated by rectal examination. The results of these evaluations combined with laboratory data should provide the etiology of infertility in the SCI patient.

Laboratory evaluations should include a urinalysis as well as urine culture and sensitivity tests and biochemical determinations of serum testosterone, luteinizing hormone (LH), and follicle stimulating hormone (FSH) concentrations. To detect retrograde ejaculation, a post-ejaculatory urine specimen is examined for sperm. If semen is obtained, it should be evaluated according to the parameters listed in Table 1, on two occasions, separated by at least 1 mo. Variations greater than 20% between the values obtained indicate the need for further semen analyses.

Mean and median sperm counts, in a random sampling of normal males, have been found to be 107 million and 83 million/mL, respectively (*40*). However, the values given in Table 1 represent levels usually accepted as the lower limits of fertility in men. Lower counts may prove adequate in the SCI male who uses adjunctive means of insemination.

Erectile Dysfunction

The incidence of erectile dysfunction after a spinal-cord injury depends on several factors, including the level of spinal-cord injury and whether the cord lesion is complete or incomplete. Spontaneous erections appear to occur more frequently after higher spinal lesions, being found in about 50% of patients suffering a sacral cord lesion compared with 93% of those with a cervical injury (*11,24*). In all cases, the quality as well as the quantity of erections maintained are diminished. Obviously, erectile dysfunction plays a significant role in the patient's ability to

Table 1
Minimal Adequate Values for Semen Analysis

A. Volume 2.0–5.0 mL	
Sperm density	20 million/mL
Morphology	60% normal (head and tail)
Motility	60% with good forward progression (2, scale 1–4)
B. Absence of significant:	
1. Pyospermia	
2. Bacteria	
3. Sperm agglutination	
4. Hyperviscosity	

father a child. Fortunately, this problem, although common in SCI patients presenting with infertility, lends itself to surgical correction through the use of penile prostheses. For a review of these prostheses, the reader is referred to other chapters in this book.

Ejaculatory Dysfunction

The process of ejaculation, which is a separate entity from erection or orgasm, is twofold. First, prostatic fluid, seminal fluid, and sperm are expressed into the posterior urethra; then, this fluid is expelled from the urethra through a series of rhythmic contractions (*27*).

In a recent review of ejaculatory dysfunction, Thomas (*36*) further subdivided this twofold process into three distinct phases. The first phase, emission, appears to be controlled by the sympathetic nervous system and involves the transport of seminal fluids from the prostate and seminal vesicles combined with sperm into the posterior urethra. In the second phase, adrenergic input causes a pressure chamber to develop in the prostatic urethra by closing the bladder neck. This pressure also contributes to the expulsion of semen, the third and final phase, which occurs when the external sphincter opens and the bulbocavernosus, ischiocavernosus, and perineal muscles contract simultaneously. Neurologic stimulation of these muscles is brought about via the pudendal nerve and, in the intact urogenital system, results in the rhythmic explusion of approximately 2–5 mL of semen from the urethra.

The two major problems that can occur in patients who suffer a spinal-cord injury are (a) loss of the ability to ejaculate or (b) ejaculation resulting in the retrograde expulsion of sperm into the bladder rather than out of the urethra—so-called retrograde ejaculation. These conditions can occur either alone or simultaneously. Infertility in the SCI male with a complete deficit is probably caused by one or both of these problems.

Obviously, the clincian must first address the patient's inability to ejaculate. Once ejaculation has been achieved, then a semen specimen should be collected and analyzed, and the patient evaluated for retrograde ejaculation. The ultimate goal is to obtain a sufficient quantity of viable sperm to inseminate the patient's wife, either naturally or artificially.

Loss of Ejaculation

In a review of infertility in SCI men, Brindley (*7*) noted the presence or absence of ejaculation in 604 SCI men by combining data from several large studies. Of the patients with complete lesions of the lower thoracic or lumbar cord, 90% failed to ejaculate, compared to 96% of those with complete cervical lesions. Patients with incomplete lesions usually were ejaculatory.

Obviously, the lack of ejaculation was the most common cause of infertility in SCI males in this large review. The inability to ejaculate must be diagnosed and treated before further evaluation and/or therapy aimed at achieving a pregnancy can proceed. In such patients, especially if they experience an orgasm, one must also rule out retrograde ejaculation as outlined below. Then, one can attempt to artificially elicit an ejaculation. The three methods used to stimulate ejaculation in SCI men are

1. Vibratory stimulation
2. Electrostimulation
3. Intrathecal neostigmine injection.

Vibrator Ejaculation

This method of stimulating ejaculation was first introduced by Sobrero et al. (*34*) in 1965. Years later, it was popularized in France by Francois et al. (*14*), who introduced it to that country in 1980. Brindley introduced the procedure in England in 1981 (*7*). Vibrator application relies on stimulaing the glans or frenulum with an electric vibrator to induce reflex ejaculation.

In the technique reported by Brindley, the patient is placed in the supine position, and if his SCI lesion is at or above the T5 level, his blood pressure is monitored. This precaution is necessary because there is always the possibility that vibratory stimulation may cause severe headache or systolic hypertension. If the latter exceeds 200 mm Hg, the patient is immediately raised to a vertical position, a maneuver that rapidly restores blood pressure to normal. A Ling 201 vibrator with an 80-Hz frequency and 2.5 mm pull-to-peak amplitude is placed under the frenulum for 3 min. After a 1- to 2-min rest period, the procedure is repeated for a total of four cycles, or until ejaculation is induced. Brindley reported 49 successes in 93 SCI patients. However, the technique usually failed if it was attempted within 6 mo after the SCI, and always failed if reflex flexion of the hips could not be induced by scratching the sides of the patient's feet. The absence of this reflex implies damage between L2 and S1 cord roots. Of 62 patients with reflex flexion of the hips who had been injured more than 6 mo prior to testing, 48 (77.4%) were successfully treated by this technique, which led to a total of seven pregnancies when vibrator stimulation was combined with artificial insemination. In these cases, the semen specimen was injected into the vagina with a syringe, or if less than 0.5 mL of semen was obtained, it was injected directly into the cervix by means of a cannula. Autonomic dysreflexia was noted in seven of the 93 SCI men treated; six were tetraplegic and one had a lesion at the T2 level. Dysreflexia occurred just after ejaculation and, in most cases, was relieved by postural treatment.

The advantages of vibrator application to induce ejaculation include the production of better semen than that produced after electroejaculation. Furthermore, most specimens are expelled in an antegrade fashion, free from contamination with urine. The production of partially retrograde specimens, as evidenced by a very low volume of ejaculate, is uncommon with vibratory stimulation. Ejaculations were external in 46 (94%) of 49 patients. Sperm counts in seven of these patients demonstrated at least 50 million motile sperm/ejaculate; 11 expelled semen containing from 5 to 50 million motile sperm/ejaculate, whereas semen from 12 contained from 500,000 to 5 million motile sperm/ejaculate. Semen from the remaining patients contained less than 500,000 motile sperm. Three patients demonstrated retrograde ejaculation.

Electroejaculation

Electrical stimulation by means of an electrode inserted into the rectum has been used to induce ejaculation in domestic animals since 1936 (*6*). This technique was first applied to humans by Horne et al (*19*) to treat infertility in SCI men. Since that presentation, several authors have described various methods of inducing ejaculation by electrical stimulation. (Table 2).

Table 2
Electroejaculation

Name of authors	Method	No. of patients	Ejaculated	Pregnancy
Horne, et al. (*19*)	28 curved urethral sound to S.V. + prostate × 4, sex massage. S.V., + prostate with urethra 45–60 m amps total	18	11 (61%)	—
David et al. (*11*)	Rigid bipolar electrode 15–60 V, 4–8 ms, freq. 140/s over S.V. + prostate × 5–10 min. or until ejaculation	16	4 (25%)	—
Francois et al. (*15*)	Details not reported	31	13 (42%)	1
Martin et al. (*27*)	Bipolar platinum electrode on plastic rectal probe 20Hz sinusoidal frequency not to exceed 0.37 mA/mm² applied for 2 s	15	8 (53%)	—
Brindley (*7*)	Gloved-finger electrode, small cathode, large anode, battery stimulator supplies 100 ms pulse duration, net current less than 0.1 mA at varying voltages and frequencies, stimulation over obturator point	154	97 (63%)	3
Perkash et al. (*30*)	Bipolar platinum electrode or plastic rectal probe 20 Hz sinusoidal frequency not to exceed 0.37 mA/mm² applied for 2 d	30	22 (72%)	—
Bennett et al. (*2*)	Polyvinyl chloride probe with ventral electrodes, ave. 30 stimulations, ave. 15.6 volts, 315 mamps, sine wave summation applied	37	22 (59%)	4

In these techniques, electroejaculation results from the direct stimulation of efferent sympathetic fibers innervating the vas deferens, prostate, and seminal vesicles by the application of an electric current across the rectal mucosa (*6,11*). Horne et al. (*19*) originally used a curved 28 French urethral sound, insulated except for its tip, to deliver a 4-second current over the area of the seminal vesicles and prostate, which were then massaged. The urethra was finally milked for semen. These investigators noted ejaculation in 11 of 18 (61%) patients treated by electrostimulation.

David et al. (*11*) used an electric current over the same area, employing a rigid bipolar electrode, with less success; four (25%) of 16 patients so treated ejaculated. Interestingly, three of the 16 patients had incomplete cord lesions and could ejaculate spontaneously. Francois et al. (*15*) reported a 42% success rate in 31 patients. These authors also reported the first term pregnancy using electrostimulation and artificial insemination. Martin et al. (*27*) achieved a 53% success rate in 15 patients using a bipolar platinum electrode on a rigid rectal probe. In a later publication, these authors (*30*) reported a 63% success rate, using the same electrode to treat 30 patients. The bipolar electrode used by Brindley (*6,7*) consisted of a narrow cathode and two large anodes attached to a gloved finger. A battery powered stimulator supplied the current, which was directed over the obturator areas to elicit ejaculation. Brindley reported a 63% incidence of successful ejaculation in 154 patients with three associated pregnancies.

Side effects were infrequent and mild. Francois et al. (*15*) noted perspiration, headache, and transient hypertension only during the first attempts at stimulation, whereas Brindley (*6*) reported local heating of less than 0.5°C. Five patients underwent sigmoidoscopy immediately after electrostimulation, and the mucosa was found to be normal. After 256 stimulations, blood-tinged stools were noted on only two occasions with the next defecation. Hypertension, with or without headache, occasionally occurred in patients with lesions above T4, and generally diminished after placing the patient in a vertical position. In 15 patients treated by Brindley (*7*), electrostimulation caused intolerable pain, and the procedure had to be discontinued. The eight failures in the Perkash (*30*) series also may have been associated with intolerable pain. Although not expressly stated, most ejaculation failures after electrostimulation appear to have occurred in men unable to tolerate the procedure.

In Brindley's series, of the 97 patients in whom electrical stimulation induced ejaculations, semen expulsions were antegrade in 69 (70%) and retrograde in 28 (29%) (*7*). Brindley also found that electrostimulation caused ejaculation in patients treated during the first 6 mo after

SCI. In contrast, vibrator stimulation was rarely successful during this period. However, poor sperm motility was noted in electroejaculates. Furthermore, only 11 of 690 patients with antegrade ejaculations expelled semen containing 5 million or more sperm, whereas no semen specimens from 28 patients with retrograde ejaculations contained 5 million or more sperm/ejaculate. These results are poor when compared with those reported for vibratory stimulation more than 6 mo after SCI (*7*). Although Perkash et al. (*30*) reported total sperm counts of over 40 million in 18 of the 22 patients they treated, 27 (77%) of the 34 semen specimens they examined showed sperm motility of less than 20%. Francois et al. (*15*) reported that sperm motility in 13 of the patients was greater than or equal to 30%.

The cause of the low numbers of motile sperm seen in electroejaculates is difficult to identify. Histologic studies of biopsies from 18 patients treated by electrical stimulation by Horne et al. (*19*), varied from complete testicular atrophy to normal. Perkash (*30*) noted normal testicular tissue in six of 13 biopsies, and mild tubular atrophy with normal Sertoli cells and interstitial morphology in three of the remaining seven patients. These authors postulated that the poor motility of sperm in electroejaculates may be related to either a chronic low-grade infection, chronic antibiotic therapy, or a combination of the two. They also suggested that endocrine as well as isolated abnormalities in testicular and/or sperm morphology should be ruled out. However, the marked reduction noted in sperm motility appears to be a feature of most semen specimens following electroejaculation. Therefore, sperm obtained by that method would be inappropriate for artificial insemination. On a more optimistic note, several investigators have noted that semen parameters improved with successive electroejaculations (*5,30,7*).

In a recent review, Bennett et al. (*2*) utilized electroejaculation in 37 SCI men. These authors performed anoscopy prior to and after electrostimulation. A polyvinyl chloride bipolar probe was utilized for the stimulation. Patients were also catheterized after stimulation to recover sperm ejaculated in a retrograde manner. Although these authors reported a high mean total sperm count (182 million with a range of 5.4–1,415 million), the average motility was again noted to be low (22%, range 0–55%). Interestingly, the authors reported the results of artificial insemination in 10 spouses with 4 (40%) achieving pregnancies. The authors did not find the sperm penetration assay helpful in predicting pregnancy outcome.

In summary, electrostimulation would appear to be a relatively successful method for inducing ejaculation in SCI males. However, the markedly decreased motility of sperm associated with electroejaculation suggests that this method should only be used after other techniques have failed. Every attempt must be made to optimize sperm motility by avoiding deleterious agents, such as urinary tract infections or antibiotic therapy, and by counteracting the effects of urine on sperm. This latter caution is especially important because most specimens obtained by electroejaculation are contaminated with urine. The pain sometimes associated with ejaculation induced by rectal probe stimulation is not an absolute containdiction to the procedure, since it can be performed under general anesthesia, with successful ejaculation (*6*).

Intrathecal Neostigmine-Induced Ejaculation

Neostigmine, injected intrathecally, has also been used successfully to induce ejaculation in SCI men. In a recent review of infertility in paraplegic men, MacMahon et al. (*24*) commented on their use of intrathecal injections of neostigmine in five patients, each of whom received 0.3–0.5 mg of neostigmine bromide (Prostigmine, Roche). All patients had spinal-cord lesions ranging from the level of C4,5 to T12. Four of the five men (80%) ejaculated after the injection, and the sperm recovered were used to inseminate their spouses. Three of the four patients had antegrade emissions and one retrograde. This latter patient had been placed on a urinary alkalinization regimen before ejaculation was induced; no pregnancies resulted.

Of the five patients treated, three developed autonomic dysreflexia, which was controlled with nitroprusside given by continuous intravenous drip at a rate of 0.5–10 μg/kg/min. One of the five patients developed persistent sinus tachycardia and was found to have an underlying cardiac disorder. Because of the high incidence of dysreflexia, treatment was administered in the intensive-care unit where patients could be closely monitored with arterial and intravenous lines in place. Other common side effects included nausea, vomiting, drowsiness, and urinary retention. No sensory changes were noted; however, transmission through motor arcs was decreased, as were muscle tone, reflexes, and voluntary power.

Although erections were noted in 60% of the patients treated, interestingly, ejaculations did not occur for several hours after treatment. Multiple ejaculations were a common phenomenon, however. The mechanism whereby neostigmine results in erection and ejaculation is unknown. The drug may act directly on the anterior horn cells. Nevertheless, because of the high incidence of autonomic dysreflexia associated with this procedure, it has not become very popular. The authors of this review caution that the technique probably should not be used in patients with severe cardiovascular disease or with a history of stroke.

Retrograde Ejaculation

As stated earlier, semen specimens must be collected and analyzed for fertility potential and ultimately used to impregnate the patient's wife. In most cases, this is easily done by collecting either the specimen in an appropriate container as it exits the urethra, or by milking the urethra. Frequently, ejaculations are expelled in a retrograde fashion into the urinary bladder (*7*). Over 40% of the ejaculations induced in SCI men by electrostimulation are retrograde, compared with a 1.5% incidence in infertile men who do not suffer from SCI (*41,7*).

Retrograde ejaculation in the SCI patient probably results from lack of adrenergic stimulation to the bladder neck at the time of ejaculation. Thus, the bladder neck fails to close, altering the path of least resistance from normal—i.e., through the urethra—to retrograde—i.e., into the bladder. Any process that interferes with normal bladder neck contraction can also interfere with or cause retrograde ejaculation. For example, transurethral resection of the bladder neck for urinary retention is a potential anatomic cause of retrograde ejaculation. Medications such as alphamethyldopa, dibenzyline, and guanethidine can interfere with the normal bladder neck mechanism (*41*). Causes less frequently seen in the SCI patient, but which can affect bladder neck competency, include diabetes mellitus, previous bladder neck surgery such as Y-V plasty, posterior urethral stricture, previous transurethral or suprapubic prostatectomy, or bilateral sympathectomy or retroperitoneal lymph node dissection.

Retrograde ejaculation is diagnosed by examining the first urine specimen voided after ejaculation. SCI patients may have to be catheterized to obtain the specimen. Also, it may be difficult at times to distinguish between patients who ejaculated into the urethra and those with a partially retrograde ejaculation. Obviously, when the ejaculate is less than 1.0 mL, retrograde ejaculation is suspect, and the patient must be evaluated. However, ejaculates containing a diminished concentration of sperm also suggest retrograde ejaculation. Consequently, the first 15–20 mL of urine should suffice to wash out most of sperm that may have collected in the urethra and should be collected separately. If the remainder of the urine also contains a high concentration of sperm, then retrograde ejaculation is the most probable diagnosis.

The treatment of retrograde ejaculation can be divided into two main categories. The first comprises attempts to close the bladder neck either using sympathomimetic drugs such as phenylpropanolamine, brompheniramine, or neosynephrine (*41*), or by surgical reconstruction of the bladder. Pharmacotherapy has been reported to be only rarely successful (*16,24,41*), and surgery is not often a viable alternative. The second category of treatment involves attempts at retrieving sperm from the bladder. Noteworthy problems include the deleterious effect of urine on sperm, potential trauma to sperm caused by the introduction of catheters into the bladder, infections introduced with foreign bodies, and damage caused by techniques used to concentrate the sperm and separate them from urine.

Urine has long been known to be harmful to sperm (*10,16*). Brindley (*7*) noted markedly decreased motility of sperm contaminated with urine, apparently caused by both the pH and osmolality of urine (*10,16*). Crich and Jequier recommended replacing the urine with glucose or Ringer's lactate, alkalinizing the urine with oral agents such as sodium bicarbonate, and washing the specimen with a nutrient solution after it is voided spontaneously or obtained by catheterization (*10*). Furthermore, it is noted that sperm from urine with an osmolality higher than that of sperm had poor motility, which improved as the osmolality of urine approached that of serum (*10*). These findings were also reported by Mahadevan et al. (*26*). Interestingly, Crich and Jequier found that, in able-bodied patients with retrograde ejaculation, ejaculation could be converted to antegrade by having the patients ejaculate with a full bladder (*10*). This technique has been applied to patients with SCI lesions as described in the preceding Chapter 21.

Techniques for the Treatment of Retrograde Ejaculation

As noted before, several different techniques are available for retrieving and treating sperm after retrograde ejaculation, each of which has met with varied degrees of success. Based on knowledge of the effects of urine on sperm, a reasonable technique is one that attempts to achieve the following goals:

1. The Partner. Evaluate the patient's partner before an involved invasive regimen is undertaken to procure, process, and inseminate sperm. The patient's wife must be evaluated to ensure ovulation and identify the optimal time for artificial insemination.
2. Alkalization. Alkalinize the patient's urine by administering 12–15 g of oral sodium bicarbonate for 2–3 d before sperm are to be retrieved.

3. Urine pH and osmolality. Instrument the bladder as little as possible. Encourage the patient to void spontaneously; otherwise catheterization is required. Urine pH and osmolality are then determined; the optimal pH of urine is 7.4 and osmolality is 300 mOsm. If the values of the test samples deviate widely from the optimal values, treat the patient with hydration, water fasting, or supplemental bicarbonate. Alternatively, if the sample is obtained by catheterization, 20 mL of normal serium albumin can be instilled into the bladder before the catheter is removed.
4. Ejaculation. As stated earlier, the least invasive method of inducing ejaculation should be used. If the patient is unable to ejaculate, vibration stimulation can be tried. Only when this method fails to induce ejaculation should electrostimulation be instituted.
5. Collection of sperm. Immediately after ejaculation, the patient voids or is catheterized to empty the bladder. The pH of urine is then adjusted to 7.4 with 5% sodium bicarbonate.
6. Sperm preparation for insemination. The semen is washed with BWW (*8*) or other nutrient buffer, and is then centrifuged at 2500 rpm for 10 min. The supernatant is discarded, a pellet of sperm is resuspended in nutrient buffer, and the process is repeated. The final pellet is resuspended in 1 mL of the nutrient buffer to be used for insemination. A small aliquot of this final specimen can be examined microscopically and the quality and quantity of the sperm can be determined.
7. Insemination. The patient's wife is placed in the lithotomy position, and the sperm solution injected directly into the vicinity of the cervix using a 3.0 mL sterile syringe. A cervical plug can be used as an alternative. The patient should remain in the supine position for a period of 2 h. Many variations of the technique described have been used (*7,8,41*). However, certain tenets must be adhered to, regardless of the technique used. These are: (a) urine should be alkalinized and uninfected, (b) attempts should be made to limit, as much as possible, contaminating the sperm with urine, and (c) the effect of urinary contamination must be minimized by instrumenting the urinary tract as little as possible and treating the retrieved sperm in a fashion that optimizes their fertilizing potential.

A review of several data reveal that most of the success reported with artificial insemination using sperm retrieved from the bladder occurred in patients whose retrograde ejaculation was caused by factors other than SCI. Notably, Zelikousky (*41*) reported a 66% pregnancy rate among 24 patients with retrograde ejaculation. The patient population, however, was mixed, but the author unfortunately did not report the percentage of success in SCI patients or whether any of the pregnancies achieved were in these patients. One must therefore assume that, although it appears to be feasible for treating SCI men with retrograde ejaculation, the ultimate success of this technique is relatively low.

Often specimens retrieved from SCI patients with retrograde ejaculation either demonstrated that sperm counts were too low or contained too few sperm with acceptable motility (*7,8*). Cameron and Gilbert (*8*) used meticulous pH adjustments and washing with nutrient buffer to optimize motility. Another technique that can be used to isolate sperm with the best motility and, one hopes, the best chance of fertilizing the ovum, is the swim-up technique. In this process, a centrifuged specimen of sperm is resuspended and nutrient buffer is layered on top of the suspension, which is incubated. It is hoped that the most viable sperm will swim up into the top layer and be retrieved for insemination. The application of this technique to the SCI patient awaits further investigation.

If the total number of motile sperm retrieved is too small for insemination, further options are available. However, deciding when the sperm count is too small may be a problem. Sperm counts of 1 million/mL are usually required for artificial insemination when the specimen is injected in the vicinity of the cervical os. However, Brindley demonstrated a pregnancy with concentration of 50,000–500,000 motile sperm/mL (*7*).

If the combined use of the techniques described above results in too few motile sperm for artificial insemination into the vagina or through the cervix, one can consider the use of in vitro fertilization. Although this technique is costly and involves invasive manipulation of the female partner, it allows the removal of most of the barriers to fertilization and, therefore, requires many fewer viable sperm. Use of in vitro fertilization for severely obligospermic men is only recently being studied. Its success in the treatment of SCI patients awaits further clinical investigation.

Recently, investigators have attempted to aspirate sperm directly from the vas or the epididymis for artificial insemination or in vitro fertilization. Such methods would bypass many of the difficulties seen with SCI patients who have retrograde ejaculation. Silber et al. (*33*) recently demonstrated that sperm could be aspirated from the most proximal epididymis and successfully used in in vitro fertilization (WF) with a term pregnancy in one patient. Although the method was applied to men with obstructive azoospermia resulting from congenital absence of the vas deferens, this may be applicable to the SCI patient as a direct method of obtaining sperm for IVF. A major difficulty is the need for surgical exploration of the scrotum for every attempted cycle. Wide-spread use of this technique awaits the results of larger studies.

Couples going through in vitro fertilization (IVF) may need emotional support and counselling to minimize trauma in case of failure.

Primary Testicular Disease

Testicular biopsies have shown that infertility in the paraplegic male can result from testicular damage in from 8 to 50% of the cases. Either an absence of spermatogenesis or maturation arrest was observed in testicular biopsies from 50% of 57 paraplegics studied by Leriche et al. (*20*). These authors also reported interstitial sclerosis with necrosis of the germinal epithelium and tubular obstruction in 64% of their 57 patients. These observations were confirmed by MacMahon et al. (*24*) and David et al. (*11*), who found that spermatogenesis was severely depressed in most SCI patients. Histologic evidence of spermatogenic arrest was obtained by Bors et al. (*4*) in two of 34 paraplegics, whereas testicular biopsies in the remaining patients showed tubular fibrosis in seven and secondary atrophy—defined as greatly reduced cell populations with generalized pyknosis of all cells and the complete absence of mitotic activity in germ cells—in 22 patients. Spermatogenesis was normal in only three of these 34 paraplegics. Furthermore, of the seven patients biopsied by Horne et al. (*19*), testicular histology was normal in two, and germinal epithelium was completely absent or maturation arrest was severe in four. Atrophy of the left testis, but a histologically normal right testis, was found in the remaining patient.

The mechanism whereby SCI leads to testicular damage is unclear, and undoubtedly further investigations are needed. However, some suggest that decreased sympathetic innervation leads to testicular atrophy with subsequent impaired spermatogenesis as a likely cause. This can be diagnosed histologically.

Hormone Levels in Spinal-Cord-Injured Men

Bors et al. (*4*) and Leriche et al. (*20*) could find no correlation between the duration of SCI and the testicular histologic findings. They also found no apparent relationship between infection of the ureter or prostate and testicular biopsies. Hence, in an effort to explain the effects on spermatogenesis, serum androgen and gonadotropin levels were evaluated by several investigators (*4,11,15,20,25,30*). The conflicting results of these studies can be summarized briefly as follows:

1. Serum testosterone levels in 42 patients evaluated by Leriche et al. (*20*) were elevated in 26 and depressed below normal in 16; Perkash et al. (*30*) reported elevated androgen levels in all 30 of their SCI patients compared with controls, whereas Madduri et al. (*25*) could find no significant differences between testosterone levels in age-matched controls and those in six paraplegic men, and David et al. (*11*) reported normal androgen levels in all 16 SCI men they studied.
2. Luteinizing hormone (LH) levels in 24 SCI men studied by Leriche et al. (*20*) were high in six, depressed below normal in nine, and normal in nine; Perkash et al. (*30*) reported levels significantly higher than controls in 30 SCI men; whereas levels in 16 SCI men studied by David et al. (*11*) and in one studied by Francois et al. (*15*) were normal.
3. Follicle stimulating hormone (FSH) levels were high in nine, below normal in eight, and normal in seven of 24 SCI men studied by Leriche et al. (*20*); Perkash et al. (*30*) found no significant difference between FSH levels in 30 paraplegics and normal controls; FSH levels were normal in 16 SCI men studied by David et al. (*11*) and in one studied by Fancois et al. (*15*).
4. Estrogen levels in 30 SCI patients evaluated by Perkash et al. (*30*) and six paraplegics studied by Madduri (*25*), were not significantly different from controls, but were elevated in 30 of 34 men studied by Bors et al. (*4*).
5. 17-Ketosteroid levels in serum were normal in 54 SCI men studied by Leriche et al. (*20*), but were elevated in nine of 34 paraplegic men evaluated by Bors et al. (*4*).
6. Prolactin concentrations were measured by Perkash et al. (*30*), who found no significant difference in 30 SCI men compared with controls.

Based on the data summarized, it is impossible to draw any conclusions about the relationship between serum androgens or gonadotropins and the testicular failure sometimes seen in SCI men. In fact, serum hormone levels and testicular biopsies have been evaluated in the same patients, but no correlation was found between the results of the two studies.

Testicular Biopsy: Indications

The first step in the infertility evaluation of an SCI male is to examine the ejaculate, whether it is antegrade or retrograde. If sperm are consistently absent, impaired spermatogenesis is the most likely cause. However, because SCI patients have a high incidence of acute or chronic urinary tract infections, obstructive azoospermia must also be entertained. A serum level of FSH three times normal is diagnostic of testicular failure, obviating the need for testicular biopsy. On the other hand, in the presence of a normal serum FSH without marked testicular atrophy on physical examination, a testis biopsy is indicated since azoospermia in the presence of biopsy evidence of spermatogenesis is characteristic of obstructive azoospermia.

Obstructive Azoospermia

As stated earlier, azoospermia in the paraplegic male is most often the result of ejaculatory dysfunction, primary testicular failure, or both. Nevertheless, in a population of patients prone to infections of the urogenital tract (*4*), azoospermia may at times be caused by an obstruction in the genital tract. Typically, the patient will demonstrate the absence of sperm in the ejaculate and in the bladder after ejaculation. Testis biopsy will reveal spermatogenesis to the spermatozoan stage. In such patients, congenital and acquired causes of obstructive azoospermia must be explored.

Congenital Causes of Infertility

Congenital obstruction is usually caused by agenesis of the vas deferens. This paired structure is derived embryologically from the Wolfian (mesonephric) duct, which also gives rise to the ureter and the body and tail of the epididymis. The seminal vesicle arises from the distal outpouching of the mesonephric duct destined to become the most distal portion of the vas deferens. Since the seminal vesicles are the only source of fructose in semen, the presence of this sugar in either antegrade ejaculates or ejaculates recovered from the bladder is evidence that the distal vasa deferentia and seminal vesicles have developed normally and that the genital tract is patent through the ejaculatory ducts.

However, if the test for fructose is negative, either the seminal vesicles are absent bilaterally, signifying vasal agenesis, or the ejaculatory ducts are blocked. The former condition is not amenable to treatment at the present time. Transurethral resection of the ejaculatory ducts corrects the latter. This procedure, although not complicated, should only be performed by an experienced endoscopic surgeon.

The patient's ability to father children prior to spinal injury rules out congenital causes of obstructive azoospermia. It is then necessary to locate the point of the acquired obstruction, by scrotal exploration and vasography, which should be performed only under direct vision. Attempts at blind cannulation of the vasa can lead to injury and further points of obstruction. Also, plans should be made to proceed with microsurgical repair at the time of vasography. Most andrologists believe that this type of reconstructive surgery is best performed using microsurgery, especially if it becomes necessary to connect the vas deferens to the epididymis. A detailed discussion of the techniques and equipment necessary for such surgery is beyond the scope of this chapter, but several good reviews of microsurgery as it applies to reconstruction of the vas deferens and the genital tract are available (*23,32*).

In the technique used by the author, each hemiscrotum is approached separately through an anterior incision, and the testicle and cord structures are delivered. The epididymis is examined for signs of dilatation, which may signify obstruction. The vas deferens is then palpated for areas of obstruction, and if none is located, the vas deferens is then hemitransected sharply at the junction between the straight and convoluted vas. The lumen is cannulated with a catheter from a 23-gage angiocath, and 10 mL of sterile saline are gently injected through the lumen. If the saline flows through without resistance, then the vas deferens can be assumed to be patent into the prostatic urethra. If any question remains, a formal vasogram can be performed by injecting full-strength Renografin, and taking an X-ray film of the pelvis and genitalia.

At the time of hemitransection, the fluid that drains from the testicular side of the vas is collected on a clean microscope slide and examined off the field for spermatozoa. If the vasogram is consistent with obstruction, the areas of obstruction are explored and bypassed using standard microsurgical techniques for vasovasostomy. Once patency has been assured through the prostatic end of the vas, then sperm must be sought at the testicular end of the vas. If there are no sperm seen, the epididymis is explored to find the tubule proximal to the point of obstruction, which can be anastomosed to the vas deferens. This is done by transecting the epididymis, beginning at the tail of the epididymis and proceeding proximally. At each point, the cut surface of the epididymis is examined for a tubule from which sperm are seen to efflux. When this loop is found, the vas is anastomosed to this epididymal tubule microsurgically.

The chances that vasoepididymisostomy may lead to successful ovum fertilization and pregnancy are greater as more of the epididymis can be salvaged. However, statistics on pregnancies following vasoepididymisostomy are based on patients with an otherwise normal, functional genital tract. The chances of success in a population of SCI men must be poorer, especially if ejaculatory dysfunction is also a problem. This guarded prognosis must be discussed with the patient before the reconstructive microsurgical procedure is undertaken. However, for the motivated patient suffering from these problems, the above approach may provide the only hope of genetically fathering a child. A detailed discussion of the alternate means of fathering a child, as presented below, should be undertaken prior to embarking on surgical therapy.

Urinary Tract Infections

Before clean, intermittent catheterization became routine, SCI patients with a concurrent neurogenic bladder were treated either with an indwelling catheter or by operative intervention to create incontinence (*1*). However, chronic indwelling catheters, whether they are per urethra or suprapubic, are associated with a high incidence of complications. These include infection, calculus formation, and squamous cell carcinoma of the bladder. Hence, every effort must be made to keep the patient free from all indwelling catheters. This is best accomplished by clean, intermittent catheterization (*1*). However, even with this technique, asymptomatic bacteriuria can be seen in up to one-third of some patient populations *1*). The offending agents in most of these infections seem to be normal skin and urethral flora. These same agents could conceivably contaminate semen.

Recent studies have shown a lack of correlation between bacteriuria with such organisms and a decrease in fertility, as measured by small sperm counts and motility (*28*). However, this finding contrasts with data from earlier studies implicating such infections in infertility (*13*). Other investigators demonstrated that infections of seminal and prostatic fluid with coliform bacteria may be associated with sloughing of early spermatids into the ejaculate and an increase in seminal leukocytes (*9,39*).

It is evident that bacterial infections must at least be suspect contributors to infertility. Furthermore, *Chlamydia trachomatis* and *ureaplasma urealyticum* have been implicated as causes of infertility in men (*3,28*). However, the relationship of these organisms to male infertility is still controversial (*12,18,38*). Therefore, it would seem appropriate to look for urogenital infections in the SCI patient who appears to be at a greater risk because of urinary stasis and/or urethral instrumentation.

If urogenital infections are present, they must be treated appropriately, and attempts must be made to maintain the sterility of urine, especially in patients being treated for retrograde ejaculation. High-dose antibiotic therapy can be deleterious to the patient's semen. Both nitrofurodantoin in high doses (*29,35*) and the sulfa drugs (*37*) have been shown to cause reversible germ-cell depletion. In fact, many of the antibiotics used to treat acute or chronic urinary tract infections may have a deleterious effect on the patient's fertility potential. Consequently, it would seem prudent to treat bacteriuria in SCI men who want to father children with acute courses of antibiotics other than those mentioned above. Antibiotic suppression therapy should be avoided, and efforts should be made to minimize urinary stasis by striving to sterilize urine and to properly use clean intermittent urinary catheterization.

Intrascrotal Temperature Changes

Robinson et al. (*31*), in 1968, noted that a rise in scrotal temperature depressed and then caused a rebound rise in sperm counts. These investigators heated the scrotum by placing a 150-W light bulb in the vicinity of the scrotum, causing its temperature to rise 0.5 to 2.7°C. The process was repeated for 30 min each day for 14 d in 14 SCI men. Sperm counts were found to be depressed in few men. Although this effect was not significant, the authors noted a trend toward oligospermia. Brindley (*5*), in 1982, invaginated the scrotum around a thermometer to measure scrotal temperature in 13 normal subjects and 23 paraplegics in sitting positions. Normal subjects had a mean scrotal temperature of 35.27°C, whereas that for the paraplegic men was 36.15°C. These results were statistically significantly different ($p > 0.001$), and the higher temperatures in paraplegic men were associated with poor sperm motility.

The association between an elevated intrascrotal temperature and poor-quality semen is not only evident in paraplegics. Zorgniotti and Macleod (*42*), in 1973, reported scrotal temperature in 35 control and

50 patients with varicoreles as well as 44 patients without varicoceles; all subjects were infertile. When measured by wrapping the scrotal skin around a bulb immersion water bath thermometer, significant temperature differences of 0.6–0.8 °C were noted between control and varicocele patients in both the standing and supine positions.

To counteract the effects of scrotal hypothermia on spermatogenesis, Zorgniotti et al. (*43*) used a testicular hypothermia device in six infertile men with poor-quality semen and increased testicular temperature. The device, consisting of a scrotal support, a water reservoir, and an automatic pump, caused scrotal hypothermia by evaporation. The water was pumped slowly and allowed to drip onto the scrotal support so that it remained damp. Used for 24 h daily for 2 w, this technique was associated with a 50% pregnancy rate and improved semen quality in five of the six infertile patients treated. Although it has been used in SCI patients, results have not been reported as yet. It may be of value in selected patients with large numbers of retrievable sperm with poor motility, who also have an increased intrascrotal temperature. However, further studies in SCI men are necessary.

Donor Insemination

It is obvious from the above discussion that treatment of infertility in the SCI male is at best difficult, costly, and lengthy, and at worst, impossible. Further, the infrequent rate of success may discourage all but the most highly motivated couples from persevering. This chapter, therefore, would not be complete without a discussion of the alternatives available to these couples.

If the gynecologic examination of the female partner is normal, one can consider artificial insemination with donor semen (AID). This technique allows the couple to benefit from the use of banked sperm to achieve their goal of obtaining a pregnancy and offspring. Sperm banking has become popular around the country, and there is usually no difficulty in obtaining donor semen. Concern about communicable diseases, such as hepatitis and AIDS, may change this in the future. Guidelines concerning the proper surveillance and handling necessary to guard against transfer of the agents in the semen are presently in a state of flux, and one should seek the most recent recommendations before prescribing such therapy.

Couples going through in vitro fertilization (IVF) may need emotional support and counselling to minimize trauma in case of failure.

Adoption

For couples in whom AID is not acceptable or not applicable, there remains adoption. Adoption in the United States is regulated by state law. Preadoption requirements, adoption procedures, and legal finalization processes vary from state to state. Public agencies may charge minimal or no fees. The waiting time depends on a variety of factors, the most important of which is the availability of the child requested.

The Child Welfare League of America has over 400 member agencies. In addition, Catholic Charities, Lutheran Social Services, and others arrange for child placement. The department of social services in every state has listings of these agencies. The North American Council on Adoptable Children (NACAC), an organization of adoptive parents, has provided information and assistance to adoptive applicants, adoptive families, and agencies involved in adoption since 1974. For the directory of approximately 250 member groups of NACAC, write to: NACAC National Office, 1346 Connecticut Avenue, NW, Suite 229, Washington, DC 20036.

Child adoption by an SCI couple (one partner is able-bodied) is a new alternative for those wanting a "complete" family. It is advisable to have one member of the family physically able to care for a child properly (*21*). The adopting couple should have the following prerequisites:

1. A desire to adopt
2. A sound socioreligious background
3. Physical and economic stability and
4. Outside support systems.

Inlaws or other extended family members or social agencies must be available to render some form of child-family support services if an emergency arises. Some support groups, such as *Resolve*, cannot only help the couple deal with the psychologic and emotional trauma of infertility, but also alert the couple as to what possible avenues are open. For further information regarding special-needs and/or black children, contact: Elizabeth Cole, North America Center on Adoption, Division of the Child Welfare League of America, 67 Irving Place, New York, New York 10003, (212) 254-7410. For older couples in which the husband is a quadriplegic, it is most advisable that they not act as full-time parents, but instead apply as foster parents.

Intercountry Adoption

After World War II, children from Europe were brought to the United States for adoption. After the Korean and Viet Nam Wars, Americans began to adopt oriental and South American children. During the last two decades, an average of 4000 foreign-born children were placed with American couples or single persons. International adoption requires three simultaneous processes: obtaining a homestudy, securing documents necessary for US Immigration requirements, and the requirements of the child's country of origin. To aid in making an informed decision about which country and which agency to apply to, there are two important publications. Both are available from their authors: Foreign Adoption Resources, Anna Marie Merrill, 911 Cypress Drive, Boulder, CO 80303; and Now to Adopt Internationally, Jean Nelson-Ericksen and Heino R. Ericksen, 919 West 28th Street, Minneapolis, MN 55408.

Conclusions

This chapter has discussed those factors that are primarily responsible for infertility in the SCI male. These factors include: anejaculatory states, retrograde ejaculation, primary testicular failure, obstruction azoospermia, urinary tract infections, and intrascrotal temperature changes. The incidence with which these factors bring about infertility is much higher in the SCI male population than in the general infertile male population. A coordinated diagnostic evaluation, including indications for ancillary studies, is presented. Therapeutic alternatives for each condition are discussed, along with methodology where appropriate. It is hoped that the diagnostic approach outlined above coupled with the proper therapeutic intervention will improve the ability to obtain a pregnancy in this particular patient population.

References

1. Anderson, R. U. (1986) Urinary tract infections in spinal cord injury patients, in *Campbell's Urology*, 5th Ed (P. C. Walsh, et al. eds.) Saunders, Philadelphia, pp 886–899.
2. Bennett, C. J., Seager, S. W., Vasher, E. A., and McGuire, E. J. (1988) Sexual Dysfunction and electroejaculation in men with spinal cord injury: Review. *J. Urol.* **139**, 453–457.

3. Berger, R. E., Alexander, E. R., Monda, G. D., Ansell, J., McCormick, G., and Holmes, K. K. (1978) Chlamydia trachomatis as a cause of acute "idiopathic" epididymitis. *N. Engl. J. Med.* **298**, 301. (F and S **42(1)**, 107).
4. Bors, E., Engle, E. T., Rosenquist, R. C., and Hollinger, V. H. (1950) Fertility in paraplegic males. A preliminary report of endocrine studies. *J. Clin. Endocr.* **10**, 381–398.
5. Brindley, G. S. (1982) Deep scrotal temperature and the effect on it of clothing, air temperature, activity, posture and paraplegia. *Br. J. Urol.* **54**, 49–55.
6. Brindley, G. S. (1981) Electroejaculation: Its techniques, neurological implications and uses. *J. Neurol. Neurosurg. Psychiatry* **44**, 9–18.
7. Brindley, G. S. (1984) The fertility of men with spinal injuries. *Paraplegia* **22**, 337–348.
8. Cameron, M. C. and Gilbert, W. R. (1985) The recovery of sperm, insemination, and pregnancy in the treatment of infertility because of retrograde ejaculation. *Fertil. Steril.* **44**, 844–845.
9. Couture, M., Ulstein, M., Leonard, J. M. and Paulsen, C. A. (1976) Improved staining method for differentiating immature germ cells from white blood cells in human seminal fluid. *Andrologia*, **8**, 61.
10. Crich, J. P. and Jequier, A. M. (1978) Infertility in men with retrograde ejaculation: The action of urine on sperm motility, and a simple method for achieving antegrade ejaculation. *Fertil. Steril.* **30**, 572–576.
11. David, A., Ohry, A., and Rozin, R. (1977–8) Spinal cord injuries: Male infertility aspects. *Paraplegia* **15**, 11–14.
12. DeLouvois, J., Harrison, R. F., Blades, M., Hurley, R., and Stanley, V. C. (1974) Frequency of mycoplasma in fertile and infertile couples. *Lancet.* **1**, 1073.
13. Fowler, J. E., and Kessler, R. (1983) Genital tract infections, in *Infertility in the Male.* Lipshultz, L. I. and Howards, S. S. eds.) Churchill Livingstone, New York, pp. 283–298.
14. Francois, N., Lichtenberger, J. M., Jouannet, F., Desert, J. E., and Maury, M. (1980) L'ejaculation par le vibromassage chez le paraplegique a propos de 5 cas avec 7 grossesses. *Ann. De Medicine Physique.* **23**, 24–36.
15. Francois, N., Maury, M., Joreannet, D., David, G., and Vacant, J., (1978–1979) Electroejaculation of a complete paraplegic followed by pregnancy. *Paraplegia* **16**, 248–251.
16. Glezerman, M., Lunenfeld, B., Potashnik, G., Oelsner, G., and Beer, R. (1976) Retrograde ejaculation: pathophysiologic aspects and report of two successfully treated cases. *Fertil. Steril.* **27**, 796–800.
17. Greenburg, S. H. Lipshultz, L. I., and Wein, A. J. (1978) Experience with 425 subfertile male patients. *J. Urol.* **119**, 507.
18. Gump, D. W., Gibson, M., and Ashikuza, T. (1984) Lack of association between genital mycoplasmas and infertility. *N. Engl. J. Med.* 310–937.

19. Horne, H. W., Paull, D. P., and Munro, D. (1948) Fertility studies in the human male with traumatic injuries of the spinal cord and cauda equina. *New Engl. J. Med.* **239**, 959–961.
20. Leriche, A., Berard, E., Vauzelle, J. L., Minaire, P., Girard, R., Archimband, J. P., and Bourret, J. (1977–78) Histological and hormonal testicular changes in spinal cord patients. *Paraplegia* **15**, 274–279.
21. Leyson, J. F. J. (1986) Spinal cord patients and family. Personal communication.
22. Lipshultz, L. I. and Howards, S. S. (1983) Evaluation of the subfertile male, in *Infertility in the Male* (Lipshultz, L. I. and Howards, S. S. eds.) Churchill Livingstone, New York, Chapter 9, pp. 187–206.
23. Lizza, E. F. and Nagler, H. M. (1987) Microsurgical applications in urology. In *New Techniques in Urology* (deVere White, R. W. and Palmer, J. M., eds.) Futura, Mount Kisco, New York, Chap. 25, pp. 375–394.
24. MacMahon, R. G., Lee, R. D., and Lipshultz, L. I. (1984–1985) *Infertility in the paraplegic male, Current Therapy of infertility*, pp. 199–202.
25. Madduri, S. D., DeSalvo, E., and Seebode, J. J. (1979) Plasma androgens and estrogens in paraplegic men. *Urology* **13**, 178–181.
26. Mahadevan, M., Leeton, J. F., and Trounson, A. D. (1981) Noninvasive method of semen collection for successful artificial insemination in a case of retrograde edjaculation. *Fertil. Steril.* **36**, 243–246.
27. Martin, D. E., Warner, H., Crenshaw, T. L., Crenshaw, R. T., Shapiro, C. E., and Perkash, I. (1983) Initiation of erection and semen release by rectal probe electrostimulation (RPE). *J. Urol.* **129**, 637–642.
28. Naessens, A., Foulon, W., Debrucker, P., Devroey, P., and Lauwers, S. (1986) Recovery of microorganisms in semen and relationship to semen evaluation. *Fertil. Steril.* **45**, 101–105.
29. Nelson, W. O., and Bunge, R. G. (1957) The effect of therapeutic dosages of nitrofurantoin upon spermatogenesis in man. *J. Urol.* **77**, 275.
30. Perkash, I., Martin, D. E., Warner, H., Blank, M. S., and Collins, D. C. (1985) Reproductive biology of paraplegics: results of semen collection, testicular biopsy and serum hormone evaluation. *J. Urol.* **134**, 284–288.
31. Robinson, D., Rock, J., and Menkin, M. F. (1968) Control of human spermatogenesis by induced changes of intrascrotal temperature. *JAMA* **204**, 80–87.
32. Silber, S. J. (1984) Microsurgery for vasectomy reversal and vasoepididymostomy. *Urology* **23**, 505–524.
33. Silber, S. J., Balmaceda, J., Borrero, C., Ord, T., and Asch, R. (1988) Pregnancy with sperm aspiration from the proximal head of the epididymis: A new treatment for congenital absence of the vas deferens. *Fertil. Steril.* **50**, 525–528.
34. Sobrero, A. J., Stearne, H. E., and Blair, J. H. (1965) Technic for the induction of ejaculation in humans. *Fertil. Steril.* **16**, 765–767.
35. Steinberger, E., and Nelson W. D. (1957) The effect of furadroxyl treatment and x-irradiation on the hyaluronidase concentration of rat testes. *Endocrinology* **60**, 105.

36. Thomas, A. (1983) Ejaculatory dysfunction. *Fertil. Steril.* **39**, 445–454.
37. Toth, A. (1979) Reversible toxic effect of salicylazosulfapyridene on semen quality. *Fertil. Steril.* **31**, 538.
38. Toth, A., Lesser, M. L., Brooks, C., and Labriola, D. (1983) Subsequent pregnancies among 161 couples treated for T-mycoplasma genital tract infection. *N. Engl. J. Med.* **301**, 505.
39. Ulstein, M., Capell, P., Holmes, K. R., and Paulsen, C. A. (1976) Nonsymptomatic genital tract infection and male infertility. *Human Semen and Fertility Regulation in Men* (Hafez, E. S. E., ed.) Mosby, St. Louis, pp. 335–369.
40. Whorton, M. D., and Meyer, C. R. (1984) Sperm count results from 861 American chemical/agricultural workers from 14 separate studies. *Fertil. Steril.* **42**, 82–86.
41. Zelikovsky, G. (1984–1985) *Retrograde ejaculation. Current therapy of infertility*, pp. 202-204.
42. Zorgniotti, A. W., and Macleod, J. (1973) Studies in temperature, human semen quality, and varicocele. *Fertil. Steril.* **24**, 854–863.
43. Zorgniotti, A. W., Sealfon, A. I., and Toth, A. (1980) Chronic scrotal hypothermia as a treatment for poor semen quality. Preliminary communication. *Lancet* **1**, 904.

23

Sociosexual and Marital Relationships

Jose Florante J. Leyson

Introduction

Humans are social creatures who generally seek the same or opposite sex to satisfy sociobiological or economic needs, as well as the need for companionship. Recent data have revealed that in the younger age groups whether disabled (physically challenged) or able-bodied, companionship is in fact most preferred (*1,21,28*). Since 1945, there has been a tremendous surge of interest in the sexuality of SCI patients, as evidenced by a marked increase in the number of publications, lectures, and seminars on the subject (*2–4*). Unfortunately, before World War II, both physicians and the lay public tended to believe that with paralysis or "deviations from normal physical posture," individuals became asexual. They ignored the fact that these people had brains, were otherwise functioning normally, and retained many pleasant memories of their sexual experiences in the their "recall centers" (*4*). Perhaps physicians were ill at ease, or the social milieu was such that they felt inhibited about, discussing sexuality with their patients. With the liberated social climate of the 1980s, patients at last became more assertive. Today, in the 90s, they can freely ask explicit questions about sex and are willing to relearn facts about sexuality and sexual relationships (*1,3,4*).

Sexual Rehabilitation of the Spinal-Cord-Injured Patient
Edited by J.F. Leyson, © 1990 The Humana Press, Inc.

Clinical Neurologic Classification of Sexual Functioning

To facilitate different levels of sexual potentials, Comarr categorizes the types of post-trauma sexual dysfunctions into two main classes (*1,7–9,11–13*):

1. Reflexogenic sex: complete or incomplete
2. Areflexogenic sex: complete or incomplete

The above typology is based on whether or not reflex activity is present through the S2-S4 spinal cord segments via the pudendal-pelvic nerves and cerebral reflex circuitry (*6,7*). By inference, the examiner can usually assume that, if the bulbocavernosus reflex is present through the pudendal nerve, in all probability it is also present through the autonomic nervous system (*6–9*). Comarr's data revealed that, for quads and paras with different neurologic findings, 90% of the males with Reflex Complete Sex had reflexogenic erections (*9*). Of this group, 70% were able to achieve successful coitus with gratification of the partner. However, most patients will be unable to ejaculate or achieve orgasm. Many will have what the author calls "orgastic equivalents," e.g., temporary abolition of spasticity following coitus, with a complete sense of restfulness. Psychogenic erections and the ability to ejaculate are not the rule among SCI patients, but very occasionally exceptions do occur (*7–9*).

Some type of erection occurred in 98% of males with Relfex Incomplete and 83% of the partners achieved successful coitus; 45% of the patients had psychogenic erections. Of those who were able to have successful coitus, about 36% ejaculated (*1,9,11*).

Most Areflexic Complete Sex males did not have erections of any type. They were unable to attain erection, ejaculate, or achieve orgasm; 27% attained psychogenic erections. These latter patients had lesions below the T12 dermatome. The success rate of those who attempted coitus ranged from 27 to 50%. Interestingly, those patient who had reflexogenic complete sex with lesions above the T12 segment could not attain psychogenic erections, with only rare exceptions. The percentage of those who could ejaculate ranged from 19 to 35% (*1,9*).

In the Areflexic Incomplete Sex group, 83% had psychogenic erections, and of those who attempted coitus, 75% were successful, whereas 56% were able to ejaculate and achieve orgasm (*7–9*). Female patients in general were more fortunate. Menses returned in most of those of childbearing age, and most could become pregnant and deliver vaginally. In contrast, most male patients could not ejaculate and sire children.

Female Sexuality and Male Fertility

The ability of SCI women to achieve orgasm depended on the status of sensation in the clitoris and labia. Many women, even those without genital site sensations, could reach orgasm with stimulation of other erotic zones, e.g., nipples (*3*). Many woman could fantasize and reach orgasm, which would be very difficult for males. Among the Areflexic Sex patients who ejaculated, the range of voluptuous sensation went from nearly normal to "it's better than nothing" (*3,7,9*).

The ability to sire children was studied in 529 patients. Of those with reflex incomplete sex. In the group with areflexic incomplete sex, 5.6% sired children, whereas 10% of those with areflexic incomplete sex did so. (*7–9*).

Sexual Counseling and Therapy

The author believes that sex counseling can be initiated by the SCI care giver with whom the patient has the greatest rapport. However, sex therapy should be done only by a certified sexologist. Most authors insist that whoever is selected as counselor must be well-versed not only in the anatomy and physiology of the normal patient but especially in that of the neurologically afflicted person. The counselor must also know the statistical potentials for penile–vaginal intercourse, which, for the SCI patient, depend on the level of the lesion and whether it is complete or incomplete, as well as the reflex status of the sacral segments of the spinal cord. It is unfair to counsel the SCI patient solely on substitute techniques or other sexual options without first ascertaining which potential level of penile-vaginal sexuality each has retained (*2,7,21*).

Of paramount importance is that the counselor use words and phrases that the patient can understand: the use of medical terminology is a waste of time when speaking to patients who have not had the advantages of a broad education. Many are embarrassed to admit that they do not understand what a counselor is saying. The counselor/therapist begins the conversation with medical terminology, but then picks up the patient's hesitations, grimaces, or lack of cognitive response and tactfully reverts to more understandable terms (*1,21*). If street language must be used, the counselor could not hesitate to use it. Male counselors often assume that women know the "polite terms," but my experience indicates that many do not (*4,21,28*). On the other hand, the counselor must be careful not to "talk down" to the more knowledgeable.

Individual Counseling Sessions

In our practice, SCI patients normally receive their initial invitations to counseling sessions before their first weekend pass and *Initial Group Session*, and are made aware of the opportunity when initially contacted by their psychologists and/or social workers. Patients are encouraged to participate, but are not coerced; and individual sessions are generally held in the counselor's examining room with the doors closed, thus assuring completed privacy. Female patients are accompanied by a female member of the medical staff. Most patients arrive in the examining room on a gurney, completely undressed, but covered with a sheet or blanket to expedite the neurologic examination. An hour or more is allotted for each patient.

Male and female sexual function questionnaires are utilized to provide baseline for future interviews and for research purposes. Sexual data includes: age of patient, date of injury, social and religious standards, sexual preferences, neurological level, preinjury medical/surgical history, laboratory and specialized diagnostic tests, and use or abuse of drugs or alcohol. The detailed neurological and sexological examinations performed include tests of sensory levels, status of residual local and central reflexes, and such additional psycho-psychiatric studies as may be indicated. The full battery of sexological specialized tests are discussed in the chapters on male and female sexual diagnostics, respectively.

The patient begins to hear about sexuality when he or she is first contacted by the psychologist, the socialworker, and the physician following admission. All members of the rehabilitation team report to one of the three alluded to above, particularly if he or she feels that early contact with the patient is indicated. (*1,9*).

Every six weeks, Initial Group Sessions are held for one hour. Announcements of these Sexuality Meetings are posted and patients are invited to attend in their wheelchairs or beds, if they are bedridden (*1*). Hospital policy requires that those under 18 years of age must have the written consent of a parent before they are allowed to participate. The parents, a spouse, and/or sexual partner are invited. The two hour lectures are geared toward the patient's level, and nonmedical terminology is used insofar as is possible (*7*). The lectures provide an opportunity for discussions of the interrelationship of the bladder, the bowel, and sex, while explaining the innervation of the triad. Large drawings showing the connectivities of the spinal cord and cord equina to the bladder, bowels, and sex, as well as cross-sections of the spinal cord are used. These sessions have proved to be the best way to introduce the subject of sexuality in a gradual, nonthreatening manner, especially to those who are timid or hesitant about discussing it (*1,7,9*). Patients are frequently asked questions to ascertain whether they understand the lecture material and to stimulate their interest and input.

From the beginning, patients are told that no two SCI individuals are alike; the lectures cover the material in general terms, and the participants are urged to request Individual Counseling Sessions with complete privacy. Patients are invited to return to the subsequent Group Sessions as often as they wish, both during their hospital stay and after they are discharged.

Post-injury inquiries concerning erections are also addressed to determine whether these are psychogenic and/or reflexogenic, i.e., stimulation; what percentage of the time the patient can attain either a psychogenic or reflexogenic erection; how long the erection lasts; is the erection firm or semifirm; is the partner satisfied; and can the patient ejaculate and/or have an orgasm? Obviously, spontaneous comments made by the patient, describing unusual findings, are noted. Lastly, there is a sheet for pre- and post-marriage status dealing with the patient's age at the time of marriage, the date of marriage, children, adoptions, artificial inseminations, compatibility, living together, and divorces (*2,4,21*).

Female patients are also given a neurologic examination that emphasizes the sacral segments, including the endocrine systems (*5*). (Females are routinely examined in the presence of a female coworker). Also, inquiries are made concerning pre- and post-injury menses, contraceptives used, marriage, pregnancy, types of deliveries, sexual experiences, and ability to reach orgasms (*21*). One of the queries concerns religion and is of major importance. Although most patients tend to be liberal, the sensitivities of the devout must be respected. Our approach to the latter group is extremely subtle. Over the years, in fact, many ministers have called the author for an appointment, during which the patient, the minister, and the author have discussed sexuality with excellent cooperation from the clergy (*21*).

Only after the patient has been examined and interviewed does the counseling session begin. Counseling covers the topics listed in Table 1. At the end of each individual session, each patient is reminded that he or she is welcome to ask any member of the team for further discussions at any time before discharge from the hospital. After discharge, patients are welcome to make an appointment with the Sex Clinic of the Outpatient Spinal Cord Injury Service. These followups have proven to be of paramount importance both for single and married persons. (*2,4,21*).

Table 1
Topics Covered in Relationship and Sociosexual Counseling

I. Choice of being sexual or asexual (*12*)
  a. Heterosexuality and homosexuality
  b. Other sexual options
  c. Sexual phobias

II. Sexual anatomy
  a. Perineal areas and hypersensitive sites
  b. Delineation of erotic zones and foreplay

III. Socialization techniques (*12*)
  a. Explanation of how to cope with the four stages of psychological reactions post-cord-injury
  b. Building of self-image and future relationships
  c. How to establish the first social contact
  d. Identification of interests and revival of hobbies
  e. Finding friends and job opportunities
  f. Learning how to enjoy being alone—meditation
  g. Avoiding things that compound loneliness
  h. Pros and cons of getting a pet (for quadriplegics, specially trained pets may be expensive).

IV. Stress management
  a. Treatment of pain and spasms
  b. Relaxation techniques and peer group meetings
  c. Family support and community services
  d. Learning self-reliance and biofeedback
  e. Financial planning and social allotment (utilization)

V. Communication techniques
  a. Exploration of each other's sociosexual needs
  b. Specificity of mutual sexual satisfaction

VI. Sexual positioning (*23*) in relation to:
  a. Level of injury
  b. Incompleteness or completeness
  c. Spasticity and flaccidity
  d. Urinary devices, ostomies, and assistive braces
  e. Pressure sores
  f. Other complications (contractures, arthritis, etc.)

VII. Sexual activity and potentials—"Fantasy and sex dreams"
  a. Prognostication of the types of erections
  b. Oral sex and different orgasmic responses
  c. Stuffing (penis) techniques (*12*) and masturbation
  d. Clitoral stimulation and other erotic zones
  e. Perineal-vaginal muscle exercises
  f. Vibrators, dildoes, and other sexual aids
  g. Hormone therapy and drug complications

Table 1 (Continued)
Topics Covered in Relationship and Sociosexual Counseling

h. Papaverine penile injections or chemoerection complications (*28*)
i. Surgical therapy, penile implants (*24,25*), and erection pacemakers
j. Electrostimulations for erection, ejaculations, and orgasm (*28*)

VIII. Autonomic dysreflexia during coitus (*1*)
a. Presexual bowel and bladder preparations
b. Complications and management

IX. Precautions against sexually transmitted disease
a. Use and abuse of illegal drugs
b. AIDS
c. Avoidance of other venereal diseases

X. Fertility and contraception
a. Fatherhood possibilities (*10,15–17,19*)
b. Female personal hygiene, menses, pregnancy, and types of deliveries (*1,5,6,12,18,20*)
c. Child adoption and step-parenting
d. Artificial insemination
e. Sperm banking and embryo implants

Abbreviated Sex Therapy (BST)

In patients with incomplete lesions or those whose sexual recovery is up to 85%, and for the sexual (significant other) partners, a brief sex therapy (BST) is prescribed. Instead of a 45–60 minutes session, Ferris modified the standard sex therapy to consist of four 15-minute office therapy visits for non-SCI patients (*29*). This author has further modified this technique to a 20–30 minute BST session. Ferris' procedures are:

1. Sex re-education: Teaching SCI patients the male and female sexual response cycles. It is stressed that females need much longer time for their sexual arousal and there may only be a mini-orgasm, not the so-called true "explosive" orgasm. Sexopharmacology: explaining to the couples that certain medications can affect their sexual responses.
2. Teaching sensate-focus techniques: Defining extragenital erotic zones; emphasizing bowel and urinary bladder preparations.
3. Assigning homework exercises (sexual) for one hour twice per week. Patients are encouraged to study the "genital map," and

to try to be comfortable about examining each other's partner. They are advised to keep a diary and scoring record with the scale of 1–10 in terms of pleasure and arousal. Reading references are also provided.

4. Encouragement to rekindle the "romance" a couple may have experienced during an earlier phase of the relationship (*29*).

The average BST lasts about 10 sessions. If there are no tangible results after the BST, the couple is referred to follow-on individual or group therapy sessions.

Subsequent support group sessions and/or counseling are conducted once every two weeks. The third group session is devoted to assertiveness/training. Furthermore, these group sessions serve as an adjunct to individual therapy.

Personal and Sociosexual Relationships

Choosing the right "love" or marital partner is the most important personal decision in one's life (*30*). Before taking that giant step for a permanent commitment, Bassell suggested use of the "love test," which consists of two measurement tools: 1. An "emotional" maturity rating form and 2. a "romantic attraction" questionnaire (*30*). A combination of emotional maturity and romantic (sexual) attraction to each other suggests that the framework of a suitable partnership exists. The results of the "love test" are scored by the Scabs (a psychologist) method, and are recorded in the personal "love profile," i.e., individual scores for awareness, relating, competence, and integrity. For further elucidation, the differences between sexual attraction and emotional maturity (*30*) are given in the following table.

Sex	Emotional maturity
1. Primitive, biological urge	1. Social intercourse with coping ability, self-discipline, and high standards of behavior
2. Temporary satisfaction lacking respect and dignity	2. Continuous satisfaction with respect, dignity, and caring
3. Interest can be one way or mutual and short-lived	3. Interest is usually mutual with strong desire and a determination to continue
4. Can be boring if without romance	4. Interest build up as the relationship grows
5. Primary purpose is procreation via pleasure	5. Pleasure, responsibility and successful adjustment to life

For a successful emotionally mature relationship, one should observe Bessell's ten rules of togetherness (*30*):

1. Never guess or assume. Develop the habit of asking. Talk it out.
2. Do not consider your partner a sex object. Try to understand that the partner is a human being, like you. Sexual roles and lovemaking are only part of your relationship
3. Teamwork makes love work. Partners should work together as a team pulling their resources together
4. Give the four (4) A's every day:
   Attention is recognition and care
   Acceptance is inclusion and telling someone as special
   Approval is reinforcing what he or she does
   Affection is an affirmation that you really care
5. Build common interests. Some common hobby you can enjoy and share. Example: a 27-year-old quadriplegic male got divorced after only six months of marriage because he claimed the couple had no common interests beyond marital union
6. Learn to be a better lover. Keep experimenting and learning to improve oneself in the marital bed. Don't be too embarrassed to ask for what pleases your partner
7. Don't play games. Avoid making each other jealous, using the silent treatment, keeping score, bargaining, or even trying to buy love with gifts
8. Take risks for more intimacy. You must allow your partner to come within your personal boundaries.
9. Be polite, gentle, and show respect. Provide help around the house or in other activities. Show affection by being polite.
10. Give as much of yourself as you can. Give all you can to your partner—an unconditional surrender of one's love to your loved one

As relationship grows, love prescriptions are ordered toward a happier marriage (*30*):

1. Forget about fighting. Discuss your problems
2. Try really listening
3. Build trust
4. Communicate—never underestimate the power of the spoken or written word
5. Be sensitive to your partner's mood
6. Be honest even though it may hurt
7. Share one to one time

8. Let your partner/lover support your efforts toward maturity
9. Show respect and give unconditional love and loyalty
10. Share some common interests and give attention, approval, acceptance, and affection

Sociosexual Interactions and the Art of Meeting People

Socialization with new men or women for the physically challenged (disabled) person is one of the major sociophysical barriers that must be overcome. A majority of SCI persons not only lose the physical control of their bodies, but also suffer from socioemotional disruption of their relationships with their lovers, their friends, and their families. However, instead of waiting for that someone special to approach you or sulking in bed or wheelchair, there are some things an SCI person can do (*31*):

1. Maintain a kempt appearance and healthy look. It's better to be a pearl in the oyster, than a grain of sand in a silver platter or wheelchair.
2. Be approachable, but not too aggressive. Be relaxed, wear a smile, speak with a pleasant voice and a genial manner.
3. Change the channel. Don't dwell in the past or harbor negative feelings about your injury or shortcomings. Look towards the future with projects, hobbies and be energized with new acquaintances.
4. Make facial contact (eye contact may be difficult if someone is in a wheelchair).
5. Go for the fun of it. If you feel stagnant, get moving (keep on wheeling). While at a party get some chips (food), joke with some friends. Be an active listener. Sometimes, one may go "wheelchair" dancing.
6. Find mutual interest in drawing the other person out. Example: a 22-year-old quadriplegic male first met his wife while going fishing (the woman loved fishing too).
7. Show genuine interest in the other person. Be honest.
8. Make genuine compliments. Avoid remarks that may sound like "come ons."
9. Have a good time and just enjoy their company. Don't be disappointed if these few encounters do not turn to friendship, but just acquaintanceships.
10. Respect the other person's personal and emotional space.

11. Show sensitivity to the other person's emotional rhythm, pace, and sociosexual moods.
12. Practice a good sense of humor. A "wheelchair comedian" is better than a "walking curmudgeon."

Furthermore, in order to uncover a patient's personal brand of attractiveness, confidence and self-esteem can be enhanced by following these tips (*32*):

1. Magnify your personal assets by focusing on your best features. If your are fat, why not dress to accent those curves. "Dress to cheer, not to scare."
2. Explore your interests and turn them into full-scale enthusiasms. Even though you are depressed from other personal problems including your disability, show some "zest" for life. Indulge your passions; you may find somebody who will share these passions.
3. Set realistic goals for personal growth. Take self-improvement or avocational courses. These will further boost your self-esteem and may lead to an additional source of personal income.

Psychophysical Fitness and Personal Reenergizing Techniques

The non-acceptance of one's disability is one of the causes of chronic depression often resulting in mental fatigue. However, there are about nine to ten million physically normal people who are suffering from chronic physical fatigue. In order to overcome recurrent tiredness we frequently advise the following reenergizing techniques (*28*):

1. Schedule the activities of daily living according to priority. Organize your day with a less cluttered agenda, including a doctor's visit. If chronically busy, try to make fewer appointments.
2. Think positive. Adopt an optimistic attitude towards life and its problems. Ask yourself "Is it really worth doing?"
3. Find extra support. Stress is lighter when caring friends and family provide emotional support.
4. Exercise regularly. Regularity of active and passive physical exercises by a disabled person can allay depression, anxiety, even lessens pains or spasms. Schedule your sexual activities along with the other activities of daily living. Unlike able-bodied persons, spontaneity in lovemaking may result in embarrassing "urinary and bowel accidents."

5. Learn to relax. Anytime you feel tense or angry, slowly take a full, deep breath and then exhale equally deeply and slowly. Try to massage your arms or legs for two minutes. If you are a quadriplegic, 2-3 minutes of breathing exercises will make you feel refreshed.
6. Eat energy-rich foods. A balanced diet should consist of high-protein, low-fat foods (chicken and fish) together with vegetables to provide bulk for better bowel movements/care. A multivitamin/mineral supplement taken weekly will also provide extra help in maintaining proper body metabolism.
7. Avoid smoking, alcohol, and dependency on sleeping pills or "strong" pain medications. The chronic use of tranquilizers and sleeping pills can be habit-forming and may distort the normal cycle of sleeping and dreaming.
8. Reduce caffeine and other chemical stimulants and avoid illegal drugs. The caffeine present in coffee, tea, and certain soft drinks can cause fatigue by overstimulating the mind, thus reducing the amount and quality of rest or sleep.
9. Keep a controlled environment. Make sure your bedroom temperature, humidity, and noise levels suit your comfort. Choose a comfortable bed that is also designed to prevent the development of pressure sores/ulcers.
10. Maintain a good biorhythm. If possible, always rise and retire at the same time. This program will keep your biological clock in proper working order: thus every morning you will arise refreshed and full of energy.

In most states (USA), a majority of different religious sects, i.e., Catholics, Protestants and Mormons) offer or require premarital "couple" sessions or pre-nuptial (pre-canon) counseling, with the hope of reducing divorce rates in marriages among their faithful. Although these premarital assessement/counseling sessions are mainly tailored to able-bodied couples, SCI marital candidates can also reevaluate and learn more about their emotional maturity and decision-making abilities by attending them. The question whether a prenuptial agreement between SCI couples is beneficial or not still remains controversial.

Marital Status and Marriage

The immobility that follows SCI may hinder the patient from engaging fully in various types of social and personal interchanges. Once the patient has passed through the denial and depression stage, the psychosocial resources and defenses of these patients might be so overwhelmed that they prefer to avoid all social contact. However, during the final phase of learning to accept his/her cord trauma/disability, the patient often seeks social interaction, companionship, and love, all of which may lead to marriage.

Marriage fulfills many needs, some of which are emotional, economic, social, and love/companionship (*2,4*). However, to find a partner, one must first establish a relationship. Therefore, SCI patients must be encouraged to rebuild their self-esteem, re-educate themselves for social interaction, and sharpen their communication skills. Some patients are direct and some are subtle. Although there are different service organizations that cater to various groups of handicapped persons (video dating, resource networking, and telephone introduction services), friends and acquaintances are the best reference source (*21,28*).*

In choosing a spouse, most able-bodied persons surveyed indicated that glamour and security are important prior to marriage (during the courtship phase). After marriage, fulfillment, companionship, and maturity become vital to the success of the union (*4,21,22*). The handicapped person considered trust, maturity, love, and companionship—not necessarily in the order cited—as the most important factors in a marriage. Consequently, SCI men must be made to realize that many women do not need to reach orgasm, but achieve emotional satisfaction through warmth, affection, and a caring attitude. To an older or even a young person, marriage often depends on the sociopsychological makeup (value system) of the cord patient. Factors that may influence the success of a marriage depend on: (a) similarities between partners in terms of socioeconomic status, personality, age, and intelligence; and (b) similar interests, attitudes, and religious beliefs. On the other hand, factors, that may predict marital failures are (a) conflict during courtship, (b) extremely dissimilar values, (c) character disorders (neurosis or psychosis); (d) intense jealousy or mistrust; and (e) sexual incompatibility (*26*). However, in some personality disorders (sadomasochism) both partners may complement each other.

In order to maintain a "sexiting" (erotic) marriage, the following are ten cardinal rules that will help make passion burn brighter (*33,34*):

1. Remember that good sexual encounters begin while your clothes are on. It may be a striptease or a playful and gradual undressing as part of bowel and urinary bladder preparations. This process of "getting into the mood" constitutes a prelude for both psychosexual and physical nonsexual closeness between partners.

---

*Ed note: In Ireland, because of the high immigration rate of young people, the government and some social organizations sponsor marriage "encounter arrangements" for both able and disabled persons.

2. Take time to think about yourself as a sexual being. Condition yourself and your partner to the notion that sexuality is not just a fragment of one's life; it is part of the total process of life and living in a relationship.
3. The marriage comes first, while the rest is second. Make regular time for togetherness with your partner. Invest ample time in your marriage and sharing each other, either discussing or relaxing.
4. Use love techniques: listen, observe, verify, and empathize. Talk about sex with your partner. Discuss what you and your partner like and dislike among sexual activities—foreplay, interplay, and postplay.
5. Take responsibility for your own sensual pleasures; "supersexuality" depends upon accepting the erotic cycle that emerges between two persons over time. Learn to coordinate your partner's and your own sexual needs with bowel and bladder care. Give compliments to your partner's loving care and "good sex."
6. Don't let sex become routine. Unlike bowel and bladder care, which should be done by schedule, different tempos and different times (time of day, night or early morning) should be used for sexual encounters. Don't be trapped into thinking that sex must always include intercourse to be gratifying. Lovemaking can include: massaging, feathering, and playful sensual touchings. Experiment with different positions in bed and out of bed. For paraplegics, one may try in-wheelchair mounting. Introduce new sensual options such as mutual sex fantasies, masturbation, erotic video-watching. However, the use of "sex toys" maybe limited to those who are knowledgeable about sexual, bowel, and urinary anatomy and its complications in SCI patients. Initiate sexual opportunities with unexpected kinds of invitations. Exchange sexual roles. Try switching roles, alternating turns at being the passive or aggressive partner. With quadriplegics, however, the able-bodied partner must take the aggressive role.
7. Use fantasy as a prelude to whetting your sexual appetite. A word of caution must be stressed: some people become depressed when they reminisce about their pre-injury sexual abilities.
8. Don't go to bed or have sex when angry. The best way to handle this problem is to minimize the amount and duration of anger. Recognize its source and try to talk it out while it

is still at the level of hurt or frustration–before bitterness or total resentment sets in.

9. Avoid overemphasizing the mechanical aspects of the sexual act. Recognize that supersex in marriage is something one must earn over a period of time. Sex is more a matter of priorities than are genitals, bowel, and bladder problems, including pain and social commitments. An erotic marriage is developed by sharing dreams with and attention to each other, and by learning that the relationship is lasting, comforting, and with fulfilling love (*21*).
10. Keep some romance in your life. We must love creatively as though there is only now. A plain old-fashioned thoughtfulness, a surprise gift, and doing something special can go a long way. Expect to adjust to constant change. We must learn to remarry a different and changing person several times during marriage. Remember, an aging SCI patient undergoes more emotional and physical changes (pains, contractures, cardiorespiratory, and renal problems) than do abled-bodied persons.

Being a "wheelchair (SCI) person" can be lonely, let alone fraught with the difficulties of overcoming architectural barriers. Loneliness can affect people in even the best of relationships or marriages. In order to avoid loneliness and boredom in "wheelchair" marriages, the following tips may help:

1. Paraplegics may take a brief but separate vacation such as visiting parents or relatives for a few days. For quadriplegics, a day of separate social outings will help restore the personal appreciation of each partner.
2. Share your goals, work, and pride in success whether they are in household chores or in business.
3. Take on a major work project with your spouse. A quadriplegic can help decide the color or design for the kitchen flooring or wallpaper in the bedroom.
4. Try to pursue separate interests or hobbies, so that you have something new to talk about and avoid boredom.
5. Talk frankly about your feelings of loneliness and pay attention to what your partner is saying.
6. Share your innermost feelings (personal secrets) thus making each partner feel closer to the other, and thereby allaying loneliness.

7. Bring fun back to your marriage by being playful. Intimate play includes touching—an affectionate or gentle tap by a quadriplegic hand or a hug from a paraplegic spouse.
8. Surprise each other by doing something unexpected—a gift even though there is no special occasion.
9. Laugh together. "Laughter is the best medicine." Couples who laugh at the same jokes seemed to remain together longer.
10. Be sensual and make love at different times during the day or week. A quadriplegic male can undress his partner by using his or her teeth or stimulate the other spouse with his tongue (*21,35*).

Marriage between a physically challenged (disabled) and a physically able person requires much commitment and energy. In order to provide a feeling of profound connectedness and fullness of a vibrant long-term relationship, the couple should learn how to make love to their spouses. Furthermore, these techniques may even prevent extramarital affairs (*27,36*):

1. Keep the marriage alive emotionally by being intimate, tender, and offering daily compliments and attentiveness. Remember birthdays and other special events.
2. Engage in periodic physical (pleasuring) and spiritual enrichment. Know how to touch sensually and keep sexual anticipation alive. Make a commitment to sexuality—meaning accepting yourself as a sensual being who enjoys giving and receiving pleasure. Convey to your spouse that you are truly interested in "sexual celebrations." Many spouses complain that their spouses (especially the older ones) are lukewarm or too inhibited about sex. Be honest to each other. Avoid faking sexual satisfaction. Tell your spouse what makes you feel sexy. Limit intake of "gas-producing vegetables" if you are a quadriplegic with a tendency to pass flatus during sexual activity.
3. Take time and know how to play. It's okay to laugh in bed. Don't have too rigid rules about what sex should be. Try to relax, experiment, improvise and have fun as much as possible.
4. Define and accept the need for open communication. You can still talk to your spouse while engaging in other activities. Sexually satisfied couples tell each other about their fantasies and turn-ons.
5. Develop a more secure self-concept by overcoming fear of physical inadequacies (*27*). One of the strongest sexual fears

for both sexes is simply not being desirable enough. The majority of SCI patients is uncomfortable with their bodies because of imperfections, whether they are pre- or post-injury deformities or disabilities. Feeling comfortable with your own disability and residually functioning body is simply a prerequisite of feeling comfortable with your partner.

6. Defend against any form of exploitation and take time to plan lovemaking (*27*). In this hurried and stressful world, an SCI patient and her/his partner need to set aside the time for presexual preparations, a moment to understand each other and talk about the things that make the relationship work. Remember that the heart of every successful marriage is respect, love, communication, understanding, and commitment (*21*).
7. Lastly, the couple should remain lovers, even as parents, or as step- or foster parents. Parenthood should not prevent a couple from enjoying unhurried and uninhibited sexual celebrations (*35*). SCI couples should never stop using their assets, their senses of humor and imagination, to refresh their physical and emotional relationship.

The aforementioned marital counseling usually follows individual and group session sex counseling and/or therapy. Intensive Marital Therapy is given to couples with unresolved marital and sexual problems. Family Therapy is also offered to SCI families with marital and child-rearing difficulties, including child adoption, step- or foster parenting, and the prevention of child abuse and spouse violence.

Divorce and Remarriage

After a divorce, 30–35% of the younger age group of SCI couples tries to remarry. In order to increase the incidence of success for second marriages, the confidentiality of several matters regarding one's first marriage must be maintained, including (*37*):

1. Sexual ability: Whether the first husband/wife was disabled or not, a lousy lover or not, your new spouse deserves a chance. If he/she isn't a good lover, he/she needs help by gentle words and touch.
2. Looks: The new spouse may not be good looking, but beauty after all is more than skin deep.
3. Romantic nature: If the new spouse is not as thoughtful as

the first one, try behaving romantically; he/she might feel compelled to reciprocate.

4. Sense of humor: Acknowledge your spouse's good humor if he/she is blessed by one.
5. Career: Make your lover feel important as long as he or she cares, loves you, or provides a comfortable living for you.
6. Personality: Be thankful when he or she is not a perfectionist.
7. Charisma: If the new lover is not outgoing, be satisfied with his or her simple and honest virtues.
8. Sensitivity: If your new spouse is not as sensitive as your ex, accept him or her as is; try to speak about self-improvement tactfully when necessary.
9. Parents: Remember that your marriage comes first. However, avoid making offensive comments about in-laws; a spouse's fragile sense of self-worth may depend on strong family ties and support.
10. Effects on you and your relationship: What matters most in successful marriages is mature love and respect. Most people want to hear that they are special. But above all, know your second spouse and how to make him or her feel good (*37*).

Divorce Statistics

A large study of male veterans by Comarr in 1962 showed that the divorce rate was higher among those married before than those married after they had been injured (*4*). Patients married for the first time after they were injured had the lowest divorce rate. In fact, the rate in this latter group was far lower than that in the general population. It is safe to assume that the high divorce rate among those married before they had been injured was a result of the fact that the injured individual was no longer the same person. Comarr agrees with Crewe et al., who stated that the disability was something that neither of the partners had bargained for as part of their marriage agreement; perhaps most couples do not marry "for better or worse" (*14*).

The SCI patient frequently initiated the divorce. Some actually instigated the divorce for a variety of reasons, whereas others wanted a divorce soon after they had been injured and were still in the stages of depression and/or denial (*4*). Their physical inadequacies often cause them to accuse their wives of infidelity, an accusation that was usually unfounded. This stresses the importance of psychotherapy during the early post-injury period (*4,21*). The least number of divorces occurred among patients who had not been married prior to their injury, for reasons that are self-evident; the women were accepting their new mates "as is," with their eyes "wide-open." Crewe et al.'s (*14*) statement that "in the post-injury marriages, the disability was an accepted or at least an acknowledged part of the relationship," is apparently quite accurate.

It is interesting that the conclusions reached by Crewe et al. and by Comarr are very similar, even though the latter study involved veterans, whereas the former investigator studied non-veterans (*4,14*). It is also interesting that Comarr's publication appeared 17 years earlier; evidently changes in the social milieu since that time did not appear to affect the divorce rate. Recent studies revealed that coital ability played a role in the divorces of some SCI patients, but was not as important as one might anticipate (*4,21,28*). The following review of data has revealed that romantic attraction and emotional maturity are the main ingredients for a successful relationship in able-bodied couples.* However, acceptance, understanding about the disability of one partner or both, plus romanticism and emotional maturity seem to be the right formula for a happier marriage. Someone has remarked that love is a miniorgasm, while marriage is a symphony of love and respect.

Living Together

In the primeval forest, cohabitation without the blessings of marriage was practiced by our ancestors to aid in food gathering and personal protection. The ancient Greeks' institution of marriage was mostly ceremonial in nature. However, the Hebrews, and other subcultures headed by a sultan or king, instituted formal marriage to minimize the legal problems of property division and inheritance upon the death of the spouse. Although monogamy and the marriage institution have survived and are once again becoming more popular as the 21st century approaches (*21,28*), there is still an estimated twelve million unmarried couples living together in the US (*38*). Of the 250 SCI couples from seven states (California, Illinois, Pennsylvania, New Jersey, New York, Connecticut and Virginia) interviewed by the author, about 0.5–1% were living together; in all cases one of the partners had a T_1 paraplegic or lower-level injury. The average age was thirty-nine (39), and most of the cohabiting couples had been living together before the cord injury and continued to do so for economic and personal (family) reasons even after post-trauma rehabilitation. As of this writing, only

*Ed note: In some cases, the attitude and relationship with in-laws can play havoc with the relationship/marriage and may lead to divorce.

two of the couples living together pre-injury and one couple post-injury two to thirty years post-trauma got married, probably for economic reasons. The advantages and disadvantages of living together depend on the needs of the couple concerned. Most relationship experts (sex therapists) believe that cohabitation does not necessarily assures a successful marital union (*38*). However, it is advisable that, when the SCI patient has no economic security and plans to have children, she/he should have a "palimony contract" drawn to protect them and the children from economic disaster should the relationship dissolve. If one partner is much older, divorced or richer, a prenuptial agreement, although unromantic, may help prevent many economic heartaches and also constitutes an acid test of one's true marital intentions. Furthermore, if one of the partners has no ambition to work to help out the couple's "much needed" family income, the following suggestions on how to encourage gainful employment may defuse anger, unlock his or her desire for such employment, and/or help stimulate other productive pursuits (*39*):

1. Let him/her know that anger or resentment is inappropriate, that it's better for him/her to channel "hostile energy" to work on "constructive energy" such as applying for a job.
2. Don't overnuture your partner; and show him/her your personal approach to maintaining a positive attitude.
3. Give praise, if he/she takes some action, encourage his/her talents, and boost you partner's morale.
4. Let him/her make mistakes and laugh about them. Some may feel exposed or embarrassed; it can prove helpful to encourage them to work for a living. A heart-to-heart talk is always helpful.
5. Suggest job-placement or networking resources and provide your partner with leads or information.
6. Finally, suggest guidance counseling, in the hope that your partner will allow a third party to liberate his/her dormant work energies.

Conclusions

The physical disability following spinal cord trauma does not significantly alter the innate biological urge to make sociosexual contact with other human beings. Although architectural barriers may prove temporary hindrances to such emotional and physical interactions, any resourceful SCI person will establish a short- or long-term relationship whether by living together or marriage. The success of an SCI relationship is mostly determined by the emotional maturity of each partner, their love/respect ratio, the presence of an open dialog, and the establishment of a deep commitment. Furthermore, divorce rates are reduced, especially when the marital partner of an SCI understands and accepts his/her post-injury shortcomings. Although the physical malfunction hampers one's mobility, any relationship is sustainable if the previously defined sociosexual and marital suggestions may be put to practical use.

References

1. Bors, E. and Comarr, A. E. (1960) Neurological Disturbances of Sexual Function with Special Reference to 529 Patients with Spinal Cord Injury. *Urological Survey* **10**, 191–225.
2. Braddom, R. (1976) *Sexual Function in Spinal Cord Injury.* pp. 1–4, Ohio State University.
3. Bregmann, S. (1975) *Sexuality and the Spinal Cord Injured Women.* Sister Kenny Institute, Minneapolis.
4. Comarr, A. E. (1962) Marriage and Divorce among Patients with Spinal Cord Injury I, II, III, IV, V, in *Veteran Administration* Proceedings of the 11th Annual Spinal Cord Injury Conference. Bronx, New Your, pp. 163–215.
5. Comarr, A. E. (1966) Observation on Menstruation and Pregnancy among Female Spinal Cord Injury Patients. *Paraplegia* **3**, 263–272.
6. Comarr, A. E. (1966) Interesting Observations among Females with Spinal Cord Injury. *Medical Services Journal, Canada* **22**, 651–661.
7. Comarr, A. E. (1970) Sexual Function among Patients with Spinal Cord Injury. *Urologia Internationalis* **25**, 134–168.
8. Comarr, A. E. (1973) Sex among Patients with Spinal Cord and/or Cauda Equina Injuries. *Medical Aspects Human Sexuality* **7**, 222–238.
9. Comarr, A. E. (1978) Sex Classification and Expections among Quadriplegics and Paraplegics. *Sexuality and Disability* **1**, 252–259.
10. Comarr, A. E. and Bors, E. (1955) Spermatocystography in Patients with Spinal Cord Injury. *Urol.* **73**, 176–178.
11. Comarr, A. E. and Gunderson, B. (1975) Sexual Function in Traumatic Paraplegia and Quadriplegia. *Am. J. Nurs.* **75**, 250–255.
12. Comarr, A. E. and Vigue, M. (1978) Sexual Counseling among Male and Female Patients with Spinal Cord and/or Cauda Equina Injury. *Am. J. Phys. Med.* Part I **57**, 107–122, Part II **57**, 215–227.
13. Cressey, J. M., and Comarr, A. E., Gangsei, D. L., and Coffman, R. J. (1981) Sexuality and Spinal Cord Injury. *SCI Digest*, Department of Education, Rehabilitation Services Administration (HEW), National Research Data Center (Phoenix, Arizona) **3**, 23–30.

14. Crewe, N. M., Athelston, G. T., and Krumberger, J. (1979) Spinal Cord Injury: A Comparison of Preinjury and Postinjury Marriages. *Arch. Phys. Med.* **60**, 252–256.
15. Curtis, W. (1980) Personal Communication.
16. El Masri, W. S. (1980) Personal Communication.
17. Frankel K. (1982) Personal Communication.
18. Griffith, E. R. and Trieschmann, R. D. (1975) Sexual Functioning in Women with Spinal Cord Injury. *Arch. Phys. Med. Rehabil.* **56**, 18–21.
19. Guttman, L. and Walsh, J. J. (1971) Prostigmin Assessment Test of Fertility in Spinal Men. *Paraplegia* **9**, 39–50.
20. Hite, Shere (1976) *The Hite Report.* (Dell, New York).
21. Leyson, J. F. J. (1983) Sexual Enhancement in Marriage. Presented at the Asso. of Phil. Practicing Physicians in America Meeting. Houston, Texas, August 10–14.
22. Mace, D. R. (1982) Love Before and After Marriage. *Med. Aspects Human Sexuality* **16**, 73–85.
23. Mooney, T. D., Cole, T. M., and Chilgren, R. A. (1975) *Sexual Options for Paraplegics and Quadriplegics.* (Little Brown, Boston, 1st edition.
24. Scott, F. B., Bradley, W. E., and Timm, G. W. Management of Erectile Impotence: Use of Implantible Inflatable Prosthesis. *Urology* **2**, 80–82.
25. Small, M. P., Carrion, H. M. (1975) Penile Prosthesis: New Implant for Management of Impotence. *Florida Med. Assn. J.* **62**, 21–25.
26. Todd, J. (1982) Predicting Marital Success or Failure. *Med. Aspects Human Sexuality* **16**, 69–81.
27. Voth, H. M., Perry, J. A., McCranie, E. J. and Rogers, R. R. (1982) Viewpoints: How Can Extramarital Affairs be Prevented. *Med. Aspects Human Sexuality.* **16**, 63–74.
28. Leyson, J. F. (1988) Sex Odyssey 2001. Presented at the Annual Meeting of Phil. Physicians in America. Long Beach, CA, July 26–31.
29. Ferris, R. (1988) Brief Sex Therapy or The 15 Minute Hour. Brief Guide to Office Practice. *Medical Aspects Human Sexuality* **22**, 49–56.
30. Bessell, H. (1984) The Love Test. Morrow, New York, New York.
31. Bhaerman, S., and McMillan, D. (1988) A Unique Way to Meet New Men. *Woman Magazine* (Aug) **9**, 30,80.
32. Goodman, S. (1988) What Makes a Woman Sexy? (Sex Appeal). *Woman Magazine* (Aug) **9**, 36, 37.
33. Masters, W., Johnson, V., and Kolodny, R. (1988) The Too Passionate Affair. *Woman Magazine* (Aug) **9**, 46, 47, 85.
34. Pearsall, P. (1988) How To Maintain an Erotic Marriage. *Reader's Digest* (March) **133**, 39–44.
35. Zilbergeld, B. (1989) What Happy Couples Say About Sex. *Reader's Digest* (Feb.) **134**, 13–16.
36. Penney, A. (1988) How to Make Love to Your Husband. *Reader's Digest* (Oct.) **133**, 33–38.

37. Amatenstein, S. (1988) Ten Things You Shouldn't Tell Your Second Husband (about your first marriage). *Woman Magazine* (Aug.) **9**, 66, 85, 96.
38. Living Together (1988) NJ Network. Oregon Public Broadcasting System. The European Journal. Cologne, W. Germany.
39. North, G. (1988) I Love Him But He Has No Ambition. *Woman Magazine* (Aug.) **9**, 26, 27.

24

Salvaging One's Sexuality

The Patient's Viewpoint

J. Dahlberg and J. M. James

Introduction

Throughout this book, the clinical effects of spinal-cord injury on sexuality have been competently addressed. Equally important are the personal concerns of the patients.* The issues often raised by newly injured individuals encompass such physical questions as, "Will I be able to achieve an erection?" or "Will I be able to conceive (or father) a child?" However, often overshadowing such easily answered concerns are the issues involving the psychological assault on a person's sexuality. Not so readily answered, these concerns are raised by both males and females. Question, such as, "Who will want me now that I must use a wheelchair?" or "Will I be able to attract a partner?" seem simple, yet are significant because they affect all areas of an individual's life. As helping professionals, we must educate ourselves regarding these issues, stay alert to what they mean to our patients, and exhaust the available resources to resolve them. Because it is often difficult to maintain a patient's perspective, the following exercise, implemented by Dr. Ted Cole, may help you define what some of the basic concerns are from the patient's viewpoint. Recall your most recent sexual experience in as much detail as possible. Recreate the time and the location. Try to remember everything about your partner—the warm sensations, your body's reactions, how you responded to touch. What techniques did you use to make it particularly pleasurable? What

*Mr. Dahlberg is quadreplegic; Ms. Taggie (James) is paraplegic.

Sexual Rehabilitation of the Spinal-Cord-Injured Patient
Edited by J.F. Leyson, © 1990 The Humana Press, Inc.

positions? As you wander through your recollection, imagine yourself in that experience as a quadriplegic. You are deprived of any sensation lower than your chest area. Become aware that your breasts and genitals no longer respond spontaneously to stimulation. Parts of your hands and arms are numb to the touch and, moreover, fail to respond adequately to your commands to touch and explore. Recall how you needed assistance to undress and get in bed. As you lie there, pockets of worry form in your consciousness. You worry about whether your urinary catheter and leg bag might be a turn-off to your partner. Your worry that an involuntary bowel movement might mar an otherwise memorable experience. You also worry that your flaccid muscles or atrophied legs make you less attractive and less sexual.

Bringing your self back to the present, analyze what thoughts and feelings you have as a result of the above fantasy. List all the things you think would have changed from that first recollection of the recent sexual encounter. Does this provide you with a different perspective? We all will have slightly different responses to the fantasy, because our sexual experiences and conditioning vary from individual to individual, but the fact remains that most people come up with a similar list of concerns. Priorities may vary, but the most common responses include fear, self-doubt, and frustration. So, too, will our patients vary in their concerns based on their past history and biases, but most experience the same reactions, in varying forms, that you had. They may even add a few more to the list.

If we take a look at some of the more frequently occurring concerns, we will see that they appear most often in the following descending order of importance. Before examining them more closely, however, keep in mind that you may encounter variations on these themes, since each individual has had experiences unique unto himself.

"Who Would Want Me?"

Whether the newly injured person is single or married, male or female, his or her self-concept takes a beating. Concerns about wheelchairs, braces, or mobility give way to an overwhelming sense of worthlessness. As counselors, we invariably hear a variation of the question, "Who would want we (find me attractive, and so on) now that I'm in a wheelchair?" This rather simply phrased question is but the tip of a vast iceberg of underlying fears. Married patients may suggest that their partners "find someone better"; this often reflects their sense of worthlessness. It may also be an attempt to be reassured by the spouse that they do not want to leave. This testing of the marital waters often reflects feelings about sexual inadequacy, changed family roles, or concerns about dependence. Whether the family roles were as traditional as breadwinner or homemaker or whether they varied from the norm, each person, depending upon the level of injury, must deal with changes in his or her life patterns. Invariably, these changes attack the established sense of self.

Likewise, persons who are single or not involved with a significant other face what appears to them to be an insurmountable obstacle of finding a partner. Understandably, the risk-taking involved in initiating any new relationship becomes compounded when a sense of self-worth has been threatened because of an acquired disability. Traditional methods of meeting people often have to be modified to avoid the possibility of built-in failure. A competitive situation such as one encounters in a singles' bar, for example, might not be the best experience for a newly disabled person. Success is more likely to occur in safer situations, such as special-interest or hobby groups where the emphasis shifts from dating to special activities. However, even when some of the risk factor is eliminated, patients often remain fearful and question why someone would want to date (much less marry) a "cripple."

Even when a person succeeds in attracting a new partner, both men and women can frequently be faced with the worry of "what will their parents think?" Whether this concern is well-founded or not, some patients are anxious about meeting a new partner's parents or family, thinking the family might disapprove of a potential relationship with a person who is "less than whole." These fears can diminish, however, with a strengthened self-concept.

As a patient progresses and becomes more self-confident, the initial fears cited above may disappear or, at least, can be kept in perspective. The issues that are longer lived, however, crop up despite solid relationships or successful risk-taking. Many people express fears and self-consciousness about body image. The values of today's society stress physical beauty. The media is full of examples of the ways we should look, smell, or act. A spinal-cord injured person faces a number of changes in direct conflict with these standards. Muscles in the paralyzed areas atrophy, and body functions change. So, in spite of a return to a sense of self-worth, many of our patients are concerned about the changes in their body image for a long period of time—perhaps years. The situation is further complicated because of the presence of "extraordinary" devices such as leg bags, catheters, and other urinary devices, as well as such equipment as wheelchairs and braces, which are continually present and which affect a person's sense of his/her sexuality.

Further problems with self-image can also be related to standards prevalent in our twentieth-century society. In addition to the concerns about a "body beautiful," many people find that definitions of what is "masculine" or "feminine," as well as definitions of what are acceptable family and community roles, can affect their concepts of sexuality. Male quadriplegics, for example, have expressed anxiety upon meeting new people because they have been led to believe that a firm handshake reflects other masculine virtues. Some males also resent the disadvantage at which they are place by continually being forced to look up at someone during conversation. Furthermore, "looking someone straight in the eye" is impossible for someone sitting in a wheelchair. Such situations may cause feelings of inferiority or dependence, both of which are undesirable masculine characteristics according to the cultural dictates today.

Because women have usually been the shorter of the two sexes, they seem to express less concern with the foregoing issues, although they do find that constantly looking up at people can be a "pain in the neck." Feelings of dependence or inferiority are less of an issue to many women. Rather, some report greater frustration with having to monitor assertive behavior; which is still not completely acceptable as a feminine characteristic in our society.

Another issue is that many women feel frustrated in trying to remain feminine and attractive while surrounded by shiny chrome and rubber. Additionally, some women feel that disabled men have more options for expressing their masculinity than disabled women have for displaying their femininity. Sports and athletics provide an opportunity not only to develop remaining body function, but also to express competitive or assertive feelings. Women seem to feel they have fewer options. Additionally, many women feel that societal standards allow men to get by if they have "personality," whereas women are victims of a bias that emphasizes beauty and physicality as a gage of worthiness.

One final consideration that is predominately feminine is a concern about dressing to accommodate the disability. Urinary appliances such as leg bags and catheters make wearing dresses or skirts difficult for many women. Certain impracticalities in feminine dress manifest themselves during transfers or just simply in living from a wheelchair. Since our manner of dress often reflects aspects of our sexuality, some women feel the frustration of having further limitations placed on their sexual expression.

If we take a moment to summarize at this point, we can see that the assault on an individual's self-esteem following a spinal-cord injury has numerous subtleties. Concerns most often expressed by individuals cross all gender lines and are directly related to their intrinsic feelings of sexuality. Initial fears often reflect questions about physical function, but these questions can usually be answered simply, providing the care-giver has the correct information available. Concerns that are more difficult to resolve and that have an ongoing effect on a spinal-cord-injured individual envelope the issues of self-concept and the broader definitions of sexuality. However, since some of the physical functions are interrelated to feelings of self-concept and worth, we will take a moment to investigate what those issues are in the following section.

The Psychology of Physiology

One of the first areas usually addressed about sexuality and spinal-cord injury regards physical function. Any health professional can readily become acquainted with the correct information, keep current with new findings, and relay that information to the patient. It is important, however, to recognize that questions that arise about such basics as erection, orgasm, or fertility often mask more serious concerns about self-worth. As professionals, we must be careful to consider all possibilities, rather than "playing it safe" with textbook answers to medical questions.

With this in mind, we will see that the concerns in this area are both masculine and feminine, with only slight variations because of anatomy. Unfortunately, in our society, males are often led to believe that the size and frequency of erections are direct correlates of their masculinity. Equally unfortunate is the fact that most complete spinal-cord-injured males lose the ability to achieve an effective erection. Especially with older or more traditional patients, loss of erection signals feelings of failure at "being a man." Many men express concerns that they will no longer be able to satisfy their partners or even complete an act of intercourse. Since a large percentage of males who become disabled have seldom been taught alternate expressions of their sexuality, the health professional faces a unique challenge of helping the male patient reestablish his sense of masculinity.

Although women, on the other hand, do not have the same concerns about the overt physical expression of their sexuality as the men, they also fear the physical sexual repercussions of spinal-cord injury. Even though intercourse is not necessarily affected, women experience frustration at loss of sensation and inability to return their partner's thrusting movement. Often, women may have some difficulty with lubrication, and many care-givers think they have solved the problem by suggesting use of certain jellies or lubricants. However, the problem is certainly more intrinsic to the woman's sense of sexuality than it might appear, and care should be taken that the female not be overlooked in the more significant areas of self-worth because her physical problem may seem to be more easily solved, at least on the surface.

Both genders raise question about fertility and their ability, or inability, to reproduce. Many women are surprised to learn that child-bearing is still an option, and it is important not to overlook this issue with them. In addition to addressing the physical considerations of pregnancy, do not forget that this issue has hidden concerns as well. A desire by some women to have children may be overshadowed by concerns for mobility during pregnancy or even the ability to care for a child from a wheelchair. On the other side of the issue, if a woman is not desirous of having a baby, it is just as important to discuss contraceptive alternatives in order to diminish any fears of becoming pregnant, which might further complicate a sexual encounter already fraught with anxiety.

It is also important to note at this point that the inability to father a child by a spinal-cord-injured male is one of the critical issues for the younger patient, especially if he has never had a child prior to his injury. Many men feel "incomplete" because of this inability and, interestingly, report than these feelings can persist even if alternate methods of child-bearing, such as artificial insemination by donor sperm or adoption, are pursued.

Many patients also question whether or not they will be able to experience orgasm again. Much has been written on this subject and should become familiar to every professional, especially the information on fantasy orgasm. Some less obvious concerns can be hidden behind this question, however, Some patients—usually with the higher levels of injury—have difficulty adjusting to a more dependent position during intercourse, especially if they have been used to the more dominant role in their sexual pattern. This, plus decreased sensation, is likely to raise the anxiety level or prevent an individual from taking the risks necessary to reestablish a successful sexual life. As care-givers, we may find it easier merely to provide the patient with information, but we must be careful to explore all aspects of the issue, since merely having a map does not always insure a pleasant journey. Patients may also be concerned about their partner's orgasm, fearing they may no longer be able to meet the needs of their significant others. This can, in turn, rekindle feelings of insecurity or a sense of diminished self-worth.

All in all, questions about physiology can provide opportunities to explore many areas of sexuality as a whole. Routine questions can give insight into deeper areas of concern, as well as provide a basis upon which health professionals can build to help patients reestablish a strong sense of self-worth.

Professional Strategies

The obvious question now arises, "How can we, as helping professionals, assist our patients in overcoming these concerns?" High on your list of priorities should be to acquaint yourself with the basic information available. Books, seminars, and journals can provide a solid foundation in this area. By being aware of all aspects of the questions about sexuality, it is possible to establish a rapport with your patient that will enhance the education/counseling process. However, before we can adequately provide that information, we need to examine our own attitudes toward sexuality as well as disability. We must be aware of any personal biases regarding these issues. We all have them, and we all carry them into our professional encounters. By being alert to their existence, we can take care to minimize their effects on the concerns of our patients.

Where and how we got our early messages on sexuality has a long-lasting effect on how we deal with our own sexuality, as well as those with whom we interact. Did our early learning experiences leave us feeling positive and open or negative and judgmental in some ways? How will our attitudes about certain sexual acts or sexual preferences affect our ability to help a patient who may choose to practice these acts? Also, since our patient's early learning will have affected his or her thoughts and feelings regarding sexuality and the choices he or she makes, we need to be alert to those biases as well as our own.

The other side of this double-edged sword is our early learning and later experiences regarding physical disabilities. Again, have we grown up feeling positive and open about disability, or do we harbor some negative, judgmental attitudes about that as well? How will this affect our ability to interact with our patients and assist them in their sexual adjustment? Additionally, what subconscious messages did our patients bring into their spinal-cord injury regarding disabled persons? Will that make it harder for them to see themselves as productive and sexual beings?

Conclusions

The areas of concern surrounding sexuality can certainly be complicated. However, with the right approach, a successful solution to the problems is possible. Many patients' questions and concerns can be resolved by informing them what specific changes they can expect sexually after their spinal-cord injury. This should include information on anatomy and physiology of sexual response for both able-bodied and spinal-cord-injured persons. This information can be delivered individually or in group settings, and can be augmented with written material and movies.

Sexual counseling should be offered to all patients and their significant others to help them sort out the myriad changes encountered following a spinal-cord injury. Individual, group, and couple counseling are all effective means of meeting these needs. Peer counselor can also be very helpful at times in counseling sessions. Some patients, because of premorbid sexual problems or extreme difficulty in coping with their disability, will need intensive therapy. If a qualified sex therapist is not available on the staff of the hospital or clinic, a relationship should be developed with one in the community. Fortunately, few patients will need this level of treatment, since most will be able to reintegrate their sexuality through education and counseling.

The most important thing we can remember is to try to see the issues from the patient's perspective. By being aware of the concerns and by providing the correct information, we can help each SCI individual achieve a rehabilitated sense of sexual self. We are certainly not suggesting that the material or the order in which it has been presented in this chapter is all-inclusive or a textbook formula for problem-solving. You will find that variations are as numerous as the individuals with whom you work. However, keeping an open mind and a listening ear, as well as considering some of the things we have suggested, may help you be one of the factors that help salvage the sexuality of your patients.

25

The Forgotten Others

Partners of the Spinal-Cord-Injured

Robert J. Neumann

Introduction

For the spinal cord injured themselves, the right to be a sexual person is a battle largely won. In a random sample of 154 able-bodied persons in a large midwestern city, Albrecht (*1*) found that only 27% agreed with the statement "I wouldn't let myself fall in love with a person who is paraplegic." Occasional vestiges of old ways remain, as when a few years ago a Roman Catholic priest in the Chicago area refused to marry a paraplegic male and his fiancee because their marriage could not be consummated in the traditional manner, and children could not result. Mainstream opinion, from the medical community to Ann Landers, quickly arose to the defense of this young man and his partner, and indeed a way was found.

Within the rehabilitation profession, a considerable body of literature has accumulated in recent years documenting incidences and prevalences of physiologic sexual responses, and suggesting techniques by which the spinal cord injured may best elicit them. However, curiously little is mentioned about a spinal cord injured individual's sexuality in relation to another person. However, except for masturbation and fantasy, sexual behavior always occurs in the context of a relationship with another human being. Our present literature has precious little to say about the nature of the relationship, its special problems, and its unique rewards. It has little to say about the people who are partners of the spinal-cord-injured (SCI). These partners are truly the forgotten others.

Sexual Rehabilitation of the Spinal-Cord-Injured Patient
Edited by J.F. Leyson, © 1990 The Humana Press, Inc.

As clinicians working with the spinal cord injured, we must develop an increased sense of awareness that, when it comes to sexuality, it is the relationship that is our real patient. This premise follows Masters and Johnson's concept that there is no such thing as an uninvolved or unaffected partner in any relationship, and that an equally extensive knowledge of and attention to the concerns of each party is critical if the most effective treatment is to be delivered (*10*). As clinicians, we need to examine and challenge, if need be, some of our own assumptions. How often, for example, do we assume the partners have an easier adjustment and, therefore, can be expected to be more flexible, because after all, they are still healthy and are not the ones who have suffered an injury with devastating physical consequences? As clinicians, we need to sensitize ourselves to the specific issues that partners of the spinal cord injured express with remarkable frequency, if only we were perceptive enough to hear.

To assist in these tasks, this chapter reviews pertinent literature and presents findings from a study by the author. Clinical experience is also utilized in an effort to describe characteristics of SCI persons and types of individuals most attracted to the SCI person.

Characteristics of SCI Marriages

Relationship variables were initially introduced to the literature in the form of studies on rates of marriage and divorce for the spinal cord injured. The consensus of data reported by several researchers (*2,5,7,8*) was that marriages of SCI persons ended in divorce in rates that did not differ significantly from that of the general population. Furthermore, as DeLoach and Greer (*4*) point out, data from studies of persons with various severe disabilities, not just SCI, suggest that severely disabled persons marry at almost the same rate as the nondisabled, but later in life. The obvious conclusion is that SCI per se does not preclude either establishing or maintaining a successful marriage/relationship.

Somewhat more controversial is the question of whether preinjury or postinjury marriages are more stable. Pioneering studies by Comarr (*2*) and Guttmann (*8*) produced results indicating that postinjury marriages are somewhat less likely to fail. Comarr's (*2*) data showed that the divorce rate for preinjury marriages was 33% whereas that for postinjury marriages was only 21%. Comarr concluded it was apparently more difficult for the preinjury spouse to adjust to a spouse's newly acquired disability than to accept a spouse who the partner never knew as physically intact (*2*). Furthermore, Deyoe (*5*) also reported data showing greater stability for marriages begun after the onset of SCI.

Contrasting to the results of Comarr (*2*), Guttmann (*8*), and Deyoe (*5*), El Ghatit and Hanson (*6,7*) found no significant difference in the divorce rates of preinjury and postinjury marriages (24.4 and 23.1%, respectively). In their analysis of the data, El Ghatit and Hanson suggested some interesting dynamics of what may have occurred in these relationships (*6,7*).

In their analysis of *preinjury marriages*, El Ghatit and Hanson found 26.7% of those married at the time of injury had become divorced by the time of the study. Seventy-six percent of those who were divorced believed their injury was a major factor in the divorce. The divorce rate following SCI varied according to whether the individual had ever been divorced previous to the injury. Approximately 27% of those in their first marriage at the time of injury became divorced, whereas 42% of those who had been married more than once before the injury became divorced after the injury. The level of injury was not significantly related to the divorce rate. However, the divorce rate was higher for couples with children than for those without, which contradicted the impression that children necessarily provide a stabilizing influence. The influence of economic factors was also apparent in the finding that divorce rate was correlated with employment status. The highest divorce rate (37.7%) occurred among those men who had been employed at some time after injury, but were not able to sustain it. The lowest divorce rate (17.6%) was among those who were presently employed.

In their study of *postinjury marriages*, El Ghatit and Hanson (*7*) found the overall divorce rate of those who were single at the time of injury was 24.6%. Only 41% of the men who became divorce felt their disability was major factor in the divorce, whereas 76% of the men in preinjury marriages believed it was. For those who were single at the time of injury, the presence of children (natural or adopted) in a subsequent marriage was associated with a significantly lower divorce rate. However, for those who remarried after injury, the presence of children was not related to the divorce rate.

Although necessary and interesting, divorce rates provide only a very gross measurement—a measurement somewhat akin to analyzing health by measuring death rates. They directly reveal nothing about qualitative factors in the relationship, such as marital satisfaction, communication patterns, or social life. They tell us little about the individuals who comprise the relationship. Crewe et al. (*3*) addressed themselves to these latter issues in an excellent study of the pre- and postinjury marriages of 55 SCI persons and their partners. Not the least of the strengths of this study is that, as far as could be determined, it was the first in which partners of the SCI persons were included as an integral part of the analysis.

Crewe et al. (*3*) found consistent differences in pre- and postinjury marriages favoring the postinjury unions. Only on two variables—social life and self-rating of satisfaction—were no significant differences found. Both pre- and postinjury relationships were found to be socially active and high in self-rated satisfaction, but results on each of the other variables clearly flavored the postinjury relationship.

Based on psychological interviews, postinjury marriages were found to be significantly happier and spouses were judged to be more satisfied with their situation than were those in preinjury marriages. A trend toward better sexual adjustment in postinjury marriages was also noted. Both groups reported similar self-ratings of sexual satisfaction. However, one-third of the preinjury group claimed satisfaction with no sexual activity at all, a response made by only one of the 31 persons in the postinjury group. This appeared to be part of a general tendency for those in preinjury marriages to expect and be content with less in life. SCI individuals in postinjury marriages were judged to be more independent in activities of daily living and less likely to receive unnecessary help from their spouses. SCI persons whose marriages survived were more likely to live in small towns and rural areas, but those who were successful in locating new partners after injury were more likely to reside in large metropolitan areas.

Crewe and associates (*3*) outlined several selective factors involving partners, which may have been more favorable to postinjury relationships. They observed that preinjury partners may have faced more difficult tasks of adjustment in the sense that severe disability was something neither partner bargained for as part of their marriage agreement. However, for the postinjury partner, the disability of necessity was an acknowledged and accepted part of the relationship from the very beginning. By being in the position of making a completely free choice, the new partner may have been more likely to avoid feelings of being trapped in an unexpected and undesired situation. Also, by making a free choice, the new partner also strongly affirmed that the SCI person was desirable and lovable, thus helping to alleviate concerns about attractiveness.

Not mentioned by Crewe, but a definite possibility, is the factor that in postinjury relationships, it is not necessary for the new partner to unlearn previously acquired roles and ways of interacting. The prospective partner who meets an SCI person postinjury needs to have enough role *flexibility* to improvise satisfactory patterns of behavior where no ready-made social scripts exist to be a guide. However, unlike the partner in a preinjury relationship, there is no issue of role *extinction* for the postinjury partner, and no need to unlearn ingrained ways of relating, that the SCI may now have rendered impossible or inappropriate.

Crewe and associates (*3*) suggested that patterns established during initial hospitalization might have been responsible for the fact that SCI persons in postinjury marriages tended to be more physically independent. Those in preinjury marriages had a ready source of available assistance—the partner, who, out of compassion or a desire to minimize conflict, may have been overly helpful and thereby unintentionally prevented attainment of fullest independence in ADL skills. However, those not married at the time of injury and who lacked the ready assistance of a partner were more likely to learn to depend on themselves and indeed may later have taken particular pride in physical independence as a sign of equality in the marriage.

Reading these research studies, one could quickly be seduced into the belief that preinjury partners face insurmountable dilemmas. This would be unfortunate, mistaken, and definitely of no assistance to the couple with a new injury who are desperately attempting to make their relationship work under very trying circumstances. As clinicians, we need to keep in mind that the large majority of both pre- and postinjury marriages not only survive, but are rated satisfying by the participants in them. The major clinical value of these research studies is to provide reliable data sensitizing us to specific areas that are most likely to be issues for our clients. Another way to do this is to turn to clinical evidence itself.

Problems of Partners from a Clinical Perspective

Hohmann (*9*) has observed that the emotional distress experienced by most newly injured persons is a normal reaction to an abnormal situation. A similar observation could be made with equal validity about the partners of SCI persons. They too are undergoing a period of crisis and stress. As such, it is to be expected that they will also frequently have strong reactions to it. Unfortunately, too often in the acute medical and rehabilitation setting, the emotional needs of the partner and the relationship become lost, as we focus on ministering to the needs of the more obvious patient. True, we often give lip service to the ideal of making partner and family part of the rehabilitation process, but in practice, the partner is more typically seen primarily in tense, catch-as-can meetings with the doctor in the hallways, where he/she is given brief summaries of his/her mate's progress. Worse yet, if the partner's way of expressing concern is to behave nurturantly toward the injured spouse, that partner is likely to be labeled by hospital staff as overprotective, and thus be viewed as an enemy subverting the rehabilitation team's efforts to promote independence. In response to such a situation, the partner may be counseled to allow the patient more independence or the partner's visiting hours may be restricted; rarely are the underlying emotional needs of the partner addressed.

This focus on the patient produces feelings of isolation and aloneness in the partner, and sometimes feelings of guilt from resenting all the attention focused on the obviously needy spouse. However, focusing on the patient is not confined solely to medical personnel. The comments of friends and acquaintances of the couple invariably focus on the injured person, sometimes with unintended devastating effects on the partner. As the wife of a quadriplegic male stated, "I only recall two people who actually said 'How are *you* doing, Sue?' One was a good friend. . . . I told Tom, if I go out to a meeting and one more person asks how you are, I'm going to scream" (*11*).

As the couple begins to resume life outside the rehabilitation center, the demands for providing needed physical care and assistance may alter each partner's roles and self-concept, to the detriment of their identities as sexual persons. For some, the roles of attendant and lover are incompatible. Having to provide assistance, especially with such tasks as changing catheters and bowel programs, can remove the romance from a relationship. This can neutralize sexual attraction for both parties. As the wife of a paraplegic male related, "I became more of a mother, nurse, in-charge image. Not only to him . . . but to myself. I felt almost neuter sexually, and I still haven't recovered from that" (*11*).

For some individuals who receive validation of their own sexual identities and desirability through the physical responsiveness of their mates, the fact that accustom responses may now be impossible is very distressing. This phenomenon was insightfully described by one partner of a paraplegic male: "Even though logically I know it's not my fault he cannot have an erection, or experience an orgasm, or cannot get stimulated as he used to, I still know how he used to respond to me, and I feel less of a woman sexually because I can't get him to respond" (*11*). Clearly, the woman who made this observation could identify the logical fallacy in her equation of her husband's loss of erection with a loss of her own sexual desirability. Despite this insight, she continued to feel diminished.

Aside from the obvious core issue of sexual identity, there is also the element faced by many couples that each partner wishes the other to share a full measure of pleasure from their mutual sexual activities. This is one reason why it is especially important for the SCI person to explore which sexual activities are still genuinely pleasing, and communicate this to his or her partner. Even more, it is essential for the SCI individual to avoid developing the attitude that sex is something done just to satisfy one' partner. In sex, one-sided pleasure proves pleasing to no one.

DeLoach and Greer (*4*) outlined four factors that, although not specifically sexual issues, can put significant stresses on an SCI person's overall relationship with the partner. These factors are differences in (1) pace of life (2) temperature preference (3) income allocation and (4) social activities.

To use one example, it may take the SCI person considerably more time to complete even such basic daily activities as bathing and dressing than it does his or her partner. Furthermore, DeLoach and Greer (*4*) estimate that SCI persons may need to spend up to 36 h/wk in disability-related tasks, such as bowel programs and urinary management. Given this situation, considerable stress can be generated in the relationship unless the partner is able to develop constructive ways of utilizing the time periods her or his mate is busy with these activities.

Persons Attracted to the Spinal-Cord-Injured

DeLoach and Greer (*4*) suggested that there are several types of persons who are particularly attracted to the severely disabled: the walking wounded, the would-be dictators, the unsolicited missionaries, and the gallant gesturers. The *walking wounded* are those who have been hurt in relationships with able-bodied persons and, thus, seek out a disabled person who presumably will be more sensitive to their needs. The *would-be dictators* are those whose own insecurity is so severe that they need to have someone (the disabled person) they feel superior to and can dominate. The *unsolicited missionaries* are those who develop a relationship with the disabled individual in order to bring about that person's spiritual salvation. The *gallant gesturers* are those who really discount disabled persons as sexual beings, but have sex with them anyway to do them a favor. DeLoach and Greer conclude that sound relationships have no chance of growing from each of these types, with the exception of certain of the walking wounded.

The tone of this typology is rather pessimistic and gives little indication of positive, life-enhancing reasons why one may choose to become the partner of a SCI person. Further, no data was presented regarding how this typology was derived. Nonetheless, the descriptions are thought provoking and catchy, and clinically, it may be of heuristic value to present them to SCI persons as a device to stimulate discussion.

In a study on the caring relationships of SCI men and their partners, Neumann (*13*) found that women partners in his sample tended to score either very high or very low on self-actualization, with the high scores predominating. Self-actualization was measured by the I-scale of Shostrum's Personal Orientation Inventory. Of the 20 women partners in Neumann's sample, 43.1% scored at or above the mean for self-actualizing persons, whereas only 23.8% scored at or below the nonself-actualizing mean. These figures clearly suggest that there are many women who choose to develop or continue relationships with SCI men for reasons that are healthier and life enhancing. Perhaps the strong inner-directedness of the more highly actualized woman partner is the key. Higher levels of inner-directedness may make it more likely that a woman would choose an SCI mate, because the opinions of others have less salience to her, and because the obvious physical drawbacks are outweighted by the potential total satisfaction in the relationship. For similar reasons, it may also be that inner-directedness is a useful characteristic to have in negotiating the adjustments necessary when one's able-bodied mate becomes unexpectedly spinal cord injured.

Simmons and Ball (1984) researched the role of self-actualization in the marital adjustment of spinal-cord-injured men. Their sample consisted of 32 couples in which the husband was spinal cord injured. Both partners individually completed the Personal Orientation Inventory and the Dyadic Adjustment Scale. Both husbands and wives married *after* the injuries were found to be significantly more inner-directed and had better marital adjustment than those married *before* the injuries. Wives in the former group had better marital adjustment if they were more inner-directed, while wives in the latter group were better adjusted if they were more present-centered and capable of intimate contact. These adjustment patterns were hypothesized, but not actually found, in Neumann's study, probably because of that author's small and possible atypical sample.

Neumann (*12,13*) also investigated attitudes toward physical attractiveness in these women partners of SCI men. He found a clear majority (60%) indicated that physical attractiveness in a sexual partner was either very or moderately important to them. Only 20% rated physical attractiveness slightly important, and another 20% stated that they did not think about it. Regarding the physical attractiveness of their SCI mate, 45% felt their partner was about as attractive as they were and 35% described their partner as being *more* attractive. Interestingly, fully 80% of the women partners reported they have frequently, or at least occasionally found themselves drawn toward men who were not physically beautiful in the conventional sense, but they found them attractive anyway. Neumann concluded that, although women partners of SCI men may have defined attractiveness in idiosyncratic ways, it clearly was still important to them. This belies the popular notion that physical attractiveness does not matter to the woman who is a partner of a seriously disabled man. Not only was attractiveness important, but these women felt their SCI partner had it.

Finally, Neumann (*12,13*) measured certain sexual experiences in his group of women partners. As a group, these women did not have extensive sexual experience, either in terms of total numbers of partners *ever* in sexual intercourse (median number of partners ever = 1.0, or in terms of age at first coitus (median age = 21.0 years). Neumann explained these findings in the context of traditional patterns of psychosexual socialization, where men tend to perceive interactions in terms of the specifically sexual, and women in terms of more general love, romance, and emotional caring.

Conclusions

The emotional reactions of partners of the spinal cord injured are normal responses to an unusually stressful situation. Relationships established postinjury may have certain factors working to their advantage, but partners with high levels of self-actualization are to be found in both pre- and postinjury relationships. As clinicians, we need to be mindful of the special problems outlined in this chapter, but we also need to be aware of the rewards and opportunities for growth. As one woman partner wrote, "My husband has more self-esteem and self-confidence and has just bloomed since our marriage. My reward is just being with him, for he is a truly fascinating and lovable individual" (*12*).

References

1. Albrecht, G. L. (1976) Reducing public barriers of the severely handicapped, Northwestern University, unpublished manuscript.

2. Comarr, A. E. (1962) Marriage and divorce among patients with spinal cord injury. I. J. Indian Med. Profession. **9**, 4353–4359.

3. Crewe, N. M., Athelstan, G. T., and Krumberger, J. (1979) Spinal cord injury: A comparison of preinjury and postinjury marriages. *Arch. Phys. Med. Rehabil.* **60**, 252–256.

4. DeLoach, C. and Greer, B. G. (1981) *Adjustment to Severe Physical Disability: A Metamorphosis* (McGraw-Hill, New York).
5. Deyoe, F. (1972) Spinal cord injury: Long term follow-up of veterans. *Arch. Phys. Med. Rehabil.* **53**, 523–529.
6. El Ghatit, A. and Hanson, R. (1975) Outcome of marriages existing at the time of a male's spinal cord injury. *J. Chron. Dis.* **28**, 383–388.
7. El Ghatit, A. and Hanson, R. (1976) Marriage and divorce after spinal cord injury. *Arch. Phys. Med. Rehabil.* **57**, 470–472.
8. Guttmann, L. (1964) Married life of paraplegics and tetraplegics. *Paraplegia,* **2**, 182–188.
9. Hohmann, G. (1972) Considerations in the management of psychosexual readjustment in the spinal cord injured male. *Rehabil. Psych.* **19**, 50–58.
10. Masters, W. E. and Johnson, V. E. (1970) *Human Sexual Inadequacy* (Little, Brown, Boston).
11. Morgan, A. B. (1980) The forgotten injured: The impact of spinal cord injury on the family. Videotape presentation. Memorial Medical Center, Springfield, Illinois.
12. Neumann, R. J. (1979) The forgotten injured: Women partners of spinal cord injured men, a preliminary report. *Sexual Disabil. J.* **2**, 287–292.
13. Neumann, R. J. (1980) The relationship of marital status and quality to correlates of self-actualization among spinal cord injured men and their partners. Doctoral Dissertation. University Microfilms International, Ann Arbor, Michigan.
14. Simmons, S. and Ball, S. (1984) Marital adjustment and self-actualization in couples married before and after spinal cord injury. *J. Marriage Family,* 943–945.

26

Male Homosexuality and Other Varieties of Sexual Lifestyles

Jose Florante J. Leyson

"I cannot procreate. You cannot procreate with me. So, what does it matter what we do with one another, the affection, the warmth we feel? It did not bring ruin to your day-to-day life or to mine. It was love, finally, and what is the ruin in love?" (*Cry to Heaven* by Anne Rice, published by Knopf, New York, 1982).

Introduction

The human male is endocrinologically a bisexual animal that secretes both male and female hormones; the masculine characteristics are determined by the predominance of androgenic hormones and sociocultural behavioral influences. Homosexuality has been practiced at least since the Ancient Greeks, and probably earlier. However, different civilizations, cultures, races, and religions have adopted various interpretations and attitudes toward homosexuals and homosexuality (*5,9,31*). Freud, in 1905, believed that homosexuality was a mental illness or sexual perversion that could be treated by hypnosis (*10*). He proposed that the symptoms of homosexuality could be suppressed through the use of transference psychoanalysis; the criterion for the cure was detachment of the cathexis from the homosexual object (*10,34*). However, in the 1980s, homosexuality was dropped from the American Psychiatric Association's list of psychiatric illnesses.

Sexual Rehabilitation of the Spinal-Cord-Injured Patient
Edited by J.F. Leyson, © 1990 The Humana Press, Inc.

There are several recent theories regarding the etiology of homosexuality: hormonal, sociobiologic, and a combination of both. The hormonal or neuroendocrine theory suggests that prenatal stress triggers the secretion of less masculinizing adrenal androgens, which compete with the testicular androgens for receptor sites in the brain. Thus, an androgen deficiency in a genetic male during the prenatal (critical) period of brain maturation gives rise to a predominantly female orientation, resulting in postpubertal homosexual behavior (*37*). On the other hand, Bell believes that homosexuals are born as normal males and become homosexual because of influences from abnormal or adverse life experiences particularly from their parents (*38*). This sociobiologic theory also labels homosexuality as a "developmental deviation" (*38*). The purely biologic (hormonal) theory is challenged by Bell et al., who proposes the so-called combination theory in its place (*38*). This theory proposes that homosexuality evolves from an altered biologic precusor with a mixture of sociopsychological aberrations. Bell et al. concluded that homosexuals are gender nonconformists, and believe that homosexuality is but another human behavioral variant, rejecting the kind of therapy that "converts" homosexuals to heterosexuals (*38*).

The sociobiologic theory is also supported by Green, who suggests that reparative mechanisms operate among those feminine boys who did not have close relationships with fathers and male peers. This "male-effect starvation feeling" may motivate these "sissy boys" to search for love and affection from males (*39*). Other authors propose that homosexuality arises for several reasons: pre-adolescent ignorance of sex/gender roles, fear of change, and a deviation from or sociopolitical statement about traditional sociosexual values (*40*). However, for the SCI person, male homosexuality is sometimes a matter of sexual adaptation—a necessary adjustment to an adverse social climate in which there is a lack of heterosexual partners. Most women are not attracted to men on wheelchairs; for example, a 38-year-old, divorced, paraplegic male who had been heterosexual for five years post-SCI injury later became a bisexual and presently practices homosexuality because he finds only male friends in his social circumstances.

The dominant Judeo-Christian culture still does not condone homosexuality on the grounds that it is unnatural: such behavior does not lead to procreation, which is viewed as the only legitimate reason for intercourse. In the world of Islam, homosexuality is totally unacceptable behavior and is punishable by death. Eastern cultures, in contrast to those of western world, have mixed attitudes (*1,5,31*), depending on the particulars of early religious group's beliefs. In the Orient, i.e., the Philippine Islands, homosexuals are considered meek (feminine) and less aggressive or assertive than other males. With the sexual revolution, however, European and North American homosexuals have become vocal and aggressive (assertive) (*1,25*). The Gay Liberation movement was conceived in New York City in 1969 (*25*) to establish a visible platform from which gay men and women could demand equal human rights (*1,25*). However, as of 1988, most church groups still consider gays a community health hazard. Capitalists view them as unemployable while communists see them as decadent capitalist backsliders and believers in the nuclear family almost everywhere categorize them as products of birth defects and threats to their children's sexual development (*25*).

It is estimated that 1–2% of females and 3–6% of males are homosexuals, and perhaps as many as 33% of all persons will have had some kind of homosexual experience during their lifetimes (*11*). In 1983, about 17 million Americans were believed to be practicing homosexuality (*21,24,25*). No significant differences were observed in terms of ethnic groups (*11,25*). Eight varieties of homosexual expression are known: preferential or obligatory, developmental homoerotic, pseudohomosexual, situational, exploitive, enforced, variational, and finally ideological or political (*11*). Observations by other authors (*11*) and personal interviews have revealed that the most probable type of homosexuality in SCI men is either situational or political, although a minority are of the preferential type and practiced homosexuality prior to their SCI. It is estimated that the incidence of SCI in the United States is about three per 100,000 per annum, so that there probably were about a quarter of a million such affected individuals as of 1983 (*8*).

The incidence of homosexuality in the SCI population is presently not known. However, because of the sexual revolution and the tragedy of acquired immune deficiency syndrome (AIDS), these patients are now more vocal and visible. A survey of 90 males and 12 females revealed 1.5% and 0.3% as homosexuals, respectively. There were no hormonal abnormalities seen in any of these subjects, even in one 60-year-old female who suffered hirsutism. Both female and male homosexuals complained of extreme difficulty finding a sexual partner (sometimes even with a sexual surrogate) because of psychosocial and architectural barriers.

Data have suggested that there is some similarity between those brain regions that control aggression and those concerned with sexual behavior (*18*). Furthermore, bioamine mechanisms that increase testosterone are associated with aggressive behavior in both male and female animals, including mice (*18*). It is known that SCI usually occurs in aggressive, adventurous, and athletic-oriented men, 18–32 years old (*8*). Is it, therefore, possible that masochistic sexual activity is still practiced in post-cord trauma gay men by virtue of their aggressiveness? Our studies of 110 SCI men did not show any increase in testosterone levels postrauma. Interviews with five SCI men did not reveal sexual aggressiveness or violence, although all of them displayed personality disorders, probably from anger, frustration, and depression associated with their disabilities (*31*).

Etiology and Diagnosis of Sexual Dysfunction

As discussed in the preceding chapter on the diagnosis of sexual dysfunction, most SCI "straight" (heterosexual) men suffer from neurogenic organic erectile and ejaculatory impotence. On the other hand, desire/arousal disorders are usually psychogenic in origin, although in a small minority, the cause may be organic. Our limited clinical data on gay patients revealed similar findings in the "straight" cord victims (*31*). However, we are inclined to believe that the sexual problems of SCI gay men with incomplete lesions seemed to be associated with a psychogenic overlay more often than those in nongay SCI men. It must be stressed that the gay population contains a subgroup of illicit drug users in whom pharmacologically induced sexual dysfunction should be ruled out (*4*). The diagnosis of sexual problems in the SCI gay population should not significantly deviate from the routine SCI sexual evaluation procedures, as presented in their respective chapters.

The insertor, i.e., the partner who acts as the male and inserts his penis or dildo into the oral or anal orifice of his sexual partner, should undergo sexual diagnostic tests for the corresponding problems, such as impotence or ejaculatory dysfunction. The insertee, i.e., the partner who acts as the female and is the recipient of the penis or sexual object, should be evaluated for sexual problems like the SCI female, except for vaginal pressure transducer–sexual response monitoring. The insertee (or vice versa if the partners exchange sex roles) who complains of a poor or weak orgasmic genitoanal sexual muscular contractile response can be evaluated using an anal probe. The orgasmic probe monitoring device is similar to the vaginal pressure transducer and quantifies sexual anal muscular responses (*2*).

The probe (plug) is equipped with a pressure transducer and a photoplethysmograph that monitors pelvic or rectal muscle tension and vasocongestion. The plug can register the degree of anal sphincter contraction pressures (normal pressure = 150–300 cm H_2O (*2,26*), and probably detects the amount of anal lubrication. Although the quantity is minimal during sexual activity (*26*), as a diagnostic aid it can determine the incidence of anal incontinence in patients with low-normal anal sphincter pressures during orgasmic phases or the depth and frequency of penile thrusting to avoid rectal pressure buildup. Dartos (scrotal) and ischio- or bulbocavernosus electromyography may help to identify localized sacral lesions. Both partners should undergo a routine sexological medical history and physical examination, with emphasis on the genitoanal and oral areas.

Oropharyngeal examination (with oral cultures) and rectosigmoidoscopy, with or without stool culture and biopsy, must be done in SCI gays with persistent sore throats, diarrhea, and other clinical symptoms. Serotyping for specific bacterial, fungal, and viral toxins may be indicated in selected suspect cases. Dream analysis may be helpful for patients with orgasmic pleasure–response problems.

Management of Sexual Dysfunction

The treatment strategy for converting homosexuals to heterosexuals was initiated by Freud in the 1900s and preached by Socarides until the early 1980s, especially in cases where the adolescent withdrew from sociointerpersonal contacts and engaged in homosexual fantasies (*10,34*). Recently, however, Masters and Johnson suggested that homosexuals should be treated for their sexual problems and their behavior considered an alternative lifestyle (*26*). The general attitude toward the disabled in the ancient and developing worlds has been one of rejection (*30*). In Third World countries, being homosexual and handicapped is even worse. However, when the United Nations declared 1980–1990 the International Decade for the Disabled, countries of the industrialized world (i.e., Japan, USA, etc.) and the developing nations (i.e., Philippines) took steps to recognize the rights of the handicapped, although each of their cultures still resist fully recognizing the sexual expressions of the disabled.

Arousal Dysfunctions

The three most common causes of arousal problems in able-bodied persons are: alcohol and drug abuse, aging, and marital monotony (*14*). However, in the SCI patient, and even in the handicapped gay, depression is the most common. Chemically (i.e., drug) induced endocrine neurotransmitter deficiency should be ruled out (*4*). Sexual counseling should include stress- and depression-reducing techniques, sensory amplification, and hypnosis (*20,31*). Sensory amplification can include aerobic/anaerobic warm-up of the body by both partners, holistic massage, or feathering. Sensual body lubrication massages or bathing is also advised. Depression must be treated with minor tranquilizers to avoid adverse drug side effects. Diazepam (Valium) is a clinically useful drug in the management of spasticity syndromes, but may aggravate depression. However, Johnson claimed that prolonged (chronic) use of Valium can decrease sexual performance in able-bodied males, because it can precipitate hypotestosteronemia and hypoestrogenemia (*32*). Our clinical study of 50 SCI men did not reveal hormonal changes; Diazepam in average doses of 30 mg/d are being given even to the elderly (*31*). Pain from various causes is another source of arousal problems in both the able-bodied (*23*) and the disabled straight and gay SCI populations. The posterior coital approach (Fig. 1) is advised for patients with painful arthritic or contracted joints. Appropriate nonaddicting analgesics, acupunture, alternative coital positions, or sometimes minor ablative neurosurgery may be required to relieve this frustrating problem. The use of marijuana for the treatment of pain and spasticity remains under investigation.

Erectile and Ejaculatory Impotence

One of the most difficult problems a gay man must overcome post-trauma is not only architectural barriers, but personal relationships, e.g., finding a sexual partner or lover and "marital"/household companion. Interviews with five gay cord patients revealed that three of them retained their preinjury relationships. The remaining two homosexuals are starting life anew by employing the "old techniques" of socializing with people, i.e., going to parties and social gatherings or meetings. At times, gay singles bars pose an architectural barrier, and nondisabled gays look up, not down, for the "perfect" guy. Physical disability or a wheelchair image is a negative signal for both social and sexual encounters in the gay world. Although it is believed that mild violence or roughness is usually associated with nonSCI gay sex, our data suggest the contrary, especially in both disabled and nondisabled gays who have stable one-to-one relationships and those in "married" or household-couple situations (*31*).

Erectile and ejaculatory dysfunctions of the able inserter (sexual partner of the SCI gay) are usually psychogenic, and probably are caused by anxiety or the fear of hurting the partner because of paralysis.

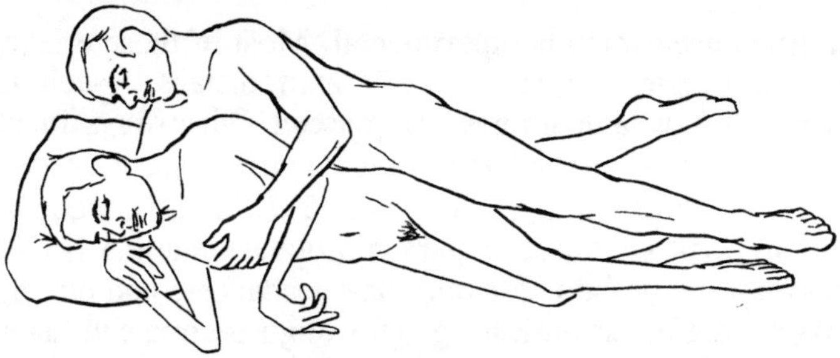

Fig. 1. The insertee (quadriplegic) lies on his side with a pillow supporting his neck. The partner (insertor) penetrates from the rear, while stimulating other erogenous zones. This position can be utilized as an alternative approach by heterosexual couples with contracted extremities.

Ejaculatory problems can be treated with training sessions designed to make the patient recognize his preejaculatory sensations (*6,29*). The therapeutic formats include: (a) penile manipulation, minimizing demand performance and practice to control or anticipate preejaculatory sensations (*6,29*); (b) substituting another form of extra-anal or oral stimulation; (c) erotic foreplay or stimulation can be bypassed, and carefully graduated levels of anal or oral penile containment introduced as soon as this option is acceptable to both partners.

Other masturbatory techniques and vibrators can be used to achieve good ejaculatory control through experimentation. Posterior coital entry is suggested (Fig. 1), so that the inserter can control thrusting. Squeeze or withdrawal techniques are used when necessary. The insertor is counseled to use lots of lubricant in an empty anal canal, and to gradually dilate the canal with calibrated dildos or fingers before penile penetration to prevent mucosal tears and lacerations. It must be stressed that the insertor's (either the sexual partner or the SCI gay himself) penis may incur several types of sexually transmitted lesions. The most frequently encountered are: (a) viral diseases (herpes genitalis)—herpes virus type-2 lesions are characterized by edematous pruritic wheals surrounded by blisters or vesicles (*16,35*). Our clinical experience with acyclovir (Zovirax) has demonstrated that the medication is 90–95% effective in eradicating the lesions. (b) Erythemas—angry erythematous rashes of the foreskin and penis may be associated with diabetes mellitus. Treatment consists of diabetic control, local or oral antibiotics, and circumcision when necessary if the lesion is persistent. (c) Fungus infection—*Candida albicans* lesions are angry, red, pruritic, and covered by white cord-like flecks. These lesions may occur in patients exposed to chronic antibiotic therapy and those with diabetes mellitus (*15*).

The etiology of erectile impotence in SCI men is usually organic (neurogenic), but in a minority of cases it can be a mixed problem (*31*). The pharmacologic management of organic impotence is evolving rapidly and most drugs used remain experimental. Most of these erectogenic medications fall under the category of "aphrodisiacs," such as cantharis (Spanish fly), volatile nitrites, and ginseng. Other drugs are utilized both to enhance sexual arousal and to regain potency, e.g., dopamine-like preparations, bromocriptine mesylate (5–7.5 mg/d), a dopamine* agonist for hyperprolactinemia; parachlorophenylalanine (PCPA), a serotonin synthesis inhibitor for migraine headaches; and clomiphene citrate (50–200 mg/d), an antiestrogen for oligospermia and Laennec's cirrhosis (*4*). Furthermore, some alpha-adrenergic antagonists and beta-2 agonists have been used to treat impotence. Morales et al. (*28*) revived the use of yohimbine HCl (Yocon), an alpha-2 adrenergic antagonist, to manage organic (vascular and neurogenic) impotence. However, our clinical data show that yohimbine did not produce significant effects when given orally in a total dose of 44 mg/d to organically impotent gays. Our recent clinical experience with intracorporeal injections of papaverine (40–60 mg), with or without phenoxybenzamine (3–6 mg) demonstrated a 90–95% positive responses.

Those few young patients with vascular occlusive disease may benefit from percutaneous transluminal laser (penile) angioplasty. It must also be emphasized that the implantation of a penile prosthesis should be entertained only as a last surgical alternative in the management of organic and therapy-resistent psychiatric impotence.

Retrograde ejaculation can be treated with alpha-2 adrenergic stimulants, such as ephedrine sulfate, 50 mg orally, four times a day. This drug is contraindicated in patients with hypertension, and its effectiveness is limited. Clonidine (Catapres) a centrally active antihypertensive, may be tried in patients with incomplete SCI lesions. However, no control studies are as yet available. Another alternative is electro-ejaculation for nonejaculators; for details, see specific chapters elsewhere in this volume.

Other Associated Sexual Risks

Oroanal Problems

Oral sex by patients with poor genital/oral hygiene and ammoniacal macerated penile skin caused by infrequent (urinary condom) uridom changes, can result in secondary oral as well as genital infections. Partners must be cautioned not to—and resist the urge to—bite the penis, especially at the height of orgasms. We treated two of our patients, 21

*Ed note: There are an estimated 750,000 IV drug abuser Americans. Gay heroin addicts with impotence from hyperprolactinemia may be treated with bromocriptine (methadone therapy).

and 41-yr-old paraplegics who had sustained deep dental penile wounds caused by human bites, by inserting a Foley catheter and administering oral antibiotics and tetanus toxoid. If bacterial, viral, or fungal infections develop, the patient must be treated appropriately and orodental hygiene must then be reemphasized.

Sex-related anorectal and gastrointestinal problems are not uncommon in the gay population. Local rectal problems, such as anal fissures and hemorrhoids, can be aggravated by poor bowel care and vigorous penile thrusting in the presence of a dry anal mucosa and spastic anal sphincter. This spasticity may be reduced by diazepam (Valium), amyl nitrate (*19*), or gradual dilation with a dildo during foreplay. Amebiasis, giardiasis, and shigellosis must be ruled out in gay patients with persistent diarrhea. Other causes include constipation in the presence of chronic ororectal infection and/or suppuration. Syphilis and gonorrhea must also be included in the differential diagnosis (*7,17*).

Brachioproctic Eroticism (BPE)

Lowry and Williams reported a new form of sexual pleasuring called "brachioproctic eroticism" (BPE): handballing or fistfucking (*41*). This form of sexual penetration involves the insertion of the hand/arm into the rectosigmoid colon of the sexual partner for sexual pleasuring. This non-SCI data have shown that most males experience intense pleasure and some revealed mixed responses of pain. Relaxant drugs and analgesics were used by 37% of the subjects to reduce any discomfort. In SCI patients, BPE can trigger autonomic dysreflexia, especially in quadriplegics (if hand/arm insertion is forceful against a full urinary bladder or rectum, and spastic rectal sphincters), or can result to mucosal rectal tears and bleeding. Our clinical experiences reveal that no muscle relaxant is safe enough to reduce rectal sphincter spasticity without producing generalized muscle weakness. Thus, it behooves the sex therapist to advise the sexual partner to empty the urinary bladder/rectum, lubricate both rectum and hand or arm, and to sound a caution regarding the hazards of handballing.

There are approximately 20 million homosexual Americans who may seek new sexual experiences such as "gerbilorgasm." This novel (animalistic) sexual expression involves a gerbil—a jerboalike rodent belonging to the mouse family, which is declawed and inserted into the rectum via a "habit trail" conduit. The erratic motion of the (confused) gerbil inside the rectal ampulla will initiate sexual excitement. In SCI patients, gerbilorgasm can be experienced only by those who have intact pelvic/rectal sensations or whose "feelings" have returned.

However, in SCI, the dangers of rectal bleeding, perforations, and even sympathetic hyperreflexia must be reemphasized.

Acquired Immune Deficiency Syndrome (AIDS)

The decade 1960–1970 was characterized by a tremendous change in lifestyles and sexual behavior, change accompanied by an increase in the population of male and female homosexuals (*25*). The lesbian lifestyle is generally quieter and less ostentatious than that of gay men. The Center for Disease Control (CDC) in Atlanta has conducted studies revealing that gay men engage in sexual activity with a thousand anonymous partners or strangers during a lifetime (*24,25*). This promiscuity has predisposed the male homosexual to AIDS with an estimated relative risk of 5 in 100,000 (*17,22*). In 1989, there were about 103,000 and 148,000 cases of AIDS in the USA and worldwide respectively. Nearly 73% of these cases involved male homosexuals. Approximately 65,000 or more have already died of the disease. In 1992 there will be an estimated 390,000 AIDS victims in the United States, and the incidence of disease carriers is expected to rise to 3 million. The greatest concentrations of AIDS patients are found in New York City, San Francisco, Miami, Newark, and other large urban centers. In addition to male homosexuals, other groups at high risk are intravenous drug users (17%), hemophiliacs (1%), and others, including heterosexuals and others who are recipients of multiple blood transfusions.

As of March 1990 about 38 gay SCI men had been reported to have AIDS. HTLV III or human retro-virus has been identified, which is believed to be a weak and slow-growing pathogen. The following precautions, if observed carefully, may reduce the risk of contracting AIDS: (a) limit sexual partners to two or fewer, and only to acquaintances, (b) avoid the intravenous use of drugs or blood transfusions, prolonged kissing with open lesions, and reduce stress, (c) shower or wash before and after sex, (d) avoid exchange of body fluids or rough oral sex contact with AIDS victims, (e) maintain good health habits through daily exercise, proper bowel care, and the use of "thicker" self-sealing with 9-nonoxydol condoms. The key to prevention, as with hospital precautionary measures, is to avoid sexual contact with AIDS victims (especially anal sex) and to practice cleanliness or safe sex (*22*). It should be stressed that the passive gay sexual partner or the nonpromiscuous gay may also be infected with AIDS (*22,24*). Furthermore, gay SCI men with renal disease or kidney transplants are also at risk, for AIDS aggravates the renal problem, both directly and indirectly. The disease is rare in Asia and the Middle East. Dr. L. Montagnier of France has predicted that by the year 1998, there will be about ten million people affected with AIDS; the large majority will be North Americans, Africans, and Brazilians.

Orgasm and Relationships

In the young, sexual assertiveness may enhance sexual contact for the gay SCI population. However, in the elderly population, physical loss of beauty and physiological functional deceleration take a toll on the previously active and "lustful" gay sexual life. Aging produces structural and metabolic changes in the brain and neurotransmitter–receptor systems(*3,36*). Thus, sex counseling is geared toward understanding the delayed sexual responses (*12,31,36*) with associated cardiorespiratory problems. The resumption of sexual activity postmyocardial infarction can make patients feel better about themselves. Using nitroglycerine or calcium channel blocker tablets or chest patches prophylactically before coitus appears to be beneficial. A less stressful coital position is also suggested (Fig. 2). Interviews with three SCI gay men revealed that they cherish the sensual embrace or touching–kissing as intensely as orgasm during sexual celebration (activities). It is the essence of belonging (bonding), reassurance, and open communication that constitute a stable relationship—sometimes a substitute for miniorgasms.

Data from studies conducted in Washington, DC and other major cities have shown that the interpersonal problems of the homosexual relationship are similar to those found in heterosexual couples. Some believe that relationships between gay couples are actually more stable and happier than those among the general population (*31,33*). Couples who experience problems in their relationships should be referred for marriage (couple) counseling (*12,21,31*). The marriage (which is legal in Denmark) of one SCI gay to an able partner, may benefit him psychosocially and financially.

Counseling SCI Gay Patients with AIDS

Sexologists and therapists treating HIV positive and gay-SCI AIDS patients are faced with a number of concerns in meeting the immediate and extended needs of these persons. An important component in counseling is knowledge of the patient's religious beliefs since these may considerably affect their responses to AIDS. Some belief systems may in fact lead to a possible resolution of long-standing conflicts about the gay lifestyle and may result in a greater sense of personal comfort and ease about the course of the limited life span. Regardless of the

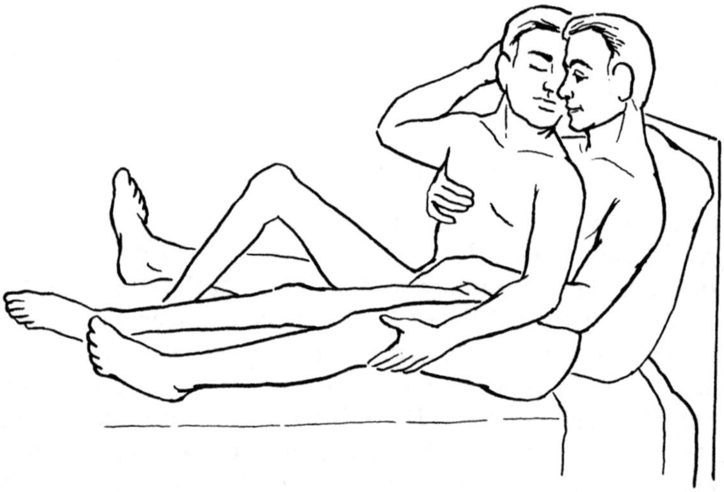

Fig. 2. The insertee (paraplegic) is cradled and supported by his partner, and this position is less demanding.

degree of religious affiliation, the gay-SCI AIDS patient lives in a culture that is the spiritual inheritor of more than two thousand years of Judeo-Christian prejudice (*42*). Once reiterated to the patient then, the following suggestions may prove helpful to him in facing the mounting psycho-sexual pressures and the spiritual dilemma:

1. Be sensitive to the patient's religious beliefs in relation to AIDS and his anticipated emotional and sexual problems.
2. Teach the patient coping mechanisms to deal with the issues of death and dying and with the negativistic attitude toward homosexuality and AIDS exhibited by many segments of our society.

Transvestites and Transsexuals

Cross-dressing has been a theatrical practice employed by actors since the time of the pagans, both for entertainment and religious reasons. Sexual overtones with transdressing is not the same as transexuality. *Tootsie*, a 1982 American film about a transvestite, drives home a point—a reenactment of some important life scenes, an insight into troubling conflicts, and a profound catharsis for personal, marital, and sexual problems (*13*).

Transvestites (TV) have several reasons for their behavior, including:

1. Erotic pleasure from cross-dressing
2. A personal response to gender issues—a social red-signal against stereotyping of men's clothiers.
3. A political statement favoring a sociosexual identity in which TV gain a new kind of acceptance for their alternative lifestyle (*43*).

An incontinent SCI male transdresser may have a few problems: (a) hiding a urinary leg bag beneath a low-cut dress and (b) atrophic and unattractive legs post-SCI can be a negative signal for socialization. On the other hand, the female SCI transvestite who dons jeans or pants should not have similar problems. Sexual counseling should be tailored to each person's specific problems. Most therapists believe that cross-dressers don't want to be relieved of their feelings. They simply want their partners to accept them and their cross-dressing as a woman. They don't want to change. They just want society to accept them as is.

A major problem for TVs is that the average male feels threatened when he meets a male dressed like a woman, let alone a disabled male. He is confused, oftentimes angry, because his macho image is challenged. The able-bodied male psychologically and physically looks down on the wheelchair-bound handicapped (*43*).

There are as many as 150 support groups for able-bodied TVs, but the handicapped (physically challenged) person has only limited option: an understanding sexologist/therapist. For further help and counseling there are few organizations able to cater to SCI patients, such as the Renaissance Education Association in Pennsylvania, Delaware, and New Jersey, the Society for the Second Self and the Androgyny Unlimited Clinic, both in New York City.

Transsexuals

Transvestitism (TV) seems to be solely a behavioral aberration, but transexualism (TS) arises from a more deep-rooted psychosexual problem. Bullough et al. revealed that the lack of interest in sports was as a marker for feminine behavior that correlated with transsexual identity. They also reported that TS report more unhappiness as children and less academic achievement in their school days (*44*). Furthermore, Green suggested that TS emerges in its mature form only when subjective gender discontent persists into late childhood or early adolescence (*39*).

During the 1970s, transsexual surgery seemed to be a panacea for the management of transsexual dysfunctional syndromes. However, a decade later, researchers at Johns Hopkins University demonstrated that transsexual operations do not cure or relieve the psychosexual problems of transsexuals (27). Currently, society is still generally reluctant to accept transsexuals, and employers consider them to be counterproductive. Some pilots, public officials, and police department personnel have probably been fired because they are transsexuals. It must be emphasized that most spinal cord injuries occur in aggressive and adventurous men. Thus, a male transsexual who suffers a cord trauma was probably a female surgical convert. These patients take testosterone postoperatively to accelerate the acquisition of masculine physical characteristics. But, the important question is: do androgenic hormones trigger aggressiveness and adventure-seeking when administered to mature women? Able-bodied transsexual "females" usually retain some feeling in and around the newly formed vagina, but the neoclitoris possesses normal sensation because it was fashioned from the original penile shaft or glans penis. Spinal cord trauma, depending on the type or level of cord lesion(s), would probably produce genital sexual problems similar to those of the normal female. However, the loose neovaginal introital muscles are probably more lax (due to paralysis) than those of the normal vaginal pubococcygeus (PC) muscles. In patients with incomplete lesions, pelvic muscle tone sexercises, a personal or vaginal perineometer* (clinical trainer), or biofeedback therapy can be tried. Sex counseling should include a variety of options for sexual positions (Fig. 3).

In transsexual "males" the neopenis usually has an implanted (solid) penile prosthesis with compromised postoperative erotic sensations; thus, erectile dysfunction should not exist. These patients do not need to ejaculate, but the scrotal sac, newly fashioned from the labia majora, can be erotically sensitive, depending on the degree of SCI recovery or type of lesion. Finally, before definitive sex therapy or surgical alternatives (use of artificial neovaginal sphincter) are offered, the suggestions given in Table 1 should be considered during sex counseling.

There are few organizations that offer counsel to transsexuals (TS) on the educational services, on research, on medical and psychiatric referrals, and on peer pre-operative and post-operative adjustment. Further TS counseling and referral may, however be obtained from the following: Renaissance Education Association of Pennsylvania, Delaware, and New Jersey, and Transsexual (TS) Counseling in San Francisco, California.

---

*Farrel Instruments, Inc., PO Box 1037, Grand Island, NE 68802

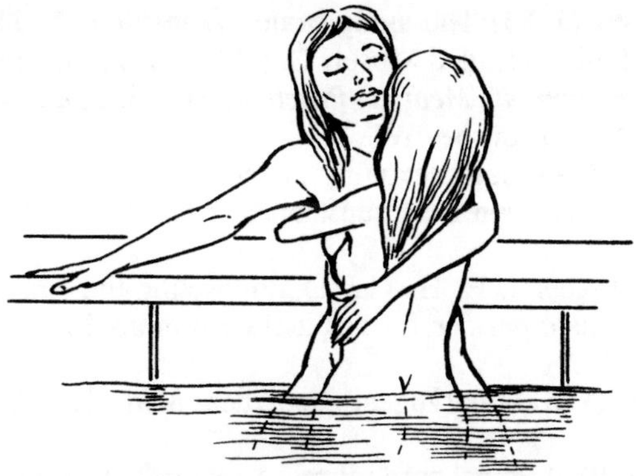

Fig. 3. The transsexual (quadriplegic) is held by her/his partner, while they float at the edge of the swimming pool or tub and by multidirectional motion stimulate erogenous zones to orgasm(s).

Table 1
The Ten Commandments (Cautions) of Sexual Counseling

1. Don't get people into trouble with their God or morality.
2. Don't hang your morality on the patient.
3. Don't force the patient to talk about sex.
4. Don't threaten the patient with your sexuality.
5. Don't make sex an all-or-none experience. There is no substitute for love or an understanding relationship.
6. Don't assume that, once sexuality has been discussed, it is forever resolved for that patient.
7. Don't assume that there is only one way to convey sexual information.
8. Don't expect too much from spouses/partners in their ability to change roles.
9. Don't forget that all relationships, especially that most intense of all relationships—marriage, require compromise.
10. Don't hide facts or truths. Let him/her face reality in subtle ways. Sex is not the only ingredient of a happy life.

References

1. Bogen, I. (1981) Sexual myths and politics. *J. Sex Ed. Ther.* **7**, 7–15.

2. Bohlen, J. G. and Held, P. J. (1979) An anal probe for monitoring vascular and muscular events during sexual response. *J. Psychophysiol.* **16**, 319–323.

3. Bondareff, W. (1983) The aging brain. *Transition.* **1**, 21–32, 37–40.
4. Buffum, J., Smith, D., and Moser, C. (1981) Drugs and sexual function, in *Sexual Problems in Medical Practice,* 1st ed. (Lief, H. I., ed.) pp. 211–121, AMA, Monroe, WI.
5. Collins, J. P. Male homosexuality in Japan. Presented at the American Assoc. of Sex Education and Counselors and Therapists, Oct. 16–20, 1983, Honolulu, HI.
6. Crist, T. and Kenan, E. H. (1981) Counseling the spinal cord injured female and female partner for a spinal cord injured male. *J. of Sex Ed. Ther.* **7**, 29–33.
7. Evrard, J. R. (1981) Pharyngeal gonorrhea. *Med. Aspects Hum. Sexual.* **11**, 31–32.
8. Fonseca, J. (1983) Spinal cord injury. A medical and sociological assessment. *VA Lett.* **15**, 1.
9. Foster, A., and Foster, F. M. (1983) The mahu and the gay: polynesian homosexuality and its implications for an existential theory of homosexuality. Presented at the American Assoc. of Sex Educators, Counsellors and Therapists. Oct. 16–20, 1983, Honolulu, HI.
10. Freud, S. (1905) Three essays on the theory of sexuality. *Standard Ed.* **7**, 125–244.
11. Gadpaille, W. J. (1981) Understanding the varieties of homosexual behavior, in *Sexual Problems in Medical Practice,* 1st ed. (Lief, H. I., ed.) pp. 71–82, AMA, Monroe, WI.
12. Gochros, J. S. Marriage counseling when one partner is gay. Presented at the American Assoc. of Sex Educators, Counsellors and Therapists. Oct. 16–20, 1983, Honolulu, HI.
13. Henderson, H. (1983) Tootsie and Dr. Moreno–Next slide, please. *Sex. Med. Today.* **7**, 22.
14. Jacobson, A. S., ed. (1982) Arousal: The most fragile link in human sexual response. *Sex. Med. Today.* **6**, 4–13.
15. Jacobson, A. S., ed. (1983) After myocardial infarction: Restoring male sexuality. *Sex. Med. Today.* **7**, 26–30.
16. Jacobson, A. S., ed. (1983) Herpes: Truth and consequences. *Sex. Med. Today.* **7**, 6–16.
17. Jacobson, A. S., ed. (1983) Facing AIDS. *Sex. Med. Today.* **7**, 6–10.
18. Karczmar, A. G. (1980) Drugs, transmitters and hormones and mating behavior; in *Modern Problems of Pharmacopsychiatry. Drug Treatment of Sexual Dysfunction.* (Ban, T. A. and Freyhan, F. A., eds.) Ch. 1, 1–52 S. Karger, Basel.
19. Labataille, L. M. (1975) Amyl nitrate employed in homosexual relationship. (letter) *Med. Aspects Hum. Sexual.* **9**, 122.
20. Levitt, E. E. (1983) Hypnosis in the treatment of sexual dysfunctions. An update. *J. Sex. Ed. Ther.* **9**, 23–27.
21. Lief, I. H. (1981) Sexual problems in medical practice. 1st ed. AMA, Monroe, WI.
22. Loo, M. H., Davis, J. M., Metnoka, C., and Yurt, R. W. (1983) Kaposi's sarcoma and the AIDS patient. *Infect. Surg.* **2**, 865–872.

23. Maruta, T. (1982) Chronic pain patients. Expect marital and sexual disruption. *Sex. Med. Today.* **6**, 20–27.
24. Marx, J. L. (1982) New disease baffles medical community. *Science.* **217**, 618–621.
25. Morganthau, T., Carey, J., Raine, G., McCormick, J., and Friendly, G.: Gay America. *Newsweek.* Aug. 8. 1982, pp. 30–40.
26. Masters, W. and Johnson, V. (1966) Human sexual response. Little, Brown and Co., Boston, MA.
27. Money, J. (1981) Johns Hopkins University. Personal Communications.
28. Morales, A., Surridge, D. H., Marshall, P. G., and Fenemore, J. (1982) Nonhormonal pharmacological treatment of organic impotence. *J. Urol.* **128**, 45–47.
29. Morse, W. I., and Morse, J. M. (1981) Coital premature ejaculation with masturbatory ejaculatory incompetence. *J. Sex Ed. Ther.* **7**, 3–7.
30. Odebiyi, A. I. (1983) Handicaps and the handicapped in ile-ife, Nigeria: A socio-cultural disease. *J. Social Worker.* **10**, 152–154.
31. Romo, M., and Leyson, J. F. J. (1977) Homosexuality and spinal cord injury: cultural prospectives and sexual dysfunctions (Unpublished data).
32. Schiller, P., and Watsa, M. C., eds. (1983) Valium decrease sex performance in men. International counsel for sex education and parenthood news and views by Dr. G. T. Johnson. **1**, 11.
33. Silverstein, C. (1981) *Man to man: Gay Couples in America.* Morrow, New York.
34. Socarides, C. W. (1978) *Homosexuality.* Jason Aaronson, New York.
35. Summers, J. L. (1981) Penile rashes. *Med. Aspects Hum. Sexual.* **15**, 67–68.
36. Vassilchenko, G. S. (1980) Age aspects of the male sexual activity. *J. Sex Ed. Ther.* **6**, 10–14.
37. Dörner, G. (1979) Hormones and sexual differentiation of the brain. In *Sex, Hormones, and Behavior.* Ciba Found. Symp. (Excerpta Medica, Amsterdam) 81–101.
38. Bell, A., Weinberg, M., and Hammersmith, S. (1981) Sexual Preference: Its development in Men and Women. Indiana University Press, Bloomington, IN.
39. Green, R. (1987) Toward a developmental sexology—The sissy boy syndrome as the development of homosexuality. Yale University Press, New Haven, CT.
40. Robinson, P. (1989) Portrait of a family—Sexuality: Homosexuality. NJ Network, Channel 8 WNJN, Feb. 11.
41. Lowry, T., and Williams, G. (1983) Brachioproctic eroticisms. *J. Sex Ed. Therapy* **9**, 50–52.
42. Slowinski, J. (1988) Persons with AIDS and religion: A clinical viewpoint. *J. Soc. Sex Therapy Res.* **6**, 4.
43. Francouer, R. (1989) Personal communications.
44. Bullough, V., Bullough, B., and Smith, R. (1983) A comparative study of male transvestites, male to female transsexuals and male homosexuals *J. sex res.* **19**, 238–257 (Aug. issue).

27

Female Homosexuality

Concetta J. Panzarino

Introduction

Hermaphroditism in invertebrates is a natural phenomenon. In the lower animals, gender role reversal is quite often the rule, not the exception. For instance, in some species of birds, the female lays the eggs, and the male hatches and attends the young. In the primeval forest, the fabled "Amazons" established a homogeneous (female) society both for protection and survival. As society and people changed, (female) homosexuality (lesbianism) has become a biological need, adaptation, or (choice) an alternative lifestyle. However, the prejudice and homophobia common in society make it very difficult for anyone to be a lesbian, let alone someone with a disability.

Just as disability cuts across cultural, racial, socioeconomic, and religious backgrounds, so does lesbianism. Just as disability isolates, so does lesbianism. Lesbianism, however, is pleasurable, whereas disability is not, although societal mores may make lesbianism a disability of sorts.

There are as many myths about lesbianism as there are about disability. Lesbians are a threat to the family structure since they do not remain dependent on men. Disabled women often threaten the idea of family, because they may alter the woman's role in a family system. For instance, it may be more productive for a disabled mother to work in the world and have her husband do the work of child rearing. Disabled women who are not able to do housekeeping may exchange traditional roles of caretaking for other careers. Lesbians are often labeled "man haters" because they give their energies to other women instead of men. Not all lesbians hate men, and not all lesbians want to be like men. Many lesbians are mothers with children. Woe to the individual who bears the burden of this double stigma.

Sexual Rehabilitation of the Spinal-Cord-Injured Patient
Edited by J.F. Leyson, © 1990 The Humana Press, Inc.

Within the lesbian culture, the disabled lesbian is freer to take on any role she chooses, because there are no designated roles. This is not to say that there is no prejudice within the lesbian community regarding disability. Most lesbian social activities are inaccessible, often up many steps in hidden-away places. Few of the events can afford to be sign-language interpreted or have brailled programs. Inaccessibility of events makes it difficult to find sexual partners. Able-bodied lesbians view disabled lesbians with the same "ableist" prejudices as the rest of society. They see them as sexless, mindless, dependent objects to be taken care of.

Why does a disabled woman become a lesbian? Some women become lesbians because they fall in love with other women. Others say they were born lesbians, and still others say they become lesbians as a political statement. Some have no interest in politics at all. We could argue at this point the validity of homosexual preference. Is it an illness? Is it a choice? Is it a predisposed genetic occurrence or an adaption to adverse socio-physical alterations? We know that at least 10% of all populations is homosexual. We know the American Psychiatric Association acknowledges that homosexuality is not an illness. The "why" of lesbianism is a moot point. The "how," in terms of how to live and be a whole, disabled person with any sexuality, let alone homosexuality, is more the point. For the 10% of disabled women who are lesbians, acknowledgment of their sexual preference in a homophobic structure is dangerous to their survival.

R., a lesbian with spina bifida, said in an interview:

> To be a disabled lesbian means that when your caseworker comes to the door at 8 o'clock in the morning to evaluate the care you're receiving from the home attendant and tells you how you should socialize and you shouldn't live alone, you have to lie. If you say, as some disabled lesbians have, that you live with a woman who is your lover, you risk harassment. If you say you live with a friend, they ask where she sleeps, since there is only one bedroom. The County Social Service feels that to provide attendant care for someone with your sexual perversion would be to support . . . your, immorality.

To be a disabled lesbian means that, if one is in the hospital, in intensive care perhaps, one's family is allowed to visit, but not the lover with whom she has lived for 15 years. To be a disabled lesbian means that one may be more vulnerable to attack from men who are threatened by her choice and want to teach her a lesson. Being a lesbian and disabled means that, if one is blind or cannot turn pages because of quadriparesis, there are few available to read her lesbian literature, newspapers, or love letters in privacy. Government-sponsored readers or page turners may refuse to provide materials that they consider "perverted." It is inappropriate to ask a friend to assist in intimate correspondence. People who generally will assist a paraplegic woman up an icy curb turn away from a woman who openly displays her lesbianism. Many disabled lesbians survive by hiding or denying their sexuality. These negative cultural attitudes often obliterate the positive self-concept that so many disabled people struggle mightily to maintain.

There is a strong, courageous group of lesbians who have not denied their sexuality, although they are disabled. They are surviving by educating their lesbian community about disability, and the larger community about disability and lesbianism. These women are learning coping mechanisms to fight the hate and fear that surround them. Some lesbians who became disabled later in life felt that they were able to use the coping skills they had learned in dealing with their lesbianism and apply them to the new stigma of disability. The same is true for disabled women who later became lesbians. Whether someone is denied service in a restaurant because she is lesbian or because there is no room for her wheelchair, she must still choose to fight her oppression or succumb to it. Disabled lesbians can survive only by realizing that they have a right to the service, a right to life, and a right to love. These rights must be protected and fought for by all..

What does the right to sexuality or sexual preference mean? Lesbian and heterosexual women understand the meaning of the word "sexuality" in different ways, as do disabled women and able-bodied women. The societal view of women's sexuality is shifting, although slowly, from one limited by a primary focus on intercourse to a more realistic concept of multidimensional pleasure. Orgasm is a word that is used, misused, over- and underestimated. It is a part of the pleasuring process. Lesbians are interested in achieving and exploring pleasures between women. Sexual pleasure between women can be nurturing, comforting, and secure, usually inviting both partners to be active participants.

> "How can a quadraplegic be active?" asked an able-bodied lesbian. S. said, "There are many ways to be active. I can be with my lover by talking, by moving my head, my mouth. I can watch her be active and be involved in that process. Haven't you ever made love with someone who's using all their parts, but their minds and hearts are not really there?"
>
> "Yes. It was like that for me more with men."

Often disabled women who are unattracted to men are told that they are not dealing with their sexuality. These women spend a lot of energy attempting to kindle an attraction for men that is simply not there. In reality, many of these women are lesbians who are attracted to women in an atmosphere where this is not permitted.

There are books on lesbian sexuality, and there are books on sexuality and disability. There is much research being done on the pleasuring of women. A disabled lesbian is a woman. She knows her own feelings, and yet, she is different because she is disabled. In all pleasuring, we must be open to our partners. Love-making between lesbians is usually a joint effort. When sexual partners are able to communicate their sexual needs and desires freely, lovemaking is enhanced. The nature of disability requires more communication. Therefore, closeness can be increased through disability.

Disabled Lesbians Enjoy Many Types of Pleasuring

Some enjoy genital sex: some do not. Orgasm can be of primary importance to some, minimal importance to others, and be nonexistent to still others. Sexual pleasuring for disabled lesbians grows with the ability to communicate one's pleasure and to enjoy the pleasuring without guilt. It is difficult to engage in intimacy without confusion.

The heterosexual model that pervades the media, as well as many of our earliest memories, is often associated with the power or dominance of man over woman. The woman is not expected to acknowledge or discuss her sexuality, be it pleasurable or painful. In fact, many women learn to feel guilty if they achieve or acknowledge their pleasure. This is a major burden to the quadraplegic who may only be able to express her pleasure vocally, against all societal conditioning.

The disabled woman, often filled with physical and psychological pain, must use many mechanisms to deny or minimize her pain. In doing so, she often loses the ability to feel any pleasure. Other disabled women, because of spinal cord injury, have lost actual sensation in various parts of their bodies, often including their genitalia. It is crucial for disabled lesbians to begin sexual pleasuring by building on what is already pleasureful. For some, this may mean fantasy or pleasant thoughts. The largest organ of pleasure that we possess is the skin. If one is visually oriented, mirrors and proper lighting are crucial. If one can see a lover touch a part of one's body that has lost tactile sensation, much excitement can be felt by the mind. If smell is a primary sense for another, there are wonderful oils and incense. For many, the voice is an instrument of the goddesses.

The disabled woman often feels guilty about her body. She may feel guilty about not being able to live up to the image of the beautiful American woman portrayed in the media. In her isolation, she cannot realize that even most able-bodied women fail to match the Miss Americas or the Twiggies or whatever the "in" ideal woman is at the moment. Women suffer from low self-esteem and poor self-image, and the disabled woman suffers more so.

The lesbian ideal frees women from much of this. However, within the lesbian community there has developed another type of ideal woman—the "super dyke." These are not supposed to be smooth-skinned or frail and dependent, as in the male culture. Instead, they are required to be physically strong and totally independent.

The disabled lesbian becomes an enigma on both sides of these value scales. She is at once strong in that she is a survivor, and yet depends on appliances, medications, guide dogs, catheters, bed pans, sign language interpreters, and/or attendant care. Somehow amidst the extreme denial, pain, invalidation, and depression, the disabled lesbian learns to achieve sexual pleasuring with another woman and feel good about it.

Each disabled lesbian with her own specific disability, her own tastes, likes, and dislikes, has her own obstacles to sexual pleasuring. A woman with arthritis may have difficulty with positions. The deaf SCI lesbian needs light to communicate with her partner, who may be very shy and want the lights off. The blind SCI lesbian may not know when it is safe to hold her lover's hand, because she cannot see if anyone is watching. The woman with a hidden disability such as epilepsy may avoid sexual pleasuring for long periods of time for fear that the stimulation could cause a seizure. The lesbian with a heart condition resists telling her partner of her physical disability, anticipating that her partner's fear may cause rejection; better to pass as able. There are even more variables at play when both lovers are disabled, although this may increase the degree of validation.

It would be a very wonderful thing if there were a book outlining how to deal with every situation and every physical problem that arises for the disabled lesbian. This is a very remote possibility. Even intercourse between able-bodied men and women varies from partner to partner. The disabled lesbian, as well as the heterosexual woman who may seek to pleasure herself, must read through male-oriented, pro-penis ads for information on vibrators and their attachments. The disabled lesbian is left to seek advice on pleasuring women in the chapters for disabled men in various publication. What she finds there she usually already knows because she is a woman. Lesbian creativity, combined with disabled creativity in an atmosphere of openness and love, provides an atmosphere for the invention of novel devices and adaptations of pleasuring techniques and personal relationships.

Lesbians disabled by spinal-cord injury must learn to use what resources they have. One woman, using only her voice, tells a fantasy of what she would really like to do with her lover. Another leaves candles lit in her room, which provide more intimacy and romance than an electric light bulb and yet allows her to see her lover touching her. One quadriplegic uses a paintbrush held in her mouth to stimulate her lover. The possibilities are endless. In counseling the SCI homosexual, the following suggestions may help the client enhance her sensualities:

A. *Sensory amplification*: The method used by some disabled women to achieve the most pleasure and satisfaction from a sensory input is simply the act of thinking about a physical stimulus, concentrating on it, and amplifying the sensation in the mind to an intense degree. This technique makes it possible to achieve a higher level of satisfaction, and possibly even a mental orgasm. Some who have lost physical sensation in the genital area are able to substitute or transfer sensations from areas of the body that have retained some feeling, such as the inside of an arm, the neck, breasts, buttocks, or around the anal area. By transposing these sensations mentally or by using the imagination to create a fantasy, you may find intense satisfaction (*1*).

B. *Oral sexual techniques*: A commonly used means of sexual expression for the spinal-cord injured person is the use of the mouth to excite and give pleasure to . . . her partner. You may find that you receive more pleasure with this option, partly because your lips and tongue, which have not been impaired by your injury, are more sensitive to touch and temperature than any other part of your body. In addition, the sensations you receive from the smell, taste, and texture of your partner's skin are heightened and could be quite a turn-on for you. The act of kissing and caressing many areas of your partner's body in a sensuous, tender way will enhance the feelings of togetherness. When you and your partner are caressing and using your mouths on each other at the same time, or even if one of you is passive, the sensations can be tremendously pleasing. The sensations you receive from your partner's tongue caressing or sucking a sensitive area, such as your ear, neck, wrist, breast, or genital area, can be transposed to another part of your body that has less sensitivity.

Oral–genital sexual activity can be done mutually by two partners who position themselves in a way that makes each partner's genitals easily available to the other's mouth. If possible, the Foley catheter should be removed. Because of your difficulty in changing positions quickly, your partner might have to be the one who does the shifting and positioning. Either through your verbal directions or the refined communication of touch, you can develop a style of lovemaking that is beautifully tender and passionate. Whether you use oral stimulation for transposing sensation for arousal in foreplay or you and your partner simply enjoy it, remember that any part of the body can be made clean enough for oral contact. So do not be hesitant to try oral stimulation in any way you may want to. It can be enjoyable and fun for you and your partner. Keep in mind that the . . . (clitoris) and vagina are highly sensitive to receiving pleasure and that the hands with their high degree of dexterity and the mouth with its great sensitivity have great capacity for giving pleasure. Paraplegics and quadriplegic who choose this enjoyable option find that the old jokes and myths that surround oral–genital sex are just that and have little validity.

Each of us receives taste and smell in a different way. Everyone has . . . her own individual scent and taste. As you know, the odor from any part of the body is caused by normal secretions of the skin. Once the area is clean, there is no odor other than the natural scent of the individual. In a reasonably clean and healthy person, the vagina or (clitoris) has no more harmful germs than, and is not very different in taste from, a person's mouth. It should be noted, however, that in some instances the mouth can transmit a type of yeast infection to the genital area that can cause an irritating rash. The soap, oil, or other substance you use on each other will add to or change the taste you receive when you use oral stimulation (*1*). With the AIDS pandemic, it may now be advisable to use a vaginal "plastic" shield if one engages in oral–genital stimulations (2).

C. *Manual Stimulation Alternatives*: Manual stimulation of your partner is the use of any part of your body other than your genitals or mouth (feathering) to stimulate and please your partner. A finger, thumb, wrist, elbow, knee can be enough of a protrusion to stimulate the clitoris. It is rubbing and stroking the sensitive areas of the . . . vagina and clitoris that brings a . . . woman to orgasm. Depending on your ability to move, you can let your partner supply the rhythm and motion or increase your enjoyment by trying it yourself (*1*).

D. Miscellaneous Physico-Sexual Problems:
   1. Discomfort and pain: Any physical pain can dampen the pleasure or joys of sexual celebrations. Specific therapy should be utilized to treat this pain syndrome. Other therapeutic options include different medications, acupunture, psychotherapy, biofeedback, transcutaneous neurostimulations, selective nerve block/rhizotomy, and even dorsal (spinal cord) column stimulation (*2*).
   2. Contractures and muscle spasms: In patients with arthritic and post-injury (SCI) contractures, positional coital techniques is advised to make the patient and his/her partner comfortable (*2*). Dose adjustment of muscle skeletal relaxants, i.e., dantrolene sodium (Dantrium), baclofen (Lioresal), diazepam (Valium), or in combination is suggested. Sometimes surgical frozen-joint release procedures are resorted to.
   3. Urinary and bowel incontinence: In most rehabilitation institutions, it is a routine discharge policy to educate the patients and their health assistant aides regarding urinary and bowel care prior to social and sexual activities.

      If the patient complains of urinary leakage during orgasms, even after urinary catheterization, a trial of oxybutynin HCl (Ditropan) at 5–10 mg orally 30 min prior to sexual activity is advised (*2*). Post-auricular skin scopolamine patch (Trans-derm scop) can be applied 3–6 hours prior to sexual celebration both to prevent urinary leakage and reduce motion sickness while lying on a water mattress (*2*). Furthermore, if manual bowel emptying does not prevent fecal incontinence during sexual celebration, a surgical implantation of an "artificial urinary (urethral) sphincter" around the rectal ampulla is another management option. However, patients with an implanted rectal "artificial urinary sphincter" may have difficulty inserting large dildoes during anal sex.
   4. Coital autonomic dysreflexia (hyperreflexia): It is not unusual for a patient with thoracic fourth (T4) injury to experience headaches from autonomic hyperreflexia during

intercourse or masturbation. In case this problem occurs, it is wise to stop and rest until the symptoms disappear before resuming sexual celebration. To prevent coital autonomic hyperreflexia, a calcium channel blocker or a nitroglycerine patch may be applied to the chest half an hour before lovemaking along with proper bowel and bladder care preparations. Lesbianism is a sexual option for pleasuring that has built-in birth control. In addition, the incidence of venereal disease is significantly lower for lesbians than for any other sexually active group. Why do disabled women become lesbians? Why not?

Global Awareness and Assistance

In 1977 an organization called the Disabled Lesbian Alliance (DLA) was formed to provide support among disabled lesbians and to work toward the elimination of attitudinal and architectural barriers within the lesbian community and in the community at large. In 1980 in Michigan, there was a national conference for disabled lesbians. The Alliance is now networking throughout the world. It has provided a way for disabled lesbians to be less isolated from one another. For further information and assistance, DLA can be contacted by writing to: Ms. C. Panzarino, M.A., Rd. 1, Box 98, Monticello, New York 12701 USA.

References

1. Mooney, T. O., Cole, R. M. and Chilgren, R. A. (1975) *Sexual Options for Paraplegics and Quadriplegics,* pp. 73, 82, and 84 (Little, Brown, Boston).
2. Leyson, J. F. (1988) Updates in Sexual Medicine. Presented at the annual winter meeting, Association of Physicians (Phil.) in America, Philippine Convention Center, Dec. 14–17, 1988, Manila, Philippines.

28
Diabetes Mellitus and Other Metabolic Disorders

Kowit Danviriyasup
and
Robert L. Winer

Introduction

Patients with spinal-cord injury (SCI) may have or develop the same diseases, including a variety of metabolic disorders, as their still-ambulatory counterparts. The complications or sequelae of these conditions may compound or aggravate those related to the SCI itself. Impotence is a common complication of many metabolic disturbances, especially diabetes mellitus, and since diabetes is quite a prevalent disease, sexual dysfunction related to it may be a serious problem for SCI patients. This article will address the impact of diabetes mellitus, liver disease, and several miscellaneous metabolic disorders on sexual function.

Diabetes Mellitus

Incidence and Clinical Manifestation

Potency may be defined as the ability to initiate, sustain, and successfully complete the act of coitus, and impaired potency is quite

Sexual Rehabilitation of the Spinal-Cord-Injured Patient
Edited by J.F. Leyson, © 1990 The Humana Press, Inc.

prevalent in diabetes mellitus, occurring in as many of 50% of male patients (*5a,18,22,25*). The true prevalence may be higher than this, since most reports have relied upon the patients' subjective evaluation. Also, diabetes is present in over one-third of patients presenting with erectile dysfunction (*19a*). Although the incidence of impotence increases with age (*22,25*), there is no direct correlation between the duration of diabetes and the presence of impotence (*18,25*). An occasional patient may have impotence as the initial manifestation of diabetes (*8*), and some patients may experience reversible impotence as a function of the degree of metabolic control (*22*).

The characteristic manifestation of impotence in diabetic men is the loss of erectile ability with respect to both initiation and maintenance, but little or no decrease in libido. Since libido, orgasm, and ejaculation are generally unaffected, the term "erectile impotence" has been suggested (*18*). Generally, when libido or orgasm is disturbed, a psychogenic component should be considered.

Typically, the onset of impotence is gradual and progresses over a period of several months to a year, with an interval during which the firmness of erection is decreased. The occurrence of impotence is not correlated with requirements for insulin therapy or known complications such as peripheral vascular disease, hypertension, retinopathy, or nephropathy (*18*). However, impotence is more prevalent in diabetic men with neuropathy compared to those without neuropathy (*10,18*).

In SCI, the pattern of sexual dysfunction is different from that in diabetes mellitus. Although erectile capacity is retained, the ability to ejaculate is lost (*5,27*). Except when a complete upper-motor-neuron lesion is present, SCI patients may be able to experience an orgasm (*5*).

When the diabetic SCI patient has sexual dysfunction related to diabetes itself, the major manifestation should be erectile impotence. If the patient has a finding other than that, e.g., retrograde ejaculation, then it is not the result of diabetes, and another etiology should be sought.

Etiology of Sexual Dysfunction

Sexual dysfunction resulting from diabetes mellitus itself appears to occur primarily in male patients. There are very few studies of female sexual function, and they have been based on subjective data about sexual arousal and response. The sexual response in diabetic women appears to be unaltered, with the frequency of sexual intercourse and orgasm being comparable in diabetic and nondiabetic patients (*9*). Even though there are no studies of sexual function in female diabetics with SCI, it is likely that the findings in ambulatory patients would apply equally to SCI.

In order to better understand the pathogenesis of impotence in diabetes mellitus, the physiology of normal penile erection should be appreciated. Penile erection is a vascular phenomenon brought on by neurological reflex with little direct voluntary control (*5,7,30*). Erection is considered to be psychogenic if stimuli result in arousal of the erotic centers within the brain, although it is considered reflexogenic if either the genital region or nearby visceral structures are stimulated (*7,30*). The term stimulative erection has also been used when there is direct tactile stimulation of the genital areas. Normally, erection depends on adequate penile blood pressure, blood flow, and an intact autonomic nervous system. Several factors that may affect normal penile physiology have been considered in the genesis of erectile dysfunction in diabetes mellitus, including hormonal, circulatory, and neuropathic abnormalities.

Since diabetes mellitus is an endocrine-deficiency state, a hormonal basis for impotence had long been suspected. Shoffling and colleagues (*25*) found that diabetic men with impotence had decreased urinary excretion of gonadotropin and increased excretion of ketosteroid, with the latter being the result of the presence of weak androgenic metabolites. They suggested that the impotence was related to hypogonadotropic hypogonadism. However, plasma levels of testosterone were measured by several groups of investigators and were found to be normal (*11,15,18*). Furthermore, the finding of normal testicular histology (*11*) and the absence of a response to testosterone therapy (*9a*) suggest that hypogonadism is not present in diabetic men.

When pelvic circulation is compromised, as in patients with severe vascular disease and the Leriche syndrome, erectile impotence usually results (*6*). Since severe atherosclerosis and arteriosclerosis are frequent complications of diabetes mellitus, it is reasonable to suggest that vascular disease may cause diabetic impotence. In two uncontrolled studies, penile blood pressure was found to be abnormally low in impotent diabetics (*1,12*). However, the significance of vascular disease itself in the genesis of diabetic impotence has not been proven and requires further investigation.

The final, and probably most important factor, is neuropathy. Peripheral and autonomic neuropathy is a common complication of diabetes mellitus, and if the process affects those nerves controlling erection, then erectile impotence may result. The control of bladder and erectile function are mediated by the same nerve group, and thus, dysfunction in one might be accompanied by an abnormality in the other. Ellenberg evaluated bladder function in 47 impotent and 30 potent diabetics, and found that 79% of the former and only 10% of the latter had a neurogenic bladder (*9a*). When the study was expanded to 200 diabetic men, the impotent patients had a higher incidence of neuropathy (82%) than the potent ones (12%). Similar findings have been confirmed by others (*15,18*). Interestingly, histologic evidence of neuropathy involving neural fibers in the corpora cavernosa has been demonstrated (*18*). Thus, the available data strongly support the theory that neuropathy is the major factor responsible for erectile impotence in diabetes mellitus.

Evaluation

Most SCI patients retain erectile capacity, either reflexogenic or psychogenic, except when their lesion is of the complete lower-motor-neuron type (*5,27*). If this latter group of patients is excluded, then the presence of erectile impotence should suggest a superimposed factor, either psychogenic and/or organic.

During the evaluation of impotence, there are several areas that should be carefully investigated and that may help in the differentiation of psychogenic from organic causes (*23*).

1. If possible, the onset of impotence should be documented, and the presence of any specific life events should be noted. Organic impotence tends to be progressive and not temporally related to psychosocial events. It should be noted that impotence may occur early in the course of SCI, but this usually improves with time
2. The pattern of erection should be described. Most SCI patients, except those with complete lower-motor-neuron lesions, maintain reflexogenic erection, although those with superimposed diabetes mellitus have neither psychogenic nor reflexogenic erection. Impotence that is episodic implies a psychogenic determinant
3. If nocturnal erection with adequate turgidity is present, then diabetes mellitus is probably not the cause of sexual dysfunction
4. Patients with psychogenic impotence often have diminished libido, although those with organic impotence do not
5. SCI patients may have impotence from organic causes other than diabetes mellitus.

Finally, a number of medications may cause impotence, e.g., various antihypertensive agents (*19a*), estrogens, alcohol, morphine and other opiates, cocaine, and amphetamines. Although the medical and sexual history of the patient may help to differentiate psychogenic from organic causes and one organic cause from another, it should be recognized that for many patients both psychogenic and organic factors coexist.

A thorough neurologic examination is mandatory, particularly with respect to the level and completeness of the SCI. More than 90% of patients with complete upper-motor-neuron lesions have reflexogenic erections, whereas only 25% of those with complete lower-motor-neuron lesions have erections that are of the psychogenic variety (*5*). Patients with incomplete lesions do better, with over 90% having reflexogenic and/or psychogenic erections (*5*). Similar studies in Japanese SCI patients have yielded a smaller percentage, but trends and patterns were similar (*27*). The physical examination should also include a careful search for vascular disease. Diabetic peripheral neuropathy may be difficult to diagnose when SCI is present. However, diabetic patients with high cord lesions may have absent knee and ankle reflexes, rather than hyperreflexia, when diabetic peripheral neuropathy is present.

Obviously, all SCI patients with sexual dysfunction, especially impotence, should be screened for the presence of diabetes mellitus, and the diagnosis should be confirmed with a glucose-tolerance test. When the diagnosis of diabetes mellitus is established in the SCI patient with impotence, additional specialized tests may help in determining the causative factor(s) for the impotence such as:

1. *Nocturnal Penile Tumescence.* Two or more episodes of nocturnal penile rigidity and tumescence (NPTR) normally occur especially during REM sleep. NPT can be readily quantitated, and may be an objective index of erectile ability. Men with organic impotence, as in that resulting from diabetes, have decreased or absent NPT (*16,17*), whereas those with psychogenic impotence have normal NPT. During the period of spinal shock, there is decreased or absent NPT, which returns to normal with recovering or incomplete lesions. However, even patients with complete lesions who have reflexogenic erections may have weak or short bursts of NPT activity (Leyson, J. F., personal communication). Normal NPT in an impotent SCI patient with diabetes mellitus suggests that the impotence is unlikely to be the result of diabetic (and SCI) neuropathy.
2. *Penile Blood Pressure.* SCI itself does not cause a decrease in penile arterial blood pressure, unless associated with underlying vascular occlusive diseases. On the other hand, diabetes mellitus associated with arteriosclerosis can cause a decrease in penile blood flow and blood pressure. Diabetic vascular insufficiency is probably responsible for impotence when penile blood pressure is low in the SCI patient with diabetes.
3. *Bulbocavernosus Reflex.* This reflex may be evaluated either by direct physical examination or electronically. The response

to stimulation is penile rigidity, which can be assessed visually, or the efferent nerve impulses may be monitored by surface electrodes. This reflex is delayed in diabetics with impotence (*14*), whereas it is normal or increased in SCI patients unless there is a sacral-cord lesion. In that case, the reflex will be decreased because the reflex arc is interrupted.

4. *Pudendal Evoked Response.* This noninvasive technique assesses the integrity of the afferent limb (pudendal nerve) of the erectile reflex arc. Electrical stimuli are applied to the penis, and responses are recorded over the spine at the L1 vertebral level. Patients with SCI above the lumbar level have normal pudendal evoked responses (*13*), whereas diabetics with peripheral neuropathy have an abnormal spinal evoked response (*14*). This technique may help to detect diabetic neuropathy in SCI patients and determine its role in the genesis of impotence.

A summary of differential diagnostic features, based on the above tests, for SCI and diabetic patients is given in Table 1. However, the data available are limited, and there is need for further investigation before definite differential points can be firmly established.

Management

Successful management of the SCI patient with diabetes mellitus and impotence requires an integrated approach involving the patient, the family, and the health care team. Most of the patients will have both organic and psychogenic determinants for their impotence (*4,19,20,24*). Thus, sex counseling, as discussed elsewhere in this book, may be a very helpful therapeutic agent for these patients with impotence. In some patients, peripheral vascular disease may be responsible for the impotence, and confirmation by arteriography might be necessary, since good results have been reported from inferior epigastric-penile artery vascular grafts, especially in younger men with incomplete lesions (*21*).

Erectile impotence resulting from diabetic neuropathy is irreversible, and if the patient desires sexual intercourse, then surgical implantation of a penile prosthesis may be indicated (*26*). Of course, before any surgical procedure is considered, the patient must have a careful psychological evaluation. Available devices include the Small-Carrion prosthesis and the inflatable penile prosthesis, each of which has its own advantages and disadvantages. If surgical correction is elected, then

Table 1
Differential Features of Impotence in Diabetes Mellitus and Spinal Cord Injury*

	Diabetes mellitus	Spinal-cord injury
Type of erection		
Reflexogenic	↓	→ ↓[1]
Psychogenic	→ ↓	→ ↓[1]
Penile blood flow	↓	→
Nocturnal penile tumescence	↓	→[1]
Bulbocavernosus reflex	↓	→[2]
Pudendal evoked response	↓	→[2]

*→ normal, ↓ abnormal.
[1]Pattern depends on level and completeness of injury.
[2]May be abnormal with lower-motor-neuron lesions.

the type of prosthesis used should be based on careful medical and psychological evaluation of the individual patient, as discussed in the chapter on surgical treatment of impotence.

Liver Disease

Sexual dysfunction is frequent in patients with chronic liver disease and cirrhosis. A common feature in many patients with chronic liver disease is alcohol consumption. Chronic alcoholism is probably at least as prevalent in SCI patients as in the general ambulatory population and complications from alcohol abuse, including sexual dysfunction may also be present.

Sexual dysfunction in cirrhotic patients is characterized by loss of libido, decreased spermatogenesis and testosterone production, testicular atrophy, and gynecomastia (*2*). The clinical features are similar to those in the patient with androgen deficiency and estrogen excess. Several endocrinologic studies have demonstrated alteration in sex hormones associated with hepatic cirrhosis (*2*). Although circulating testosterone is low, estrone, estradiol, and prolactin are elevated. The hypogonadism of liver disease is felt to be both primary and secondary in nature (*29*). A primary gonadal defect is suggested by the impaired testicular testosterone response to gonadotropin stimulation, the histologic demonstration of testicular atrophy, and elevated LH and FSH levels. Secondary hypogonadism is suggested by the decreased hypothalamic response to clomiphene citrate, with two-thirds of cirrhotic patients failing to produce a 50% increase in gonadotropin.

Alcohol itself may directly interfere with gonadal testosterone production. The main acute effect of alcohol relates to its central nervous system depressant properties. Although alcohol may decrease inhibition of sexual expression, making sexual overtures easier, it also reduces the sensitivity of central nervous system centers essential for sexual performance. Women may fail to achieve orgasm, whereas men may experience erectile impotence and retarded ejaculation, which may be in part the result of associated peripheral neuropathy.

Successful management of sexual dysfunction in SCI patients with a history of heavy alcohol intake depends in great part on the degree of irreversible liver damage. If there is severe hepatic dysfunction, then therapeutic efforts will probably be to no avail. Those with less impairment of liver function may benefit from abstinence from alcohol. Psychological support and counseling should be provided. Although a clear-cut benefit has not been demonstrated, some SCI may respond to testosterone therapy, especially if the circulating level is very low (*28*). However, exogenous androgen may lead to gonadal suppression and persistent gynecomastia, perhaps related to increased peripheral conversion of testosterone to estrogen. Clomiphene citrate may increase gonadotropin release and, thereby, improve testosterone production (*3*). Although some patients have had a favorable response, the long-term effects of clomiphene have not been well characterized, and its use is still considered investigational.

Miscellaneous Conditions

There are other endocrine and metabolic conditions that may have an adverse effect on sexuality (*19*). Both hypo- and hyperthyroidism can cause sexual dysfunction, as can acromegaly and adrenal insufficiency. If there is a clinical suspicion for the presence of any of these diseases, then appropriate laboratory tests will confirm the diagnosis. Correction of the endocrinopathy should improve sexual function.

Conclusions

A variety of metabolic disorders may contribute to sexual dysfunction in SCI patients, as well as the general ambulatory population. Two very common conditions are diabetes mellitus and chronic liver disease associated with alcoholism. The former causes erectile impotence, which probably is the result of the neuropathy of diabetes, whereas the latter causes sexual dysfunction, which may be related, in part, to hormonal imbalance. Although sexual dysfunction in these two groups of patients appears to have a strong organic component, psychological factors also play a role. In addition to specific forms of therapy for selected patients, e.g., penile prosthesis implantation in diabetic erectile impotence, the treatment plan should also include psychosocial evaluation and appropriate sex counseling.

References

1. Abelson, D. (1975) Diagnostic value of the penile pulse and blood pressure: A doppler study of impotence in diabetics. *J. Urol.* **113**, 636–639.
2. Baker, H. W. G., Burger, H. G., de Krester, D. M., Dulmanis, A., Hudson B., O'Connor, S., Paulsen, C. A., Purcell, N., Rennie, G. C., Seah, C. S., Taft, H. P., and Wang, C. (1976) A study of the endocrinologic manifestation of hepatic cirrhosis. *Q. J. Med.* **45 (177)**, 145–178.
3. Bjork, J. T., Varma, R. R., and Borkowf, H. I. (1977) Case Reports: Clomiphene Citrate therapy in a patient with Laennec's cirrhosis. *Gastroenterology* **72**, 1308–1311.
4. Bohannon, N. J., Zilbergeld, B., Bullard, D. G., and Stoklosa, J. M. (1982) Treatable impotence in diabetic patients. *West J. Med.* **136**, 6–10.
5. Bors, E. and Commar, A. E. (1960) Neurological disturbances of sexual function with special reference to 529 patients with spinal cord injury. *Urol. Survey* **10**, 191–222.
5a. Braunstein, G. D. (1987) Impotence in diabetic men. *Mt. Sinai J. Med.* **54**, 236–240.
6. Canning, J. R., Bowers, L. M., Lloyd, F. A., and Cottrell, T. L. C. (1963) Genital vascular insufficiency and impotence. *Surg. Forum* **14**, 298–299.
7. de Groat, W. C. and Booth, A. M. (1980) Physiology of male sexual function. *Ann. Intern. Med.* **92**, 329–331.
8. Dutsch, S., and Sherman, L. (1980) Previously unrecognized diabetes mellitus in sexually impotent men. *JAMA* **244**, 2430–2432.
9. Ellenberg, M. (1971) Sex and the female diabetic. *Med. Aspects Hum. Sex.* **11**, 30–38.
9a. Ellenberg, M. (1971) Impotence in diabetes: Neurologic factor. *Ann. Intern. Med.* **75**, 213–219.
10. Ellenberg, M. (1980) Sexual function in diabetic patients. *Ann. Intern. Med.* **92**, 331–333.
11. Faerman, I., Vilar, O., Rivarola, M. A., Posner, J. M., Jadzinsky, M. N., Fox, D., Lloret, A., Berstein-Hahn, L., and Saraceni, D. (1972) Impotence and diabetes: Studies of androgenic function in diabetic impotent males. *Diabetes* **21**, 23–30.

12. Gasket, P. (1971) The importance of penile blood pressure in cases of impotence. *Can. Med. Assoc. J.* **105**, 1047–1051.
13. Haldeman, S., Bradley, W. E., and Bhatia, N. N. (1982) Evoked responses from the pudendal nerve. *J. Urol.* **128**, 974–980.
14. Haldeman, S., Bradley, W. E., Bhatia, N. N., Glick, M. E., and Ek, A. (1982) Neurologic evaluation of the bladder, bowel and sexual disturbances in diabetic men. Proceedings of the International Symposium on Diabetic Neuropathy and its Treatment, pp 298–301 (Excerpta Medica, Belgium).
15. Jensen, S. B., Hagen, C., Froland, A., and Pedersen, P. B. (1979) Sexual function and pituitary axis in insulin treated diabetic men. *Acta. Med. Scand.* **S624**, 65–68.
16. Karacan, I. (1980) Diagnosis of erectile impotence in diabetes mellitus: An objective and specific method. *Ann Intern. Med.* **92**, 334–337.
17. Karacan, I., Salis, P. J., Ware, J. C., Dervent, B., Williams, R. L., Scott, F. B., Attia, S. L., and Beutler, L. E. (1978) Nocturnal penile tumescence and diagnosis in diabetic impotence. *Am. J. Psychiatry* **135**, 191–197.
18. Kolodny, R. C., Kahn, C. B., Goldstein, H. H., and Barnett, D. M. (1974) Sexual dysfunction in diabetic men. *Diabetes* **23**, 306–309.
19. Levine, S. B. (1976) Marital sexual dysfunction: Erectile dysfunction. *Ann. Intern. Med.* **85**, 342–350.
19a. Lipson, L. G. (1984) Treatment of hypertension in diabetic men: problems with sexual dysfunction. *Am. J. Cardiol.* **53**, 46A–50A.
19b. Maatman, T. J., Montague, D. K., and Martin, L. M. (1987) Erectile dysfunction in men with diabetes mellitus. *Urology* **29**, 589–592.
20. Meyer, J. K. (1977) The treatment of sexual disorders. *Med. Clin. N. Am.* **61**, 811–823.
21. Michal, V., Kramer, R., Pospichal, J., and Hejhal, L. (1977) Arterial epigastricocavernous anastomosis for the treatment of sexual impotence. *World J. Surg.* **1**, 515–519.
22. Rubin, A. (1967) Sexual behavior in diabetes mellitus. *Med. Aspects Hum. Sex.* **1**, 23–25.
23. Schiavi, R. C. (1979) Some problems in the differential diagnosis of erectile disorders. *Sexuality Disability* **2**, 66–70.
24. Schiavi, R.C. (1980) Psychological treatment of erectile disorders in diabetic patients. *Ann. Intern. Med.* **92**, 337–339.
25. Schoffling, K., Federlin, K., Ditschuneit, H., and Pfieffer, E. F. (1963) Disorders of sexual function in male diabetics. *Diabetes* **12**, 519–527.
26. Scott, F. B., Fishman, I. J., and Light, J. K. (1980) An inflatable penile prosthesis for treatment of diabetic impotence. *Ann. Intern. Med.* **92**, 340–342.
27. Tsuji, I., Nakajima, F., Morinoto, J., and Nounaka, Y. (1961) The sexual function in patients with spinal cord injury. *Urol. Int.* **12**, 270–280.
28. Van Thiel, D. H. and Lester, R. (1977) Therapy of sexual dysfunction in alcohol abusers: A Pandora's box. *Gastroenterology* **72**, 1354–1354.

29. Van Thiel, D. H., Lester, R., and Sherins, R. J. (1974) Hypogonadism in alcoholic liver disease: Evidence for a double defect. *Gastroenterology* **67**, 1188–1189.
30. Weiss, H. D. (1972) The physiology of human penile erection. *Ann. Intern. Med.* **76**, 793–799.

29
Renal Disease and Sexual Dysfunction

Robert L. Winer
and
Kowit Danviriyasup

Introduction

Renal functional insufficiency often develops in patients with chronic spinal-cord injury (SCI), is associated with substantial morbidity, and frequently progresses to end-stage renal disease (ESRD). As renal function deteriorates, virtually all organ systems are adversely affected. Over the past ten years, there has been increasing interest in the abnormalities of sexual and reproductive function that occur in patients with ESRD (*20a*). The main focus of this chapter will be the impact of advanced renal failure on sexual function. Even though chronic dialysis has become more widely available, including an expanded capability for patients with SCI and renal failure, there have been no systematic observations of sexual function in patients with both SCI and advanced renal failure. Although our comments are based on observations in able-bodied patients with ESRD, there is no *prima facie* reason why these cannot be extended to the SCI patient with renal failure.

Incidence

Almost all of the available data rely upon patients' reports of sexual function, and most studies involve populations that are heterogeneous

Sexual Rehabilitation of the Spinal-Cord-Injured Patient
Edited by J.F. Leyson, © 1990 The Humana Press, Inc.

with respect to age, severity, and duration of renal disease, duration and course of dialysis or renal transplant, and medication status. Although statistical analysis is difficult, there are definite patterns and trends. Levy (*20*) noted that 48% of male and 26% of female patients had the appearance or actual worsening of sexual problems as renal failure progressed, with 35% of the male and 25% of the female patients suffering still further deterioration in sexual function after dialysis was initiated. Clinical manifestations include a decreased frequency of sexual intercourse, altered potency in the men, and impaired orgasmic ability in the women. Fifty-nine percent of male hemodialysis patients reported partial or total impotence, compared to 15% before the development of uremia.

Interestingly, 43% of male renal transplant patients reported partial or total impotence, compared to 16% before the onset of uremia. Thus, even with successful management or elimination of the uremic milieu, these patients continued to experience substantial impairment of sexual function. Although others noted some improvement in overall sexual function among renal transplant patients, the level of functioning was still less than that prior to the onset of their illness (*28*). Procci et al. (*27*) reported that 40–50% of male uremic patients had erectile dysfunction with reduced frequency of sexual intercourse and that hemodialysis had no beneficial effect. In a study of 32 male patients, Abram et al. (*1*) noted that 45% had reduced sexual potency after onset of their kidney disease and that an additional 35% suffered reduced potency after beginning dialysis treatment. Of the 19 patients who received a renal transplant, only 40% reported an improvement in potency. Another marker of sexual activity was the frequency of sexual intercourse per month, which was 10.4 before the onset of uremia, 5.7 during the uremic period before hemodialysis, 4.0 during dialysis, and 7.5 after successful renal transplantation. Finkelstein et al. (*11*) studied 77 married patients, and also observed a decline in the frequency of sexual intercourse after the beginning of dialysis therapy. Forty percent of the patients reported having no intercourse, although prior to the onset of renal disease, more than 70% had intercourse at least two times per week. Sixty-five percent of the male patients had difficulty initiating and maintaining an erection, and 39% had difficulty with ejaculation. Fifty-three percent of the female patients had difficulty with sexual arousal and achieving orgasm.

In addition to the changes in libido, potency, and ability to ejaculate or achieve orgasm, there are other alterations in sexual and reproductive function, including gynecomastia, reduced gonadal size, and decreased spermatogenesis in male patients, and decreased fertility, menometrorrhagia, secondary amenorrhea, and ovarian cystic disease in female patients. Excessive menstrual bleeding may aggravate the anemia of ESRD in female patients. In many patients, the abnormalities in sexual and reproductive function may produce a profound psychological impact, particularly with respect to self-esteem and body image.

Etiology of Sexual Dysfunction

The etiology of sexual dysfunction in renal disease is probably multifactoral, involving the complex interaction of a variety of pathophysiologic mechanisms, including psychogenic as well as organic factors (Table 1). The multiplicity of factors and their interactive effects will have an impact on evaluation of the patient, as well as the design and implementation of a rational treatment strategy.

The patient with ESRD is subjected to a variety of stresses that may have psychological sequelae. There is often a decreased sense of physical well-being associated with impairment of physical activity and rehabilitation, the latter including an inability to return to gainful employment. There are conflicts related to passivity and dependency. The renal disease itself, which may be complicated by other intercurrent medical conditions, often leads to a heightened awareness of individual mortality, frequently resulting in an overriding fear of death. The absence of urine output, especially in the male, and the presence of a blood access for hemodialysis or a peritoneal catheter for continuous peritoneal dialysis (CAPD) may contribute to a distorted body image. The importance of psychological factors is underscored by the above-mentioned observations that sexual activity may remain depressed or worsen, even though there has been substantial somatic improvement as the result of dialysis or successful renal transplantation. Although the renal allograft may be functioning well, the patient is still subjected to a multitude of stresses, including fear of allograft failure and subsequent return to dialysis, dependency on medications, fear of intercurrent and occasionally fatal illnesses, serious complications of drug therapy, and altered body image. The role of depression in the genesis of altered sexual function in renal failure patients has been stressed (*11,20*). However, this has recently been questioned by Procci et al. (*27*). Even though 43% of their patients were found to be depressed, there was no difference with respect to complaints of erectile difficulty or frequency of sexual intercourse in those with or without depression.

There are multiple endocrine and metabolic abnormalities in patients with ESRD, including defects related to gonadal function. Inter-

Table 1: Etiologic Considerations in the Sexual Dysfunction of Patients with Renal Failure

Psychological factors
Hormonal and metabolic abnormalities
Neuropathy
Associated diseases
Medications and dialysis therapy

pretation of these hormonal abnormalities, particularly with respect to therapeutic implications, must take into consideration hormone kinetics, including production, secretion, degradation, and end-organ sensitivity. This is particularly true with respect to potency, since Hagen et al. (*13*) found no correlation between blood levels of hormones and the patient's ability to achieve or sustain an erection.

In male patients, there is evidence for gonadal hypofunction manifested by impaired spermatogenesis and decreased testosterone production (*9,13,15,21,30*), and the plasma testosterone level has been found to correlate with the glomerular filtration rate (*15,19,21*). Decreased functional capacity of the testes has been shown by hyporesponsivity to hCG or clomiphene citrate (*15,29,30*). In experimental models of uremia, gonadotropin stimulation results in impaired testosterone and cAMP* responses, perhaps related to a decrease in the number of gonadotropin binding sites on the Leydid cell (*5*) or a cellular defect in adenylate cyclase (*18*). LH levels are increased in only about 50% of patients. The absence of an increase in LH when serum testosterone is markedly decreased suggests an abnormality in the hypothalamic–pituitary feedback response to testosterone dysfunction (*9,15,19,21*). In male patients, FSH levels are normal or occassionally increased. Prolactin levels are markedly elevated (*21,23*) and since this hormone has an antigonadotropic action at the gonadal level, it has been suggested that altered libido and sexual activity in renal failure may be related to prolactin. Bommer et al. (*4*) and Ramirez et al. (*29a*) found that bromocriptine, a dopaminergic agonist, reduced prolactin levels and improved sexual function in male patients with renal failure. However, Lim et al. (*21*) noted that male patients treated with clomiphene, an antiestrogen, had improvement in libido and testosterone levels without a reduction in prolactin.

In a recent autopsy study of chronic SCI patients with ESRD testicular examination revealed marked atrophy with decreased or absent spermatogenesis and marked peritubular and interstitial fibrosis (*1a*). We have found decreased testosterone levels in a group of ten male

*cAMP: Cyclic Adenosine Monophosphate.

patients with SCI and ESRD when compared to a cohort of able-bodied patients with ESRD, although there were no differences in LH, FSH, or prolactin levels (*32*).

Alterations in menstrual function tend to increase as glomerular filtration rate falls, and with ESRD, virtually all female patients will have abnormal menses, often with galactorrhea. Estradiol and progesterone levels may be decreased or normal, but there are no cyclic increases (*22,26*). LH levels may be increased in the follicular and decreased in the luteal phase with no ovulatory spikes (*22,31*), suggesting a hypothalamic derangement in the regulation of gonadotropin secretion. The failure of LH to increase after administration of ethinyl estradiol was interpreted by Lim et al. (*22*) as an ovarian dysfunction in renal failure that may be the result of an alteration in the positive feedback effect of estrogen on gonadotropin-releasing hormone secretion by the hypothalamus. Although most of the data suggest a central defect, the presence of elevated gonadotropin and decreased or normal estrogen levels in some patients implies end-organ resistance as well. Also, in an experimental model of uremia, female rats had decreased ovarian cAMP and estradiol responses to gonadotropin (*17*). Although prolactin is elevated in most patients, there appears to be no correlation between its level and amenorrhea or libido (*26*). Although hemodialysis may have no effect on hormonal abnormalities, menstrual changes are variable, and patients with amenorrhea frequently develop menorrhagia or polymenorrhea. CAPD may be associated with more regular menstrual cycles than hemodialysis (*12*). Renal transplantation may reverse some of the abnormalities, and successful pregnancy has been reported.

The uremic state itself may be associated with other hormonal and metabolic abnormalities that could affect sexual function. Massry et al. (*25*) suggested altered calcium metabolism as a factor, based on observations that several uremic patients had improved sexual function after parathyroidectomy or treatment with the active form of vitamin D,1,25-dihydroxycholecalciferol [1,25-$(OH)_2D_3$]. Kreusser et al. (*17,18*) found that pretreatment of uremic rats with 1,25-$(OH)_2D_3$ markedly improved ovarian and testicular cAMP responses to gonadotropin; however, the results were independent of the serum calcium level, and the presence or absence of parathyroid tissue. The practical value of these observations is questionable in view of the finding by Blumberg et al. (*3*) that uremic patients treated for 2–4 mo with 1,25-$(OH)_2D_3$ had no improvement in sexual function, even though the serum level of parathyroid hormone fell and calcium rose. Prostaglandin metabolism is altered in uremia, and this may affect gonadal function. In their ex-

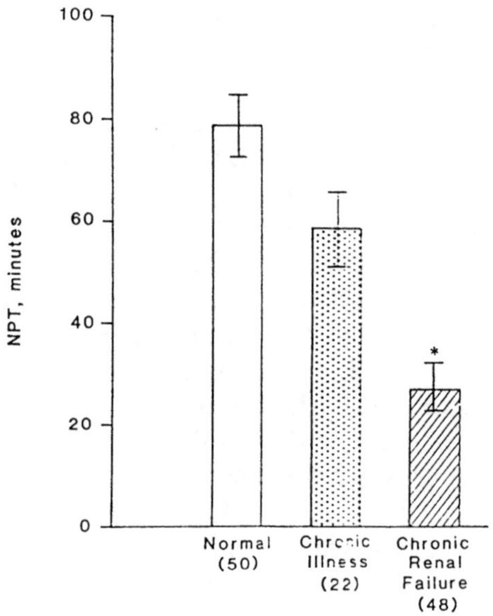

Fig. 1. Nocturnal penile tumescence (NPT), defined as 13 mm change in circumference, in three patient groups: normal, chronic illness with normal renal function, and end-stage renal disease. Those with renal failure have lower ($^*p < 0.01$) NPT values than the other two groups. The data, expressed as mean ±SE, were taken from Fig. 1 of Procci, W. R., Goldstein, D. A., Adelstein, J. and Massry, S. G. (1981) Sexual dysfunction in the male patient with uremia: a reappraisal. *Kidney Int.* **19**, 317–323, with permission.

perimental studies, Kreusser et al. (*18*) found that indomethacin, a known prostaglandin synthetase inhibitor, further impaired the ovarian cAMP response to gonadotropin, whereas in vitro incubation of ovarian tissue with PGE_1 and PGE_2 markedly improved the basal and stimulated cAMP response. Cellular zinc deficiency has been reported in uremia and has been related to sexual dysfunction. Mahajan et al. (*24*) treated a group of patients with zinc, and noted an increase in testosterone and sperm count, decrease in LH and FSH, and improved potency, libido, and frequency of intercourse. An additional metabolic consideration is the nutritional status of the patient, and many uremics have evidence of poor nutrition.

Peripheral neuropathy is a major complication of advanced renal failure, and there is increasing evidence that the neuropathic process also involves the autonomic nervous system (*7*). Penile erection normally results from impulses in the parasympathetic nervous system from the sacral segment, but impulses may also originate in the brain with efferent pathways to the genitalia via the sympathetic nervous system. The pudendal nerve carries sensory information from the penis as well as motor innervation to the bulbocavernosus muscle. Based on studies of pudendal evoked responses, Haldeman et al. (*14*) have stressed the importance of an intact pudendal pathway for normal erectile function. These electrophysiologic studies have not been done in patients with renal failure, and they would be most helpful in evaluating the degree of pudendal nerve involvement as a result of the uremic state. Measurement of nocturnal penile tumescence (NPT) has been proposed as an objective means of assessing erectile ability (*16*). Because most NPT* occurs during REM sleep, it may result from CNS impulses, and thus be a marker of autonomic nervous system dysfunction. Procci et al. (*27*) found that approximately 50% of uremic men had decreased NPT, and that the values were significantly different from normal controls and patients with chronic illness but without renal failure (Fig. 1).

There also was a direct correlation between NPT and the frequency of sexual intercourse. Further studies on the relationship between erectile and autonomic nervous system dysfunctions have recently been reported by Campese et al. (*6*). They assessed the intactness of the autonomic nervous system by the Valsalva ratio, which is a measure of the integrity of the baroreceptor reflex arc, and erectile function by NPT. Both indexes were significantly lower in the uremic patients than controls, with 44 and 48% of uremic patients having abnormal NPTs and Valsalva ratios, respectively. Interestingly, NPT and Valsalva ratios were correlated, as were Valsalva ratios and frequency of intercourse per month. The correlation suggests a shared disturbance in efferent sympathetic pathways. However, an abnormal reflex sacral parasympathetic pathway could also explain the decreased NPT in uremia. Regardless of which pathways are involved, the bulk of evidence strongly suggests that autonomic neuropathy plays an important role in the erectile dysfunction of male uremic patients.

When discussing the etiology of sexual dysfunction in uremic patients, one should consider the impact of associated diseases and concomitant drug or dialysis treatment. Other illnesses may have a direct or indirect effect on sexual function, and some of those to be considered in the uremic population include diabetes mellitus and atherosclerotic vascular disease. The aging process itself is also associated with decreased sexual activity. Some investigators have suggested that the presence of chronic illness may have an impact on sexual function. However, Procci et al. (*27*) showed that patients with chronic illness and normal renal function had NPT scores similar to the normal control group.

Hypertension is very common in patients with renal failure and many of the medications (e.g., guanethidine, methyldopa, clonidine, propranolol, and prazocin) may interfere with sexual function. One should

*NPT = the same connection with. NPTR = tumescence plus rigidity.

also be aware of medications that may affect or alter the hypothalamic pituitary regulation of gonadotropin or prolactin secretion, such as methyldopa, reserpine, clonidine, and phenothiaznes. Finally, the dialysis process itself may adversely affect sexual function. There may be marked shifts in extracellular fluid volume with subsequent hemodynamic effects, and some patients complain of being tired, weak, or "washed out" after the dialysis session. For patients on peritoneal dialysis, the presence of the peritoneal catheter in the anterior abdominal wall may be a barrier to normal sexual function.

Evaluation

Disturbances in sexuality related to the renal disease itself tend to occur only when advanced renal functional insufficiency is present. Although this has not been carefully investigated, the glomerular filtration rate, as assessed by endogenous creatinine clearance, is usually below 15–20 mL/min. Serum creatinine by itself may not be a good marker of renal function in SCI patients, especially when muscle atrophy is present. Also, the blood urea nitrogen (BUN) level may be affected by nonrenal factors. Evaluation of the SCI patient with advanced renal failure and sexual dysfunction must take into consideration psychological, physical, and metabolic factors.

Information regarding sexual dysfunction will primarily be generated by interviews with the patient or patient-administered questionnaires, and the most frequent manifestation of such dysfunction will be a decrease in the frequency of intercourse. This is a reflection of decreased libido and/or decreased ability to perform, with the latter manifesting itself as impairment in initiation and maintenance of erection in the male, and problems with sexual arousal or orgasmic ability in the female. As stressed by Finkelstein and Finkelstein (*10*), we must differentiate sexual difficulties from sexual problems, since the presence of dysfunctional symptoms *per se* does not necessarily imply that the emotional component of the relationship is poor. The therapist should try to ascertain the actual and desired levels of sexual activity both at the present time and prior to the onset of illness, and whether the level of activity is satisfactory or poses a problem for the patient. Also, the patient's physical and psychological problems should be put in the context of interpersonal, marital, and family relationships.

With respect to the physical examination, there are no distinctive features that would permit a differentiation of sexual dysfunction caused by renal failure or that related to the SCI. The diagnosis of advanced renal functional insufficiency should be based on the aforementioned laboratory finding of a low creatinine clearance. There are very few other laboratory tests that may be of value in assessing the patient. The plasma testosterone level is usually not helpful unless it is extremely low. Based on our current state of knowledge, and when there is no contrary indication, we do not recommend measuring levels of other hormones, e.g., parathyroid hormone, estradiol, gonadotropins, or prolactin. As in all patients with renal failure, it is important to assess the nutritional status, and markers such as the serum albumin level may be helpful in this regard. For some patients, particularly those on hemodialysis, determination of the plasma zinc level may be considered.

For the male patient, determination of NPT may permit quantitation of erectile potency (*16*), and differentiation of organic and psychogenic factors. The value of NPTR determination has been demonstrated by Procci et al. (*27*), who found a significant and direct correlation between NPT and the frequency of intercourse in male uremic patients. In female patients, measurement of vaginal pressures with special transducers may be considered. Electrophysiologic studies might also provide another objective parameter.

Management

The successful approach to the SCI patient with advanced renal failure and sexual dysfunction must incorporate both psychological and organic factors as etiologic possibilities. There should be an initial consultation by the physician to review the patient's medical status carefully and make appropriate adjustments. Psychiatric or psychological consultation may be in order for patients with depression or overt psychological symptoms. Finally, there should be referral for sex counseling when indicated.

With advancing renal failure, aggressive medical management of the uremic milieu will have to be replaced by dialytic therapy, either hemodialysis or peritoneal dialysis. As mentioned previously, although the patient's overall physical well-being may improve with dialysis or successful renal transplantation, sexual function frequently continues to deteriorate, emphasizing the role of psychological or unidentified organic factors. It is unlikely that SCI patients with ESRD will receive a renal transplant because they have a high prevalence of urinary tract and other infections, and there is potential danger to such patients when immunosuppressive therapy is used. If the patient's course on dialysis is punctuated by episodes of hypotension, disequilibrium, or a "washed-out'' feeling, then efforts should be made to make the dialysis process smoother. Most patients are very anemic, and efforts to improve the hematocrit should be made if the patient is symptomatic. Patients with advanced renal failure frequently have evidence of protein–calorie malnutrition, and thus, careful dietetic counseling is in order. Multivitamin and folic acid supplementation is routinely given to patients on dialysis, and such therapy should also be given to those whose creatinine clearance is less than 15 mL/min. There probably is no role for vitamin E in the treatment of these patients. The results of zinc therapy are encouraging (*24*). However, more extensive studies are necessary before zinc supplementation can be recommended. A careful review of all the patient's medications must be made, since a number of antihypertensive agents may have adverse effects on sexual function. Furthermore, the use of oral zinc (in patients with low zinc levels) in combination with dopamine (levo-dopa, 500 mg, p.o. 4x/d for 4–6 wk) seems to be promising, but remains investigational (Leyson, J.F., personal communications).

Since there is no correlation between the severity of sexual dysfunction and the magnitude of testosterone suppression in male patients, androgen therapy intended specifically to improve sexual function is not indicated unless the testosterone level is extremely low. Although no direct benefit has been demonstrated, estrogen therapy may be tried in selected female patients. The use of 1,25-$(OH)_2D_3$, clomiphene, and bromocriptine is still considered experimental. In some very carefully selected patients, implantation of a penile prosthesis has been of value (*8*). For patients on CAPD, placement of the peritoneal catheter on the lateral, rather than the anterior, abdominal wall might make face-to-face intercourse easier. With respect to coital positioning, the female on top and rear entry approach for males with penile prostheses is also advised. Finally, after identification and treatment of organic factors and evaluation of psychological factors, specific counseling may be in order. This employs the comprehensive treatment modalities of sex therapy and modifies them for use in patients who have limitations secondary to disability such as SCI and superimposed illness, such as ESRD (*2*).

Conclusions

Renal functional insufficiency, often progressing to end-stage renal disease, is frequent in SCI patients. Of the many complications associated

---

Ed. note: The use of chemorection (papaverine and prostaglandin E_1) has been effective in selected cases.

with advanced renal failure, disordered sexual and reproductive function are very prevalent, and do not appear to improve with dialytic therapy. The etiology of these abnormalities is complex, and includes psychological as well as multiple organic factors. The treatment approach must be individualized, and should take into consideration the diversity of etiologic possibilities and their interaction.

References

1. Abram, H. S., Hester, L. R., Sheridan, W. F., and Epstein, G. M. (1975) Sexual functioning in patients with chronic renal failure. *J. Nerv. Ment. Dis.* **160**, 220–226.

1a. Barton, C. H., Vaziri, N. D., Gordon, S., and Eltorai, I. (1984) Endocrine pathology in spinal cord injured patients on maintenance hemodialysis. *Paraplegia* **22**, 7–16.

2. Berkman, A. H. (1978) Sex counseling with hemodialysis patients. *Dial. Transpl.* **7**, 924–927.

3. Blumberg, A., Wildbolz, A., Descoeudres, C., Hennes, U., Dambacher, M. A., Fischer, J. A., and Weidmann, P. (1980) Influence of 1,25 dihydroxycholecalciferol on sexual dysfunction and related endocrine parameters in patients on maintenance hemodialysis. *Clin. Nephrol.* **13**, 208–214.

4. Bommer, J., Del Pozo, E., and Bommer, G. (1979) Improved sexual function in male haemodialysis patients on bromocriptine. *Lancet* **2**, 496–497.

5. Briefel, G. R., Tsitouras, P. D., Kowatch, M. A., Harman, S. M., and Blackman, M. R. (1982) Decreased *in vitro* testosterone production by isolated Leydig cells from uremic rats. *Endocrin.* **110**, 976–981.

6. Campese, V. M., Procci, W. R., Levitan, D., Romoff, M. S., Goldstein, D. A., and Massry, S. G. (1982) Autonomic nervous system dysfunction and impotence in uremia. *Am. J. Nephrol.* **2**, 140–143.

7. Campese, V. M., Romoff, M. S., Levitan, D., Lane, K., and Massry, S. G. (1981) Mechanisms of autonomic nerve dysfunction in uremia. *Kidney Int.* **20**, 246–253.

8. Carrion, H. M., Demos, J. S., and Politano, V. A. (1980) Impotence in chronic renal failure. *Dial. Transplant.* **9**, 357–358.

9. Distiller, L. A., Morley, J. E., Sagel, J., Pokroy, M., and Rabkin, R. (1975) Putuitary-gonadal function in chronic renal failure: the effect of luteinizing hormone-releasing hormone and the influence of dialysis. *Metabolism* **24**, 711–720.

10. Finkelstein, F. O., and Finkelstein, S. H. (1981) Evaluation of sexual dysfunction of the patient with renal failure. *Dial. Transplant.* **10**, 921–924.

11. Finkelstein, F. O. and Steele, T. E. (1978) Sexual dysfunction and chronic renal failure: A psychosocial study of 77 patients. *Dial. Transplant.* **7**, 877–878.

12. Galler, M., Spinowitz, B., Charytan, C., Kabadi, M., and Freeman, R. (1983) Reproductive function in dialysis patients: CAPD vs. hemodialysis. *Periton. Dial. Bull* **3** (Suppl.), S30–S32.
13. Hagen, C., Olgaard, K., McNeilly, A. S., and Fisher, R. (1976) Prolactin and the pituitary-gonadal axis in male uraemic patients on regular dialysis. *Acta. Endocrin.* **82**, 29–38.
14. Haldeman, S., Bradley, W. E., and Bhatia, N. (1982) Evoked responses from the pudendal nerve. *J. Urol.* **128**, 974–980.
15. Holdsworth, S., Atkins, M. B., and DeKrester, D. M. (1977) The pituitary-testicular axis in men with chronic renal failure. *N. Engl. J. Med.* **296**, 1245–1249.
16. Karacan, I., Dervent, A., Cunningham, G., Moore, C. A., Weinman, E. J., Cleveland, S. E., Salis, P. A., Williams, R. L., and Kopel, K. (1976) Assessment of nocturnal penile tumescence as an objective method for evaluating sexual functioning in ESRD patients. *Dial. Transplant.* **7**, 872–876.
17. Kreusser, W., Mader, H., Haag, W. D., and Ritz, E. (1982) Diminished response of ovarian cAMP to luteinizing hormone in experimental uremia. *Kidney Int.* **22**, 272–279.
18. Kreusser, W., Spiegelberg, U., and Ritz, E. (1979) Hypergonadotropic hypogonadism in renal failure—a defect responsive to 1,25$(OH)_2D_3$, in *Vitamin D. Basic Research and Its Clinical Application* (Norman, A. W., and Schaefer, eds.) pp. 763–765 (Walter de Gruyter, Berlin).
19. Krolner, B. (1979) Serum levels of testosterone and luteinizing hormone in patients with chronic renal failure. *Acta. Med. Scand.* **205**, 623–627.
20. Levy, N. B. (1973) Sexual adjustment to maintenance hemodialysis and renal transplantation: National survey by questionnaire: Preliminary report. *Trans. Amer. Soc. Artif. Int. Organs* **19**, 138–143.

20a. Lim, V. S. (1987) Reproductive function in patients with renal insufficiency. *Am. J. Kidney Dis.* **9**, 363–367.

21. Lim, V. S., and Fang, V. S. (1976) Restoration of plasma testosterone levels in uremic men with clomiphene citrate. *J. Clin. Endocrin. Metab.* **43**, 1370–1377.
22. Lim, V. S., Henriquez, C., Sievertsen, G., and Frohman, L. A. (1980) Ovarian function in chronic renal failure. Evidence suggesting hypothalamic anovulation. *Ann. Int. Med.* **93** (Part 1), 21–27.
23. Lim, V. S., Kathpalia, S. C., and Frohman, L. A. (1979) Hyperprolactinemia and impaired pituitary response to suppression and stimulation in chronic renal failure; reversal after transplanation. *J. Clin. Endocrin. Metab.* **48**, 101–107.
24. Mahajan, S. K., Abbasi, A. A., Prasad, A. S., Rabbani, P., Briggs, W. A., and McDonald, F. D. (1982) Effect of oral zinc therapy on gonadal function in hemodialysis patients: A double-blind study. *Ann. Int. Med.* **97**, 357–361.

25. Massry, S. G., Goldstein, D. A., Procci, W. R., and Kletzky, O. A. (1977) Impotence in patients with uremia: A possible role for parathyroid hormone. *Nephron* **19**, 305–310.

26. Morley, J. E., Distiller, L. A., Epstein, S., Katz, M., Gold, C., Sagel, J., Kaye, G., Pokroy, M., and Kalk, J. (1979) Menstrual disturbances in chronic renal failure. *Horm. Metab. Res.* **11**, 68–72.

27. Procci, W. R., Goldstein, D. A., Adelstein, J., and Massry, S. G. (1981) Sexual dysfunction in the male patient with uremia: A reappraisal. *Kidney Int.* **19**, 317–323.

28. Procci, W. R., Hoffman, K. I., and Chatterjee, S. N. (1978) Sexual functioning of renal transplant recipients. *J. Nerv. Ment. Dis.* **166**, 402–407.

29. Rager, K., Bundschu, H., and Gupta, D. (1975) The effect of HCG on testicular androgen production in adult men with chronic renal failure. *J. Reprod. Fert.* **42**, 113–120.

29a. Ramirez, G., Butcher, D. E., Newton, J. L., Brueggemeyer, C. D., Moon, J., and Gomez-Sanchez, C. (1985) Bromocriptine and the hypothalamic hypophyseal function in patients with chronic renal failure on chronic hemodialysis. *Am. J. Kidney Dis.* **6**, 111–118.

30. Stewart-Bently, M., Gans, D., and Horton, R. (1974) Regulation of gonadal function in uremia. *Metabolism* **23**, 1065–1072.

31. Swamy, A. P., Woolf, P. D., and Cestero, R. V. M. (1979) Hypothalamic-pituitary-ovarian axis in uremic women. *J. Lab. Clin. Med.* **93**, 1066–1072.

32. Winer, R. L., and Danviriyasup, K.: The pituitary-gonadal axis in end-stage renal disease associated with spinal cord injury. (Personal observations.) 1989.

30

Sexual Rehabilitation of Patients with Brain Damage and Spinal-Cord Injury

Sofjan Lamid

Introduction

It is well known that the sexual rehabilitation of patients with both brain damage and spinal-cord injury is more difficult and complex than that of patients with a spinal-cord injury alone. In this chapter, problems related to the sexual rehabilitation of SCI patients who have also suffered a closed head injury and/or anoxic encephalopathy are addressed. Evaluation of sexual function, counseling, and treatment for the brain injured have been neglected by most professionals (probably because of the lack of published data and clinical knowledge) in the rehabilitation setting. Thus, most multidisciplinary team members in rehabilitation trauma centers treat brain-injured patients as though they were asexual. An estimated 2.2 million new cases of traumatic head injury occur each year (*4*). Most occur in the 15–24-year-old age group, and these patients are badly in need of sexual counseling.

Why is the evaluation of sexual function and counseling for the brain-injured patient difficult or unique? Several factors make sexual counseling difficult (*5*):

1. Physical limitation such as spasticity, loss of proprioceptive sensation, impaired balance, speech disorder, and visual field

Sexual Rehabilitation of the Spinal-Cord-Injured Patient
Edited by J.F. Leyson, © 1990 The Humana Press, Inc.

deficit may cause problems in the sexual rehabilitation of patients with brain damage
2. The most limiting factor for sexual counseling in these patients is assumed to be impaired cognitive function, such as memory loss (*9*)
3. Other sequelae of brain damage, for example, agitation and hostilities, may add to the complexities inherent in sexual rehabilitation (*10*).

Sexual Function and Brain Damage

It can safely be assumed that psychogenic erection is mediated through the brain, and is initiated by visual, olfactory, auditory, and tactile stimulations. These sensory inputs are considered to be coordinated by the limbic system. The descending pathways from the central (brain) to the peripheral (thoracolumbar and sacral segments) centers are the lateral columns of the spinal cord. The anterior cingulate gyri and septal area are considered important for sexual behavior. Furthermore, Heath (*3*) has demonstrated that the septal nuclei are responsible for cerebral sexual stimulation without any form of external reinforcement. In addition, electrical stimulation of the lateral medial hypothalamus, inferior thalamic peduncle, and even the putamen have been shown to elicit erections (*8*). Strub and Black (*7*) have also shown that the more lateral regions of the limbic system are responsible for the nonvoluntary inhibition of sexual behavior. Any trauma or damage to the above cerebral structures can greatly modify libido, and secondarily impair the patient's ability to initiate penile/clitoral tumescence and orgasm. Changes in mental (psychosexual) perception (frontal lobe lesions) may alter vaginal proprioception with decreased lubrication and possibly other male/female sexual responses.

Examination of Patients with Brain Injury

A patient with a closed-head injury or anoxic encephalopathy is usually admitted to a trauma center or community hospital, where physicians and other health professionals make every effort to save his/her life. Many of the survivors have a physical and mental disability. When the patient's condition is medically stable, he/she will be transferred to the rehabilitation ward for further care. The patient will be seen by multidisciplinary team members of the rehabilitation facility. A complete physical examination is given, and includes neurologic and visual field examinations to determine the severity of the patient's disability. He/she will be seen by a speech pathologist for speech and language evaluation, a psychologist for neuropsychologic testing, and by other members of the rehabilitation team, such as a physical/sex therapist, social worker, vocational rehabilitation counselor, and an educational therapist.

Evaluation of Sexual Dysfunction in the Brain Injured

A history of pre- and postinjury sexual activities and marital status should be obtained from the patient or his/her spouse, and the patient medical record reviewed for concurrent medications, such as antihypertensives, tranquilizers, and so forth, that may affect sexual activity. The patient's sexual partner should then be interviewed for his/her willingness to participate in the treatment program for sexual dysfunction in the brain-injured patient. If the spouse refuses to take part in the program or does not care about it, sexual counseling will be of no value, especially for the patient with memory or other cognitive function impairment. Planning for the patient's discharge is also important. If he/she is going to be discharged to another institution, such as a nursing home, some counseling will probably be needed to avoid embarrassing sexual overtones or situations.

Before therapy is undertaken, the patient should be given a complete physical examination that includes neurologic, mental, visual field, and speech evaluations. Male patients should undergo urogenital evaluations, in which the external genitalia are examined and the presence or absence of psychogenic and reflexogenic erections is determined. Our sexologic workup also includes a nocturnal penile tumescence and rigidity monitor, papaverine penile injection (chemoerection) testing and other necessary diagnostic evaluations as stated in the chapter on "Diagnoses of Erectile Dysfunctions." In addition, the patient's ability to ejaculate is tested and semen from young patients is analyzed. Review of medications is advised.

With our limited experience with sexual evaluations of brain-injured women, we check for pelvic pathology, determine the level of erotic or basal sensation, record intravaginal temperature, and evaluate pelvic muscle tone and the bulbocavernosus reflex. Occasionally, we use somatosensory evoked potentials to delineate the true sensory level and identify "new" erotic zones in both men and women.

Sequelae of Brain Injury and Its Treatment

The permanent after-effects of brain damage include

1. Memory difficulty (especially the inability to recall recent events)
2. Language problems and hemionopsia
3. Weak extremities and/or impaired balance (loss of sensation)
4. Impaired self-care
5. Agitation/lability (uncontrollable crying or laughing).

These problems (*6*) and their treatment are listed in Table 1. The problems are evaluated and treated by professionals in the rehabilitation setting. On the other hand, sexual dysfunction and sexual counseling for the brain-injured patient have never been mentioned, and are given only limited professional attention and/or investigation.

Therapeutic Approach

Before the treatment program for sexual dysfunction is started in the brain-injured patient, goals and objectives are set for sexual counseling. These goals include

1. The development of new sexual skills and communication techniques
2. Sexual satisfaction for the patient's partner
3. Improving the quality of life for the patient and his/her spouse.

Whether sexual counseling will preserve the patient's marriage is problematical.

The therapeutic approach to sexual dysfunction depends on the type and severity of the patient's disability. If the brain-injured patient has weak extremities or balance is impaired, he/she and his/her spouse should change positions during intercourse. The usual man-on-top (missionary) position should be reversed to man-beneath or vice versa.

In patients with aphasia, a new treatment modality has been developed. This is a drug therapy based on the hypothesis that impaired spontaneous initiation of speech in aphasia may sometimes arise from reduced dopaminergic activity. Albert has advised the use of bromocriptine, a dopamine agonist in gradual increasing doses from 15 mg/d to a total of 30 mg/d for up to 4–6 wk (*13*). Leyson's clinical experience with Levo Dopa (L-Dopa) medications orally at 1.5–2 g/d in this type of patient showed significant results for 6 wk (*14*). Other nonmedical

Table 1
Aftereffects of Brain Injury and Their Treatment

Aftereffect	Treatment
Loss of recent memory	Memory retraining
Dysarthria/aphasia	Speech therapy and using nonverbal cues (oral bromocriptine)
Impaired balance	Frenkel's (coordination) exercises
Weakness of extremities	Progressive resistive exercises
Impaired self-care	Training in activities of daily living
Visual field impairment	Retraining with external visual stimulation
Impaired orgasmic response	Dopamine precursor (L-dopa)
Sexual dysfunction	Sexual counseling/therapy Readjust or change meds
Loss of sensation	Use sensate focus exercise Sensory re-orientation
Bowel and bladder incontinence	Empty bowel and bladder
Shortened attention span	Quiet and uncluttered environment will reduce distractions
Hesitancy	Partner needs cue, reassurance, and provide encouragement and feedback
Impulsiveness	Simple instructions, praise and feedback to facilitate sequencing of the sexual and other activities
Lability	Explain to partner that the uncontrollable crying and laughing is not caused by the interactions, but by the stroke itself
Fear of another stroke or heart attack	Reassure couple that an unhurried sexual activity will be less likely to cause another stroke or be harmful to the patient

therapy includes speech therapy, and the use of nonverbal cues or "body language" for sexual communication with patients having speech problems. Impaired cognitive function, such as memory deficit, is a difficult problem in sexual counseling for the brain-injured individual. Memory retraining could be tried, but the patient's spouse must participate if this is to be successful. Impaired spatial orientation may be corrected by reeducating patients to change positions with their partners during coitus, and to use proper lubrication. Psychological and psychiatric screening is important before sexual counseling begins in order to rule out inherent organic problems. A trial of psychotherapy followed by sex therapy is often advisable.

Sex counseling consists of open discussions between staff members and patients (group sessions and private meetings with patient and spouse). Booklets, pamphlets, and audiovisual tapes are provided for the sexual reeducation of patient and spouse. Advise the couple to keep distractions to a minimum and not to take warm or cold showers. Encourage them to be sexually active when rested, calm and unhurried.

Other Problems in Sexual Reeducation

Spasticity and pain are problems encountered in the sexual rehabilitation of the brain-injured patient. A waterbed can precipitate spasticity, as well as motion sickness in some quadriplegics, though these problems are treatable. Other alternatives, such as anal or manual sex, using dildoes or vibrators, erection aid rings, and stuffing techniques, are advised for some patients with insufficient reflexogenic or stimulative erections (*2*). For the younger patient whose memory is less impaired and who does not have satisfactory penile rigidity with functional manual dexterity, chemoerection (via intrapenile 30 mg papaverine injection) twice a week may be worth trying. However, if oral Levo Dopa or chemoerection therapy fails, a solid penile prosthesis is suggested. For women, alternative techniques for sexually stimulating the erogenous zones should be tried. Dosages of antiepileptic drugs must be adjusted to prevent drowsiness and undue muscle weakness, and the sexual partners of patients with temporal lobe epilepsy should be cautioned about possible hyposexual attitudes associated with aggressiveness and hypophagia (*9*).

During the past two years, the author has seen three patients who had sustained both brain damage and spinal-cord injury for sexual counseling. The following case report describes our treatment of one of these patients. Mr. W., a 56-year-old white paraplegic T4 male with postanoxic encephalopathy secondary to an explosion in which a piece of farm equipment landed on his head, back, and chest was transferred to the trauma center at our hospital for further care and rehabilitation. The patient and his wife requested sexual counseling. They had been married for 25 years and had enjoyed a good sex life.

Physical examination revealed that the patient's lower extremities were paralyzed. He had a complete loss of motor and sensory function, as well as of bowel and bladder function. He needed an indwelling Foley catheter for urinary drainage. The patient had reflexogenic, but no psychogenic, penile erections. He did not have a language problem, but did have impaired cognitive function, both recent and remote memory deficits. In addition to sexual counseling for SCI (*11*), our therapeutic approach was designed to improve memory by retraining and by using cues and signals before pleasuring and sexual intercourse. The participation of the patient's wife made sexual counseling successful.

Sexual Rehabilitation of Poststroke and Patients with Other Brain Lesions

Approximately 2 million poststroke patients survive with residual hemiplegia, hemianesthesia, homonymous hemianopia, and aphasia. A recent report in the literature revealed that male stroke survivors experienced a decreased erectile and ejaculatory ability (*12*). In contrast, menstruation and orgasm were decreased in poststroke premenopausal women (*1*). Retrospective studies have shown that the sexual desires of stroke patients did not diminish (*1*). These patients require a complete workup, which includes an evaluation of sexual function, a pre- and poststroke sexual and medical history review, and a urologic, as well as urosexologic examination.

Rehabilitation in patients with chronic organic brain syndrome of a different etiology should be directed toward restoring cognitive functions and other basic abilities necessary for physiosociologic interactions. As with the brain-injured patient, the treatment of sexual dysfunction in poststroke patients and in patients with other brain lesions depends on the type and severity of the disability. In addition, several other factors, including the patient's age, must be considered. Most survivors of strokes are more than 60 yr old, and their decreased sexual activity arises in part from the accompanying physiologic and psychosocial adjustments. Elderly SCI patients with organic brain syndrome (i.e., postoperative communicating hydrocephalus) have also been counseled, and there is at least one instance in which a patient's wife has elected nonsexual intercourse.

The National Head Injury Foundation estimates that about 10% of those who suffer cerebral trauma each year will have severe brain damage. In order to mitigate brain trauma, a group of Upjohn Company scientists have announced the synthesis of "lazaroids," a class of steroid derivatives that has been found to be experimentally effective in preventing secondary brain damage in mice. These compounds, 21-amino steroids, have been shown to inhibit further secondary brain trauma presumably caused by lipid peroxidation in both in vitro and in vivo studies. It is believed that this drug is 1000-fold more effacacious than methylprednisone, which is now routinely used to reduce cerebral edema. It is hoped that by the year 2000 these "lazaroids" could be administered at the scene of an accident or in the emergency room to mitigate the effects of brain injury or prevent the progression of stroke (*15*).

Conclusions

With our increasing awareness, openness, and expectations for the sexual rehabilitation of SCI patients, efforts must be increased to identify sexual dysfunction and provide sex counseling for the brain-injured patient. Sexual rehabilitation programs should be provided to selected patients and those who have slight or no cognitive functional impairment. In addition, sexual counseling should be regularly included in patient discharge plans. Those patients who will be going to nursing homes need predischarge nursing home sexual orientation/counseling to forestall future sexual embarrassments with staff or other residents. For SCI patients with brain damage, a combination of innovative therapeutic approaches with cerebral/motor-sensory amplification for the management of sexual dysfunction should be regularly included in every patient's treatment program.

References

1. Bray, G. P., Defrank, R. S., and Wolfe, T. R. (1981) Sexual functioning in stroke survivors. *Arch. Phys. Med. Rehabil.* **62**, 286–288.
2. Comfort, A. (1978) *Sexual Consequences of Disability* (Strickley, Philadelphia).
3. Heath, R. G. (1975) Brain function and behavior: I. Emotion and sensory phenomena in psychiatric patients and in experimental animals. *J. Nerv. Ment. Dis.* **160**, 159–168.
4. Kalsbeek, W. D., McLaurin, R. L., Harris, B. S. H., and Miller, J. D. (1980) The national head and spinal cord injury survey. Major findings. *J. Neurosurg.* **53**, 319–531.
5. Lamid, S. and Mantione, M. (1981) Sexual dysfunction in the brain injured. Tristate Scientific Rehabilitation Conference, North Chicago.
6. Lynch, W. J. and Mauss, N. K. (1981) Brain injury rehabilitation, standard problem list. *Arch. Phys. Med. Rehab.* **60**, 223–227.

7. Strub, R. L. and Black, W. F. (1981) *Organic Brain Syndrome*, p. 17 (Davis, Philadelphia).
8. Robinson, B. W. and Mishkin, M. (1968). Penile erection evoked from forebrain structures in macaca mulatta. *Arch. Neurol.* **19**, 184–190.
9. Berrol, S. (1981) Issues of sexuality in the head injured adults, in *Sexuality and Physical Disability* Bullard, D. G. and Knight, S. E., eds. pp. 203-207.
10. Lamid, S. (1984) Sexual rehabilitation in the brain injured patient. *Arch. Phys. Med. Rehab.* **65**, 657.
11. Lamid, S. (1986) Nocturnal penile tumescence studies in spinal cord injury males. *Paraplegia* **24**, 26–31.
12. Monga, T. N., Lawson, J. S., and Inglis, J. (1986) Sexual dysfunction in stroke patients. *Arch. Phys. Med. Rehab.* **67**, 19–22.
13. Albert, M. L. (1988) Aphasia is now treatable. *Hospital Practice* **23**, 31–38.
14. Leyson, J. F. (1988) *Sex Odyssey 2001*. Presented at the Annual Meeting, Assoc. of Philippine Physicians in America. Anaheim, CA. July 26–31.
15. Denler, J. and Ehrlich, J. P. (1988) Mitigate brain trauma? *Medical Tribune* **29**, 1, 6.

31

Sexual Functions in Respirator-Dependent Quadriplegics

W. H. Verduyn

Introduction

The most severely spinal injured person is the respiratory-dependent quadriplegic. This person has sensation only on the face and part of the scalp in C2, and an area of the neck in C3. Motor function allows only head movement. The high quadriplegic is totally dependent on other people for care, which includes: (a) respirator care—suctioning, tracheal care changes, respirator management, pacemaker antenna, transmitter and battery care; (b) daily living activities—dressing, bathing, brushing teeth, shaving, combing hair, eating, and taking medications; (c) personal care—bowel and bladder care, skin care, turning, getting up, getting back to bed. Once the patient is in the sophisticated electric recline sip'n puff wheelchair, he/she can move about independently and do his/her own weight shifts. With a mouth-stick, he/she can operate various electronic equipment, including a telephone, electric typewriter, computer, environmental controls, and others.

The general comments on sexual functions of SCI people are described well in many publications and would be very similar in the high quadriplegic (*1,9*). However, this chapter deals with recent research findings on the sexuality of patients with machine/pacemaker-assisted breathing.

Sexual Rehabilitation of the Spinal-Cord-Injured Patient
Edited by J.F. Leyson, © 1990 The Humana Press, Inc.

Sexual Function

The majority of spinal reflexes return after spinal shock. Sexual responses will occur on stimulation: manually, orally, vaginally, or mechanically (vibrator). In spinal-cord-injured males, stimulation will create a reflexogenic erection, which may be maintained as long as stimulation continues. In spinal-cord injured women (with sacral sparing), sexual stimulation, either manually, orally, intravaginally, or mechanically (vibrator), will result in responses close to those of able-bodied females: there will occur some lubrication, partial engorgement, and reflexogenic erection of clitoris.

Orgasm can cause autonomic dysreflexia (hyperreflexia) in any spinal-cord-injured person above the level of T6. This syndrome consists of severe pounding headaches, hypertension, and bradycardia. In addition, there are signs of sweating above the level of neurologic loss, flushing in the same area, and goose bumps below the level of neurologic loss. Hyperreflexia is usually precipitated by a full bladder and bowel (often severe constipation), or possibly any infection, irritation, fracture, kidney stone, decubitus ulcer, and so on. It is a well-known response to orgasm, and will occur during contractions in childbirth. This author recently reviewed pregnancy and delivery in spinal-cord-injured women, and found that 12 of 13 women who delivered vaginally and whose neurologic level was above T6 experienced hyperreflexia. The severest complication of hyperreflexia may be acute cerebral bleeding and death. Convulsions have also been reported during such acute episodes.

It is essential that the high quadriplegic and his or her partner become familiar with the syndrome of hyperreflexia and its treatment, so that they will be prepared to deal with it if it occurs. It must be stressed that, because of their high cord injuries, the compensatory systems of such patients are few and labile. Emergency treatment of hyperreflexia consists of correcting the precipitating causes, such as a full bladder/bowel, a blocked Foley catheter, infections in or a plugged tracheostomy tube, and a malfunctioning respiratory/pacemaker. Therapy should be directed to the specific causes and to their prevention. Immediate emergency treatment needs to be started, checking bladder and catheter drainage, putting the patient in the upright position, and checking for injury (skin, bone, and so on). The following drugs are helpful: our first choice is Nifedipine, amyl nitrate, and others include Nitrobid Ointment, anticholinergics, and for the unresponsive, intravenous antihypertensives (alpha-adrenergic blockers and spinal anesthesia).

Some quadriplegic males have orgasms but do not ejaculate, whereas others do so occasionally. A majority of quadriplegic women have "mental" orgasms, but lubrication may sometimes be impaired. In order to delineate the true and salvageable sexual response of these patients, a battery of diagnostic tests should be done (as discussed in the preceding chapter) and the patient interview should be systematic.

Patient Review

With this basic background information, several respiratory-dependent quadriplegics (on respirator or phrenic pacers) and their partners were interviewed. Important areas of management were discussed:

1. *Bladder Management.* Several individuals had suprapubic catheters. One used a condom catheter. Although there were no respirator-dependent quadriplegic women in this group, we do find that many spinal-cord injured women prefer a suprapubic catheter to an indwelling catheter, especially when sexual relationships are important.

2. *Respiratory Management.* Several individuals were on respirators utilizing a metal tracheal tube that gave them the ability to speak. There were also individuals who were on permanent pacers; one patient no longer had a tracheal tube. Time since injury varied from 8 mo to 6½ yr.

Frequency of Sexual Relationships

Frequency was very different for different couples, but would vary from once every 2–3 wk to twice a wk. Time spent together generally varied from 1 to perhaps 2 h/session. Intercourse was usually initiated after the spinal-cord-injured person was placed in bed in the evening, or still in bed in the morning. It was stated that this reduced the need for extensive preparations, such as undressing and bathing, since these were already taken care of. Erections, orgasm, and occasionally ejaculations were reported. Ejaculation was reported by one individual who had significant sensory sparing, especially in the rectal, penile, and scrotal area. None of the couples reported the use of vibrators. One couple developed an orally held dildo by folding soft rubber tubing, which the paralyzed male partner held between his teeth.

During discussion of oral sex, it was brought out by one of the women that, because of discomfort with oral sex preinjury, it can be very difficult in the sexual relationship postinjury. Erections were reported on direct stimulation, as was expected. Some maintained erections as long as needed, in others, loss of erection was a problem. The individual with significant sensory sparing also reported ejaculations at times.

The spinal-cord-injury individuals reported sexually sensitive areas of the face, neck, and ears, but also reported the importance of seeing the touching of their bodies by the able-bodied partners. Being able to touch their able-bodied partner with their mouth and face is an important means of contact for spinal-cord-injured individuals. Partners need to communicate with each other about what areas to touch and how to position so they can touch. All able-bodied partners mentioned the loss of embrace as a very important deprivation, one that sharply decreases the sense of bonding.

Relationships

These personal/marital relationships varied from divorce to divorce with remarriage. (This latter individual expressed feelings of surprise about the development of a new relationship.) One relationship was still intact 6½ yr postinjury. It appears that this is not unusual compared to other people with spinal cord injuries (*7,10*).

In counseling couples, it is important to be nonjudgmental. It is often very difficult for the abled-bodied person to stay in the relationship. These difficulties are generally caused by the tremendous drain on all resources—not only the physical and emotional resources, but also the financial resources—i.e., the lack of time, the need for assistance, the inability to find the proper support system. Many relationships cannot be maintained under the added burden of a significant disability. We need to realize that, even in the relationship of two able-bodied people, separations often occur because of a lack of communication, support system, and so on. However, it is interesting, and encouraging, to note that even respirator-dependent quadriplegics continue to develop new relationships, including sexual relationships and marriage, after the paralysis has occurred.

Diaphragmatic (Phrenic Nerve) Pacemaker Patients and Their Sexuality*

The few surviving high (C4 above) quadriplegics are maintained by nonportable or small LP_6 respirators. The recent clinical applica-

*This section was written by J. F. J. Leyson.

tion of phrenic (diapharagmatic) nerve pacemakers in these patients has mobilized and freed them from trache connections and cumbersome mechanical ventilators (Fig. 1) (*3,6,*). During the early days of any respiratory rehabilitation, both the physician and patient are concerned with the basic necessities of living, including nutrition, skin care, and psychological status. Although most SCI health-care-team members are hesitant to discuss sexuality, and often consider these patients as asexual, our Sex Clinic Therapy Team (VA Medical Center, East Orange, NJ) usually initiates sex topics in a subtle way. This initiation therapy is usually done at least 2 wk before the first home pass. As previously discussed (if the patient is receptive), the first sexuality session consists of basic sex education and the implications of changes postinjury. The second session consists of offering sexual alternatives and counseling. We believe that the first session should be limited to the patient only, and be designed to make the patient feel comfortable with his/her "changed" sexuality and to give patients time to reevaluate their feelings before confronting the problem with the sexual partner. During the subsequent sessions, the wife or "significant other" person should be included. The third and followup sessions then consist of film/videotape (sexual options) showing surgical management of impotence and/or sexual surrogate therapy (*4*). Before sexual counseling or therapy is initiated, the sexual partner and all family members should be taught emergency lifesaving measures in case a respirator/pacemaker failure occurs.

There are approximately 250 patients alive today with phrenic nerve (PN) pacemakers. Of the five patients interviewed, it took them almost a year or more post-PN pacemaker implantation before they would experiment with sex, because of their fear of dying. Their sexual activity depended mostly upon their sexual value system. For instance, a 21-year-old black male would not engage in oral sex because he considered it disgusting and filthy. His desires were for sensual touching, pleasuring, and sometimes intercourse with reflexostimulative erection. Other patients have tried oral sex, but their sexual partners must first be cautioned not to block the mouth or the tracheostomy orifice directly. A "dildo-stick" or extra-long vibrator (erection equalizer) can be utilized as a modified or tongue-extensor stimulator for their sexual partners. The partners may hold the hands of the patients to touch their erotic parts as a form of a reciprocal embrace. Holistic massaging is also advised as an option. The full details of this sensual touching is elaborated elsewhere. In younger patients with absent or ineffective erections who desire penile–vaginal intercourse, implantation penile prostheses is advised. However, it is essential that preop pulmonary and cardiac stress

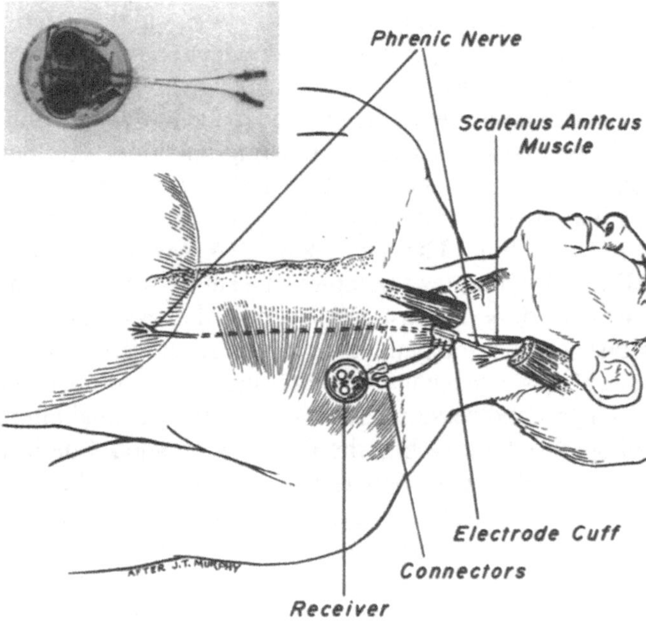

Fig. 1. Schematic diagram showing subcutaneously placed phrenic-nerve pacemaker components. The receiver (insert) is connected to the electrode cuff, which is wrapped around the phrenic nerve.

tests be done before such surgery is undertaken. Any patient who has poor cardiopulmonary stress tolerance and is beyond 55 years old is considered a poor surgical risk. Papaverine-induced intrapenile injection for impotence is not advisable because it can cause cardiac and hypertensive problems. Because of very limited motion, it is difficult to check for the presence of priapism in the patient; this may lead to the delayed implementation of therapy, which might in turn cause serious complications.

It is vital that both partners be encouraged to communicate their anxieties and sexual needs. All airways (nose, mouth, and tracheostomy) must be unobstructed during *sexual celebrations* (pleasuring, intercourse, and so on). All coital positions must be comfortable and energy-conserving. When the patient is supine, the sexual partner must not lie or apply pressure on the chest, that may compromise pulmonary and diaphragmatic functions, or dislodge (PN) pacemaker dermal antenna (Fig. 2). All medications that numb the sexual response must be adjusted accordingly. Pain treatment with transcutaneous nerve stimulation (TNS) must be used with caution, because it can aggravate sphincter-detrusor dyssynergia (*5*). Male patients with sphincters–detrusor (urethral

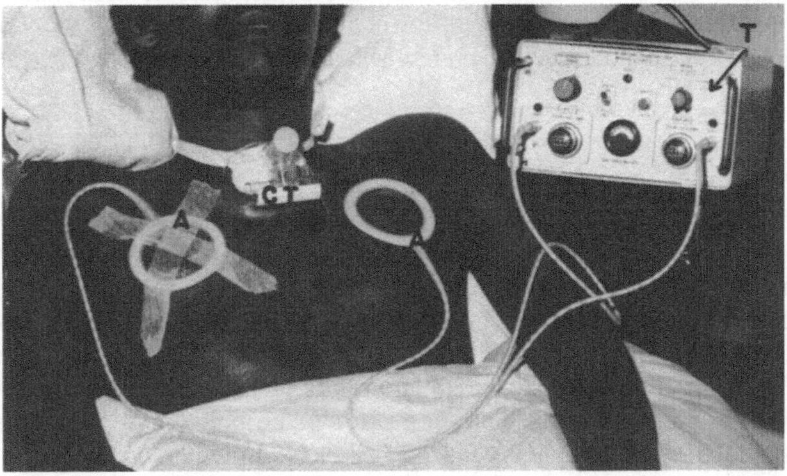

Fig. 2. Patient breathing with respiratory (PN) pacemaker. (A) Antenna, (CT), cuffed tracheostomy tube with phonation attachment and (T) external battery-powered transmitter.

sphincter–urinary bladder incoordinations) dyssynergia should be managed with surgical sphincterotomies, because PN pacing can precipitate urinary bladder dysfunction resulting in high residual urines and recurrent infections (*6*). It is also suggested that women who have poor urinary bladder rehabilitation (urinary drainage by Foley catheter) should have a suprapubic cystostomy or continent vesicostomy (for paraplegics-intermittent catheterization), because these urinary diversion/Foley drainage catheter cause ''awkward'' vaginal intercourse. However, a prototype of intraurethral tube draining may obviate the need for surgical urinary diversion or even Foley catheter drainage. (*4A*).

Fertility and Contraception Control*

Recent publications and personal communications indicate that vibrator stimulation will cause ejaculation and increase the sperm counts to appropriate levels even in SCI males (*2*). However, the use of electroejaculation should be tempered with caution, since prolonged and repeated use may cause aberrant electrical malfunction or interference (*5*). The spinal-cord-injured woman can become pregnant, and if pregnancy is not desired, proper birth control measures are needed (*8*).

*This section was written by W. H. Verduyn.

Our preference is the birth control pill, if there are no contraindications (tendency to or history of thrombophlebitis). Other types of conception control are discussed under the fertility and contraception chapter.

Conclusions

In preparing this chapter, it became obvious that no other publications on this topic were available. In our discussions with individual patients, we were impressed by confirmations of our feelings that sexual relationships remain very important to the severely handicapped person. We find that people will undertake considerable experimenting in order to have sexual relationships.

It is most important that the respirator/phrenic nerve pacemaker-dependent quadriplegic be approached as a whole person, one who is also a sexual being and who, in most cases, is either in a relationship or will in the future develop a relationship. Given that understanding, it is clear that sexual matters must be discussed with them. Practical advice should be given, particularly by encouraging SCI patients to practice their communication skills and to experiment creatively in their sexual relationships.

References

1. Cole, T. M. and Cole, S. S. (1982) *Krusen's Handbook of Physical Medicine and Rehabilitation.* 3rd ed., (W. B. Saunders, Philadelphia, PA), pp. 889–905.
2. Dahlberg, J. and Dahlberg, C. (1983) Personal communication.
3. D'Agostino, J. S. and Welch, P. L. (1979) The phrenic pacemaker. A promise of new breath and new life for respiratory patients. *Nursing '79*, **9**, 41–49.
4. Leyson, J. F. J. Sexual surrogate: A new sex therapy alternative. *J. of Multiple Sclerosis Quarterly*, 12–15 (1982).

4A. Leyson, J. F. J. (1988) Sex odyssey 2001, presented at the Asso. of Phil. Physicians in America Meeting, Long Beach, CA. July 26–31.

5. Leyson, J. F. J., Stefaniwsky, L., and Martin, P. F. (1979) Effects of transcutaneous nerve stimulation on the vesico-urethral function in spinal cord injury patients. *J. Urol.*, **121**, 635–639.
6. Leyson, J. F. J. (1982) Urodynamic profiles of spinal cord injured patients with phrenic nerve pacemakers. *Phil. Am. Med. Bulletin*, **10**, 5–9.
7. Heslinga, K., (1974) Not Made of Stone, (C. C. Thomas, Springfield, IL).

8. McClure, S. Contraception and the Spinal Injured Woman, Paper presented at Sexuality and Physical Disabilities: Medical Aspects and Clinical Care Seminar (University of Michigan Medical Center), November 1980.
9. Sha'ked Ami (1981) Human Sexuality and Rehabilitation Medicine (Williams and Wilkins, Baltimore, MD).
10. Trieschman, R. (1980) Spinal Injuries (Pergamon).

The discussion regarding obstructive sleep apnea (OSA) and Sexuality is discussed in Appendix D.

32

Sexual Surrogation for the SCI Patient

A New Sex Therapy Alternative

Jose Florante J. Leyson

> And Abraham took Hagar his wife's handmaid to bear for him a child, for Sarah his wife is barren (Genesis 16:1–6).

Introduction

Since time immemorial, substitution or surrogation for someone (something) has been acceptable (depending on the individual's and/or society's moral and sexual value systems) as long as the ultimate goal is achieved. The 20th century heralded the women's liberation movement, and in today's atmosphere of troubled unions and divorces, people seem to be more reluctant to settle down into marriage, or to establish permanent socioemotional relationships and commitments (*3*). At the advent of the 21st century, there are many "significant other" persons, mistresses, and prostitutes serving as part-time "wives," lovers, and/or sexual partners.

Sexual dysfunction can be treated medically, surgically, and/or by sex therapy techniques. In the early 1960s, Masters and Johnson advocated both single and couple sex therapy. It has also been proven clinically that sex therapy is more effective when instituted with a spouse or a romantically involved sexual partner. However, those who have no significant other as a therapy partner posed a therapeutic problem. Thus, in late 1960, Masters and Johnson introduced and trained sexual surrogate therapists for those able-bodied singles (unaccompanied adults)

Sexual Rehabilitation of the Spinal-Cord-Injured Patient
Edited by J.F. Leyson, © 1990 The Humana Press, Inc.

with psychogenic sexual dysfunction (*7*). Since maternal surrogates are beginning to be accepted both medically and sociolegally, training centers for sexual surrogates have mushroomed in most major cities, especially those in California and New York (i.e., Center for Sensory Learning, Tarzana, CA). The field of sexual surrogate therapy (especially for disabled persons) is still evolving, and no state has as yet set up licensing standard guidelines. Thus, in early 1970, the International Professional Surrogates Association (IPSA) was established. This organization, consisting of 30 original members, has the only authority to set up appropriate ethical standards for the training and evaluation of qualified surrogates. According to the IPSA, a sexual surrogate is a member of the three-way therapeutic team (supervising sex therapist, client, and surrogate) who acts as partner to a dysfunctional client in the sex therapy program. Sex surrogates participate in experiential exercises, involving sensual and sexual touching, as well as social and sexual skills training. A sex surrogate is a substitute for social and sensual–sexual training skills to reverse psychological sexual dysfunction, and enhance the pleasure of sexuality and enjoyment in patients with organic sexual problems. They differ from prostitutes or call girls (pleasure technicians) because sexual surrogates have to undergo intensive "paramedical," psychosocial, and sexual–sensual skills training before being qualified to "treat" patients or help clients overcome their sexual dysfunction (*3,6*). Prostitutes are goal and genital-oriented (sex right away and prompt gratification). If the customer cannot have an erection, that person pays to go. "Our [prostitute's] time is limited." On the other hand, the sexual surrogate (sensual therapist or pleasure–sexuality consultant) takes time to communicate and relax (*6*). Sex is not the end point, and one of the therapist's goals is to let the client revive his/her self-image and be able to resume social–emotional intercourse. Most prostitutes are young, poorly educated, and suffer from psychological problems and immaturity. Though some people consider prostitutes more beautiful than the sex surrogates, the latter are more educated, have some established relationships, are mature, and possess self-respect. Thus, the surrogates' ages range from 28 to 50 years.

Therapeutic sex sessions usually start with an initial meeting of the therapeutic team (supervising therapist, client, and sex surrogate) to establish and delineate goals. The goals cover such areas as self-image revival, allaying social fears of failure, reestablishing pleasure sensations, and reinforcing sexual–social skills. The progress of sex therapy is periodically reviewed by a certified sex therapist or sexologist. The therapeutic meeting may consist of 3–10 sessions for able-bodied and 15–20 sessions for disabled clients, depending on the severity of sexual dysfunction and the goals set (*3*). Each session usually lasts for approximately 2 h (*6*). A maximum of 2 h is set because the sessions tire the sex surrogate, who gives a great deal to the client both physically and psychologically. Ethically, sexual surrogates must not become involved with their clients either emotionally or romantically. Sometimes the sex therapy sessions may entail daily sessions for 1–2 w. This therapy may be required once or twice a week or from 1–6 mo, depending on the goals.

Therapeutic Process with Sex Surrogates in the United States

Initial or First Session

Architectural barriers must be removed to provide easy physical accessibility to the surrogate's therapy room. Intercurrent psychological and medical problems must be reviewed and treatment reevaluated before therapy. This initial meeting is geared toward relaxing the patient (client) and making him/her more comfortable. A brief paramedical–sexual history is taken, including medications and recent operations, or significant medical problems. This time may also be used to help clients get in touch with their own feelings. Clients are encouraged to ventilate their doubts, inhibitions, and fears through analytic (talk) therapy. This process may be coupled with behavioral (touch) therapy, and a simple, basic explanation of sexual anatomy and functions may be introduced. Sometimes practical pointers are given on "how to" attract the opposite or same sex and avoid embarrassing moments. Techniques designed to improve self-image (bring out the inner beauty) and to provide reassurance are also taught. Autonomic hyperreflexia is reviewed (especially by surrogates with advanced training).

Touching therapy is introduced and is more elaborate for the physically handicapped whose sensory perception is erratic. Tactile sensations may sometimes be felt as pains or lightning shocks, and sometimes as tingling or erotic sensations. Holistic or sensual massaging techniques, feathering, and bathing usually produce a soothing feeling, and help reinforce the surrogate–client relationship. To avoid embarrassing accidents, urinary and bowel care is again reviewed. If possible, such care should be done before each session. However, sometimes the surrogate has to double-check urinary bladder and bowel status (*3*). Recurrent loss of sex drive is explored. If the surrogate is a certified physical therapist, an extra charge may be imposed for additional therapy to build good muscle-anatomy contour, strength, and sometimes control. Most first and second sessions with surrogates are held with both parties clothed. The patient should be cautioned that this therapeutic approach proceeds at a measured pace to avoid unanticipated difficulties and build confidence in the patient (*6*).

Second Session

After physical cleansing and psychosocial resistances have been dealt with, sensual touching is advanced to sensate focus therapy. Body language and communication skills are reassessed and reinforced. Erogenous zones are identified in completely paralyzed patients and explored to trigger erotic sensations with the hope of precipitating such stimulations to para- or true orgasms (*4*). Lubrication and nongenital intercourse is allowed. Sometimes, oral sex is permitted with a client who has overcome most of the psychosocial barriers. Patients with skin pressure sores (lesions) may be dressed or taught personal hygiene. The use of perfume, atmosphere relaxation techniques, and the choice of beds (waterbeds may occasionally cause motion sickness and some quadriplegics may suffer muscle spasms) are also reviewed (*4*). Foley catheter care and removal are taught at the juncture. Depending on the sexual surrogate's training, therapy for ejaculatory problems is offered to SCI patients with incomplete lesions. Orientation to the artificial openings (osteotomies) and tubings (peritoneal dialysis) is done in preparation for the third and subsequent sessions. This technique will help ease the anxiety of both the patient and the surrogate, when genital and nongenital sex are later initiated. If intimate sexual contact or exposure to body fluids is anticipated, safe sex is advised to reduce the spread of AIDS (*8*). A female surrogate may try a female condom or vaginal-cervical sheath.

Third Session

Sexual intercourse or oral sex is usually introduced during this phase of therapy. Experimentation with sexual positions (with reference to contractures of extremities and painful joints) is initiated and tried. The use of body language and the wearing of erotic clothing are employed in concert with seductive communications and music. Some clients act as "peeping toms," while the surrogate pretends to change to an evening gown or takes an erotic bubble bath or shower. Reassurance during sexual and sensual stimulations is continued, even though penile erection or vaginal–clitoral anesthesia is absent or minimal. Physical and psychological sharing is also learned. Perianal or anal sexual stimulation/stroking is tried or initiated to facilitate penis–clitoral/vaginal sensuality (*3*). Homosexual eroticism and masturbatory training is reinforced in homosexual clients. Sexual aids are also introduced with sensory amplification. At this time, goals are assessed. If the client is comfortable and interacts confidently with the outside world, handles sexual frustration easily, achieves satisfactory erection and lubrication and/or orgasm(s)—psychosexual pleasures—then the therapy is considered a success and is terminated. Followup therapy sessions may be necessary for "problem" clients and for intercurrent social (psycho)—sexual inadequacies with the approval of the treating sexologist (*3*). The avoidance of intimate kissing, and the use of gloved hands, and condoms may minimize any significant risks of AIDS transmission. *It must be emphasized that all sex surrogate referral must be done through a certified sex therapist or sexologist (5)*. Surrogate sex therapy may be short-term, averaging about 15–20 sessions. Fees vary according to a surrogate's experience, qualifications, and economic status. They range from $85–$100/session of 1–2 h. Intensive daily therapy may cost up to $800–$1000 (total) in each case, including diagnostic tests.

Sex Surrogates in Europe and Other Countries

In most European countries, the medical community is now establishing formal organizations or referral centers for sexual surrogate therapy. Certified sexologists who are members of the World Congress of Sexology may be able to provide referrals. "Nonprofessional" sexual surrogation is usually provided by "educated" call girls, masseurs, and "classy" prostitutes. Though prostitution is legal in Holland and Japan, similiar services may be obtained from escort services or from sophisticated call (geisha) girls (*3*). In Tokyo, the Junior Health Club provides advanced sex-training school courses for newlyweds with special arrangements for the disabled. It has different "female instructors," and sex training–therapy is done (most often) with pants on and guidance provided by the club director. The total charge per session is about $350 (80,000 yen).

In the Philippines* sensual massage and "informal" sex surrogate therapy are provided by trained masseurs and "therapists." For shy patients, blind masseurs offer holistic massage. No sex is involved, and the charge is $10/h. Sensual therapists offer sensual therapy and massage

*This study was partly supported from a grant by the Philippine Association of Sexologists in America (PASA), Randolph, N.J.

or clinic (hot springs) at a total cost of $20–$35. "Educated" call girls provide sauna–sexual massage. Homo-heterosexual intercourse is also allowed. The average cost per person is $60 (1200 pesos). However, because of cultural prohibitions, oral sex is still not widely practiced, for it is considered dirty or religiously "unnatural."

Candidate Selection and Referrals

Prospective candidates must be screened by a sex therapist or counselor. Therapy should be tried in single (paraplegic) patients for at least 6 m before referral is made. In quads, early referral is done once the depression phase has mellowed. Because these patients have limited resources, including physical accessibility, house-call referral should be provided. Candidate selection should also include evaluation of economic status, personality, and marital situations. Patients with personality disorders should be dealt with accordingly. All intercurrent marital and medical problems should be treated or be under control before sex surrogate therapy is suggested. The spouses must be informed and involved regarding the therapy. Married patients should be given a 3–6-mo trial period prior to referral. If one of the spouses does not agree with sex therapy, it is the duty of the treating sex therapist to offer alternatives, or to suggest pastoral counseling.

For nationwide referrals, all inquires should be directed to: International Professional Surrogates Association (IPSA), PO Box 74156, Los Angeles, CA 90004, (213) 469-4720. Most major US cities have sex surrogates who are known to certified therapists (sexotherapists). For Philadelphia, Connecticut, New Youk, and New Jersey, sexual surrogates for both homo- and heterosexual disabled clientele can be contacted through A. R. Services, 782 W. End Avenue, Apt, -82, New York, NY 10025. House-call contracts are available within a 50-mile radius. SHARE (Sexuality Has a Right Everywhere), PO Box 188, Palisades Park, NJ 07650, provides house calls and weekend services up to a 100-mile radius (*3*).

Results and Implications

Personal interviews with 31 clients and six surrogates have shown that they (the clients) benefit a great deal by regaining their self-confidence, enhancing their self-images, and having fewer complaints about "paralyzing" pains (*2*). These clients grow much happier and easier to get along with, and become more cooperative in their medical and rehabilitation therapy programs. Two (single) patients have had their parents request sex surrogate referrals. Pulmonary compliance in a quadriplegic who was on a respirator improved after surrogate therapy, because the surrogate had incorporated breathing exercises as part of the treatment format. He was able to go home on a weekend using a portable respirator, and needed less pain medication.

The psychosocial impact of the above therapy is still not well documented. My interviews with 103 professionals and paraprofessionals (60 physical therapists, 25 nurses, 15 physicians of most specialties, and 3 technicians), most of them embrace the Judeo-Christian ethic, revealed that 68% considered sex surrogate therapy morally acceptable if medically indicated. Of the 68% affirmative responses, 42% were physical therapists and the remainder (26%) nurses and doctors. Most of the physicians and clinical psychologists interviewed by Malamuth et al. (5) would make referrals if its therapeutic status were to be clarified as legal. However, in 1975 Masters and Johnson advocated doing away with the services of surrogates, claiming that they undermined therapeutic relationships and goals. But it must be stresses that the above surrogate therapy was utilized for able-bodied patients. These patients (clients) have few intercurrent problems, for they do not have to overcome physical–architectural barriers, surmount recurrent urinary and bowel dysfunction, and even try to survive in the face of their own precarious cardiorespiratory function. With physical disabilities and their frequently accompanying economic disaster, the SCI patient needs all the resources and support he/she can get just to live in the presence of dwindling and friable psychological backup mechanisms. Therefore, any warm touch, tender caress, or whisper of hope may be enough to provide a ray of light in his/her dark and lonely world. A qualified and moral sexual surrogate may be able to provide companionship and comfort to these patients.

Contraindications for Surrogate Partner Sex Therapy

In Women, Homosexuals, and Transsexuals

1. The patient's moral and socioreligious conflicts constitute the primary contraindication. A majority of women, including lesbians, feel that having sexual contact with a male or another woman outside a romantic relationship is immoral or wrong.
2. Sex surrogate therapy is contraindicated in most women and especially in transsexuals with a history of childhood sexual abuse. This

previous sexual experience associated with violence and mutilation can trigger the re-experiencing of feelings of exploitation and powerlessness during the therapy sessions.

In Men

Adult Male Virgin Syndrome (AMVS). Men with AMVS who lack social skills have difficulty in generalizing their sexual competency with a surrogate to other relationships.

Both Men and Women

1. A majority of sex surrogates believe that the above sex therapy is inappropriate when the patient is married, although surrogate partners in California, Nevada, New Jersey, and New York areas do "treat" married patients/clients.
2. Psychological problems—Depressive Disorder patients suffering from major depression because of the lack of a relationship do not do well in the therapy sessions when compared to patients whose depression stems solely from loneliness and pure lack of sexual experiences.

The possible complications of this type of therapy may include: (a) emotional involvement of the patient, in which case therapeutic goals would be undermined, causing the patient to lose his/her independence; (b) exploitation and power manipulation by the surrogate, which would drain the patient economically and psychologically; (c) deception and misinformation from poorly trained and unqualified surrogates, which would give false reassurance that the therapy would provide a complete cure to the sexual dysfunctions; (d) ambivalent patient goals—the patient may not have the patience to work hard and may demand quick and unattainable solutions; (e) therapeutic abuse—the patient may regard this therapy as merely an easy way to have sex. Gross medical/health care mistakes can add more injury to the already compromised health (improper bowel care and traumatic catheterization can result in bleeding). The medicolegal drawback in sexual surrogation involves the surrogate's denial of a license by a medical or paramedical review board. In my interviews with sex qualified surrogates, I found that they still needed further instruction in the pathophysiology of the SCI and training in bowel and urinary bladder care, along with the identification and treatment of minor cardiopulmonary problems and autonomic dys (hyper) reflexia. IPSA members must be informed that the sole purpose of licensure by a medical review board is to make sure that appropriate medical supervision, instruction, and training are included in the training curriculum. I also believe that members of the review board must be either qualified surrogates or physicians certified by the American Board of Sexology or American Association of Sex Educators, Counselors and Therapists (AASECT). The legal status of surrogates is still undefined. Although no criminal charges have been filed against a surrogate (*3*), the most probable accusation by a client is prostitution. According to my research this possibility is very remote. I do hope that IPSA will be more receptive to the idea of state review board licensure.

Conclusions

The morality of using sexual surrogates in the sex therapy of SCI patients is still unsettled. However, it is my firm belief that the informed individual's (patient and therapist) conscience will decide whether this form of sex therapy is moral. If the patient cannot arrive at a decision as to whether to try such a therapeutic option, pastoral counseling is advised (*1*). This new sex therapy alternative for SCI patients seems to be logically and medically sound, but longterm evaluation is needed before a definite conclusion can be drawn.*

References

1. Kukura, J. (1983) Personal communications, New Jersey.
2. Leyson, J. F. (1980) The management of sexual (female) dysfunctions in multiple sclerosis. *M. S. Quarterly*. **Fall** 4–10.
3. Leyson, J. F. (1983) Sexual surrogate: A new form of sex therapy alternative. *M. S. Q. Journal* **Summer**, 3–7.
4. Leyson, J. F. and Powell, R. (1979) Counseling the female spinal cord injured patient. *Med. Aspects of Human Sexuality*. **16**, 59–61.
5. Malamuth, N., Wanderer, Z., Sayner, R., and Durrell, D. (1976) Utilization of surrogate partners: A survey of health professionals. *J. Behavior Therapy Experimental Psychiatry*. **7**, 149–150.
6. Jacobs, M., Thompson, L., and Truxaw, P. (1975) The use of sexual surrogates in counseling. *J. Counseling Psychologist*. **5**, 73–76.
7. Rodriquez, R. (1983) Sex surrogate confidential. *FORUM* **March**, 31-36.
8. *Private Practices: The Story of a Sex Surrogate*, CINEMAX Jan and Feb. 1988.

---

*Ed note: SCI sexual surrogation is still in its infancy and going through clinical trial. It is, therefore, prudent that a thorough patient and surrogate evaluation must be done. It is also advisable to do detailed record keeping.

33

Pharmacosexology

Sexual Side Effects of Medications and Other Drugs

Jose Florante J. Leyson
and
Robert T. Francoeur

Introduction

Until recently, few physicians and patients were aware that common medications can, and often do, adversely affect sexual responses. If the matter was discussed, the physician often had little if any specific information available. Before the 1980s, sexual dysfunctions of patients taking medications and recreational drugs were a minor concern for both the physician and the patient, because sex researchers/therapists reported that only 5–10% of all sexual dysfunctions were caused by organic or physical causes, whereas 90–95% were psychogenic in their origins. Today these same sex therapists have reevaluated their conclusions as a result of the recent rapid progress in sexology. It is now estimated that between 50–70% of all sexual dysfunctions have major organic or iatrogenic (i.e., drug-induced) etiologies. This new insight, coupled with growing awareness of the wide variety of potential adverse side effects associated with all medication, has raised many questions about the adverse sexual side effects of medications and drugs. The most common sexual side effects reported are reduced sexual desire in both men and women, erectile dysfunctions, and the inability to achieve orgasm in both sexes.

Sexual Rehabilitation of the Spinal-Cord-Injured Patient
Edited by J.F. Leyson, © 1990 The Humana Press, Inc.

General Pharmacophysiology and Therapeutic Options for SCI Patients

In 1983 there were approximately 175,000 SCI victims in the USA. With an annual incidence of 9000–10,000 new cases, the number has almost certainly reached 500,000 by the turn of the decade. The most common age of SCI injury is 19, but the average age for all cases is 28.7 yr (*1*). The etiology and age of each individual SCI may indicate the possible complications of posttrauma medication. SCI resulting from penetrating wound injuries are more common among individuals with premorbid personalities and among drug abusers. Alcohol as a drug has been implicated in the majority of automobile injuries, accounting for about 38% of SCI cases (*1*). In young patients, the use of recreational and illegal drugs may have sensitized their body systems, so that posttrauma drug interactions may be unpredictable. In the elderly, pre-injury illnesses and medications can decrease, enhance, or complicate drug effects.

During spinal shock, a majority of neurosurgeons administer corticosteroids to reduce posttraumatic edema of the spinal cord. Others believe than an alpha-adrenergic blocker (reserpine) will minimize the release of the cathecolamines and free radicals that are probably responsible for cord damage (*16*). The short-term use of therapeutic doses of steroids does not affect sexual functions. Reserpine, if administered locally or directly into the spinal cord, also produces no sexual dysfunction. However, if reserpine is used to treat chronic hypertension, reduced libido and erectile dysfunction can result.

In the elderly SCI population, cardiopulmonary complications usually accompany spinal-cord trauma. Cardiac medications, i.e., digoxin (Lanoxin), can decrease libido and even aggravate impotence in the presence of compromised systemic and penile vascular systems (*2*). Chronic use of propranolol (Inderal), with or without smoking,* may produce impotence (*17*). Inderal, an adrenergic $beta_1$- and $beta_2$-receptor blocker (antagonist), decreases brain norepinephrine levels and may reduce penile reflexes (*13*). Because the $beta_2$-adrenergic receptors are involved in erection, any $beta_2$ antagonist can cause impotence. Terbutaline sulfate (Brethine), a $beta_2$ agonist or stimulant used as a bronchodilator for respiratory problems, has been employed intravenously to elicit erection in laboratory animals (*4*). However, our experience has not shown any improvement of impotence when used in SCI patients.

*Ed note: Nicotine is a potent vasoconstrictor, so the patient should stop smoking.

Hypersecretion of gastric acid, GI dysmotility syndromes, and upper GI ulcers have been noted in the SCI population, most commonly among quadriplegics. Histamine (H_2) blockers are needed to treat this problem and avoid disastrous complications. Cimetidine (Tagamet) is an effective antihypersecretory H_2 blocker. However, if administered for more than 3 mo, it may produce some gynecomastia, impotence, and infertility problems (*7*). Ranitidine (Zantac) is a newer and more potent (H_2 blocker) "antacid" with fewer general and sexual side effects than Tagamet (*15*). Other options, i.e., Famotidine (Pepcid) may to be taken once or twice a day. It should be noted that any H_2 antagonist taken for an extended period of time can produce some sexual side effects. However, a once-a-day drug, Omeprazole (Losec)—a gastric acid pump inhibitor—seems to be an ideal choice for 4–8 wk therapy. This drug is indicated for GI reflux and gastric ulcer diseases. It must be stressed that no antisecretory drug is devoid of sexual and other side effects if used for more than 3 months. Elevated blood pressure in SCI persons can result from either preinjury hypertension or recurrent sympathetic crisis (autonomic hyperreflexia). Adjunctive treatment of such hypertension involves diuretics, and adrenergic and ganglionic blockers. All of these medications can precipitate sexual dysfunctions. Diuretics can cause erectile dysfunction, as demonstrated by reductions in the duration of nocturnal erections through NPT monitoring (*7*). The pathophysiology by which diuretics produce impotence is still unknown. However, anecdotal reports suggest that diuretics concentrate the circulating free testosterone by contracting the intravascular volume. Our clinical experience did not show any plasma testosterone level alterations. One of the hormonal renal functions is to modulate the plasma testosterone levels. Thus, diuretics may alter the homeostatic balance between free and protein-bound testosterone. Any antihypertensive that blocks the autonomic (adrenergic) nervous system and ganglionic neuronal transmission can cause sexual dysfunctions.

In order to avoid drug-induced sexual side effects, a reduction in dosage or a change in medication should be considered. For mild hypertension, biofeedback may be tried as an alternative treatment to medication, particularly with incomplete and recovering SCI patients. Other antihypertensive therapy options include the antiangiotensin, slow calcium channel blockers, metoprolol and minoxidil. Both are almost purely $beta_1$-adrenergic blockers. Of all the antihypertensive medications, guanethedine (Ismelin) has the highest incidence of sexual side effects, 20–30%, and the $alpha_1$-adrenergic antagonist prazosin (Minipress) the lowest rate, between 1 and 5% (*21*). Our clinical experience

Table 1
Detailed Female Sexopharmacology

Neurophysiology

Dopaminergic pathways facilitate, whereas serotinergic neurosystems inhibit, sexual activities in lower animals of the male species. However, in female animals, the effects of dopamine and serotonin are equivocal.

In humans, evidence regarding the effects of dopamine and serotonin are still controversial and equivocal according to several investigators. Leyson et al. has demonstrated indirectly that dopaminergic neuroreceptors facilitate orgasmic female sensory responses (*23*).

Drug Effects on Female Sexuality (*26,39*)

Drug	*Dose*	*Effects*
Atropine	0.35 mg/KG	None on arousal, lubrication, and orgasm
Methylatropine	0.5 mg	
Bethanechol	25 mg	None on lubrication/orgasm
Labetalol	100 mg (alpha/beta blocker)	Delayed orgasm
Midodrine	5 mg iv (alpha agonist)	No effect on time of orgasm
A. Inhibitory Effects—Antipsychotics (*2,18,36*)		
Thioridazine (Mellaril)	200–600 mg	Anorgasmic-delayed orgasm intensity
Trifluperazine (Stelazine)	15 mg	Delayed orgasm
Fluphenazine (Prolixin)	450 mg	Delayed orgasm
B. Inhibitory Effects—Monoamine Oxidase Inhibitors (*23,29*)		
Phenelzine (Nardil)	45–90 mg	Anorgasmia
Tranylcypropine (Parnate)	?	Anorgasmia
Isocarboxazid (Marplan)	20 mg	Anorgasmia
C. Inhibitory Effects—Antidepressants (*24,32,33,36*)		
Amoxapine (Asendin)	150 mg	Anorgasmia
Clomipramine (Anafranil)	50–100 mg	Anorgasmia delayed orgasm
Nortriptyline (Aventyl)	60 mg	Anorgasmia
Alprazolam (Xanax)	7 mg	Anorgasmia

Table 1 (Continued): Detailed Female Sexopharmacology

Medical Management in Reversing Inhibitory Effects of Antidepressants by:

1. Cyproheptadine (Periactin—antihistamine, serotonin inhibitor) 4 mg reverses nortriptyline induced anorgasmia
2. Amoxapine-induced anorgasmia counteracted by oral doses of 15–25 mg Bethanechol (cholinergic agent)
3. Amoxapine-induced anorgasmia relieved by switching to Imipramine
4. Imipramine-induced anorgasmia relieved by switching to Desipramine

Other Drugs Effects (*30,31,34,40*):

1. Propranol	↓ Libido
2. Cancer chemotherapy	↓ Libido
3. Carbonic anhydrase inhibitors	↓ Libido
4. Cimitidine (Tagamet)	↓ Libido
5. Heroin	↓ Libido
Methadone	Anorgasmia
6. Fenfluramine (Pondimin)	↓ Libido
7. Chronic alcoholism (Alcohol)	↓ Libido/delayed orgasm

Female Aphrodisiacs (*23,24,25,27*)

1. L-Dopa and Buspirone	↑ Libido
2. Nomifensine (Merital)	↑ Libido
3. Injection of Acetylcholine in septal region (female epileptic)	Euphoria; sexual arousal; multiple orgasm
4. Chlomipramine (Anafranil)	Spontaneous orgasm

shows that metoprolol (Lopressor) and minoxidil (Loniten) produce little or no sexual dysfunction. Caution is advised with Lopressor, however, because it can cause hypoglycemia in association with diabetes mellitus. (*See* Table 2.)

The drug management of sympathetic crisis (hyperreflexia) is twofold, involving local and systemic approaches. One local (application) emergency treatment of this life-threatening condition is amyl nitrate* or calcium channel blocker. In able-bodied persons, amyl nitrate reinforces psychic sexual arousal. However, our clinical data suggest that minimal arousal enhancement, or no erectile response, is produced by local penile and anterior chest wall applications in SCI persons. Phenoxybenzamine, an alpha$_2$-adrenergic antagonist, is beneficial in the systemic treatment of hyperreflexia and in internal urethral sphincter spasticity

*Ed note: Our initial clinical trial with a 1-inch patch of glyceryltrinitrate (adenylcyclase stimulator) only produced penile arterial dilatation, but did not lead to satisfactory erection.

Table 2
The Possible Sexual Side Effects of Common Medications and Drugs[a,b]

Generic Name	Major Brands	Possible Sexual Side Effects
	Nondiuretics	
Clonidine (alpha blocker)*	Catapres	L > possible; 4–70% ER; EJ none. Breast enlargement and/or tenderness, and gynecomastia; EJ and OD (CP)
Guanethidine	Ismelin	L > in F; 29% L > in M; 4–100% ER; 2–200% EJ Decreased emissions; bizarre erotic dreams; OD (CP)
Methyldopa	Aldomet	L > in F and in 7–14% M; 2–80% ER; 7–19% EJ. Breast enlargement and/or tenderness, gynecomastia, OD (CP)
Phenoxybenzamine	Dibenzyline	ER?; 4.5–100% EJ
Propranolol	Inderal	1–4% L >; ER up to 28%. L > in F (CP)
Reserpine	Serpasil Diupres	L > 7% in M (small study); L > in F; 11–33% ER; 14% EJ; bizarre erotic dreams. OD (CP)
Hydralazine	Apresoline	ER (CP)
Prazosin	Minipres	Up to 4% ER
Metoprolol	Lopressor	None reported
Minoxidil	Loniten	None reported
Atenonol	Tenormin	0.2% ER
Timonol	Blocadren	0.6% L > in M; ER occurs
Nadolol	Corgard	L > in M, ER and EJ occur
	Diuretics	
Thiazides		9–20% ER
Spironolactone	Aldactone	L > common 4–30% ER with high doses; amenorrhea. Breast enlargement and/or tenderness, gynecomastia, menstrual irregularities (CP)
Chlorthalidone	Hygroton	Some ER occurs
Hydrochlorothiazide	HydroDiuril	Some ER problems. CP reports inhibited vaginal lubrication with some diuretics
	Antispasmodic Medications	
Isopropamide	Darbid	All three antispasmodics are re-

*Ed note: Yohmibine (alpha$_2$ blocker) when taken orally at 5.4 mg 3–6 ×/d can result in up to 35% erection in SCI with incomplete lesions. It is contraindicated in renal failure.

Table 2 (Continued)
The Possible Sexual Side Effects of Common Medications and Drugs[a,b]

Generic Name	Major Brands	Possible Sexual Side Effects
Methantheline Propantheline	Banthine Pro-Banthine	ported to cause some erectile dysfunction by DDLL
	Antidepressant Medications	
Lithium carbonate		2 cases of L > and 2 of ER reported
	Tricyclics	
Amitriptyline Protriptylie Imipramine Desipramine	Elavil Vivactil Tofranil Norpramin	All tricyclics listed may increase or decrease libido; isolated cases of ER, delayed ejaculation, EJ and delayed orgasm in women. HSK reports probably no effect on libido
	MAO (Monoamine Oxidase) Inhibitors	
Tranylcypromine Phenelzine Isocarboazid	Parnate Nardil Marplan	MAO inhibitors may increase libido in M & F possibly by countering depression; delayed ejaculation, EJ, ER, delayed orgasm in F reported. HSK reports probably none
	Miscellaneous	
Trazodone	Desyrel	Causes priapism because of its adrenergic alpha blocking activity and local vasodilation
	Tranquilizers, Antipsychotics, Sedatives, and Hypnotics	
Chlorodiazepoxide Diazepam	Librium Valium	JB reports no adverse sexual side effects; DDLL report both L < and L > in M & F, EJ, decreased testosterone level, and amenorrhea
Oxazepam Meprobamate	Serax Equanil, Miltown	DDLL report both L < and L > in M & F, decrease testosterone levels, amenorrhea, and milky breast discharge
Thioridazine	Mellaril	L > occurs (only in high dose HSK); 54% ER; 30–57% EJ
Barbituates		L < or L >; ER common
Methaqualone	Quaalude	L < or L >; ER common; ejaculation delayed with high doses (HSK)
Ethyl alcohol		L < or L >; ER common; EJ occurs

(Continued)

Table 2 (Continued)
The Possible Sexual Side Effects of Common Medications and Drugs[a,b]

Generic Name	Major Brands	Possible Sexual Side Effects
	Amphetamines	
Clorphenteramine Dextroamphetamine Diethylpropion	Pre-Sate Benzedrine Tepanil	JB reports increase in libido, some ER and some EJ with amphetamines; DDLL suggest all these drugs may cause decreased libido, especially in women, and in impotence
	Hormones	
Progestins	Duphaston Gynorest Lutocylol Ovrette Nurlutin Progestasert	L > common in both males and females; EJ occurs; 24–70% ER; HSK reports: probably none.
Estrogens	Estrace Evex Dienestrol DES Estrovarin Estratab Menrium	L > and ER common in males; EJ occurs; L < or L > may occur in females
Androgens	Delatestryl Maxibolin Cyclomen Danocrine Winstrol	L < or L > in males; < or > in erections; in females may increase libido, halt menses, enlarge clitoris, cause hair growth
	Antiandrogens	
Corticosteroids		L > and ER common; EJ occurs; delays ejaculation—HSK. None reported? (short courses)
Thyroxine		L < —HSK
Spirolactone		Occasional L > and ER possible —HSK
Lutenizing hormone		L <; arousal increases
	Other Drugs and Chemicals	
Cimetidine	Tagamet	31 cases of L > and 31 of ER; Both L > and ER may be more common than documented
Aminocaproic acid	Amicar	24% EJ

Table 2 (Continued)
The Possible Sexual Side Effects of Common Medications and Drugs[a,b]

Generic Name	Major Brands	Possible Sexual Side Effects
	Other Drugs and Chemicals (Cont.)	
Disopyramide	Norpace	2 cases of ER
Clofibrate	Atromid-S	3% ER
Thiabendazole	Minietazol	9% ER
Ketamine	Ketoject	ER occurs
Disulfiram	Antabuse	10–12% ER; delayed ejaculation —HSK
Digoxin	Lanoxin	35% report L > and ER
Phencyclidine	PCP	L < or L >; ER and EJ occur
Cancer chemotherapeutics		L > and ER occur
Tryptophan		L > and ER—HSK
Marijuana		L < within 30 min; > thereafter; ER or arousal increase, impotence, abnormal menses/ infertility
Cocaine		L >
Methadone	Dolophine	6–38% L >; 6–50% ER; 5–88% EJ
Heroine		60% L >; 39% ER; 70% EJ
Volatile nitrites	Amyl nitrite	L < and arousal increase
Levodopa	L-dopa	L <; 2 cases of EJ (?)

[a]L = libido increase (<) or decrease (>); ER = male erectile dysfunction; EJ = male ejaculatory dysfunction; AD = arousal dysfunction (erection and vaginal lubrication); OD = female orgasmic dysfunction; M = males; F = females; < = an increase in response; > = a decreased response.

[b]Sources: JB = Buffum (*2*); DDLL = De Moya, Lewis, and Lewis (*3*); HSK = Kaplan (*6*); CP = Papadoupoulos (*17*).

(detrusor-sphincter incoordination or dyssynergia), as well as being a useful adjunct in hyperhidrosis (*10*). Oral administration of this drug can cause erectile and ejaculatory problems resulting from its inherent pharmacokinetics. On the other hand, two alpha-adrenergic stimulants, ephedrine sulfate and imipramine, are used to treat retrograde ejaculation and urinary incontinence resulting from internal urethral sphincter (urinary bladder neck) weakness. Ephedrine sulfate is purely a centrally acting sympathomimetic that is contraindicated in hypertension. It can produce impotence even in patients with recovering lesions (*8*). Imipramine (Tofranil), which is also used for depression, has both central and local urinary bladder neck sympathetic stimulant effects. Chronic use of this medication can cause delayed ejaculations and orgasms in both sexes.

Genitourinary complications account for 67.2% of morbidity in SCI patients. These problems usually involve an imbalanced urinary bladder with detrusor-urethral sphincters dyssynergia(s), resulting in high residual urine with or without vesico-urethral reflux (*11*). Pharmacological manipulations consist of administering three medications singly or in combination: bethanechol chloride (Duvoid; Urecholine) as a treatment for purely hypotonic urinary bladder (*19*), and dantrolene sodium (Dantrium) and baclofen (Lioresal) to relax external urethral sphincter spasticity (*11,18,19*) and for generalized unnecessary muscle spasms. Duvoid and Urecholine are parasympathetic agonists or stimulants that have "some benefits" (30% in 30 subjects) in the management of erection in non-SCI persons (*14*). However, our clinical observations reveal no change in the reflexogenic or erectile capacity in SCI persons. Dantrium probably prevents the uptake of calcium ions in the skeletal muscle sarcoplasmic reticulum, thus producing generalized muscle relaxation (*19*). Lioresal, on the other hand, acts at the spinal-cord level by blocking or suppressing neuroreceptor transmission in hyperactive neurons (*11*). Our clinical experiences with NPT and pelvic temperature monitoring reveals that both Dantrium (350 mg/d) and Lioresal (160 mg/d) have no influence on erectile-ejaculatory functions in males or on vaginal lubrication in females (*8*). Although the PDR lists impotence as one of the side effects of Lioresal in able-bodied patients, our observation and personal interviews with SCI patients have shown that this medication sometimes augments sexual arousal and enhances orgasmic response.

Diazepam (Valium) suppresses central nervous system activity and results in muscle relaxation. It is utilized in SCI patients for the management of muscle spasticity, and as a tranquilizer. This drug does not seem to have any adverse sexual side effects. Furthermore, it does not affect the contractile voluntary function of the vaginal muscles in SCI females with either complete or incomplete lesions. However, in high doses (more than 40 mg a day), it can produce drowsiness and "paralyze" the remaining normal muscles, leading to sexual nonperformance. Methacarbamol (Robaxin), believed to be a CNS muscle relaxant, has been effective in relieving muscle pains and spasms in some chronic SCI patients (*8*). Unlike Valium, which causes occasional ejaculatory dysfunction in non-SCI patients, Robaxin and other less potent nonspecific muscle relaxants do not produce sexual side effects. Calcium (slow) channel blockers such as Verapamil were initially used to relieve coronary artery spasms.* Our ongoing clinical research with this drug has shown that it seems to reduce detrusor hypertonicity with minimal relaxing effects on the external urethral sphincter spasticity in SCI patients (*8*). No adverse sexual side effects were noted.

*Ed note: Vasodilators—"Isoxsuprine" and Pentaxifylline (Trental), which decreases blood viscosity, seem to be ineffective in this particular male population.

Antispasmodic medications are usually parasympathetic antagonists used to treat gastrointestinal spasms or pains, and hyperhidrosis. Any anticholinergic parasympathetic inhibitor can cause impotence with prolonged usage. However, in SCI patients, the use of these antispasmodics is seldom indicated once these persons have achieved proper bowel care retraining. Oxybutynin (Ditropan) is a smooth (detrusor) muscle relaxant employed to manage spastic (hypertonic) urinary bladder, especially in quadriplegics. One complication of this drug is a dry mouth, but no sexual side effect has been noted (*9*).

Antidepressants, antipsychotics, tranquilizers, and other sedatives have been used with SCI patients for other therapeutic indications. A majority of SCI patients have premorbid personality disorders and psychiatric problems, and since both tricyclics and monoamine oxidase (MAO) inhibitor antidepressants act on the brain, chronic use of these medications can produce a variety of sexual dysfunctions. Other drugs and toxins causing sexual dysfunction are summarized in Table 2 and 3. Amphetamines are used as "uppers" by drug addicts, with an initial enhancement of libido and sexual arousal (*2*). However, in drug-addicted SCI persons, sexual side effects include erectile and ejaculatory dysfunctions and occasional libidinal disorders. Intravenous chloropromazine (Thorazine) has been used to treat acute hyperreflexia (*12*). Prolonged oral use of Thorazine and of benperidol (Haldol) is reported not to cause erectile difficulties (*20*). On the other hand, chloradiazepoxide (Librium), even in small doses (20 mg), may cause ejaculatory failure (*5*).

There is no clinical evidence to suggest that chemotherapeutic and antimicrobial agents per se alter or influence sexual response and function (*7*). Anecdotal reports indicate that nitrofurantin (Macrodantin) can precipitate impotence in non-SCI men. However, Macrodantin does not cause any sexual problems in SCI patients.

Chronic pains with multifactorial origins are frustrating to both patient and physician. Prostaglandin inhibitors (aspirin and Indocin) have been used to treat such pain in SCI patients with limited success. Though prostaglandin F_2-alpha has been theorized to mediate orgasmic genital muscle contraction response, no clinical datum is available suggesting that these medications can cause orgasmic response dysfunctions (*7,8*).

Hormonal alterations produced by spinal cord trauma revert to normal after a year. Testosterone is used to stimulate the appetite and reverse certain metabolic changes in both non-SCI and SCI patients with renal failure. Furthermore, testosterone is beneficial in the management of impotence that results from hormonal deficiency states. However, prolonged use of this androgenic hormone can interrupt the hypothalamic-pituitary-gonadal feedback circuitry, and lead to impotence. The use

Table 3
Other Drug Effects on Male Sexuality (*41*)

A. Ejaculatory Inhibition or Retrograde Ejaculation	
Thioridazine	(Mellaril)
Chlorpromazine	(Thorazine)
Chlorprothixine	(Taractan)
Mesoridazine	(Serentil)
Perphenazine	(Trilafon)
Trifluoperazine	(Stelazine)
Butaperazine	(Repoise)
Butyrophenones	(Haldol)
Chlordiazepoxide	(Librium)
Amoxapine	(Asendin)
Desipramine	(Norpramin)
Chlomipramine	(Anafranil)
Amitriptyline	(Elavil)
Imipramine	(Tofranil)
Phenelzine	(Nardil)
Pargyline	(Eutonyl)
Mebanazid	(Actomol)
Iproniazid	(Marsilid)
Isocarboxazid	(Marplan)
Alpha-methyldopa	(Aldomet)
Reserpine	(Serpasil)
Quanethidine	(Ismelin)
B. Painful Ejaculation (*23,41*)	
Amoxapine	(Asendin)
Imipramine	(Tofranil)
Protriptyline	(Vivactil
Desipramine	(Norpramin)
Thioridazine	(Mellaril)
C. Priapism (*23,41*)	
Trazodone	(Desyrel)
Chlorpromazine	(Thorazine)
Thioridazine	(Mellaril)
Methaqualone	(Quaalude)
Quanethidine	(Ismelin)
Hydralazine	(Apresoline)
Prazosin	(Minipres)
Labetolol	(Normodyne)
Tolbutamide	(Orinase)
Heparin	(Heparin)

Table 3 (Continued): Other Drug Effects on Male Sexuality (*41*)

D. Industrial Pollutants (*32,43*)	
Insecticides	Impotence-libido/ejaculatory dysfunctions
Carbon disulfide	Libido/erectile dysfunctions
Nitrous oxide	Partial loss genital sensation and ejaculatory dysfunctions
E. Miscellaneous (Research Drugs/Chemicals) (*23,44*)	
Wellbutrin (Burroughs-Wellcome Co.)	Antidepressants/aphrodisiac
LY-163502 (Eli Lilly Co.)	Aphrodisiac?

of oral progesterone and estrogen derivatives in the female SCI patient is rare. Chronic intake of these drugs can cause sexual, fertility, and neoplastic complications. Topical application of a progesterone/estrogen combination cream/ointment is advisable for the treatment of dyspareunia in patients with incomplete lesions and vaginal epithelial atrophic changes. Administration of antiandrogens has been advocated as the last resort to control repeat SCI sexual offenders (*6*).

Erectiogenic drugs are usually alpha-2 adrenergic blockers and local vasodilators. The effects of these medications are discussed elsewhere. However, two vasodilators are worth mentioning: papaverine·HCl and the prostaglandin E (PGE) series. Papaverine is utilized both as a chemoerection agent and a diagnostic test reagent for venogenic erectile dysfunction. On the other hand, PGE_1 is a better local injectable penile chemoerection agent since it produces less fibrotic reaction in cavernous tissues during its prolong usage.*

Other Drugs and Chemicals

Oral estrogen (DES) has been utilized for symptomatic treatment of carcinoma of the prostate. This type of neoplasm usually occurs in the elderly, for whom organic impotence is common. Sexual dysfunctions in elderly SCI patients on chemotherapy for metastatic neoplasms are probably the result of neurogenic involvement, as well as drug toxicity itself. Aminocaproic acid (Amicar) is an adjunctive treatment for disseminated intravascular coagulation (DIC). This abnormal coagulatory problem also usually results from disseminated neoplastic disease. Any associated ejaculatory dysfunction is caused by complications from the ravages of the neoplastic cells.

---

*Ed note: Subcutaneous injections of apomorphine (dopamine agonist) have been shown to cause erection in able-bodied males. But because of serious side effects, it has limited use in SCI men.

However, there are newer types of antihyperlipidemic drugs with less or no sexual side effects. Clofibrate (Atromid-S) is used to lower high blood cholesterol levels, which can cause impotence. Cholesterol is one of the parent compounds of many steroids and hormones, and reducing the level of this necessary steroid/hormonal substrate can upset the process of normal hormone production, which is needed for normal sexual functioning and responses (*2,7*).

Addicting drugs, such as cocaine, heroin, and methadone, interfere with CNS coordination and thereby cause sexual dysfunctions. Recreational drugs, such as PCP (phencyclidine) and marijuana (claimed by some patients to be beneficial for pains and spasms), initially enhance arousal sensitivity; however, chronic users usually experience not only erectile and ejaculatory problems, but also infertility.

Levodopa (L-dopa) is one of the treatments for Parkinson's (dopamine deficiency) disease. Clinical studies from Mexico indicate that 48% of impotent non-SCI men responded to dopamine administration. Our initial study of this drug with SCI men showed promising results (*8,22*). Ejaculatory dysfunctions seen in those taking this medication may be caused by its interferences with prolactin secretions.

Conclusion

Any drug or medication that interferes with the coordination of or neurotransmission between the central and peripheral sexual centers, or that blocks neurohormonal and intercellular messenger systems—the cyclic adenosine monophosphate (phosphatidate) phospoinositide cycle mediators—can cause havoc among the sexual functions and responses. Physicians prescribing medications for SCI patients that may produce adverse sexual side effects should include inquiries about any adverse sexual side effects that may have been noticed by the patient in their followup interviews. When these occur, the medication should be reduced, discontinued, or changed if possible. Biofeedback, acupuncture, acupressure, and other nonstandard treatment modalities may offer alternatives to drug medication and thus may be tried for the management of hypertension and for pain therapy. When the physician and other health professionals have open minds and maintain a comfortable rapport with their patients, effective communications are a natural outcome despite the often negative sexual attitudes of our culture. With such an openness, patients will be comfortable talking with the healthy care professionals about any adverse sexual side effects of prescribed medications.

As the above discussion indicates, sexual side effects observed in SCI persons are not always identical with those observed during use of the same medication by non-SCI persons. The SCI patient is unique psychologically and pathologically because of multiorgan involvement, and because these patients are generally under the influence of a variety of medications and psychopharmacological compounds, the physician or sex therapist should take time to explain the wide range of individual responses to drugs. Patients should be warned about the dangers of mixing alcohol and central nervous system acting drugs. Diphenylhydantoin (Dilantin), in particular, may potentiate alcohol's effects. Thus it is probably ineffective in controlling convulsions associated with alcohol withdrawal. Furthermore, chronic use of the drug in high doses (400 mg/d) may cause impotence.

In order to minimize drug-induced sexual dysfunctions, the physician must meticulously select the proper medication and dosage, keeping in mind the importance of good sexual readjustment in the total rehabilitation of the SCI patient. A complete drug history, prior to initial sexual evaluation, is mandatory (*18*). In the majority of cases, it is the severity of the trauma, the presence of associated diseases, and the level of lesion that determines the degree of sexual recovery. The physician, the sex therapist, and the patient must all be vigilant for any unpleasant drug-induced sexual side effects. Understanding the pharmacokinetics of each medication will facilitate a rapid and pleasurable sexual rehabilitation of the spinal-cord-injured patient.

Tables 1, 2, and 3 summarize the data available on the sexual side effects of medications. The data reported are drawn primarily from clinical research on able-bodied and disabled (physically challenged) male patients, and from laboratory animals. Very little data is available on the sexual side effects of medications on female patients, though it may be assumed that their responses will be similar because of the similarities in neurohormonal factors in male and female sexual libido, arousal, and orgasmic functions.

References

1. Bringing research into effective focus. (1983) Statistical findings at the Regional Spinal Cord System *Rehab. Brief* **6**, 1–4.

2. Buffum, J. (1982) Pharmacosexology—The effects of drugs on sexual function. A review *J. Psychoactive Drugs* **14**, 1, 2, 5–44.

3. DeMoya, A., DeMoya, D., Lewis, M., and Lewis, H. (1982) *Sex and Health.* New York: Stein and Day.

4. Domer, F. R., Wessler, G., Brown, R. L., et al. (1978) Involvement of the sympathetic nervous system in urinary bladder internal sphincter and in penile erection in the anesthetized cat. *Invest. Urol.* **15**, 404–410.
5. Hughes, J. M. (1964) Failure to ejaculate with chlorthiazepoxide. *Am. J. Psychiatry* **121**, 610, 611.
6. Kaplan, H. S. (1979) *Disorders of Sexual Desire.* Bruner/Mazel, New York.
7. Leyson, J. F. J. (1981) Recent theories of male and female sexual physiology. Read at the Assoc. of Phil. Practicing Physicians in America. Anaheim, CA, Aug. 13–15.
8. Leyson, J. F. J. (1982) Sexual Options in SCI patients. Spinal Cord Injury Symposium. Kessler Institute for Rehabilitation, West Orange, NJ. April 22.
9. Leyson, J. F. J., and Manigbas, J. (1978) Use of oxybutynin in preventing autonomic dysreflexia in SCI patients. Presented at AUA Meeting, New York Section, Valentine's Award, New York, NY, April 14.
10. Leyson, J. F. J., Stefaniwsky, L., and Martin, B. R. (1978) Phenoxybenzamine as adjunctive treatment of hyperhidrosis in SCI patients. Read at the Am. Paraplegia Society Meeting. Annual Spinal Cord Inj. Conf. Northport, NY. Sept. 18, 19.
11. Leyson, J. F. J., Martin, B. F., and Sporer, A. (1980) Baclofen in the treatment of detrusor-sphincter dyssynergia in spinal cord injury patients. *J. Urol.* **124**, 82–84.
12. McGuire, E. J., and Rossier, A. B. (1983) Treatment of acute autonomic dysreflexia. *J. Urol.* **129**, 1185–1187.
13. Melman, A. (1983) Rat study shows reduced reflex in penis and propanolol use. *Urology Times* **11**, 23.
14. Meyer, J. J., Kern, A., Godec, C. J., and Cass, A. S. (1982) The response of impotent patients to Duvoid. Presented at the Am. Urol. Assoc. Meeting. Kansas City, MO. May 16–20.
15. News Briefs (1983) OK due for ranitidine vs ulcers. *Medical Tribune* **24**, 1.
16. Osterholm, J. L. (1976) Early management of spinal cord injury: Theory and practice. The vascular and cellular basis for spinal cord hemorrhage necrosis. In *Current Controversies in Neurosurgery*, Morley, T. P., ed. Philadelphia, PA, Saunders, Chap. 5.
17. Papadopoulos, C. (1980) Cardiovascular drugs and sexuality: A cardiologist's review. *Arch. Intern. Med.* **140**, 341.
18. Segraves, T. R. (1981) Psychopharmocological agents associated with sexual dysfunctions. *J. Sex Ed. Therapy* **7**, 43–45.
19. Sporer, A., Leyson, J. F. J., and Martin, B. F. (1978) Effects of bethanochol chloride on the external urethral sphincter in SCI patients. *J. Urol.* **120**, 62–65.
20. Tennet, G., Bancroft, J., and Cass, J. (1974) The control of deviant sexual behavior by drugs: A double-blind controlled study of benperidol, chlorpromazine and placebo. *Arch. Sex. Behav.* **3**, 261–271.

21. Wartman, S. A. (1983) Sexual side effects of antihypertensive drugs. Treatment, strategies and strictures. *Postgrad. Med.* **73**, 133–138.
22. Leyson, J. F. J. (1984) Use of dopaminergic drugs in the treatment of impotence. Presented at the annual meeting of Society for Sex Therapy and Research. New York City, NY. Oct. 19–21.
23. Leyson, J. F. J. (1988) Updates on sexual medicine. Presented at the Annual Winter Meeting of the Association of Philippine Physicians in America, Manila, Phil. Dec. 14–17.
24. Beaumont G. (1973) Sexual side-effect of clomipramine (Anafranil). *J. Int. Med. Res.* **1**, 469–472.
25. Bowers, M. B., Woert, M. V., and Davis, L. (1971) Sexual behavior during L-dopa treatment for Parkinsonism. *Amer. J. Psychiat.* **127**, 1691–1693.
26. Degen, K. (1982) Sexual dysfunction in women using major tranquilizers. *Psychosomatics* **23**, 959–961.
27. Freed, E. (1983) Increased sexual function with nomifensine. *Med. J. Australia* **2**, 538.
28. Gross, M. D. (1982) Reversal by bethanechol of sexual dysfunction caused by anticholinergic antidepressants. *Amer. J. Psychiat.* **139**, 1193, 1194.
29. Lesko, L. M., Stotland, N. L., and Segraves, R. T. (1982) Three cases of female anorgasmia associated with MAOIs. *Amer. J. Psychiat.* **139**, 1353–1354.
30. Malatesta, V. J., Pollack, R. H., Crotty, T. D., and Peacock, L. J. (1982) Acute alcohol intoxication and the female orgasmic response. *J. Sex Res.* **18**, 1–17.
31. Pierce, J. R. (1983) Cimitidine-associated depression and loss of libido in a woman. *Amer. J. Med. Sci.* **286**, 31–34.
32. Quirk, K. C., and Einarson, T. R. (1982) Sexual dysfunction and clomipramine. *Can. J. Psychiatry* **27**, 228–231.
33. Sangal, R. (1985) Inhibited female orgasm as a side effect of alprazolam. *Am. J. Psychiat.* **142**, 1223, 1224.
34. Shalet, S. M. (1980) Effects of cancer chemotherapy on gonadal function of patients. *Cancer Treatment Reviews* **7**, 141–152.
35. Shen, W. W. (1982) Female orgasmic inhibition by amoxapine. *Am. J. Psychiatry* **139**, 1220, 1221.
36. Shen, W. W., and Sata, L. S. (1983) Inhibited female orgasm resulting from psychotropic drugs. *J. Reproductive Med.* **28**, 497–499.
37. Souner R. (1983) Anorgasmia associated with imipramine but not desipramine: A case report. *J. Clin. Psychiatry* **44**, 345–346.
38. Souner, R. (1984) Treatment of tricyclic antidepressant-induced orgasmic inhibition with cyproheptadine. *J. Clin. Psychopharm.* **4**, 169.
39. Wagner, G., and Levin, R. J. (1980) Effect of atropine and methylatropine on human vaginal blood flow, sexual arousal and climax. *Acta. Pharmacol. Toxicol.* **46**, 321–325.
40. Wallace, T. R., Fraunfelder, F. T., Petursson, G. J., and Epstein, D. L.

(1979) Decreased libido—A side effect of carbonic anhydrase inhibitor. *Ann. Opthalmol.* **237**, 1563–1566.
41. Segraves, R., Madsen, R., Carter, S. and Davis, J. (1986) Erectile dysfunction associated with pharmacological agents. In Segraves, R., and Schoenberg, H. (eds.) *Diagnosis and Treatment of Erectile Failure.* Plenum, New York City, NY.
42. Espir, M. L. E., Hall, J. W., Schirreffs, J. G., Stevens, D. L. (1970) Impotence in farm workers using toxic chemicals. *Brit. Med. J.* **1**, 423–425.
43. Layzer, R. B. (1978) Myeloneuropathy after prolonged exposure to nitrous oxide. *Lancet* **1**, 1227–1230.
44. Crenshaw, T. (1989) Personal communication.

Flouoxitine (Prozac) has similar ''aphrodisiac-like'' benefits of (wellbutrin) Bupropion, but possesses more side effects.

Controversies and Research

34

Controversies and Research in Female Sexuality

Jose Florante J. Leyson

Introduction

Nature has genetically programmed the female for procreation. The estrus cycle of lower animals assures that the female of the species is allowed genital contact only when the ova are ripe. In the primeval forest, the sexual behavior of female homo sapiens was programmed to the estrus cycle, allowing coitus only during ovulation.

Current sexual attitudes/behaviors, as described by modern theories of the sociobiological behavior of humans, are products of the interplay between genes and sociocultural influences (*20*). Furthermore, recent data theorize that the human female ''aborted'' herself of the ''genetic-estrus cycle'' program, replacing it with a self-regulated sexual cycle and response so as to protect and ensure survival of the species. This ''sexual contract'' theory states that the female, through cerebral mechanisms, can control her menstrual cycle; thus she can determine how many times or how many partners may impregnate her within a certain period (*7*). This fertility period coincides with the harvesting of crops or the abundance and availability of game. This newly learned sexual pattern has made the female an active partner in controlling the sexual behavior of males. The female can now choose, or offer herself to, the man who is strongest and can provide the most food, thereby assuring herself of excellent offspring with a better chance of surviving.

Was sociobiology responsible for genetically locating the ovaries intra-abdominally so as to ensure the continuity of the species, even after spinal cord injuries? The procreative function of females who sustain spinal cord injuries is preserved, even though ovaries and testes

Sexual Rehabilitation of the Spinal-Cord-Injured Patient
Edited by J.F. Leyson, © 1990 The Humana Press, Inc.

are subserved by both the parasympathetic and the sympathetic nervous systems. Only the reproductive functions of extra-abdominally located testes are affected by cord trauma.

Is male infertility partly the result of circulating high levels of catecholamines that may trigger abnormalities in thermoregulatory and neurohormonal mechanisms by a disturbed autonomic nervous system? Our initial clinical data from 18 subjects have shown that catecholamine levels in 10 males and 8 females post-SCI do not differ, although the titer was slightly higher in male quadriplegics. (*22*).

Siroky (*15*) has stated that testosterone is responsible for libido in both sexes, and demonstrated that its administration to hypotestosteronemic males augmented sexual fantasizing and improved their sexual satisfaction. Limited studies of three SCI women have shown that each benefited from oral testosterone, even when one patient had pre-treatment clinical idiopathic hirsuitism.

Testosterone acts on both the spinal cord and the brain, partly to modulate responses to sexual activity in conjunction with four known neuroreceptor systems—the noradrenergic, cholinergic, dopaminergic, and serotoninergic. In the absence of cerebral trauma or disease, the adult SCI patient may experience different degrees of orgasmic responses. However, Bondareff has demonstrated significant neuron and neurofibril loss as well as structural, metabolic, and functional changes in cerebral neuroreceptor–neurotransmitter systems in the aging brain (*1*). If one subscribes to the concept of sexual dimorphism, i.e., assumes that the female brain is less well biologically adapted to visuospatial functioning than the male brain (*17*), then females with a larger cerebral splenium, resulting from a larger number of neurofibers, would have an edge in neurocerebral sexual response/orgasms compared to males. On the other hand, is it logical to administer dopamine and its derivatives (a noradrenaline precursor) to aging males with orgasmic dysfunctions and to aging females with low libido and impaired orgasmic responses if their adrenaline–dopamine levels are low?

From the limited research done, it seems that women with a spinal cord injury (SCI) are capable of experiencing sexual pleasure. There is increasing evidence that orgasmic circumvaginal muscle contractions are mediated by a neurotransmitter: prostaglandin F_2-alpha (*9*). Patients with complete spinal lesions may experience sensual sensations or pleasure and mini (para) orgasms, probably via a substance P, described as a potent smooth muscle contractor present in paraplegic animals. Leyson (*9*) believes that substance P may also be responsible for facilitating the passage of both sexual and urinary impulses across the traumatized spinal segment. The different psychosocial pattern of the

SCI woman may account for the varied physiosexual responses of both the vaginal/clitoral and the "new" erotic zone stimulations. These women will have to learn to enjoy different or new forms of stimulation and ways of responding. It is not known whether purified substance P, when it becomes available for clinical use, will enhance sensory or orgasmic responses in females with anesthesia of the genitals and "hypo-orgasmia" (*9*). *See* Fig. 1.

Grafenberg (G) Erotic Spot and Ejaculation

Whipple et al. (*18*) rediscovered the Grafenberg (G) spot and advocated that stimulation of this area, where a sensitive network of nerves is located, induces orgasm in some women. As previously mentioned, we differ from Masters and Johnson's position that there is only one orgasm or orgasmic trigger—the clitoris. Our present research and clinical experience reveal two types of orgasm, clitoral (superficial) and vaginal (deep) (*9*). Clinically, only 10% of the women the author studied achieved orgasm with G-spot stimulation, without considering how difficult it is to locate this spot. However, in SCI women, caution is required since G-spot stimulation may cause reflex micturition. Patients with sacral cord lesions may not experience a stimulatory erotic feeling.

Recently, Whipple and Perry (*19*) studied certain groups of normal female ejaculates and demonstrated that the ejaculate is chemically similar to that from males, except for the absence of sperm. However, male ejaculation is the ejection of "sex secretions" through a series of rhythmic muscular contractions, starting from the epidydimis to the vas deferens—from the testis to the musculoglandular prostate to the ejaculatory duct surrounded by the bulbocavernosus muscles. Although Mallon (*12*) has demonstrated vestigial female prostatic tissue, the primitive gland probably does not contain mature muscular components. Furthermore, the largest female secretory/lubricating (Bartholin's) gland, the female homolog of Cowper's gland, is devoid of muscular elements. Therefore, it is only logical to conclude that female ejaculation cannot occur physiologically because ejecting muscular components are absent. This phenomenon, therefore, should properly be termed female sexual-secretory expulsion. The fluid is expelled in either of two phases during sexual activity: (a) penile thrusting, when secretions are expelled suddenly from Bartholin's and other accessory glands in hypersecretor females by penile pressure in a contracting vaginal barrel, and (b) at orgasm when the secretions are squeezed between the penis and the vaginal wall, or against the congested vaginal wall itself. Clarification

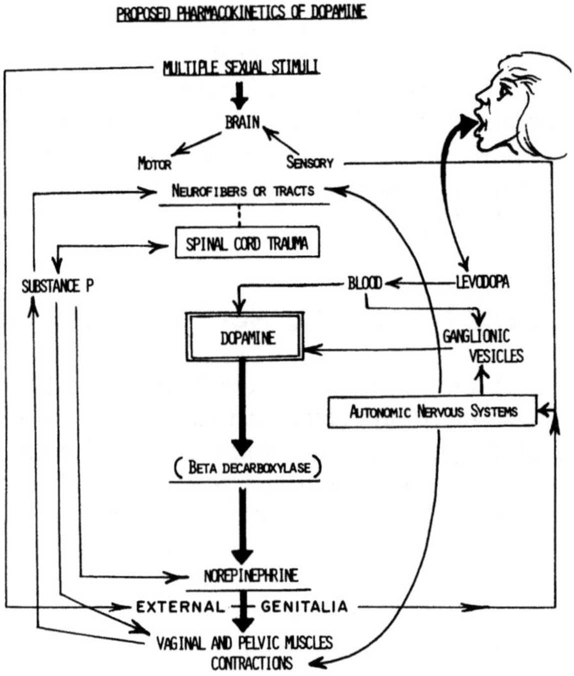

Fig. 1. Schematic diagram of the possible mechanisms by which dopamine in collaboration with substance P initiates vaginal (perivaginal) muscle contractions.

of this sexual phenomenon is vital if fear is to be allayed that a recovering SCI female is still "normal," even though she cannot expel orgasmic secretions.

Diagnosis

The diagnostic armamentarium for female sexual dysfunctions became almost ideal with the introduction of the sexplotter (SP)-300 portable physiologic recorder (Fig.2)* It might benefit from a few modifications, such as (a) the transistorization of some of its components; (b) the use of a housing permitting up to six plug-in modules with the capability of running eight diagnostic functions—bruxing, female arousal, vaginal contractions—using photoplethysmography, EMG, ECG, heart rate, biofeedback, and temperature/BP; or (c) the addition of a miniature computer to extrapolate eight signals (recordings) into four understandable data segments. One of the pressure transducers or sensor plugs should be able to act as a vibrator for stimulating or training purposes. For details of the various diagnostic steps, please refer to Chapter 11.

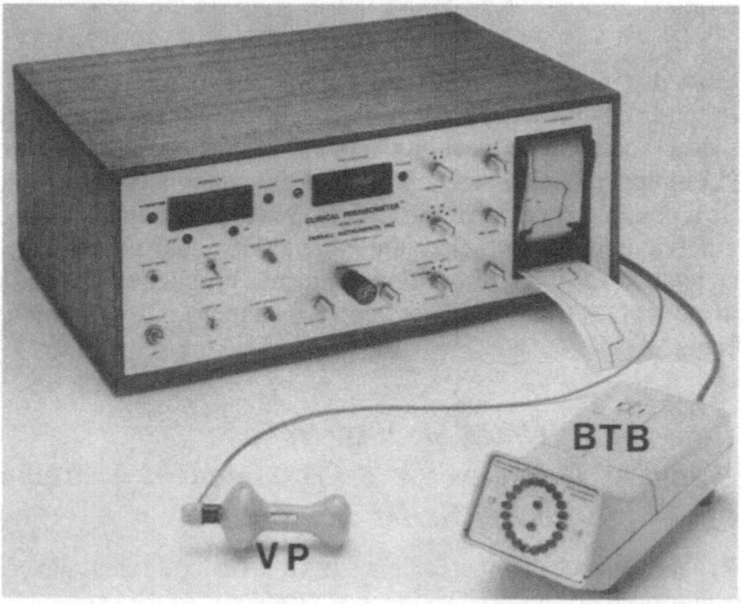

Fig. 2.* Clinical perineometer used to treat urinary incontinence and sexual dysfunction. Its attachments are a vaginal plug (VP) and a portable (personal) biofeedback trainer box (BTB) equipped with a visual light cycle feedback display and audiotone.

Genital Anesthesia and Vaginal Hypotonia Causing Orgasmic Dysfunction

Orgasm is a neurohormonal cerebral phenomenon with local pleasurable sensations from ischiococcygeal and pubococcygeal muscle contractions. Spinal cord trauma can result in both genital anesthesia and vaginal muscle atonia or hypotonia. Most SCI patients experience the return of genital sensations, but SCI females and their partners complained about the looseness of the vaginal introitus—the "empty well" syndrome (*9*). There are several options in the management of orgasmic dysfunctions caused by genital hypotonia or anesthesia and loose or absent vaginal muscle contractions: (a) medical, biophysical, and electronic rehabilitation; and (b) nerve transplantation.

* Farrel Instruments, Inc., Grand Island, NE 68802, USA.

Medical Therapy

Most drugs used to treat cord trauma are muscle relaxants that relieve spasticity. Presently, in fifty clinical trials, we have demonstrated that ''slow'' calcium channel blockers are ineffective in the treatment of SCI urethral sphincter–urinary bladder dyssynergia (incoordination) (*10*). Is it possible to utilize a ''fast'' calcium channel stimulator specific to the pelvic muscles to tighten the vaginal introitus? Our initial trial of five women for internal urethral sphincter stimulation showed that ephedrine sulfate was useless in the management of vaginal muscle hypotonia.

Other Medical Options: Dopamine Derivatives and Prostaglandin F_2 Alpha and E Series (E_1 and E_2)

Recent advances in neuroscience have revealed several new types of sexual-orgasmic neurotransmitters or receptors. At the cerebral level, parasympathetic (cholinergic), sympathetic (norepinephrinergic), and other peptidergic neurotransmitters are present. Dopamine is degraded to norepinephrine by the enzyme beta-decarboxylase in the blood and ganglionic vesicles (Fig. 1). At the level of the sacral cord and end organ—genitovaginal structures—norepinephrine is a neurotransmitter and prostaglandin E_1 (PE_1) for clitoral erections and vaginal muscle contractions. The (PE_1) and vasoactive intestinal polypeptide (VIP) initiates clitoral erection. This action is believed to be reinforced by norepinephrine. A newly identified peptidergic neurotransmitter, neuropeptide Y, possibly mediates clitoral erection and prepares the vaginal walls for orgasmic contractions. However, the relationship between this peptide and norepinephrine is still under investigation (*21*). It is believed that one of the sexual neurotransmitters, norepinephrine, acts on both levels of the cerebrospinal cord and pelvic -vaginal end organ (*8*). Dopamine, a precursor of norepinephrine, when given orally can augment the levels of norepinephrine, thus sensitizing a damaged or traumatized neuron or neuroreceptors to erotic stimulations. The author studied 15 patients, most of whom had complete chronic lesions from C5–L2 and who ranged in age from 26 to 62 yr. These patients were initially treated with a placebo, followed by oral dopamine (levodopa) at 4 wk intervals. Most of the patients had complained of genital anesthesia and a loose vaginal introitus, which hindered their orgasmic responses. Of the 15 SCI females, 9 (60%) responded to therapy after

2½ wk, while 6 improved on the placebo. The probable mechanism of dopamine therapy is illustrated in Fig. 1. Oral Levodopa (500 mg.) or Carbidopa and Sinemet* should be given for 2–3 mo and then tapered gradually. Treatment is terminated after 4–5 mo. with a 1-wk rest period every 6–8 wk. cycles. Doses are given three to four times a day, and the maintenance dose is given three times a day (*9,21*). It is also advisable to correct associated diseases and supplement such treatment with adjunctive sex counseling. The above data also demonstrated that patient with severe peripheral neuropathy and those with sacral cord lesions (conus medullaris injury) do not respond to dopamine. Major side effects are nausea, headaches, drowsiness, and muscle weakness. Future research will be geared toward the use of dopamine antagonists to determine whether depleting dopamine and replacing it with oral dopamine derivatives can restore impaired orgasmic responses (*9,21*).

The prostaglandin series labeled to act as sexual neurotransmitters are F_2-alpha (α) and (prostaglandin) E_2. These facilitate sensual sensations and maintain erotic output (PE_2) which it is hoped will lead to orgasm. Prostaglandin F_2-alpha ($PF_{2\alpha}$) initiates pelvic and vaginal muscle contractions during orgasm; while PE_2, when prepared as an ointment, can be applied to the anesthetized genitalia, providing temporary sensual sensations during sexual activity. Although PF_2-alpha has been used clinically by obstetricians as an abortifacient, it is hoped that it will soon be available in an oral preparation for the management of dysorgasmia and/or orgasmic dysfunctions associated with weak vaginal contractions.

Biophysical and Electronic Rehabilitation

It must be emphasized that the vagina is merely a potential space or canal that is usually passive until sexually stimulated. The rectal sphincter by contrast, is in tonus to maintain fecal continence at all times. Post-cord trauma, when the vaginal introitus is lax, rehabilitation of the sexual musclature should be initiated. The Kegel pubococcygeal (PC) or perineal exercises are ideal for both urinary incontinence and vaginal "looseness" in females with incomplete or recovering lesions.

For biofeedback and other forms of bionic sex therapy, the following can be used: (a) a vagitone†, and (b) a perineometer‡ (Fig. 2), both for

---

*These oral preparations are not as pure as Levodopa.

†Gyne-O-Tek, Inc., O.O. Box 29017, Portland, OR 97229, USA.

‡Farrel Instruments, Inc., Grand Island, NE 68802, USA.

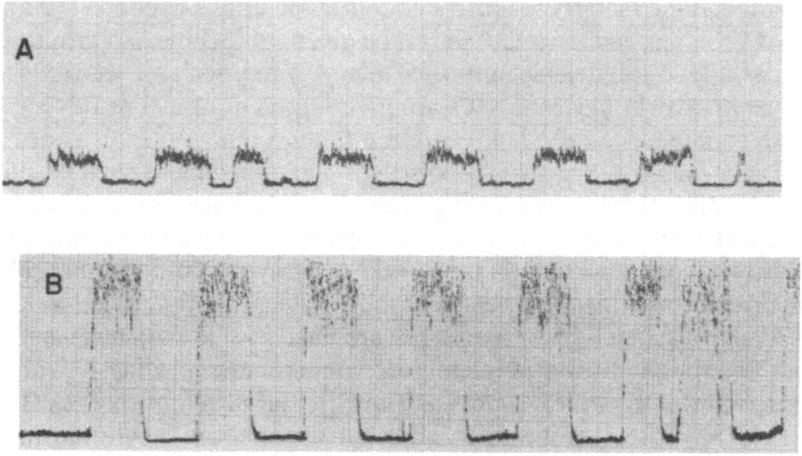

Fig. 3. Vaginal myography of a 42-year-old L2 paraplegic woman 3 mo postspinal shock (A). Postperineal training showing normal pubococcygeus muscle strength 10 mo post-trauma (B).

diagnostic–therapeutic (clinical) and self-training (personal) purposes. Vagitone is an electronic (low-voltage) muscle stimulator that has been 90% effective in curing nondisabled patients suffering stress urinary incontinence, and 65–70% effective in improving sexual or orgasmic dysfunction in incomplete and low paraplegics. The clinical perineometer has been used for diagnosis and for training. Figures 3A and B demonstrate pre- and postSCI perineal muscle training exercises. Another option for vaginal (perineal) exercises is a vaginal EMG probe or rectal probe electrostimulator, similar to those used for impotence and urinary incontinence. Interestingly, 10% or probably more SCI females with complete or sacral sparing lesions experience satisfactory vaginal orgasmic contractions.

Transcutaneous Neurostimulation (TNS)

Leyson et al. (*11*) have demonstrated that TNS can trigger external urethral sphincter spasticity in high quadriplegics, resulting in high residual urine volumes and recurrent infections. McGuire (*13*) also observed that electrical cutaneous stimulation or TNS over some dermatomes (i.e., femoral, peroneal, and tibial) produced urinary bladder sphincter (pudendal-pelvic nerve reflexes) activity. With the above premise, three dermatomes were stimulated by TNS in five patients (Fig. 4). These clinical data have shown that it might be feasible for SCI

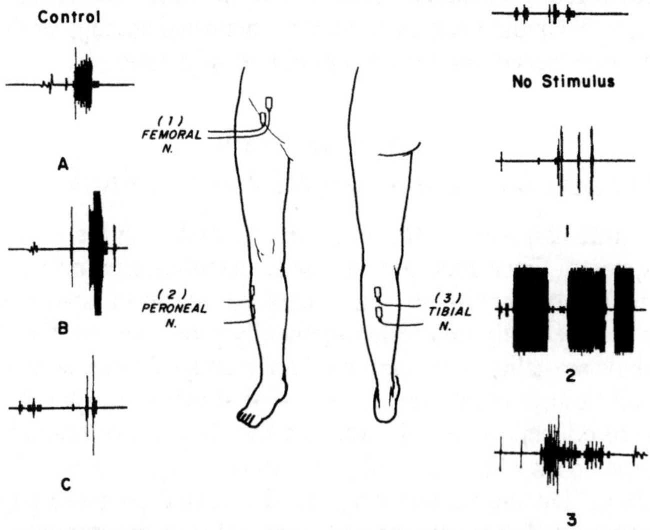

Fig. 4. Vaginal electromyographic (EMG) recording in a nonstimulated normal woman. A, B, and C tracings demonstrate vaginal contractions under volitional control. (1) EMG of a 58-year-old chronic T10 paraplegic showing minimal activity. (2) Maximal spike potentials and (3) moderate vaginal contractions following TNS of the respective dermtomes.

females to initiate vaginal contractions by electrically stimulating specific (peroneal and tibial nerves) dermatomes with a pocket-size portable stimulator (*21*).

Vaginal Contraction (Orgasmic) Pacemaker

Direct stimulation of the peripheral sexual center (S2-S4) activated both the dorsal and ventral roots, which would result in nonspecific reactions—urinary bladder and urethral sphincters, rectal and vaginal contractions—simultaneously (*16*). The pudendal nerve, which serves both sensory and motor functions, subserves the rectum, external urethral sphincter, and the lower third of the vagina. The pelvic nerves also supply the lower vaginal barrel.

Urinary incontinence devices inserted either rectally or vaginally produce pudendal–pudendal and pelvic–pudendal reflexes, causing the both internal and external urethral sphincter to contract, thereby correcting urinary loss. Thus, it may be possible to trigger vaginal contractions by stimulating the pudendal and/or pelvic nerves. To test this hypothesis, selective pudendal or pelvic branches (those supplying the low vagina) should be stimulated. The orgasmic pacemeker should have two stimulators for implantation in each of the aforementioned nerves* (Fig. 5A,B). To avoid early or premature neuronal damage or degeneration, only one nerve should be stimulated at a time.

Laser Orgasm (Transcutaneous—Genital Laser Stimulation)

Orgasmic responses differ between the male and the female of the human species. Once men are aroused, ejaculation is obligatory and orgasm is usually inevitable. This sexual-conception (sperm seeding) response is genetically and reflexogenically programmed. On the other hand, female sexuality is programmed differently. Female sexual arousal is not at all built to create the excitation that leads to orgasm, because ovulation or conception occurs whether she climaxes or not. Therefore, female orgasm may be a learned psychophysiological and reflexogenic phenomenon. During female orgasm, the sexual pleasure triggers an increased blood flow to the pelvis, especially to the genitals, leading to vasocongestion and clitoral erection. This pleasure response can easily be inhibited during childhood or adolescence as a result of sexophysical taboos, traumas, psychological problems, and disease processes. This orgasmic phenomenon can be relearned through sexual therapy, i.e., pleasuring and/or masturbation training. Later in life, this conditioned reflex may automatically trigger a peripelvic and genital blood flow when a woman becomes sexually aroused. Furthermore, pleasurable genital or sensual stimulation lead to vasodilation by both neurohormonal and psychological mechanisms.

It is believed that in some nonorgasmic women, the genital and peripelvic arteries do not adequately dilate because of suprasacral or cerebral suppressions. Furthermore, in SCI women, both sacral and suprasacral complete cord lesions can impair local sexual vasodilation or vasocongestion phenomena. As a result of alterations in both local and central sexual response centers, these types of women need a local stimulus to precondition or automatically activate their local response system when pleasurable psychic or tactile sensation is experienced.

In non-SCI females, nonorgasmia can be treated with hypnosis, masturbation, or other forms of sex therapy. A warm compress or locally controlled heat or ultrasonic energy may create local peripelvic vasodilation, but unsupervised heat application may produce skin burn in SCI females. However, in 1986 Dr. Jacques Waynberg, Director of the Institute of Sexology in Paris, introduced a new innovation—transcutaneous

*Ed note: S_2 root stimulation may lead to vaginal (vasocongestion) lubrication, a possible treatment for post-SCI vaginal dryness.

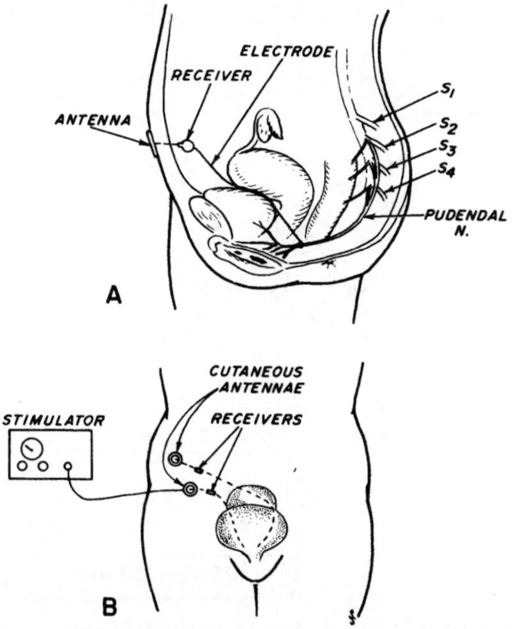

Fig. 5. Schematic representation of an electrode cuffed around one of the pudendal nerves with a transponder (receiver). Vaginal contractions are initiated by electrical stimulations via dermal antennae through electrodes (receivers) brought out behind the urinary bladder.

genital laser-stimulated orgasm. Laser (light amplification of stimulated emission of radiation) orgasm for non-SCI women is based on the principle that laser ''light'' can trigger and subsequently precondition the peripelvic region to vasodilate following pleasurable or erotic sensory experiences. To elaborate further, there are three kinds of lasers used in medicine:

(1) Soft (cutaneous) lasers, which do not penetrate beyond the epidermis; dermatologists used this type to treat warts, scars, and other skin problems
(2) Mid (transcutaneous) lasers, which penetrate deeper beyond the dermis but do not burn
(3) Power (subcutaneous or deep) lasers, which penetrate deeper into the subcutaneous layers and beyond; they burn or vaporize pathologic and even normal tissues.

Dr. Waynberg used mid lasers in non-SCI anorgasmic women, who report not feeling anything during sexual activity. He applied the laser to the genital area for 4 min, three times a week, for 6–8 wk (Fig. 6).

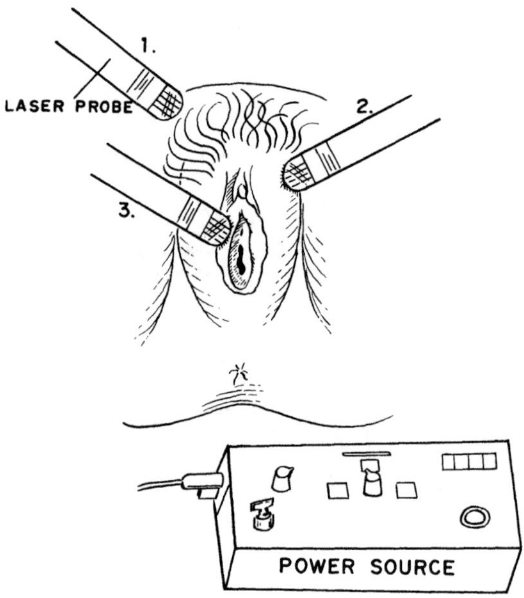

Fig. 6. A hand-held laser probe can be applied on three different genital areas to obtain maximum effect. The micro-electrophotic vibrations are presumed to create or initiate artificial and enhanced genital blood flow, facilitating sensory and psychic orgasmic responses.

The patient masturbates at night after each treatment and gradually progresses to orgasm. Of the 20 non-SCI females treated, 13 became orgasmic (cured) (*23*). The therapeutic use of lasers in SCI females with orgasmic dysfunction is still in its infancy and experimental phase. The application of mid lasers to facilitate orgasmic responses may be more effective in suprasacral lesions. Those with complete sacral cord destruction may not respond to this type of biosexotechnology because the peripelvic vasocongestion reflex may be absent (although in rare cases, orgasms may still occur through other undocumented neurohormonal or neural and psychic mechanisms).

Neurotransplantation

Advances in microsurgical techniques have made it possible to reimplant disconnected extremities and reconnect severed blood vessels and nerves. Carlsson and Sundin (*3*) have successfully restored some urinary bladder function after reconstructing efferent pathways in a paraplegic child. Recently, the above researchers were able to reinnervate the urinary bladder and restore male genital sensation after reanastomizing the S2 and S3 ventral and dorsal roots to the functioning T12 nerves in two adult paraplegics (*4*). However, it is still unknown whether it will prove feasible to restore vaginal contractile functioning post-SCI by nerve microimplantation to the remaining normal nerve roots or by transplantation of the adjacent nerves to the undamaged spinal cord segments above the lesion (*21*).

Miscellaneous

Sex therapy for both the able and disabled male sexual partner may consist of several options other than vaginal intercourse (*6*). The erect penis can be clasped between the breasts (especially in paraplegics), armpits, thighs, or inserted into the rectum. Oral sex is also advised in liberated nonrespirator-dependent quadriplegics. A revised holistic approach for a reluctant male partner may consist of a self-help sex therapy home computer teaching program (*14*).

Contraception

A detailed description of female contraception was given in an earlier chapter. However, recent innovative alternatives to contraception are worth mentioning. (a) A serotonin agonist or dopamine antagonist and GnRH (LHRF, luteinizing hormone-releasing factor) or its analog, can be given orally or by nasal spray (2). These preparations are ideal, because the effect of aerosol preparations is rapid and devoid of such serious side effects as thrombophlebitis. However, the amenorrhea caused by the LHRF analog can pose the risk of endometrial neoplasia. (b) Progesterone-like preparations can also be given as a nasal spray or slow-release skin patch (micropore). Patients using these contraceptives should have an intact hypothalamic–pituitary–gonadal axis. SCI women taking oral contraceptives should be cautioned that antibiotics, tranquilizers, antiepileptics, nonsteroidal anti-inflammatory agents, and urinary antiseptics can reduce its effectiveness (*24*).

Lesbianism

It is estimated that about 3000 females suffer from some form of spinal cord trauma annually. Thirteen percent of the nationwide population of veterans are females, as are 3–7% of the population of SCI veterans (*5*). A phone interview with 22 SCI females revealed that homosexuality occurs in 1% of the sample. It is believed that, because of the low level of testosterone in females, sexual activity is associated with less roughness or violence, unlike male gays. The use of sensate focus as part of sex therapy is crucial to delineate erotic zones in lesbian SCI women and to define hypersensitive (paresthetic–dysesthetic) or painful areas. The diameter of the vibrators used should be chosen so as not to overdistend a hyperreactive (spastic) vaginal barrel, thus forestalling a sympathetic crisis. It is also advised that vaginal tampons be changed twice a day to avoid "toxic shock syndrome." This probably occurs because of the high prevalence of recurrent or chronic urinary tract infection; thus vaginal or oral contamination (during sexual activity) with urinary tract infection; thus vaginal contamination with urinary infection is high. The colonization of different organisms in the vaginal tampon may lead to septicemia, shock, and eventually death. It must be reemphasized that sexual experimentation (with caution) remains the key to sexual happiness with fewer medical and emotional problems.

AIDS and Pregnancy (*25*)

The Centers for Disease Control lists the sources of AIDS infection in women as follows: 51% in drug abuser; 29%, heterosexual activity with an infected person; 11% blood transfusion; 8% unknown, and less than 1% from homosexual (lesbian) activity. It is estimated that about 132,000 women worldwide and 108,000 in the USA are infected with HIV, of whom 35% are expected to develop the disease within the next 5 yr.* Furthermore, CDC in Atlanta (Center for Disease Control) reveals that about 18% of the asymptomatic females in the general population are AIDS seropositive. However, the incidence of AIDS seroprevalence in SCI females is not presently known. Thus, it is advised that an SCI female infected with HTLV-III (AIDS) or HIV virus should consider delaying pregnancy until more is known about perinatal viral transmissions and its neonatal effects. For those who are already pregnant, the SCI female should not breastfeed her infant (because the virus may be secreted via milk). It is believed that about 6% of AIDS cases now occur in children. Preliminary reports have shown that, in infected women, pregnancy by artificial insemination has resulted in normal, healthy infants.

Cosmic Sexology

The Russians have sent two or more women cosmonauts into space for more than 3 mo. while the USA, the National Aerospace Administra-

*Ed note: HIV has affinity to neurons, thus AIDS will aggravate the sexo-neurological dysfunctions in SCI females.

tion (NASA) are conducting experiments in traumatic bone healing and the neuroelectrophysiology of invertebrates in relation to the human nervous system's response to trauma.

Biomedical data from the Johnson Space Center in Houston, Texas, have shown that there are definite alterations in the hematopoietic and hormonal systems if an astronaut stays in outerspace for a considerable period of time (*26*). Sexual activity for SCI females in a weightless environment should pose fewer problems than elsewhere, except for possible alterations of libido or orgasmic muscular responses. These sexual response dysfunctions might arise from thyroid and other sex hormone deficiencies. Furthermore, because of chronic paralysis (which leads to disuse atrophy), the SCI female may experience early forms of osteoporosis and anemia from alterations in calcium metabolism and hematopoiesis. Therefore, for those fortunate enough to travel in (year 2010) outer space, it is recommended that calcium, iron, vitamin C, and folate combination vitamins should be included as a supplement in the female's diet (*21*).

Conclusions

Although the neurophysiology of female sexuality needs still further in-depth study, the advances in sexual biotechnology will enhance the relationship/sexual dysfunction management of the SCI female as she lives and meets new challenges into the 21st century.

References

1. Bondareff, W. (1983) The aging brain. *Transition*. **1**, 21–40.
2. Bergguist, C., Nillius, S. J., and Wide, L. (1979) Inhibition of ovulation by intranasal treatment of a luteinizing hormone releasing hormone agonist. *Contraception*. **19**, 497–502.
3. Carlsson, C. A. and Sundin, T. (1967) Reconstruction of efferent pathway to the urinary bladder in a paraplegic child. *REV. Surg*. **24**, 73–76.
4. Carlsson, C. A. and Sundin,R. (1980) Reconstruction of afferent and efferent nervous pathways to the urinary bladder in two paraplegic patients. *Spine*. **5**, 37–41.
5. Copperthite, A. (1983) Vital statistics in the veterans administration medical center systems. Presented at the 29th American Paraplegia Society Meeting, Las Vegas, NE. Aug. 22–24.
6. Crenshaw, R. T., Martin, D. E., Warner, H., and Crenshaw, T. L. (1978) Organic Impotence in Sexual Consequences of Disability. A. Comfort, chap. 3, pp. 25–36. (Stickley, Philadelphia, PA).

7. Fisher, H. (1980) *Sexual Contract. Theories of the evolution of human behavior*. (Morrow, New York).
8. Karczmar, A. G. (1980) Drugs, transmitters and hormones and mating behavior in modern problems of pharmacopsychiatry. Drug treatment of sexual dysfunction. Ban, T. A. and Freyhan, F. A., eds., chapt. 1, pp. 1–52 (Karger, NY).
9. Leyson, J. F. J. (1983) Recent management of female sexual dysfunctions. Presented at the Asso. of Philippine Practicing Physicians in America, Annual Meeting: Houston, TX. Aug. 10–14.
10. Leyson, J. F. J., Seebode, J., Sporer, A., Wilchfort, S., and Scalera, J. (1984) Calcium channel blockers in the management of sphincter-detrusor dysfunction in spinal cord injury patients. Presented at the American Urological Association Meeting, New Orleans, LA. May 6–10.
11. Leyson, J. F. J., Stefaniwsky, L., and Martin, B. F. (1979) Effects of transcutaneous nerve stimulation on the vesicourethral function in spinal cord injury patients. *J. Urol.* **121**, 635–639.
12. Mallon, R. (1983) Demonstration of vestigal prostatic tissue in the human female: A histochemical study. Presented at the America Asso. of Sex Educators, Counselors and Therapists. Honolulu, HI, Oct. 16–20.
13. McGuire, E. (1983) Personal Communication. August.
14. Reitman, R. (1983) Home computers in self-help sex therapy for male psychological impotence. Presented at the American Asso. of Sex Educators, Counselors and Therapists. Honolulu, HI, Oct. 16–20.
15. Siroky, M. (1983) Libido and Sexuality: Endocrinologist aspects. Presented at the 78th American Urological Asso. Meeting, Las Vegas, NE. April 17–21.
16. Tanagho, E. (1983) The role of electrostimulation in neurogenic bladder rehabilitation. Presented at the 29th American Paraplegia Society Meeting, Las Vegas, NE. Aug. 22–24.
17. Utamsing-Lacoste, de C. and Holloway, R. L. (1982) Sexual dimorphism. Science. **216**, 1431–1432.
18. Whipple, B., Ladas, A. K., and Perry, J. D. (1982) The G spot and other recent discoveries in human sexuality. (Holt, Rinehart and Winston, New York).
19. Whipple, B. and Perry, J. D. (1981) Pelvic muscle strength of female ejaculators: Evidence in support of a new theory of orgasm. *J. Sex Research.* **17**, 22–39.
20. Why we do — what we do. (1977) *Reader's Digest* E. Thompson, ed. **3**, 183–185 (1977).
21. Leyson, J. F. (1988) Sex Odyssey 2001. Presented at the Annual Meeting of the Asso. of the Phil Physicians in America. Long Beach, CA July 26–31.
22. Leyson, J. F. and Sporer, A. (1986) *Hormonal Changes in Spinal Cord Patients Post-Trauma*. Unpublished data.
23. Waynberg, J. (1986) Personal communications.

24. Lipman, A. (1987) Drugs affecting oral contraceptives efficay. *Modern Med.* **55**, 189–190.
25. AIDS TODAY (AIDS Report) 1989 Infections Disease Today. 1:14 Jan.
26. Jaroff, L., Garelik, G., Nash, M., Woodbury, R. (1988) Space: Onward to Mars. **132**, 46–53 July 18 TIME magazine.

Women should wear loose-fitting cotton undergarments and diet in low simple carbohydrates to reduce groin irritation and yeast growth. For dry introitus use K-Y jelly or Replens.

35

Controversies and Research in Male Sexuality

J. F. J. Leyson

Introduction

This last chapter will try to present recent research findings and address controversial ideas/subjects in the understanding of the neurophysiology of erection and the sexual dysfunctions/diseases that plague the SCI man.

Mating and sexual activity are phylogenetically among the oldest and most important functions in animals and humans both for procreative and hedonistic reasons (*22*). Since the beginning of recorded history, men have sexosociologically dominated women. The previous chapters have indicated that for SCI men with reflexogenic or normal erections, the man-on-top (missionary) position during sexual celebrations may be preferable because it can help keep penile tumescence sustainable. On the other hand, for SCI men with chemoerections and penile prostheses, the woman-on-top position is better than the missionary position for it fulfills two purposes: first, it minimizes premature ejaculatory accidents; and second, it makes the woman or sexual partner pleasurably happy by (giving the partner full control of penile thrusting and possibly also prove stimulating to the G-spot). However, in a nonsexually liberated couple, the woman-on-top sexual position may threaten a man's macho self-image (*1*). If the patient has a conservative sexual attitude, his sexual problems will be aggravated by this apparently submissive posturing. As a result, counselling should be directed toward reducing the stressfulness of sexual encounters of such men. On an entirely different topic, it has recently been found that quadriparetics, or patients

Sexual Rehabilitation of the Spinal-Cord-Injured Patient
Edited by J.F. Leyson, © 1990 The Humana Press, Inc.

who complain of inadequate pleasureable embrace because of the loss of hand grasp (pinch), can be helped by tendon-finger transfer(s) or transplant(s) from flexer/extensor forearm tendons. With revived control of finger pinch or motion, these patients will find that their experience of genital sexual stimulation or sensual touching (feathering) will be greatly enhanced (*35*).

Cerebral–Spinal Sexual Response Circuitry

The sexual-cycle response pattern in humans is stereotypical and primarily viewed as reflexive in nature (*1,22*). However, recent data have revealed that sexual activity is a multisynaptic phenomenon involving anatomic, neurophysiologic, and neurohormonal mechanism (*43*). The limbic system—phylogenetically, the oldest part of the brain (*47*)—appears to contain most of the pleasure or hedonistic centers and, in turn, is integrated by several relay systems with the cortical and subcortical areas (*22*). These relay systems (circuitry) can be activated by the animal itself in the self-stimulation paradigm (*34*). There are at least 45 possible sites of erection zones occurring as far forward as the gyrus rectus of the frontal lobe (*12*), and including the medial forebrain bundle (MFB), which has been found to mediate copulatory behavior in rats (*37*). MacLean believes that the main effector pathway for the control of the sexual function starts from the MFB, goes to the ventral tegmental area, and turns toward substantia nigra, pons, and medulla (*30*). It is also theorized that the pons may contain detrusor central reflex mediator centers (*24*) and that morning erections in the presence of a full urinary bladder are not just coincidental, as Karacan has suggested (*19*), but a neurotransmitter overlapping phenomenon of a primitive involuntary reflex (vegetative) response. Furthermore, MacLean et al. reported that the pons–medullary areas are indirectly involved in sexual activity (*31*).

Thus, we wonder whether the changes in respiratory pattern during sexual celebration (coitus) result from a generalized sympathetic response, or a participation of the pons–medullary–limbic circuitry and its pleasure relay systems. As one quadriplegic on a respiratory (phrenic nerve) pacemaker points out, he needs more power (an increase in radiofrequency wave transmission impulses) to activate and maintain 'hyperrespiration' during sexual activity. This observation is clinically relevant in advising phrenic-nerve pacemaker patients to check the batteries before contemplating any sexual celebrations.

In the amphibia, the mating call and its recognition initiate copulatory behavior (*39*). In humans, on the other hand, the evolutionary shift from acoustic stimulation to distinct vocalization (spoken language) is equally important in sexual initiation. Is it, therefore, feasible to utilize ultrasonic devices to stimulate sexual arousal (in addition to tactile stimuli), if sensory perception is present, in quadriplegics who are blind and/or aphasic because of cerebral vascular insults or associated trauma?

Hemodynamics (Vascular) Mechanism(s) of Erection

Recent evidence revealed that an erection is the result of increased arterial perfusion of the deep penile dorsal (profunda) arteries as the primary event (*29,43*). There are several theories of the vascular mechanism of erection describing the shunting of blood through some unclear complex mechanism(s) in the flaccid state and "closure" of the shunts with diversion of the blood into the cavernous spaces during the erect state. Ercolani in 1869 and subsequently Conti in 1952 described muscular "polsters" or von Ebner's pads acting as valve-like structures (*6*) to shunt the blood flow inside the vascular systems, including the arteriovenous shunts, depending upon the type of stimuli. However, Deysach in 1939 was unable to confirm the presence of these "cushion-like pads" (*9*). Furthermore, Benson et al. concluded that the "polster-like structures" are simply the earliest manifestation of atherosclerosis occurring at branch points of the vessels (*2*) without any neurophysiologic supporting structures or innervation (*3*). In addition to the complex microvascular and neurologic arrangement of the penile arterial tree, the cavernous trabeculae are said to be lined with complex endothelial structures containing a wide array of component collagen and clusters of smooth muscles with somewhat random orientation (*43*). Wagner proposed that, in the flaccid state, these arterial cushions are contracted, resulting in an open arteriovenous A-V shunt, and the venous drainage is free (*46*). During the erect state, vessels that were previously tortuous, stretch out, and the arterial endothelial (smooth muscle) cushions relax, resulting in the closure of the A-V shunts and free (high-volume) passage of arterial blood into the cavernous spaces. The venous drainage is passively closed by the stretching of the tunica albuginea as the cavernous spaces fill up or expand (*46*).

Although controversy still exists regarding the process of erection, we propose a modified Wagner theory (*25*).

We suggest that there are five (5) major phases of erection: (1) detumescence (flaccidity); (2) latency (initial filling); (3) tumescence (initial phase of venous occlusion; (4) full erection, and (5) rigidity (*50,83*).

Phase I: Detumescence (flaccidity) is characterized by a rapid increase of venous drainage along with a gradual decrease in arterial flow until it reaches to its basal intracavernous pressure (*50*) and serves the metabolic nutritional needs of the penile tissues. Presumably this is the result of contracture of the arteriolar and cavernous smooth muscles by prejunctional (peripheral nerves) and postjunctional (local) activation of a predominantly alpha$_2$-adrenergic neuroreceptor, norepinephrine. This phenomenon is proven by the antagonistc action of alpha$_2$-adrenergic blockers, i.e., phenoxybenzamine and phentolamine that causes smooth muscle relaxation and produces penile erection (*83*).

Phase 2: The stage of latency is designated when the arteriolar blood flow peaks and the intracavernous pressure begins to rise (*50*). This is believed to be caused by the initial reactivation of beta$_2$-adrenergic and cholinergic receptors* (*43*), causing smooth muscle/sinusoidal relaxations. This event is also reinforced by a prostanoid receptor, prostaglandin E_1 (PGE_1) (*16,51*), and the cerebral–sensual feeling with local effects of dehydrotestosterone (DHT) (*33*). Meanwhile, there is a central (cerebral–spinal cord) blockade of both pre- and postjunctional suppression or release of norepinephrine.

Phase 3: Tumescence is characterized by a reduction of internal pudendal arterial flow and increasing intracavernous pressure (*50*). This stage signals the beginning of the venous occlusion that is believed to be the action of the neuroreceptors in phase 2, plus the direct cavernosal smooth muscle relaxation by PGE_2 (*51*), vasoactive intestinal polypeptide (VIP) (*16,43*), peptidergic neuropeptide Y (*43*), and prostacyclin (*52*).

Phase 4: Full erection denotes a new blood inflow/outflow equilibrium in which there is a maximal increase in venous outflow resistance in the face of arteriolar dilation (*50*). This phenomenon is caused by the continual activation of receptors in phase 2 and 3, plus the release of other vasoactive energy-rich phosphate compounds that in turn releases a cascade of neuroreactions, i.e., cyclic adenosine monophosphate (AMP) and adenosine triphosphate (*83*). PGE_2 has been reported as a sensory neurotransmitter that enhances penile skin erotic sensation with substance P, a noncholinergic and non-adrenergic sensory neuropeptide receptor that may be responsible for reflexogenic/stimulative erections in SCI men (*16,53*). VIP is also believed to help sustain the full erection to final phase of rigidity to orgasm (*16,43,83*).

*Ed note: Acetylcholine (neuromodulator) is released from the helicine art./trabecular endothelial (Weibel-Palade bodies) cells.

With the engorgement of the cavernous sinusoids, a subalbugineal venous plexus is compressed beneath an unyielding tunica and the perforating veins are obstructed, resulting in the final phase of erection.

Phase 5: Rigidity. Phases 4 and 5 can be artificially induced by chemoinjections (pharmacological chemoerections) and direct pudendal nerve stimulation, causing contraction of the ischiocavernousus muscles (*50*). During this phase, there is maximal participation of the cerebrospinal cord neuroreceptors—relay systems with a release of additional receptors or transmitters in Phase 3 and 4, plus a prostanoid, prostaglandin F_2 alpha (PGF_2). This prostanoid PGF_2 alpha can initiate ischiocavernosus muscle contraction, contract venous smooth muscles, and also trigger further catecholamine release (*52,83*). All these actions cause maximum veno-occlusive effect and in conjunction with genitopelvic muscle contractions will be experienced as a normal orgasmic psychic-musculogenital response. After orgasm, a resolution phase of detumescence follows with reactivation or release of pre- and postjunctional norepinephrine neuroreceptors. The basal stage is maintained until a sensual/erotic or stimulative/reflexogenic erection process is once again initiated. Beta-endorphins and enkephalin (pentapeptides), which are naturally occurring opiates, are not involved in (cerebral) erection *per se*, but are probably released from other limbic relay systems that may be responsible for the postcoital exhilaration or pain relief experienced by some arthritic patients (*22,25*). Cerebrally released prostacyclin may be the neurohormone that reduces systolic blood pressure in hypertensive patients post-orgasm (*25*). Therefore, it is logical to assume that a true aphrodisiac or an erection drug should have four components, i.e., dopaminergic-prostaglandic, adrenergic-cholinergic, and peptidergic in order to be effective (*25*). The diagram (Fig. 1) illustrates the interaction between central and peripheral neurotransmitters that initiates the complex process of erection.

To recapitulate, detumescence is an active state in which the endothelial cells, acting in unison, are stretched (contracted) and/or flattened, resulting in a wide (open) intraarterial (A-V shunt) lumen (Fig. 2A). The tumescence phase is a passive state in which cells that are normally robust protrude, producing a partial obstruction or temporary impedance to intraluminal flow (Fig. 2B). Thus, a high volume of blood is retained in the cavernous spaces (*25*). Furthermore, the neurophysiologic control of the penile venous system may be under separate (probably local) control, which is reciprocal to the detumescence–states of the erectile tissues, demonstrating the presence of reflexogenic or stimulative erections in SCI patients. This tends to support the theory that a tense or anxious man will have difficulty in initiating an erection

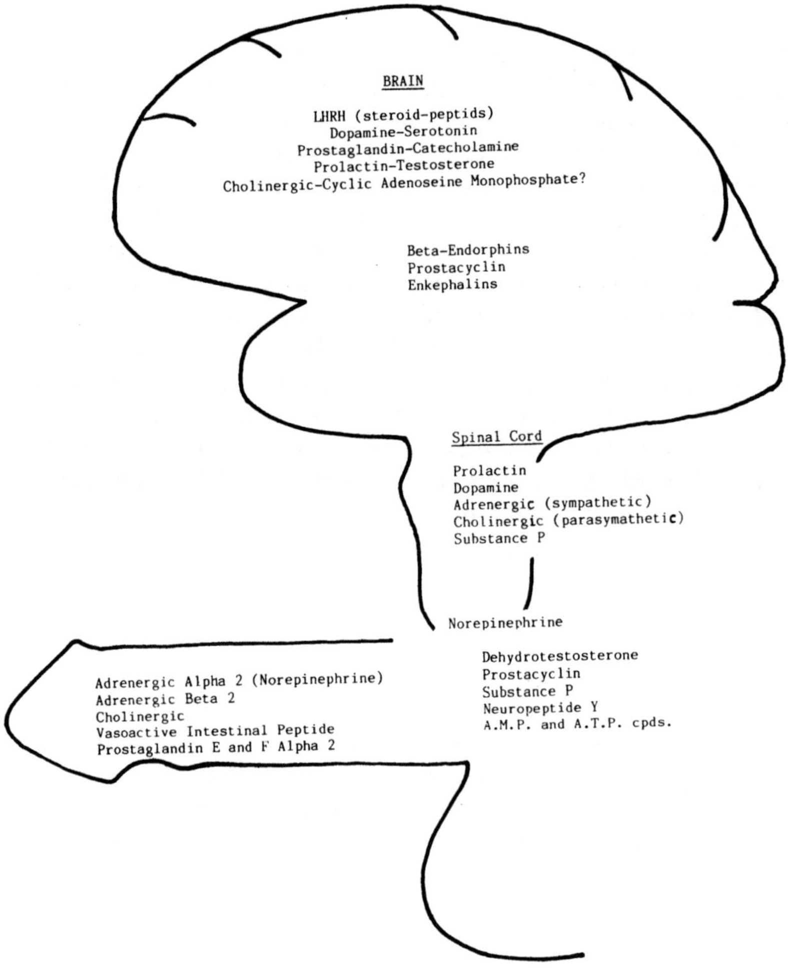

Fig. 1. The multitude of cerebrospinal and peripheral (target organ) neuroreceptor–relay systems participating in the process of erectile function: LHRH, luteinizing-hormone releasing hormone; energy-rich phosphate compounds: AMP, adenosine monophosphate and ATP, adenoseine triphosphate.

because of the hyperactivity of norepinephrine (A-V shunt open), while a relax state triggers the opposite response, causing the shunt to be closed, resulting in the desired penile rigidity.

Types of Erections

Subconscious (Basal) Erections

The phenomenon of erection is observable in both the subconscious and conscious states. Subconscious (basal) erections or nocturnal penile

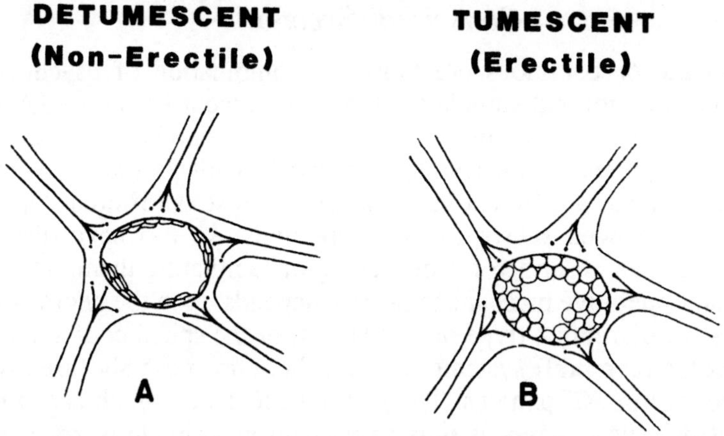

Fig. 2A. Schematic representation of one of the lumen of the cavernous trabeculae with (smooth muscle lining) endothelial cells contracting or thinned out along the basal layer. (Staining may not demonstrate these specialized cells since, during preparation, the collapsed cell walls may adhere to each other or to the basal layer in which these structures are found as one instead of several components).

Fig. 2B. The epitheloid cells reacting in unison are in their static or relaxed state producing a valve-like effect in the intraarterial or A–V shunt luminal flow.

tumescnce (NPT) usually occur during sleep; 63% are associated with rapid eye movements (REM) and the rest (37%) are associated with the non-REM phase (*20*). Karacan suggested that nocturnal erections fluctuate between 5 and 12 times in infants and young children as a physiological way of training the sexual function of the penis (*21*). As the male matures to a fully functioning sexual adult (who now controls and programs his sexual activity), his ''nocturnal'' erections normally stabilize at 3–4 times per night (*20,26*). These basal erections are usually influenced by the type of sleep—i.e., the sleeper's dream content, emotional status, and length of sleep (*25,26*). Our clinical studies have shown that, in normal patients nocturnal erections are reduced when the subject has a ''poor night's sleep'' (*25*). This type of erection is probably mediated by two different facilitatory and inhibitory pathways (*19*). Because nocturnal penile tumescence occurs when the human organism is in its basal state, it is appropriately called *vegetative erection*. Though the secretion of testosterone exhibits diurnal variation, with higher concentrations in the morning (*45*), its role in the producing the morning (wake) erection is unknown. Subconscious erections are probably caused by an internal biological (sexual) clock that primes the erection neuroreceptor circuitry in preparation for the ultimate conscious sexual response or activity.

Conscious Erections

Awake or conscious erection is a combination of psychogenic (neuroendocrine) and stimulative types. As recent literature denotes, the whole concept of purely psychogenic or purely reflex erectile mechanism(s) can be misleading in non-SCI patients (*43*). However, in SCI patients, a different situation exists. Just as different types of stimuli have been shown to elicit erections, so too have different pathways been described for producing or facilitating them. The predominant operative mechanism largely depends upon the degree of intactness or disruption (type of SCI lesion) of the spinal cord and other neurologic (cerebral) systems. Hence, there are possibly three types of erections in SCI patients. The *psychogenic type*, which is centrally mediated, usually happens in patients with incomplete or recovering lesions. The *stimulative type* occurs when the genitals are directly stimulated. Van Arsdalen et al. described this erection in normal persons as reflexogenic (*43*). The pathways are believed to be mediated by somatic fibers via the pudendal nerve transmitting the afferent impulses, whereas the efferent arm is subserved by the parasympathetic outflow located both in the S_2–S_4 cord segments (*25,43*). The *reflexogenic* type is unique in the SCI patients. This type of erection is initiated by stimulating parts of the body other than the genitalia (usually below the level of the cord lesion). The trigger impulses are probably carried by both the cutaneous afferent and efferent nerves of the (abdominal segments) sympathetic pathways (in the absence of complete destruction of the sacral cord) and by the pelvic parasympathetic components (*43*). It is therefore believed that all four (basal and awake) subtypes of erections constitute a normal penile tumescence, and can occur in SCI patients with incomplete or recovering lesions. It is interesting to note that there is no direct correlation between types of erection, level of lesion, sex dreams, bulbocavernosus reflex, and NPTR recordings.

Diagnostic Evaluation for Erectile Dysfunction

Nocturnal penile tumescence (NPT) monitoring devices have until now been considered by several investigators as the most useful adjunctive tool in the differential diagnosis of impotence (*15,43*), including that of SCI men (*26*). However, one drawback of this diagnostic aid is its inability to measure penile rigidity (*44,46*). Although the majority of erections in SCI men are either absent or fleeting (reflexogenic type), there are a few cases with incomplete or recovered cord injuries who complain only of soft erections (tumescence only, but no rigidity). In order to objectively assess penile axial rigidity, a monitor measuring both nocturnal penile tumescence and rigidity (NPTR) has been devised (*54*). There are two major kinds of ambulatory rigidity and tumescence systems: (1) Rigi-Scan (Fig. 3A); and (2) ART-1000 (Fig. 3B). Both NPTR monitoring devices have two major components: (1) an outpatient (ambulatory) penile tumescence and rigidity data-logging unit; and (2) a printer or a microcomputer for processing and printing the data. NPTR can be measured by application of two (penile base and corona) loops. The data revealed that in normal males penile rigidity was observed to rise more rapidly than tumescence. In the impotent males the tracings showed a reduction in the height and duration of rigidity and tumescence (Fig. 4) (*54*). The normal reading for rigidity is 500 g and for tumescence is 1.5 cm in height for a duration of 27–32 min. A comparative study between the two NPTR monitors reveal the significant differences as follows below:

Trade name	Sensory type	Portability	Wake-up alarm	Price, $
Rigi-Scan[a]	Active	Bulkier	None	10,000*
ART-1000[b]	Passive	Less bulky	Present	6500

[a](Rigi-Scan) Dacomed Corporation, Minneapolis, MN 55420.
[b](ART-1000) Surgitek, Racine, WI 53404.

The charts of both NPTR monitors are similiar. The "wake-up alarm" of the Surgitek ART-1000 monitor (ambulatory rigidity tumescence) enables the patient to wake-up and observe his own erection if present when the alarm sounds.

The application of laser technology to medicine has opened new vistas in the diagnostic armanentarium for impotence. However, a study by Cahill et al. (*58*) comparing laser Doppler and ultrasonic conventional Duplex Doppler penile vascular flowmetry and dynamic capillaroscopy showed no significant difference in its diagnostic value.

In non-SCI men with associated pelvic or genital vascular trauma, Abber et al. have shown that the best office screening technique for the differential diagnosis of vascular impotence is intracorporeal injection of papaverine (60 mg, in 20 mL of normal saline), compared to NPTR and penile brachial index readings (*59*).

Our clinical experience for the last 4 yr has also confirmed the value of this pharmacological testing. However, we utilized a lesser dose of

*Ed note: A portable type and a cheaper model is now available.

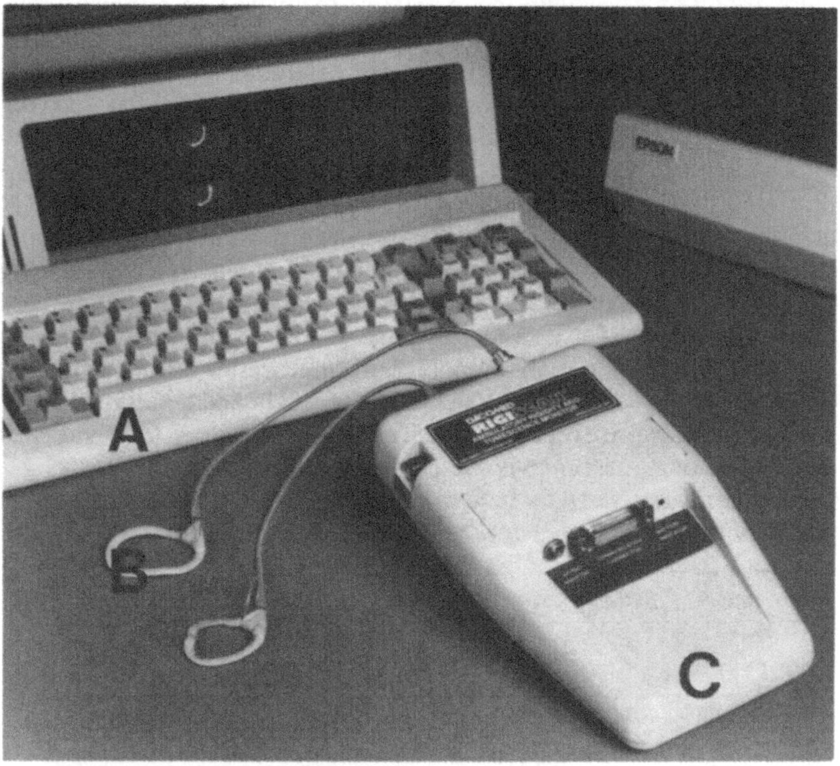

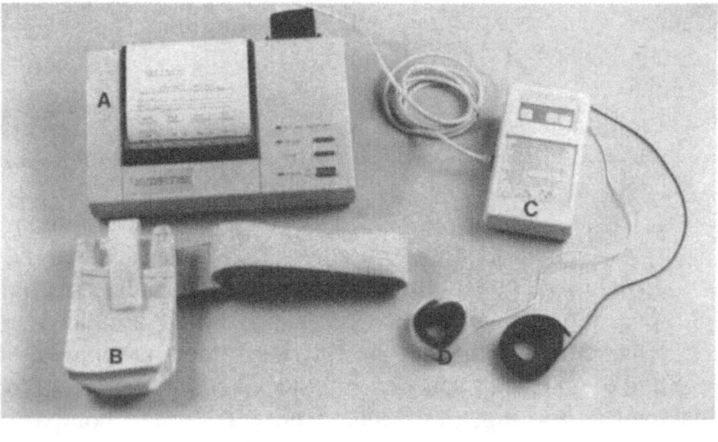

Fig. 3A. Portable penile tumescence and rigidity monitors: (A) printer and logging unit; (B) sensor loop, and (C) RigiScan.

Fig. 3B. ART-1000: (A) printer, (B) patient belt with a pocket for the monitor, (C) NPTR monitor, and (D) sensor loop.

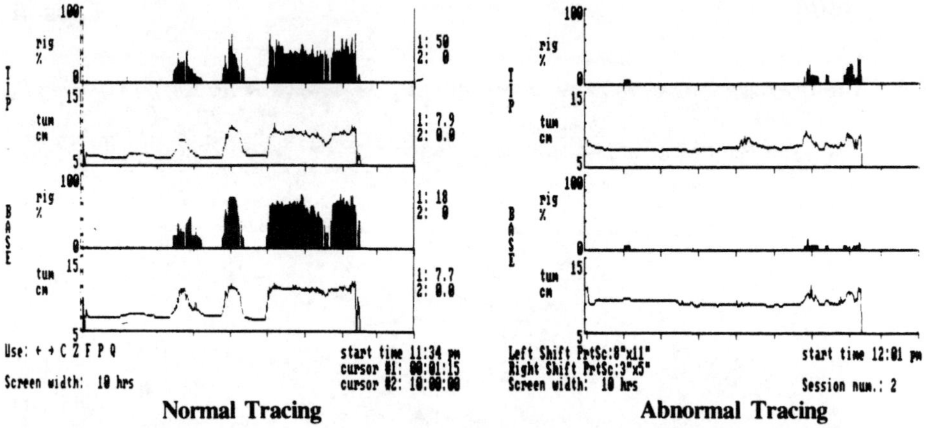

Fig. 4. NPTR tracings with normal and abnormal results. Rig.: rigidity; tum.: tumescence.

papaverine • HCl at 15 mg, and added reflexogenic stimulation (i.e., a rubbing of the scrotum, thighs, and/or suprapubic areas).

On the other hand, Wespes et al. suggested utilization of the "erectile angle" as an objective criterion to evaluate the papaverine test in impotence (*60*). The "erectile angle" is the angle (vertical axis) between the penis and the legs with the patient in standing position (equal to zero at flaccidity), which is measured before and after chemoerection (injections of papaverine). Their data revealed that, in non-SCI patients whose erectile angle is approximately 90 degrees or more, there are no vascular lesions, while those with less than 60 degree angles had evidence of vascular insufficiency. However, we must remember that in SCI patients, the paralysis prevents the subject from standing, let alone contracting their buttocks to evaluate the upward movement of the erect penis. Thus, the so-called "erectile angle" test for vascular penile integrity in SCI men is impractical.

In order to accurately diagnose correctable arterial perfusion pressure and/or venous penile pathology in young SCI men with incomplete or recovered spinal cord lesions, the use of papaverine dynamic infusion cavernosometry and cavernosography (DICC) is suggested (Fig. 5). DICC is an objective test used to quantify or record intracorporeal arterial inflow and veno-occlusive hemodynamic parameters during penile erection. The DICC procedure can determine the following three parameters: (1) equilibrium of corporal body pressure; (2) rate of fall of corporal body pressure from a control pressure over a defined-duration period; and (3) cavernosal artery systolic-occlusive pressure* (*82*) including corpora-cavernosographical readouts at a predetermined cor-

*Ed note: Abnormal occlusion pressure gradients as 20 mm Hg or more.

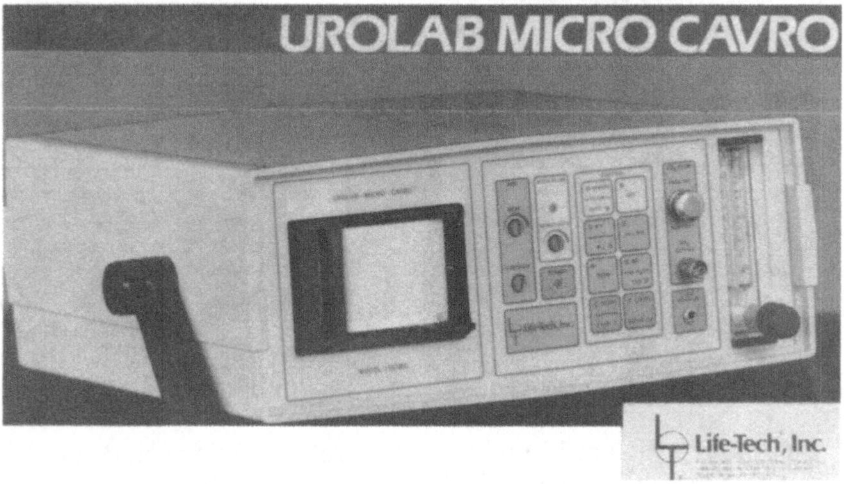

Fig. 5. Model 1151 MC Dynamic Infusion Cavernosometer with tracing paper. This monitor is used to quantify the corporal arterial inflow and venous outflow during erection.

poral penile pressure. The normal (baseline) values for cavernosometry are still controversal. It is proposed that it takes about 60–80 mL/min arterial flow (latent phase) to initiate tumescence and 100–150 mL/min flow rate to maintain rigidity for 20–30 s for a normal erection. Any deviation from these values denote arterial or venous insufficiency. However, intracorporal pressure decay (drainage cavernosography) is more accurate in detecting veno-occlusive corporal pressure defects or venous leakage. Because the majority of SCI impotence is neurogenic, the diagnostic value of DICC is limited (Fig. 6). The three diagnostic criteria of corporovenous leakage (CVL) noted in cavernosometry: 1) F_1—Normal, rigidity with a flow requirement (FR) less than 60 mL/min.; 2) F_2—Moderate CVL, rigidity with a FR greater than 60 mL/min.; 3) F_3—Severe CVL, inability to produce normal rigidity regardless of FR volume of fluid infused. Fig. 6A—Summary of diagnostic steps/therapies.

Contemporary Management of Impotence

The recent therapeutic management of erectile dysfunction is divided into five main categories:

(1) External assistive and mechanical (cylinder/ring) erection suction or occlusive devices.

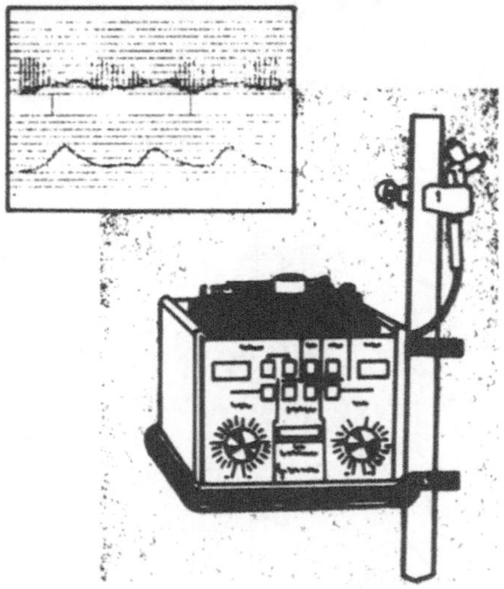

Fig. 6. Cavropump 1721 with a normal tracing (above). This monitor enables the diagnostician to perform the DICC procedure with safety and efficiency. It has also a digital readout display.

(2) Surgical: open and closed (percutaneous) vascular recanalization and implantation of penile prostheses
(3) Medical: transdermal, oral, and intrapenile injections (chemoerection) Hormonal therapy is discussed elsewhere.
(4) Electrical stimulations: vibratory genital or rectal, dermatome (segmental), or peripheral transcutaneous and direct nerve trunk/fiber or spinal cord segment
(5) Nerve fiber or trunk transplantation (for cerebral or head trauma-fetal brain or adrenal cells transplantations).

Assistive (Dildo and/or Strut) and Vacuum Constriction Devices

There are few "safe" penile external assistive and erection (suction) initiating devices that are helpful to SCI men with soft or reflexogenic erections. Aside from a dildo, a strut (Fig. 7A,B) can be used to cradle a somewhat pliant penis to aid in penetration. However, some women may complain of slight discomfort from the device (penile splint). In order to avoid such problems, we have designed a prototype for a modified "dildo" erection pneumatic device. The exposed glans penis is gently grasped by the Erecto-Aid (Fig. 8), and the erection is maintained by pumped (trapped) air inside the inner pneumatic lining splint.

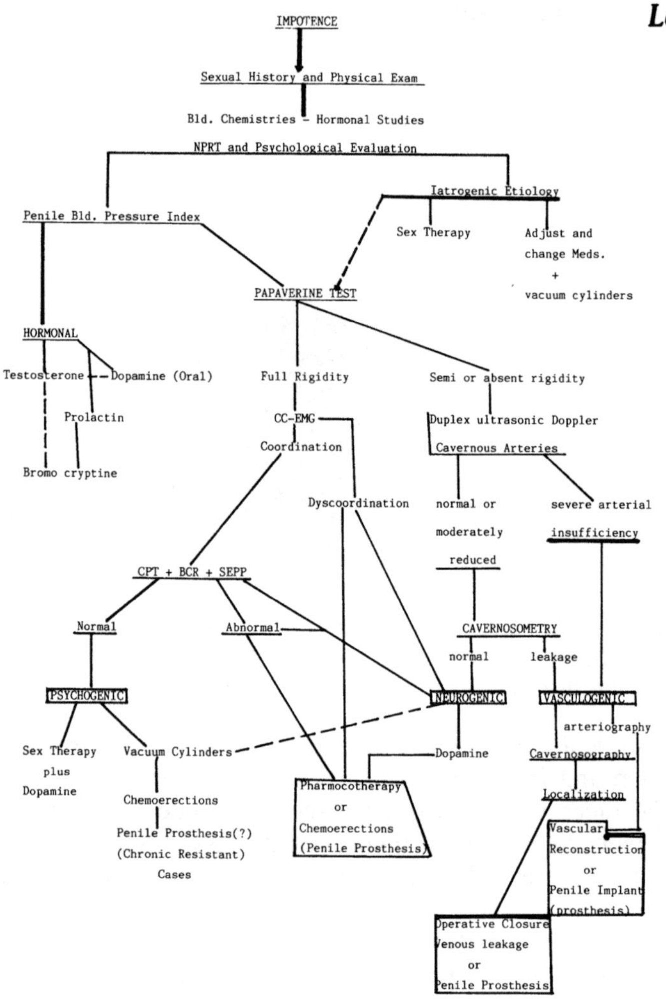

Fig. 6A. Schematic summary flow diagram of the full diagnostic battery of tests and treatment options.
Legends: CC-EMG—cavernosal corporal electromyography, CPT—cavernosal-pudendal transmission/latency test, BCR—bulbocavernosus reflex and SEPP—somatosensory evoked pudendal potentials.

The smoothed edges of the device around the glans penis will slide into a lubricated vaginal introitus with ease (*83*).

A temporary occlusive device to trap the blood in an partially erect penis is the so-called Revive system.* The Revive system consists of triple latex rings (of different diameters), a spring-pin locked cone applicator, and a sleeve. The Revive ring is applied to the base of the

*Revive System Corp., Lake Geneva, WI 53140.

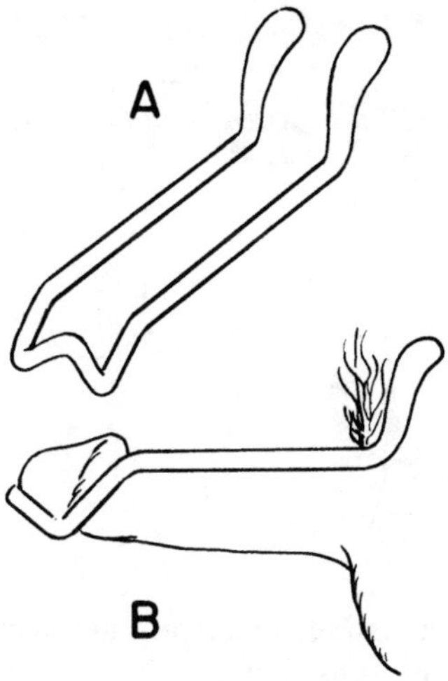

Fig. 7. (A) Empty penile splint; (B) strut cradling the semi-rigid penis.

penis with the sleeve/cone applicator after a reflexogenic erection is achieved (either by stimulation or massaging the blood from the pelvic, rectal, and scrotum regions). The Revive system is ideal for incomplete paraplegics. The ring must be left at the penile base for at least thirty minutes to avoid avascular necrosis. For those SCI men with normal ejaculation, the ring must be removed at the onset of the pre-ejaculatory sensations. Furthermore, the revive ring should also be put on the penis vertically, so that the top loop stimulates the women's clitoris making sexual activity more pleasurable.

If the patient has difficulty initiating a stimulative and reflexogenic erection, a modified dildo with suction tubing to create a vacuum for erection is suggested. This device is called the Correctaid Synergist Erection System* (Fig. 9) and is usually effective in incomplete paraplegics. However, the device (with its thinned-out tip for extra sensitivity) is not recommended for patients with poor penile sensation because erotic feeling on the glans penis will totally obliterated.

The two most popular non-invasive mechanical devices used for impotence based on the concept of blood entrapment in the penis following vacuum assisted tumescence are: Osbon Erec-Aid System† (Fig. 10) and Response (Fig. 11). The Osbon Erec-Aid System consists of a vacuum cylinder that fits over a flaccid penis; its suction effect produces an engorgement. The base of the cylinder has also an "insert"

*Smith-Collins Pharmaceutical Inc., 889 S. Matlack St., West Chester, PA 19382.
†Nu-Potent, Inc., Box 1478, Augusta, GA 30903.

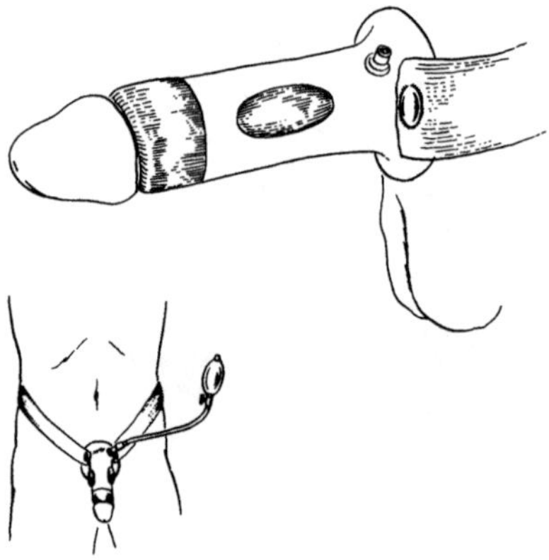

Fig. 8. This erection assistive device provides a cushioned rigidity while preserving the penile glans' sensitivity.

to make the aperture narrower or fit better for a smaller penis. In order to create a tight sealing surface rim between the base of the cylinder and the penile base, a thin coat of K-Y jelly should be applied inside the insert or cylinder's basal rim. The pubic hair should be parted before placing the cylinder firmly down against the penile base. After the penis is erect by blood entrapment, the constriction band is transferred from the cylinder to the base of the penis (Fig. 12). Once the pressure is equalized within, the cylinder is removed from the erect penis. Constriction bands should not be left on the penis for more than 30 min, and both devices require a functional hand.

On the other hand, the Response Suction Erection* device has a different vacuum pump handle (Fig. 11), and with only one type or size of constriction band. Both vacuum constriction devices cost from $390–$420 per set. Witherington has studied 1700 Erec-Aid users with mixed types of impotence, and claimed 92% achieved erection with 69% overall sexual satisfaction (*62*), with 37% penile ecchymosis and pain as the major complications. The author evaluated 75 SCI men (25 complete quads; 40 complete and 10 incomplete paras) utilizing the (Osbon) Erec-Aid system. The results showed that 50% of the complete paras, 80% of the incomplete paras, and 80% of complete quads had erections, with 72% experiencing sexual satisfaction (*53*). Complications were minor, i.e., 1% penile ecchymosis. For patients with recovered or incomplete lesions who experienced obstructed or painful ejaculation, a quick release-type of constriction band is suggested. Relative contraindication for these devices include patients on anticoagulants and

*Ed note: The "touch" type of RESPONSE device is ideal for quadriplegics, while a quadriplegic can use the POS-T-VAC device with or without assistance. (POS-T-VAC Inc., Dodge City, KA 67801).

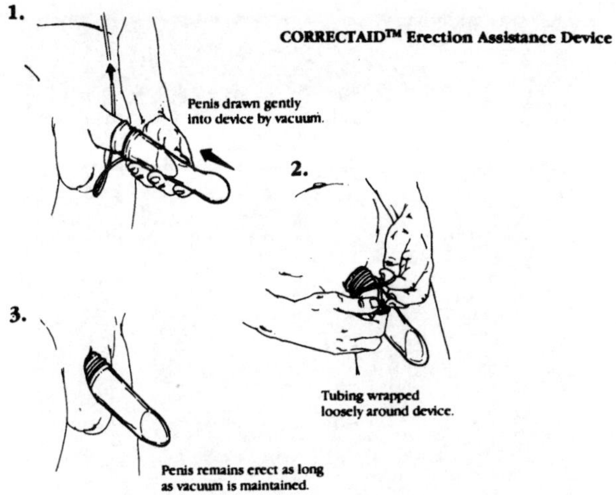

Fig. 9. Another option for an impotence corrective device is the Correct-aid. The vacuum (step 1) is created by suction with the mouth, while the device is applied around the penis. The tip of the correctaid is thin for extra sensitivity. This device is highly effective in incomplete lesions and those with low quadriplegia with residual hand function.

those with severe blood dyscrasias. In AIDS infected SCI men without additional cerebrospinal (peripheral neuropathy) involvement, the use of vacuum erection devices is a viable therapeutic option (Fig. 12A,B).

Surgical Therapy

As previously stated, the incidence of vascular causes of erectile insufficiency in SCI men is low, that open surgical arterial bypass and venous ligation are of limited use. However, with the development of fiberoptic Laser "Probe," 3–5% of stenotic arterial penile pathology can be corrected by percutaneous transluminal laser or balloon angioplasty (*67*). But studies and data from SCI patients with long-term followup results are not yet available for proper evaluation. Furthermore, open surgical venous ligation or percutaneous venous occlusion with "spring embolus catheters" for venous leakage or insufficiency is still controversial for SCI-impotent men (*68*). Nevertheless, one must be cautious about utilizing penile vascular recanalization surgery in SCI men, because the effects of the impaired autonomic and peripheral nervous system in these patients' vascular penile system are still not fully understood.

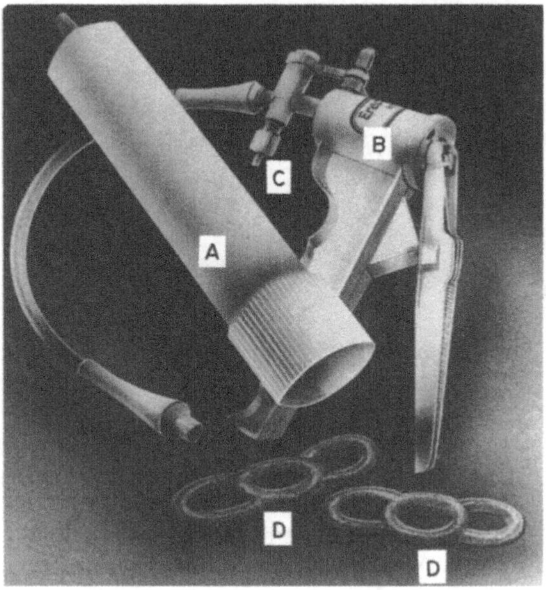

Fig. 10. ErecAid Impotence device with: A, vacuum cylinder; B, Vac-U-Pump; C, release valve; and D, constriction band(s).

Penile Bones and Sex (Penile) Prostheses

Quadrupeds (dogs) and some aquatic mammals (whales) have penile bones. In addition, male dogs have a more efficient penile vascular (venous) system, in that the glans penis swells (forming into a bulb) as a locked-in mechanism to keep the penis intravaginally, until reflexogenic ejaculation ensues. Most canine animals have normally retractile penises resulting from penile retractile muscles (*43*) and when nonerect, the penis is canceled subcutaneously. In biped mammals (man), the penis can sometimes be viewed as an oversized skin appendage. Penile bones in humans exist only in pathologic states termed *os penis*. Of all reported cases of *os penis*, none were found among SCI patients (*25*). Even if a man had penile bones, this would not assure effective post-SCI erections because, following cord trauma, most bones below the level of lesions undergo resorption as a result of post-SCI abnormal vascular exchange mechanism(s). With the introduction of internal penile (solid and inflatable) prostheses, an erect penis can be surgically fashioned. A majority of patients favor the cancelable type of prosthesis. In order to minimize the mechanical failure rate, recent models

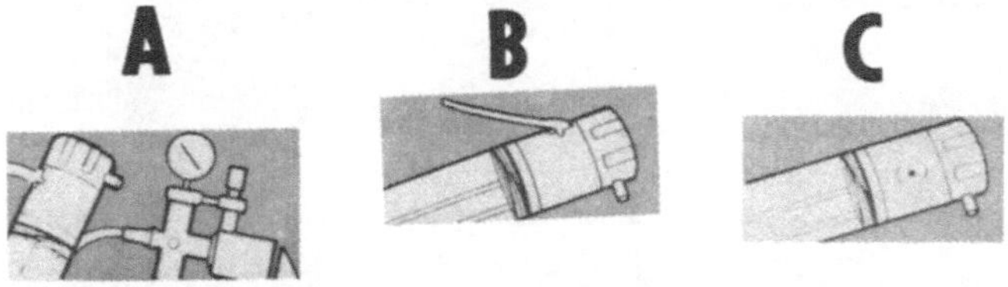

Fig. 11. Response* (standard) is another type of a vacuum-constriction device in which the mechanism to create a vacuum is by a pump, piston or touch trigger. (Inset: Three types of Response Systems) A, Piston type—used for patients who need a high rate of vacuum; B, Standard system—for controlled vacuum rise, safety, and ease of use; C, Touch rechargeable—is designed for the patient that has difficulty managing the manual pump (battery-powered).

*Courtesy from Mentor Corp., Minneapolis, MN 55411.

of the (extrapenile-contained) inflatable type have been designed with fewer accessory parts (*40*). Furthermore, the latest model (which is near ideal) is an inflatable prosthesis in which all the parts are housed inside the penis itself (*14*). There are two types of self-intrapenile-contained† inflatable prostheses: (1) Hydroflex made by American Medical (Fig. 12) Systems; (2) Flexiflate designed by Surgitek-Medical Engineering Corporation (Fig. 12F). The design and clinical advantages of the Hydroflex prostheses have been discussed in the previous chapter. The Flexiflate has a few special features compared to the Hydroflex type; its gridded tail is more flexible and bends downward, resulting in better urinary condom drainage. Furthermore, a quadriplegic man with a single functioning arm and a moderately strong pinch (plus a bending motion) can deflate the erected penile prostheses. On the other, the Hydroflex needs two functioning hands with a firm grip simultanteously to inflate or deflate the prostheses. Future developments should include a miniaturized microchip sensitive pressure value or "electronic device" specific to "some" pressure, so that just a gentle touch by a quandriplegic hand can activate the prostheses to inflation or deflation (Fig. 13). However, coital motion should not influence the status of the value/pressure device. Lewis and coworkers at Tulane University (Urology) and at the Delta Regional Primate Research Center in Louisiana are initiating a clinical trial of an external penile prosthesis. It is not a dildo

†Dynaflex (Am. Med. Systems)-type may be ideal for quads, for it can be easily deflated by one hand or by simply bending it for 10 s and releasing.

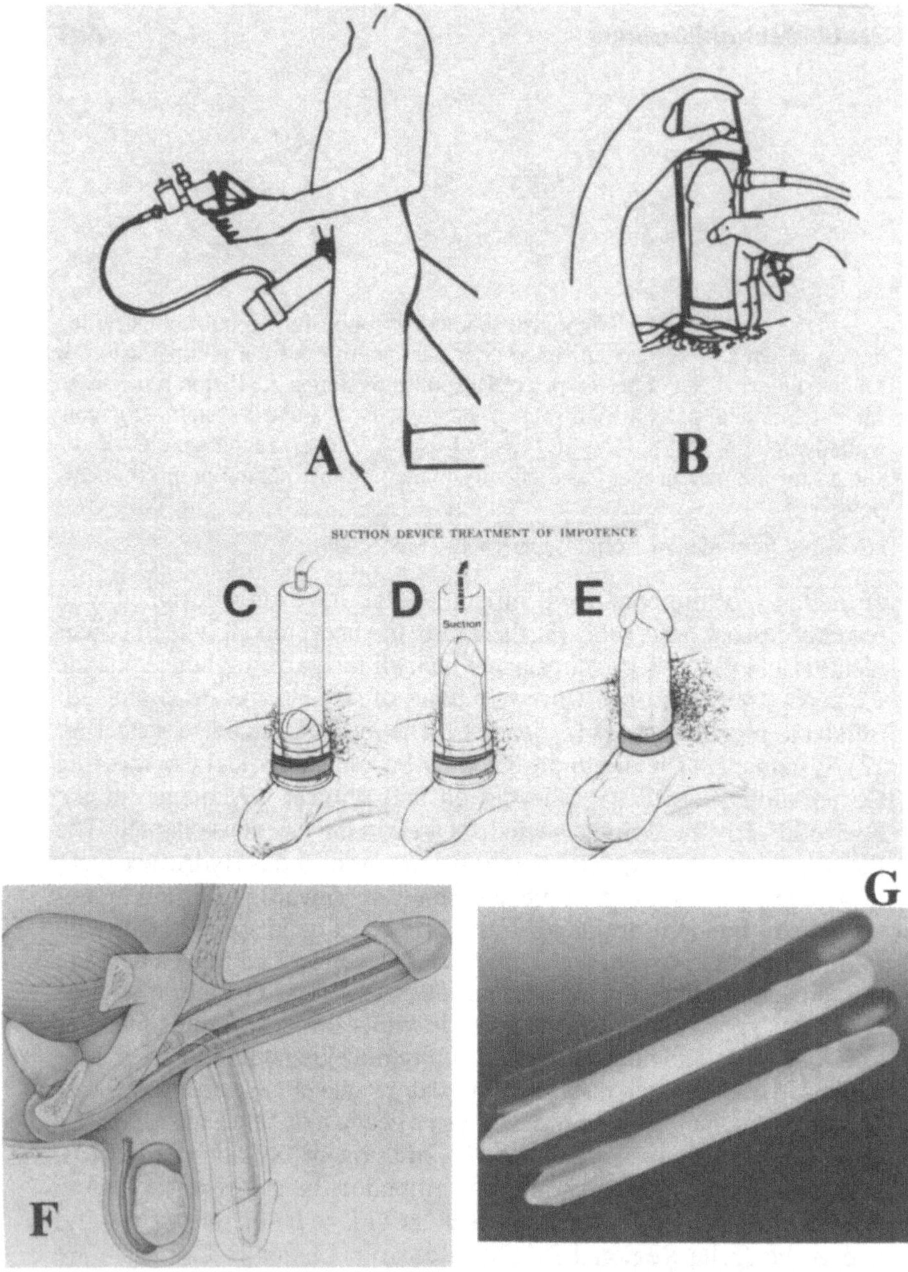

Fig. 12A. A monoparetic male gradually engorges the penis (while standing against a wall, table, or lying down) by a vacuum pump manually. B, the constriction band is slipped into the base of the penis to maintain the penile tumescence for up to 30–45 min. C & D & E, the sequence of events in the mechanical erection of the penis. Self-contained penile prostheses.

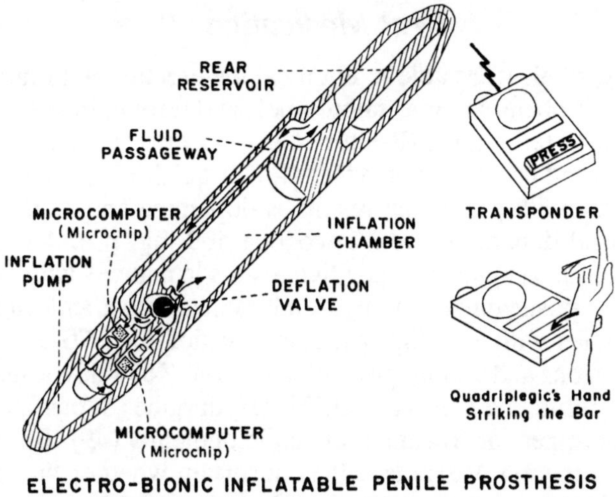

Fig. 13. A self-contained microchip bionic sex prosthesis that can be activated by a sonic beam via a transponder. The prosthesis is implanted in such a way that the portion that houses the inflation pump is located anteriorly (towards the glans penis).

(coitus assistive device), but a sex prosthesis implanted extracorporeally in a distal penile pouch, created with the existing penile skin and done as a minor operation. The possible danger with this kind of prosthesis is development of penile skin pressure necrosis with a tightly applied uridom (urinary condom).

Medical Therapy

Transcutaneous (Transdermal) Agents

There is mounting clinical evidence that although the coronary and penile arteries are of the same caliber, their vascular neuroreceptors are different. Thus, these particular arterial systems respond differently even when challenged by the same vasodilators (*83*). The author clinically tried the use of oral peripheral and cerebral vasodilators to treat SCI impotence and found these medications to be ineffective (*56*). Transcutaneous penile application of coronary vasodilators (nitroglycerine patch and prostaglandin E_1 solution) demonstrated no erection, though with the nitropatch, the patients experienced a feeling of warmth and occasional headaches (*55*).

Oral Medications

Domer, et al. were able to elicit canine erection with intravenous injection with phentolamine, salbutomol, and terbutaline (*10*). Our initial study with terbutaline (Brethine-beta$_2$-adrenergic stimulant) given orally, produced no erection in either para or quadriplegic men. Another possible drug with promising results is dopamine and its derivatives. Although oral dopamine (i.e., Levodopa 500 mg, p.o. 4 times/d for 2–3 mo) produced up to 80% positive results in patients with peripheral neuropathy, postsympathectomy, and radical proctocolectomy, our clinical studies with SCI (80) patients revealed only 70% seen in incomplete lesions and young quadriplegics (*61*). Zoler advocated the use of dihydroergotoxine mesylate (DEM) (Hydergine, dopamine agonist) as brain energizer for treatment of senile dementia (*49*). But no effect on erectile function was noted. It is uncertain whether this drug will be appropriate therapeutic option in elderly demented patients with impotence and recovering SCI lesions, but without other associated diseases.

Our comparative clinical study in 100 SCI men of 10 oral medications included: bethanechol, dopamine, genito-urinary irritant-gingseng, imipramine, terbutaline, theophylline, phenoxybenzamine, phentolamine, verapanil and yohimbine (Table 1), has demonstrated that dopamine-like drugs produced the most effective result at 55–60% after 6–8 wk of therapy. Yohimbine provided 25–30% response, while the other drugs produced insignificant therapeutic effects (*57*). Levodopa (dopaminergic agonist) was given in 500 mg doses p.o. 3 times/d for 4–5 d (to minimize nausea) and gradually increased up to 5 times/d for 3–4 mo. After 2 mo, the Levodopa dose should be reduced to a maintenance dose of 500 mg p.o. 3 times/d and discontinued at 4 mo. Levodopa therapy should have 2-wk rest periods and be resumed on a 4–6-wk cycle. It is theorized that oral Levodopa is absorbed in the bloodstream and degraded to norepinephrine by an enzyme (beta-decarboxylase) present both in the bloodstream and sympathetic ganglions. The extra quantity of pre and post-junctional released norepinephrine reinforces neurotransmission of sensual impulses and enhances the effects of catecholamines (veno-occlusive smooth muscle contractions) triggered by PGF$_2$-alpha during phase 5 in the erection cycle (*50*). The most common clinical side effects of dopamine derivatives (Sinemet and Carbidopa) are nausea, dizziness, and palpitations with or without headaches. Chronic use of dopamine derivatives without 2-wk rest periods and adequate followup can lead to depression and even psychotic complications. Because of impurities present

Table 1
Oral Vasoactive Medications
(Degrees of Erection: +1 to +5)

Drug	Mechanism of action	Effects	Duration
Bethanechol chloride	Cholinergic stimulant weak vasodilator	Elongation: +1	Avg. 1/4 h
Dopamine (Levo-dopa)	$Alpha_2$-adrenergic stimulant/peripheral and renal vasodilator	Erection: +4	Avg. 30–45 min
"Gingseng" cola	$Alpha_2$-adrenergic blocker (cardiotoxic?)	Elongation: +1	Avg. 1/4 h
Imipramine·HCl	$Alpha_1$-adrenergic blocker cerebral anticholinergic	None	None
Terbutaline	$Beta_2$-adrenergic stimulator weak vasodilator	Elongation: +1	Avg. 1/4 h
Theophylline	Smooth muscle relaxant weak vasodilator	None	None
Phenoxy-benzamine	$Alpha_2$-adrenergic (long-acting dilator)	Elongation: +1	Avg. 1/2 h
Phentolamine	$Alpha_2$-adrenergic (short-acting dilator)	Elongation: +1	Avg. 1/2 h
Verapamil	Calcium channel blocker	None	None
Yohimbine	$Alpha_2$-adrenergic blocker cholinergic stimulant	Erection: +2	Avg. 1/3 h

in these drugs (Sinemet and Carbidopa), it is suggested that Levodopa (more pure composition) is the drug of choice for oral treatment of neurogenic impotence in SCI men. Dopamine derivatives given orally also provided some return of the absent sensual penile sensation or enhance erotic dermal feelings in patients with impaired genital sensations (*56*).

Chemoerections (Intrapenile Drug Injections)

Virag reported a 50% improvement of organically non-SCI impotent men after an intrapenile (cavernous) injection of 80 mg of the smooth muscle relaxant, papaverine (*45*). Furthermore, Brinkley introduced phenoxybenzamine (Dibenzyline) intracavernosally and produced erections in 90% in organically non-SCI impotent patients (*4*). Our initial comparative study of ten (10) erectiogenic drugs using local neuroreceptive and vasoactive agents involved seventy-five (75) SCI subjects with

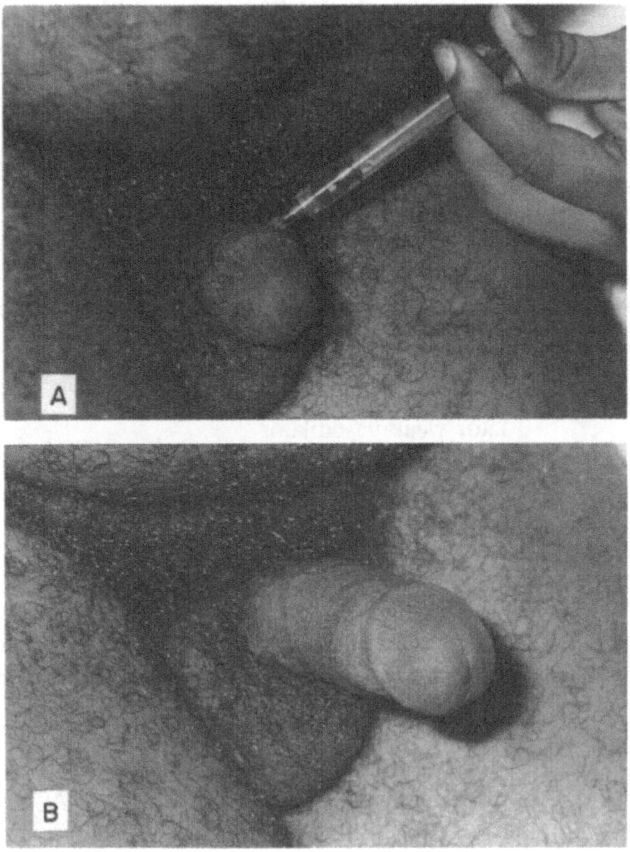

Fig. 14A. A paraplegic self-administering the erectogenic (chemical prosthesis) drug; B, penile erection 10–15 min postinjection.

possible pharmacodynamics are summarized in Table 2 (*57*). Bethanechol and theophylline (aminophylline) did not produce any erections beyond penile elongation.

Although phenoxybenzamine and phentolamine resulted in 95–98% erection rate, only papaverine produced well-sustained erections for five patients up to 6–8 h post-injection. Papaverine and phenoxybenzamine were effective in all types of SCI lesions, including those with associated peripheral vascular insufficiency (Fig. 14A,B). On the other hand, phentolamine was ineffective in patients with associated peripheral neuropathy. The vasoactive agents should be injected with a 26 or 28 gage

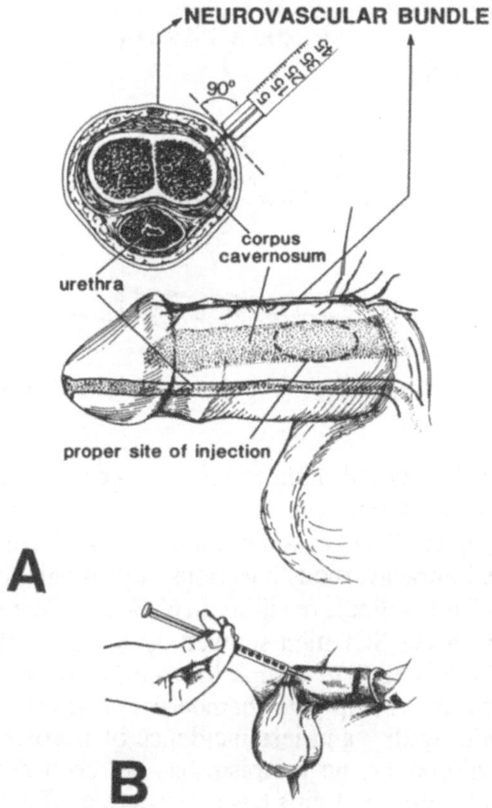

Fig. 15A. Penile topography, showing the ideal site for chemoerection; B, injection technique (with permission).

needle, an inch from the penile base on one of the lateral sides, avoiding the neurovascular bundle and urethra (Fig. 15A,B). The needle should be injected at least ¾–1 in. in depth to penetrate beyond Buck's fascia and prevent subcutaneous edema (Fig. 16). Before the drug injection, make sure to aspirate some blood to insure that the needle is in the corpora. It is also advised that these chemical penile prostheses (chemoerections) not be administered more than twice a week to reduce the risk of cavernous infection and fibrosis (*66*). Papaverine, a phosphodiesterase inhibitor, causes an increase in the level of energy-rich phosphate, cyclic adenosine monophosphate, which results in both central penile arteriolar and corporeal sinusoidal smooth muscle relaxation. Although this drug has been the most effect agent for chemoerections, its acidity (pH 3.2) and local toxic effect can lead to fibrosis of the cor-

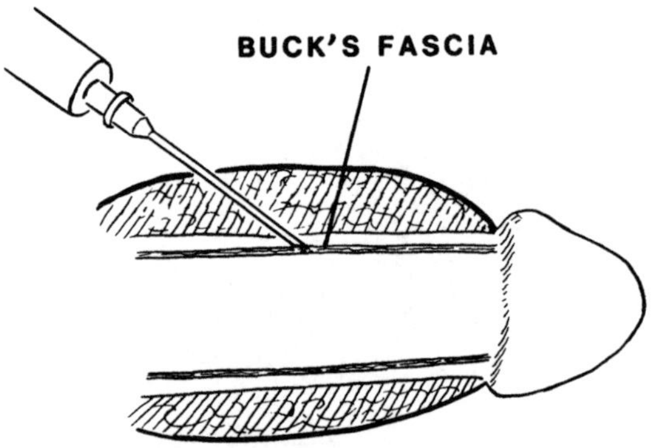

Fig. 16. Improper drug penile injection, resulting in edematous or swollen (but not erect) penis.

poreal tissue. Thus, several authors have suggested other chemicals (drugs) as therapeutic alternatives. Roy et al. advocated the use of vasoactive intestinal peptide (VIP) at 400 pmol/dose (*64*). Furthermore, Ishii et al. administered intracavernous injections of prostagladin E_1 at 20–25 mg (dissolved in 5 mL saline), resulting in 62% complete erection (*63*). Our initial study in ten SCI men showed up to 75% effectiveness.

Prostaglandin E_1 (PGE_1)* is superior to PGE_2 or papaverine in its use as a diagnostic and therapeutic chemoerection agent because it provides better penile rigidity and less incidence of fibrosis or corporeal scar formation; moreover, no priapism has yet been reported. PGE_1 also metabolizes locally, and thus has no systemic effects or reactions (*63*). Papaverine alone or in combination with other agents can cause chemically induced priapism. This local side effect is more hazardous to the SCI man because the majority of them have no penile pain or sensation. Thus, priapism can lead to fibrosis and even corporeal infection or abscess. To avoid this complication, the patient must be advised to report to the physician if an erection is sustained for more than 3 h so that appropriate therapeutic intervention can be administered. Leyson and Sayer et al. reported dopamine and epinephrine as drugs used intracorporeally to treat pharmacologically induced priapism (*57,65*). However, it is interesting to note that there are four drugs we used to detumesce, a rigid penis; recent data reveal that phenylephedrine is the safest of all chemicals (*see* Table 2, bottom), because it has the fewest systemic side effects (*82*). It is hoped that, in the future, micropore skin patches with VIP or PGE_1 and other erectiogenic drugs can be applied at the penile base to initiate or enhance a reflexogenic erection.

*Ed note: Prostin VR at 10 μg, 20, and 30 μg/mL strength. I prefer to use 20 μg at 1–1.5 mL. (Upjohn Co.).

Table 2. Intracorporeal Drug Injections (Chemical Penile Prostheses)

Drug	Mechanism of action	Effects	Duration
Papaverine*	Direct smooth muscle relaxant	Erection: +5	Avg. 2 h
Phenoxy-benzamine	$Alpha_2$-adrenergic blocker (indirect) vasodilation	Erection: +3	Avg. 1 h
Phentolamine	$Alpha_2$-adrenergic blocker (indirect)	Erection: +4	Avg. 1½ h
Bethanechol	Cholinergic stimulant (vasodilation) weak	Elongation: +1	Avg. 1 h
Theophylline	Smooth muscle relaxant (weak)	Elongation: +1	Avg. 1½ h
Terbutaline	B_2-adrenergic stimulators (vasodilation) weak	Elongation: +1	Avg. 1 h
Verapamil	Calcium entry channel blocker (vasodilation) weak	Elongation: +1	Avg. 1 h
Prostaglandin E series	Prostaglandin receptors (vasodilation) weak	Erection/ tumescence: +3	Avg. 2 h
Imipramine	$Alpha_1$-adrenergic blocker and anti-cholinergic (weak)	(Soft erection) tumescence: +2	Avg. ¼ h
Thymoxamine	(Corporal) smooth musculature relaxant? (weak dilation)	(Soft erection) elongation: +1	Avg. ½ h

Intrapenile drugs used to treat pharmacologically induced priapism:

A. Epinephrine diluted to 1 mL in 1000 mL normal saline solution
B. Phenylephedrine diluted to 10 mL in 500 mL normal saline solution
C. Metaraminol diluted to 1 mL in 4 mL normal saline solution
D. Dopamine undiluted at 40 mg per mL. Average volume per therapy: 1.0 mL.

*The majority of SCI men required a higher dose (i.e., 60 mg papaverine) for a longer and "rigid" erection in order to achieve a much "delayed" orgasmic response.

Although chemoerection therapy is absolutely contraindicated in patients† with blood dyscrasias, our clinical study of five SCI men on therapeutic anticoagulation did not show any penile bruising or ecchymosis. Therefore, it is advisable to apply finger pressure on the site of injection for 2 min and complete 3 min for men on anticoagulation therapy.

†Subcutaneous apomorphine can cause erection, but it has several side effects.

With the introduction of controlled-drug implantable delivery systems for some metabolic disease, i.e., diabetes mellitus, Leyson suggested an implantable drug delivery system (DDS) (*82*). This self-sealing device is composed of two upper and lower components (Fig. 17A,B). The upper cylinder will contain the erectiogenic drug and the lower will have the anticoagulant, in order to maintain a patent delivery tube. The patient or sexual partner can press the subcutaneously implanted DDS 15–20 min before sexual celebrations. This therapeutic modality will prevent penile edema, infection, and other complications when intracorporeal chemoerections are periodically repeated. The subcutaneous reservoir can be refilled once every 4–6 wk.

Vibro-Electrical Stimulations

Vibratory, Transcutaneous Nerve (TNS) Dermatome, and Transrectal Stimulations

Mounting behavior in male primates and the sexual-act response cycle is a sensitive hormone reflex response to tactile stimulation (*22*). Does the absence of sensory and vibratory input below the level of the lesion (i.e., in the genital area) contribute to the aggravation of erectile failure in SCI men? Edwards and Husted have demonstrated a correlation between the penile threshold for vibration and the coital frequency pattern (*13*) Herman also claimed that decreasing libido in paraplegics was probably the result of the loss of afferent input from the penile skin and other dermatomes (*18*). Recently, Meyer et al. applied vibratory stimuli (60 cps) to impotent non-SCI patients. The results revealed that patients who responded (by an increase in penile circumference) to vibratory stimuli displayed stronger erectile activity in comparison to those who had only spontaneous nocturnal erections (*32*). However, our clinical study demonstrated that, when transcutaneous neurostimulation (TNS) was applied to the penis, there was no erection beyond some insignificant penile elongation in 10 paraplegics and 5 quadriplegic (*69*). These patients also complained that their orgasmic ejaculations were less pleasurable because of traumatic postgenitalia anesthesia. Newman and Northup applied electromechanical stimulation to impotent paraplegics and were unsuccessful in inducing erection (*33*). Furthermore, a new vibrator (the Vibrector) has shown promising results both in impotence and for electro-ejaculation (Fig. 18).

Another noninvasive electro-erection technique utilizes the transrectal approach (the Biosonics Male Electric Genital Stimulator—MEGS).* Levin et al. inserted MEGS, an electrode-bearing glove that

*Biosonics Inc., Philadelphia, PA.

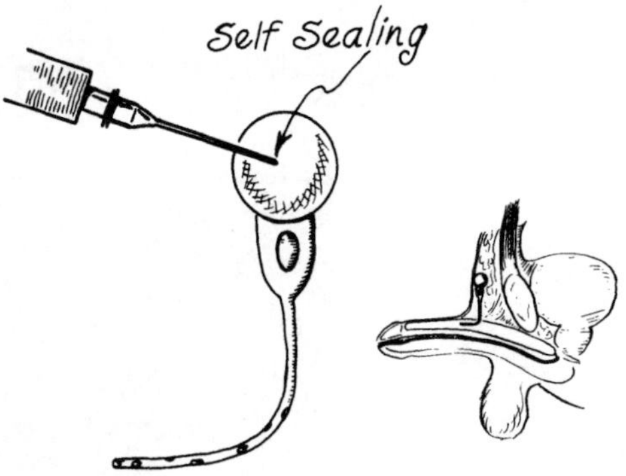

Fig. 17A. Implantable inert pouch for intermittent drug delivery; B, sagital section of the male pelvis with the implanted drug delivery system.

delivers an average of 10.5 V intrarectally, into macaca monkeys, resulting in erection (*71*). In human application, the electrical impulses are controlled by a short-range, low-power transmitter. However, this erection inducing technique has not yet been used in a significant number of SCI men. The concern is that transrectal electro-erection might cause dyasthesias and musculoskeletal spasms in quadriplegics, because the stimulation seems to be less specific and, therefore, erratic. Theoretically, this form of electro-erection will be ineffective in men with complete sacral cord injury.

Direct Erection (Pudendal/Cavernous) Nerves and Spinal Cord Center Stimulations

Experimental data have shown that indirect (transurethral) electrostimulation of the *nervi erigentes* of dogs results in erection (*70*). Furthermore, Leu et al. had successfully elicited erection in monkeys with electrostimulation of the cavernous nerve and a possible implantation of "erection pacemaker" (*29*). Our recent initial clinical data have demonstrated the feasibility of direct (percutaneous) needle stimulations of the corpus-cavernosa nerve (Fig. 19), resulting in few seconds of erection. However, in order to be more effective, refinements of the above technique should include the following: utilization of a wavelike pattern of electrical impulses, not a galvanic (or pulsating) burst of impulses; higher voltage stimulations; and a larger point-of-contact

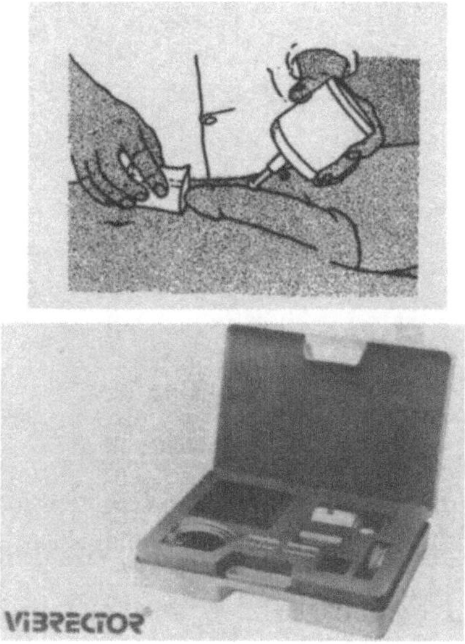

Fig. 18. Another possible erection and/or electro-ejaculation inducer would be a device using mechanical vibrations at 80–100 Hz. Ejaculation can occur in patients with high lesions even in the absence of erection.

area between the electrode and the cavernous nerve(s). Because of the difficulty of isolating the male cavernous nerve, pelvic (*43*) or pudendal nerve stimulation can be tried to produce erection (Fig. 20). It is hoped that this type of bionic sex therapy (the erection pacemaker) can be perfected in the near future and, similarly, that sophisticated intraoperative techniques to identify and isolate the cavernous nerve will be developed (probably dorsal approach).

Direct stimulation of the spinal cord to elicit erection in impotent paralyzed men is a technique still in its infancy. Khan and Choi controlled the uninhibited detrusor contractions in a post-liminectomy patient by inserting acupuncture needles in the L4 nerve root dermatome, but no erection was observed (*23*). However, electrostimulation of the ventral nerve roots (*41*) of S2-S4 has produced detrusor contractions and erections in 50% of SCI patients (*40*). With the increasing effectiveness of pain treatment by dorsal column spinal cord stimulators, it is hoped that future electrobionic S2 stimulators will be designed that specifically stimulate the spinal erection center and/or the nerve roots that may modulate or elicit erection(s). The ultimate bionic device should be equipped with at least three microcomputer channel options that will

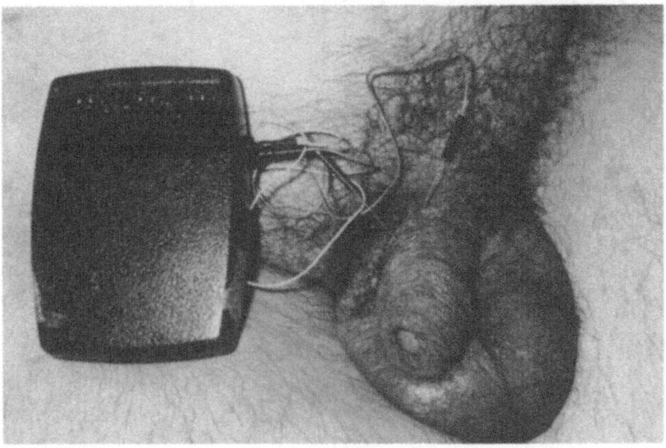

Fig. 19. A percutaneous needle placement can be reinserted to locate a maximum point of contact. The TNS personal pocket stimulator is used to deliver 10 milliohms of a pulsating electrostimulus for up to 30 min.

permit a patient to elicit voiding, pain relief, and erection at appropriate times by just a gentle touch of a button or sensor.

Cellular Surgery and Nerve Transplantation

Carlsson and Sundin have reported a restoration of the micturition reflex following anastomosis of normal T12 nerve roots with ventral and dorsal roots of S2 and S3 in sacral cord paraplegics (*5*). Although a return of penile skin sensitivity was also noted, there was no documentation of erection. The success of this operative nerve reconnection procedure may also be enhanced when nerve growth factors are isolated and become available for clinical use in conjunction with cellular microsurgery of the spinal cord and its nerve roots (*8*).

Contemporary Diagnosis and Management of Ejaculatory Dysfunctions and Infertility

Retrograde emissions and/or (absent) non-ejaculations are most probably the result of the disruption of the central (corticospinal) pathways and the peripheral (sympathetic) autonomic nervous system and decreased testicular volume (T_{12}). In some SCI lesions, both the orgasm and projectile ejaculation are preserved, although the emission disorder can be traced back to damaged sympathetic nervous pathways. However,

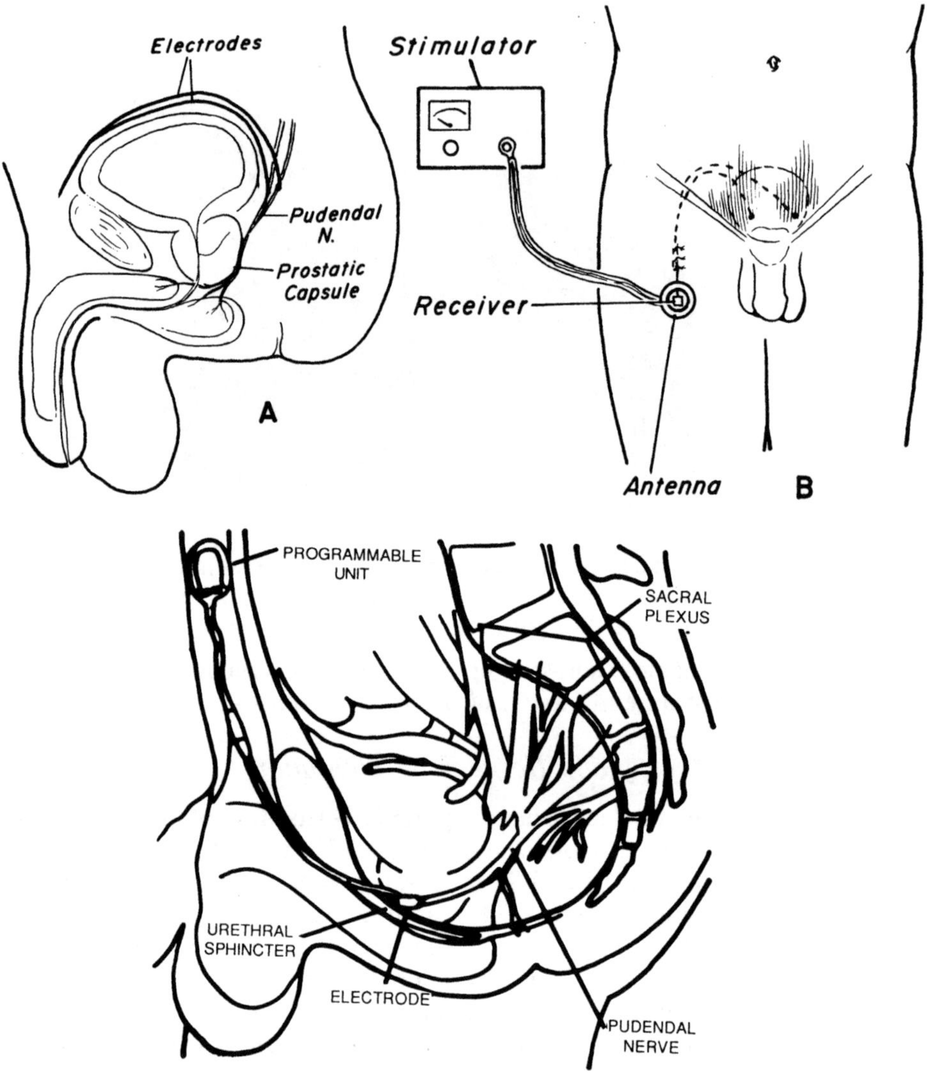

Fig. 20. Dual stimulating electrodes cuffed around the pudendal nerves along their courses down to the pelvic region and to one of terminating cavernous nerve(s) branches. B, Schematic drawing of an entire erection pacemaker setup. The stimulating electrodes' receiver is brought out from behind the urinary bladder subcutaneously either at the midthigh or suprapubically. Radiofrequency signals are picked up by the receiver via a pliable antenna pasted on the skin. The power signals of the stimulator (which can be miniaturized or pocket-sized must not interfere with the wavelengths of other pacemakers (cardiac, respiratory, and urinary bladder) that may be present in the body.

there is no clinically objective technique available to assess a sympathetic function for sexual and ejaculatory potency. Recently, Park et al. have developed a noninvasive electrophysiological test to estimate the sympathetic nervous system response to ejaculatory function (*72*). This test consists of recording sympathetic skin response, palmar and plantar-penile dorsal nerve stimulation, and bulbocavernosus reflex. Their data revealed that patients with normal ejaculation showed a plantar sympathetic skin response and those without this response lacked ejaculation or were nonejaculators (*72*). Sympathetic skin response can also be utilized to monitor treatment efficacy for ejaculatory dysfunction. The conventional therapy for retrograde ejaculations has been discussed in an earlier chapter. However, there are several medical management alternatives for reversing retrograde ejaculation: alpha$_2$-symphathomimetic drugs, i.e., Dimetapp, Extentabs, Ornade, and Sudafed (*42*). However, our clinical experience has shown that only ephedrine sulfate is 50–60% effective in higher doses (50 mg orally every 6–8 h/d). Pudendal nerve block is another alternative in preventing retrograde ejaculation during electroejaculation (*36*). Intrathecal injection of neostigmine to induce erection and ejaculation may precipitate autonomic dysreflexia in high cervical lesions (*17*). Aside from a 3-d pre-neostigmine-injection, treatment with oral Dibenzyline (40 mg/d) for three days is suggested.

Lipshultz et al. recommends nitroprusside intravenously; this is titrated with a computer and arterial pressure monitoring to manage drug-induced autonomic dysreflexia (*27*).

Subcutaneous injection of 0.2 mg of physotigmine and 40 mg of N-butylhyoscine have enhanced ejaculation, especially in patients with sparing of T_{12}.

In order to achieve maximum sperm motility, the urine pH should be above 7.0 and urine osmolarity be adjusted between 200 and 300 mOsm/kg water by dydrating the patient with an additional 500 mL of water 1 h before ejaculation. A catheterized urine/semen mixture may be certrifuged for 10 min at 2000–3000 rpm and the sperm pellet resuspended in a dextrose/Ringer's solution to a volume of 2–3 mL for sperm analysis (*42*).

The unexplained infertility of SCI men probably results from sperm autoimmunity and loss of cellular energy, as shown by a 20% motility rate measured for sperm recovered by electroejaculation (*36*). Cellular energy loss may occur because of cellular respiratory malfunction resulting from disruptions of the autonomic nervous system or from deficient neurotransmitter release of guanyl cyclase and alternations in adenosine triphosphate energy synthesis. Caffeine, a centrally acting stimulant, has been successfully used by Schoenfeld et al. to stimulate spermatozoal motility in non-SCI males; the drug was directly added to the semen sample (*38*). Our clinical experience with five paraplegics (taking caffeine orally at 2.0 g showed a 65% improvement of sperm motility after 12–14 d of therapy. However, other investigators are skeptical about its therapeutic effects. Dawson et al. reported that 1.0 g/d orally of ascorbic acid (vitamin C) has increased sperm vigor and enhanced fertility in non-SCI patients (*7*). Although in some SCI Centers, a number of patients are routinely given vitamin C to acidify their urine, no detailed study has been done regarding its effects on fertility.

Another pharmacological option to improve sperm motility is the oral intake of L-arginine tablets for 2 wk prior to sexual fertilization. This technique can be combined (with or without prior oral alkalinization) with intravaginal voiding fertilization or collection of a semen sample for artificial insemination. Our initial clinical study of the effects of adding a steroid to semen samples from non-SCI men revealed a 90% enhancement of sperm motility. However, our limited clinical trials of centrifuged mixed urine–semen samples from two paraplegics had shown 50% improvement. Future research will be geared toward studying the action of relaxin (a normal constituent of human sperm plasma) in SCI men. The study is intended to determine whether the addition of relaxin to the semen samples of SCI men with adequate sperm count will enhance sperm motility, since it has been proven to be effective in non-SCI men (*73*). In patients who occasionally ejaculate after alpha-adrenergic oral stimulations, future innovations may include the addition of oral prostaglandin-F_2-alpha, which contracts seminiferous tubules in rat testis, as a means of enhancing spermatozoal tubular transport and thus fertility (*74*).

In "non-ejaculatory" patients with incomplete SCI lesions, an allograft of tunica vaginalis as a sperm reservoir may be tried; periodic sperm harvest by needle aspiration would be used for artificial insemination. Since 1968, different artificial spermatoceles (alloplastic or with vena saphena) has produced a limited number of pregnancies, and recently this investigative work has been carried forward in SCI men in Canada and England.

Spermatozoal Antibodies

Witkin and Sonnabend have demonstrated that 56% (18 cases) of non-SCI homosexual men who swallowed the semen of their partners developed a humoral immune response to spermatozoa (*48*). From this datum, one can extrapolate that homosexual SCI patients who partake spermatozoa via their alimentary tract may possibly develop some form of infertility resulting from spermatozoal antibodies. Concern about the presence of the AIDS virus in the semen now precludes further studies in this area.

Acquired Immunodeficiency Syndrome (AIDS)

HISTORY. Human immunodeficiency virus (HIV-1) may have been affecting humans for more than 200 years, as suggested by Dr. S. Yokoyama (*76*). He believes that HIV-1 is a retrovirus related to lentiviruses found in sheep, goats, and horses that cause neurological damage and anemia. Furthermore, he pointed out that HIV-1 and the simian immunodeficiency virus (SIV) found in African green monkeys are quite similar. Whether SIV was passed to humans, where it mutated to become HIV (HIV-1), or vice versa, the precise nature of this transformation has not yet been clarified (*76*). However, the author believes that the SIV lentivirus may have been pased to humans during tribal ceremonies in either Africa or South America (Brazil) where the ritual passage to adulthood sometimes includes application of a monkey or farm animal's blood to fresh scarifications on the back of a boy or on the periumbilical areas of a girl. As these human carriers mature, the viruses might then have further mutated to HIV, which was then further passed into the western world either by sexual contact or by blood or blood-product contamination (*84*).

EPIDEMIOLOGY. The modern plague of acquired immunodeficiency syndrome (AIDS), caused by either the human immunodeficiency virus (HIV) or the human T-lymphocyte virus III, (lymphoadenopathy virus, HTLV-III/LAV), was first noted in the United States in 1978 (*75*). As of Oct. 1990, there were about 144,000 AIDS victims and over 65,000 deaths reported in USA. Worldwide, the incidence is about 192,000 cases (1990). It is projected that by 1992, there will be 365,000 AIDS victims in the USA and 6 million carriers; worldwide, there will be 500,000 cases and 5 million carriers. In 1998, there will be about 10 million cases, and by the year 2000, about 50 million cases, mostly in North America, Africa, and Brazil (*77*). By the 21st century, if no cure is discovered, it is projected there will be over 1.5 million Americans infected with the HIV virus. AIDS is no longer a disease confined to homosexual populations, but one that can infect anyone regardless of sexual orientation, race, or age. However, in the USA about 40% of all AIDS cases reported are found in blacks and hispanics (usually iv drug abusers) (*78*). Men constitute 80% of HIV sufferers (73% are homosexual or bisexual), women 16%, and children 4%.

Beyond homosexuality, predisposing factors include intravenous drug abuse, transfusions with contaminated blood or blood products, and HIV infected mothers. The incubation period of HIV infection/AIDS ranges from 30 mo to 5 yr, and perhaps as long as 12 yr. Approximately 20–50% of HIV positive individuals develop AIDS within 5 yr. Thereafter, the rate of HIV infected persons who progress to AIDS increases rapidly (*79*). The relative risk of contracting AIDS among those in the high risk group is 250/100,000, whereas among those not in a high risk group, it is 0.1/100,000. For those who practice safe sex, i.e., use condoms with a non-infected partner, the rate is estimated to be 1 in 50 million and without a condom to be 1 in 5 million.

Transmission

Heterosexual/Homosexual: There may be so-called "superinfectors," i.e, seropositive patients who are more infective than others. AIDS is a worldwide affliction with certain populations in Central Africa having the highest incidence—up to 15% testing positive for HIV antibodies. The modes of transmission are mainly through exchange of body fluids (vaginal and anal intercourse), contaminated needles, and blood products, but not casual body contact. AIDS contraction from prolonged (French) kissing is questionable. However, if there are open lesions on the oral, genital, or anal areas, kissing these areas may transfer the virus through the mucocutaneous portals such lesions afford. HIV infection is not now known to be transmitted via mosquitoes, food, water, toilets, swimming pools, sweat, tears, clothing, or telephones (*78*). The sociocultural and sexual attitudes of a country seem to determine the patterns of HIV infection (*79*):

Pattern I

North American, Europe, Australia and New Zealand: homosexual/bisexual men, iv drug abusers, and heterosexual spread.

Pattern II

Africa, Carribbean areas: blood/blood products, and heterosexual transmission

Pattern III

Asia and Middle East: Rare infection, but iv drug users and prostitutes are increasingly becoming the high-risk-group infectors. The following are the primary sources of HIV infection in humans: blood and blood products, semen, urine, cerebrospinal fluids, lymph node, brain, bone marrow, breast milk, and vaginal-anal secretions (*78*).

Virology

The HIV-1 virus is the form most commonly associated with AIDS in the US. As argued by other investigators and the author, HIV is believed to have been in humans for less than 100 years and is a recent zoonosis, not a mutant (*79*). HIV-2 virus is associated with AIDS, with one case reported in US, but is more prevalent in West Africa and in Europe. It is believed to be less virulent than HIV-1. HIV-3 is a newly described retrovirus and (HTLV-4) was recently isolated from a Nigerian patient with AIDS (*78*). The new classification system for HIV (AIDS) infection is:

NOMENCLATURE OF HIV DISEASE: NEW CDC CLASSIFICATION

Carrier	Group 2	Asymptomatic HIV seropositivity
ARC	Group 3	Lymphadenopathy
	Group 4 A	Constitutional disease
	Group 4 C2	Oral candidiasis Pulmonary tuberculosis Genital/oral herpes
	Group 4 E	Lymphoplasmocytic interstitial pneumonia
AIDS	Group 4 B	Neurological disease
	Group 4 C1	Opportunistic infections
	Group 4 D	Kaposi's sarcoma, lymphoma

HIV Testing (79)

Patient confidentiality must be guaranteed if voluntary testing is to be encouraged. Antidiscrimination laws should be passed to protect persons with AIDS and HIV-positive individuals. The most common screening methods used today are: (1) enzyme-linked immunosorbent assay (ELISA); (2) the Western blot test, which involves separation of protein components of the virus and exposure of these protein blots to test serum. Since up to 90% of initial positives by ELISA may be false, confirmation is done by Western blot analyses. Unfortunately, antibodies to HIV do not confer immunity or offer evidence of recovery from infection. ELISA/Western blot screening thus may not pick up all cases, since seroconversion can in some cases take several months. Polymerase chain reaction (PCR) analysis is particularly helpful for screening blood donors and babies born to HIV-positive mothers. This method makes use of DNA probes to identify miniscule amounts of HIV genetic material, and thus to ascertain a patient's HIV status. The HIV antigen test is useful in certain cases, especially in pediatric practice. For commercial or household use, the Recombigen test, a 3-min latex agglutination test for HIV antibody, is now available. However, this form of screening may yield more false positive, because of user error, and the individual may also lose confidentiality.

Drugs for HIV Infection

The Chinese have tried several plant extracts, but the only one that has yielded promising results to date is *Viola yedoensis.* Although the prognosis for AIDS is generally poor, Zidovudine (AZT-azidothymidine) or retrovir therapy has shown promising results in Group 3 and 4 and Subgroup C patients. Other drugs still in clinical trials are: DDI, GLQ223, Ganciclovir, and Ribavirin. Immunomodulators (immune enhancers and chemoprophylaxis) may represent the treatment of HIV infection in the future. Research into a vaccine for AIDS infection is still in its infancy, but when developed, is expected to prevent HIV virus from penetration its target cells by blocking lymphocyte and macrophage receptors (*77,79*).

AIDS and Impotence

Recent reports from the National Institute of Health in Bethesda, MD, have shown that the AIDS virus attacks specific nerve cells in the central and peripheral (spinal cord) nervous system. HIV infects the macrophage–monocyte cell population, and thus may contribute to dementia and other types of peripheral neuropathy. As of March 1990, there were an estimated 38 SCI patients with AIDS in the US. Most of these patients were either iv drug abusers prior to the injury or had become bisexuals after the cord trauma because of their limited sociosexual options. Initial clinical trials by the author in 15 neurologically impaired men (eight with AIDS only, four with multiple sclerosis, and three SCI with AIDS) with neurogenic impotence have demonstrated that 60% responded to dopamine-like oral preparations. It must be stressed that dopamine (Levo-dopa) in its purest form should be given

*Patients recovering from incomplete SCI lesions with Group 2–3 stages of AIDS usually suffer impotence from psychogenic etiologies. Organic impotence occurs in the latter stages of the disease (AIDS).

500 mg po 4 times/d for 6–8 wk to be effective. Other derivatives, such as sinemet or carbidopa, which are mixed with other chemicals, should not be offered because they rapidly lose their potency (*81*). Recent reports revealed that there is a lowering of testosterone levels in AIDS patients (*80*). The combination of dopamine derivates, testosteronem and other hormones, as a treatment for impotence caused by HIV neurological infection may be a worthwhile therapeutic option. Papaverine chemoerection and the implantation of penile prostheses can be tried on patients in remission (stable or who are HIV positive with peripheral neuropathy). However, the potential dangers of bleeding disorder and high risks of infection should be seriously considered in patient at Group 4-subgr. C_1 stage.

Prevention and Counseling (79)*

Education on the dangers of AIDS must start at a very young age, and continue through adolescence. An attempt must be made to teach those high-risk individuals still able to change their sexual practices and drug use patterns how to avoid the spread of HIV infection. For sexually active persons, the following safe sex techniques should be advised:

1. Avoid high risk partners and limit yourself to three new partners in one year.
2. Use a thick-layered condom with spermicide nonoxynol-9 or U-G 39/40 cpd. every time. For females, regular use of the diaphragm is recom mended.
3. Avoid sexual contact with persons having open orogenital or anal lesions.
4. Postpone pregnancy if the female is HIV positive.

For iv drug abusers, we offer the following advice:

1. Switch to methadone or other forms of rehabilitation treatment.
2. Always use new needles and never share needles.
3. Clean the iv needle with a 1:10 mixture of bleach and water.

COUNSELING. Sexual counseling is a vital part of the SCI patient's total rehabilitation program and are of the keys to a better quality of life. Counseling on AIDS should therefore include all the family member(s), sexual partners, and the patient. Family counseling consists of:

(1) Education (information and advice) emphasizing that living in a household with AIDS patient is safe, provided there is no sexual contact, since casual body contact does not transmit the HIV infection.

*Recent clinical data demonstrate the effectiveness of prophylactic AZT at 400–500 μg/d in HIV patients with T cells less than 500. In some centers, the therapy is combined with "septra" or "bactrim" and "pentamidine."

(2) Recommending that the patient use a separate bathroom or if, not feasible, that the toilet bowl be cleaned with 10% sodium hypochloride (household bleach of 1:10 dilution) after each use
(3) Suggesting that a separate set of dishes and utensils be used, and that these be routinely washed in hot water (dishwasher) or with 1:10 household bleach
(4) Recommending that the SCI patient restrict his or her sexual contacts.

If sexual engagement is suspected, the counselor should insist that the patient should use a "thick-walled" (polyurethane) condom (not ultra-thin ones) or a vaginal protective lining pouch to avoid HIV transmission. In the workplace or hospital, the patient should be advised to take similar precautions to those practiced at home. Health care workers should practice universal precautions, i.e., use proper gowning, wear a mask, gloves, and goggles, and avoid needle punctures. The provision of pastoral counseling, hospice care, and peer support service groups (Gay Men's Health Crisis Team) are adjunctive management modalities. For further help, the AIDS Hotline (1-800-342-AIDS) may be called.

A final note for the earthbound aging SCI male. As both males and females age,* their normal sexual responses slow down. In older able-bodied men, there is often delayed and less firm erection, with less forceful ejaculation and reduced seminal fluid volume. Older men have a longer refractory period and reduced scrotal elevation. In elderly physically challenged (SCI) men, who suffer impaired neurological sexual capabilities, the reduced level of these responses is compounded. However, with medications and sexual counseling/therapy, continued sexual activity among SCI patients in later years not only helps maintain residual functions, but mitigates many of the effects of involuntary organ changes and sex steroid deprivation.

Space Sexology

The 21st century will almost certainly open the new vista of extraplanetary travel. Weightlessness will become a much less novel experience for the able-bodied, and perhaps disabled SCI persons as well.

Since motion and transport in space are ideally suited to ease the lives of SCI patients, sexual celebrations in a weightless environment might well appear to be highly desirable. But because the human cardiovascular system is born and programmed under the influence of gravity, the heart and its hemodynamic properties are adapted to function well

*Atrophic and dry vaginas can be moistened with K-Y jelly lubricant or polymer gel (Replens).

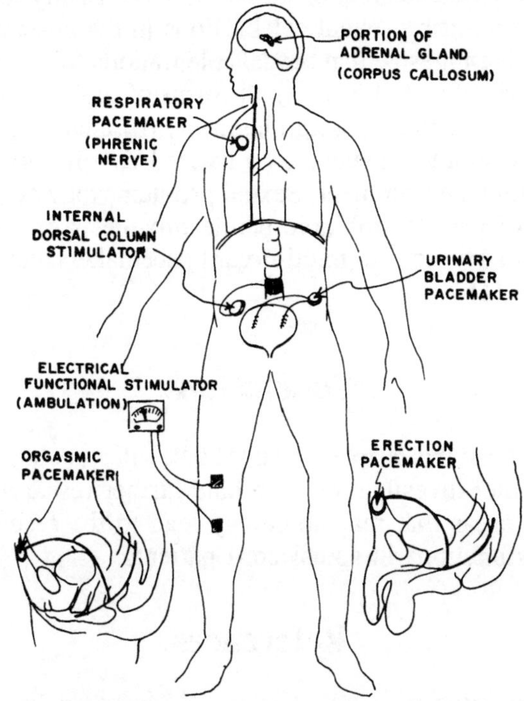

Fig. 21. A 3 million dollar spinal-cord patient with a transplanted fetal adrenal gland to provide more dopamine and respiratory and bladder pacemakers for breathing and urination. The dorsal column pain modulator relieves pain and the ambulation stimulator assists in the mechanics of walking. Both the erection and orgasmic pacemakers will hopefully enhance sexual celebration.

on earth. However, under zero gravity, the heart must pump harder; thus SCI persons with cardiac problems will be still more prone to suffer coronary dysfunction during sexual celebrations in the weightless state. It is advised that stricter criteria, beyond those of the earthbound standard tests be utilized in cardiac presexual activity screening. In recovered, incomplete, and low paraplegic SCI individuals, any minor sexual difficulties would be similar to those found in normal persons, an observation partially confirmed by the author with three chronic low paraplegics whose responses were measured while floating or playing in a swimming pool (*84*).

The spatial orientation perceived by able-bodied persons on earth, modulates her or his dermal and multireceptor-sensory systems in response to a complex reflex mechanism. An SCI male who is only capable of reflexogenic erections might have difficulty in eliciting this type of erection during sexual celebrations in the absence of gravity. As a result, it is suggested that sexual celebrations for the impotent SCI male be prescribed as follows: (a) all forms of oral sex and/or sensual touching are reasonable in weightlessness; (b) anal or penile–vaginal sexual activity should, however, be carried out in a gravity-charged and nonconfining environment. Sexual problems may be circumvented with the aid of the electrobionic penile prosthesis or other forms of urinary–respiratory–sexual (multi-organ) pacemakers and paraphernalia (*82,84*) (Fig. 21).

Conclusions

It is hoped that this chapter and this book will stimulate fresh thinking and prompt other investigators to initiate further research in these still controversial areas that may some day lead to the resolution or cure of sexual dysfunctions in spinal cord patients.

References

1. Bell, A. P., Weinberg, M., and Hammersmith, S. K. (1981) *Sexual Preference: Its development in Men and Women.* 1st Ed. (Indiana University Press).
2. Benson, G. S., McConnell, J., and Schmidt, W. A. (1981) Penile polsters: Functional structures or atherosclerotic changes? *J. Urol.* **125**, 800–804.
3. Benson, G. S., Lipshultz, L. I., and McConnell, J. (1981) Mechanism of erection and emission: Current laboratory approach, in *Sexual Rehabilitation of the Urologic Cancer Patient.* (von Eschenback A. C. and Rodriguez, D. B., eds.) Ch. 6 (G. K. Hall Medical Publishers, Boston).
4. Brinkley, G. (1983) Physiology of erection and ejaculation. Presented at the 78th American Urological Association Meeting, Las Vegas, NE. April 17–21.
5. Carlsson, C. A. and Sundin, T. (1980) Reconstruction of afferent and efferent nervous pathways to the urinary bladder in two paraplegic patients. *Spine.* **5**, 37–41.
6. Conti, G. (1952) L'erection du penis humain et ses bases morphologico-vasculaires. *Acta Anat (Basel)* **14**, 217–221.
7. Dawson, E. G., Harris, W. A., and McGanity, W. J. (1983) Vit. C. increases sperm vigor and fertility by unclumping action. *Urology Times.* **11:1** and **12.**
8. de Manizelli, L. (1983) Cellular surgery for nerve anastomosis in rats. Physician's Radio Network, News Conference.

9. Deysach, L. J. (1939) The comparative morphology of the erectile tissue of the penis with especial emphasis on the probable mechanism of erection. *Am. J. Anat.* **64**, 111-120.
10. Domer, F. R., Wessler, G., Brown, R. L. (1978) Involvement of the sympathetic nervous system in urinary bladder internal sphincter and in penile erection in the anesthetized cat. *Invest. Uro.* **15**, 404–412.
11. Dörner, G. (1979) Hormones and sexual differentiation of the brain, in *Sex Hormones and Behavior. Ciba Found Symp.* 81-101 (Excerpta Medica, Amsterdam).
12. Dua, S. and MacLean, P. D. (1964) Localization for penile erection in medial frontal lobe. *Am. J. Physiol.* **207**, 1425-1430.
13. Edwards, A. E. and Husted, J. R. (1976) Penile sensitivity, age, and sexual behavior. *J. Clin. Psychol.* **32**, 697-702.
14. Finney, R. P. (1983) New totally intrapenile inflatable prostheses for impotence. Presented at the 78th American Urological Asso. Meeting, Las Vegas, NE. April 17-21.
15. Fisher, C. Schiavi, R., Lear, H. et al. (1975) The assessment of nocturnal REM erection in the differential diagnosis of sexual impotence. *J. Sex. Marital Ther.* **1**, 277-281.
16. GU, J., Polak, J. M., Probert, L., Islam, K. N., Marangos, P. J. Mina, J. (1983) Peptidergic innervation of human male genital tract. *J. Urol.* **130**, 386-391.
17. Guttman, L. and Walsh, J. J. (1971) Prostigmin assessment test of fertility in spinal man. *Paraplegia* **9**, 39–45.
18. Herman, M. (1951) Role of somesthetic stimuli in the development of sexual excitation in man. *Arch. Neurol. Psychiatr.* **64**, 42–47.
19. Karacan, I. (1970) Clinical value of nocturnal erections in the prognosis and diagnosis of impotence. *Med. Aspects Human Sex.* **10**, 22-34.
20. Karacan, I., Hursch, C. J., and Williams, R. L. (1972) Some characteristics of nocturnal penile tumescence in elderly males. *J. Geron.* **27**, 39–45.
21. Karacan, I., Williams, R. L., and Thornby, J. I. (1975) Sleep-related penile tumescence as a function of age. *Am. J. Psychiatr.* **132**, 932-937.
22. Karczmar, A. G. (1980) Drugs, transmitters and hormones and mating behavior, in *Modern Problems of Pharmacopsychiatry. Drug treatment of Sexual Dysfunction*, Ban, T. A. and Freyhan, F. A., eds. Ch 1, p. 1-52 (S. Karger, Basel).
23. Khan, Z. and Choi, C. J. (1983) Acupuncture and Urinary Incontinence. Presented at the Urodynamic Society. American Urological Asso. Meeting, Las Vegas, NE. April 17-22.
24. Leyson, J. F. J. (1982) Urodynamic profiles in patients with respiratory pacemakers. *Phil. Am. Med. Bull.* **22**, 4-6.
25. Leyson, J. F. J. (1982) A treatise of human sexuality. Silver Jubilee Alumni Asso. Meeting: Update in Medicine. Cebu Institute of Medicine, Cebu City, Phil. June 10-12.
26. Leyson, J. F. J. and Powell, R. (1982) Comparative study of two noctur-

nal penile tumescence monitors. *J. Med. Society N.J.* **79**, 647–650.
27. Lipshultz, L. I., McConnell, J., and Benson, G. S. (1981) Current concepts of the mechanisms of ejaculation: normal and abnormal states. *J. Reprod. Med.* **26**, 499–505.
28. Lowry, T. P. and Williams, G. R. (1983) Brachioproctic eroticism. *J. Sex Ed. Therapy.* **9**, 50–52.
29. Lue, T. F., Schmidt, R. A., and Tanagho, E. (1983) Hemodynamics of erection and clinical implications. Presented at the 78th American Urological Asso. Las Vegas, NE. April 17–21.
30. MacLean, P. D. (1975) Brain mechanism of primal sexual functions and related behavior, in *Sandler and Gessa Sexual Behavior: Pharmacology and Biochemistry*, pp. 1–11 (Raven, New York).
31. MacLean, P. D., Denniston, R. H., and Dua, S. (1963) Further studies on cerebral representation of penile erection: caudal thalanius, midbrain and pons. *J. Neurophysiol.* **26**, 273–293.
32. Meyer, J. J., Godec, C. J., Kern, A., and Cass, A. S. (1982) The use of vibratory stimuli evaluation of erectile dysfunction. Presented at the 77th American Urological Asso. Meeting, Kansas City, MO. May 16–20.
33. Newman, H. F. and Northup. J. D. (1983) Problems of male organic sexual physiology. *Urol. J.* **21**, 443–450.
34. Olds, J. and Olds, M. E. (1965) Drives, rewards and the brain; in *Barrow New Directions in Psychology*, Vol. 2, pp. 327–410 (Holt, Rinehart and Winston, New York).
35. Peckham, P. H. (1983) Technical advances in upper limb rehabilitation. Presented at the 29th American Paraplegia Society Meeting, Las Vegas, NE. August 22–24.
36. Perkash, I. (1983) Electro-ejaculation in spinal cord injury patients. Presented at the 29th American Paraplegia Society Meeting, Las Vegas, NE. August 22–24.
37. Rodgers, C. H. and Law, O. T. (1967) The effects of habenular and medial forebrain bundle lesions on sexual behavior. *Psychonom. Sci.* **8**, 1–2.
38. Schoenfeld, C. Y., Amelar, R. D., and Dubin, L. (1975) Stimulation of ejaculated human spermatozoa by caffeine. *Fertil. Steril.* **26**, 158–163.
39. Schmidt, R. S. (1974) Neural correlates of frog calling. *J. Comp. Physiol.* **92**, 229–254.
40. Scott, B. F. (1983) Experience in a new inflatable penile prosthesis. Presented at the 78th American Urological Asso. Meeting, Las Vegas, NE. April 17–21.
41. Tanagho, E. (1983) The role of electrostimulation in neurogenic bladder rehabilitation. Presented at the 29th American Paraplegia Society Meeting, Las Vegas, NE. August 22–24.
42. Thomas, A. J. (1983) Ejaculatory dysfunction: Modern Trends. *Fertil. Steril.* **39**, 445–454.
43. Van Arsdalen, K. N., Malloy, T. R., and Wein, A. J. (1983) Erectile physiology, dysfunction and evaluation. Part I: Physiology of erection. *Monogr. in Urol.* **4**, 137–154.

44. Van Arsdalen, K. N., Malloy, T. R., and Wein, A. J. (1983) Erectile physiology, dysfunction and evaluation. Part II: Etiology and evaluation of erectile dysfunction. Monographs in Urology **4**, 165–185.
45. Virag, R. (1983) Papaverine for impotence. *The Lancet* p. 938. Oct. 23.
46. Wagner, G. (1981) Erection, physiology and endocrinology, in Wagner, G., Green, R. (eds.): *Impotence. Physiological, Psychological, Surgical Diagnosis and Treatment* Chapter 2, (Wagner, G. and Green, R., eds.) (Plenum, New York).
47. Weiss, H. D. (1972) The physiology of human penile erection. *Ann. Intern. Med.* **76**, 785–793.
48. Witkin, S. S. and Sonnabend, J. (1983) Immune responses to spermatozoa in homosexual men. *Fertil. and Steril.* **38**, 337–341.
49. Zoler, M. L. (1983) Dementia vs "the brain energizer". New frontiers of research. *Geriatrics.* **38**, 107–117.
50. Fournier, G. and Lue, T. (1988) *Vasculogenic Impotence: Physiology, Diagnoses and Treatment* in Monographs in Urology, Stamey, R. ed. **9**, 20–31.
51. Valji, K. and Bookstein, J. (1987) The veno-occulsive mechanisms of the canine corpus cavernosum. Angiographic and pharmacologic studies. *J. Urol.* **138**, 1467–1470.
52. Hedlund, H., Anderson, K., Fovaeus, M., Holmquist, F. and Uski, T. (1989) Characterization of contraction-mediating prostanoid receptors in human penile erectile tissues. *J. Urol.* **141**, 182–186.
53. Leyson, J. F. and Cytyrn, A. (1989) Comparative study between vacuum constrictor devices and chemoerection in the management of impotence in SCI men. Presented at the Annual Meeting of the American Paraplegia Society. April 5–7, Las Vegas, NE.
54. Bradley, W. E., Timm, G. W., Gallagher, J. M. and Johnson, B. K. (1985) New method for continuous measurement of nocturnal penile tumescence and rigidity: *J. Urol.* **26**, 4–9.
55. Leyson, J. F. J. and Cytyrn, A. (1987) Effects of transdermal and intrapenile application of vasoactive drugs in the management of impotence in neurologically impaired men. Presented at the American Spinal Injury Association, March 20–22, Boston, MA.
56. Leyson, J. F. J. (1987) Medical options in the management of impotence in the neurologically impaired men. Presented at the meeting of the American Assoc. of Sex Educators, Counsellors and Therapists. April 30–May 3, New York City, New York.
57. Leyson, J. F. J. (1987) Comparative study between oral and intrapenile vasoactive drugs in the management of impotence in neurologically impaired patients. Presented at the American Urological Association Meeting, May 17–23, Anaheim, CA.
58. Cahill, B. E., Ross, E. V., Pielet, R. W., Rice, J. C., Lewis, R. W. and Kerstein, M. D. (1988) Measurement of impotence by laser doppler flowmetry and conventional methodology. *J. Urol.* **140**, 749–750.
59. Abber, J. C., Lue, T. F., Orvis, B. R., McClure, R. D. and Williams,

R. D. (1986) Diagnostic tests for impotence. A comparison of papaverine injection with the penile brachial index and nocturnal penile tumescence monitoring. *J. Urol.* **135**, 923–925.

60. Wespes, E., Delcour, C., Rondeux, C., Struyven, J. and Schulman, C. (1987) The erectile angle: Objective criterion to evaluate the papaverine test in impotence. *J. Urol.* **138**, 1171–1173.
61. Leyson, J. F. J. (1985) Medical management of impotence in spinal cord injury. Presented at the American Spinal Cord Injury Assoc. Meeting. April 15–17, Atlanta, GA.
62. Witherington, R. (1989) Vacuum constriction devices for management of erectile impotence. *J. Urol.* **141**, 320–322.
63. Ishii, N., Watanabe, H., Irisawa, C., Kikuchi, Y., Kubota, Y., Kawamura, S., Suzuki, K., Chiba, R., Tokiwa, M. and Shirai, M. (1989) Intracavernous injection of prostaglandin El for the treatment of erectile impotence. *J. Urol.* **414**, 323–325.
64. Malloy, T. (1986) VIP: Neurotransmitter self-injection useful for impotence treatment. *Urology Times.* 14–35, Sept.
65. Sayer, J. and Parson, C. L. (1988) Successful treatment of priapism with intracorporeal epinephrine. *J. Urol.* **140**, 827.
66. Fuchs, M. E. and Brawer, M. K. (1989) Papaverine-induced fibrosis of the corpus cavernosum. *J. Urol.* **141**, 125.
67. Kuznar, W. (1987) New treatment in impotence shows hope. *Urology Times.* **14**, I, II, Jan.
68. Bookstein, J. (1989) Catheter now being used in a non-surgical impotence cure. *Urology Times.* **17**, 1, 12 Feb.
69. Leyson, J. F. and Cytyrn, A. (1986) Medical and electrical stimulations in the treatment of impotence in SCI men. Presented at the American Spinal Injury Association Meeting, March 13–15, San Francisco, CA.
70. Hashmat, A. (1985) Transurethral nervi-erigentes stimulation in dogs (penile tunes). Presented at the American Urological Association Meeting. May 12–16, Atlanta, GA.
71. Levin, R. M., Clayton, R. G., Singer, M., Strong, G., Brenman, H. S., Katz, P. and Wein, A. J. (1985) Rectal stimulation of erection in macaca fascicularis primates. Presented at the American Urological Association Meeting. May 12–16, Atlanta, GA.
72. Park, Y., Esa, A., Sugiyama, T., Kaneko, S. and Kurita, T. (1988) Sympathetic skin response: A new test to diagnose ejaculatory dysfunction. *J. Urol.* **139**, 539–541.
73. Lessing, J. B. (1986) Sperm motility may be increased by use of relaxin human treatment. *J. Reprod. Med.* **31**, 304–309, May.
74. Yamamoto, M., Hashimoto, J., Takaba, H. and Migake, K. (1987) Response of the isolated human semimiferous tubule to prostaglandins, Fla, F2a, El and E2. *J. Urol.* **137**, 345–348.
75. Meyer, A. A. (1986) AIDS: The disease and its relevance to surgeons. American College of Surgeons Bulletin. **31**, 11–16.

76. Morrison, A. (1988) HIV may be 200 years old. Infection Report. *Oncology and Biotechnology News.* **2**, 22, Sept.

77. AIDS Today (1989), *Infectious Disease Today.* **1**, 14, Jan.

78. Slim, J. (1987) Highlights in the 3rd International Conference in AIDS. Washington, DC, June 1–5, 1987. *Med. Human of Sexual Sexuality.* **2**, 8, July.

79. Kloser, P. (1988) AIDS news. Medical Aspects of Human Sexuality. **22**, 15–17, August.

80. Dobs, A. S. and Dempsey, M. A. (1988) Endocrine disorders in men infected with Human immunodeficiency virus. *Am. J. Med.* **84**, 611–616, March.

81. Leyson, J. F. (1988) Diagnoses and management of impotence in AIDS patients. Presented at the Society for Sex Therapy and Research Meeting, March 17–20, New York City, New York.

82. Leyson, J. F. (1988) Future options in impotence management. Presented at the American College of Surgeons Meeting, New Jersey Chapter. Dec. 2–4, Asbury Park, New Jersey.

83. Leyson, J. F. J. (1988) Update in Sexual Medicine. Presented at the Annual Winter Meeting, Association of Phil. Physicians in American and Philippines Med. Asso. Dec. 13–18, Manila, Philippines.

84. Leyson, J. F. (1990) Diagnosis and Management of Impotence in Neurologically Impaired Men in 2000 A.D. Presented at the Annual Meeting of the American Association of Sex Educators, Counselors and Therapists. Feb. 16–19, Arlington, VA.

Appendix A

Table 1
SCI Sexual Treatment Options

Female sexual dysfunctions	Male erectile dysfunctions
A. Sex therapy	A. Sex therapy
B. Adjustment/change of meds.	B. Adjust or change meds.
C. Alternative sexual techniques or avoidance of illegal drugs/ smoking	C. Alternative sex techniques or avoidance of illegal drugs/ smoking
D. Hormones—estrogen and androgen	D. Testosterone and zinc
E. Oral medications—dopamine-like and "brain energizer"	E. Oral medications: dopamine and yohimbine
F. Masturbation	F. Vacuum constriction device
G. Vibrators—artificial penis	G. Dildoes/assistive device
H. ? Lumbar dermatone T.N.S.	H. Chemoerection/penile injection
I. ? Laser stimulations or trans-dermal thermal massage	I. ? Laser and/or balloon arterioplasty
J. ? Orgasmic pacemaker	J. ? Vascular bypass
K. ? "Artificial vagina"	K. ? Venous ligation
	L. Penile prostheses—nonbionic or bionic (computerized)
	M. ? Erection pacemaker or stimulator

Appendix B

Table 1
Patient's Goal-Oriented Management
(After Sexological History, Physical Exam,
and Basic Laboratory Diagnostic Tests)

Female sexual dysfunction	
Group I	(Not interested in treatment, only information) Sex Education/Counseling and no further workup
Group II	(Not interested in medical treatment, but needs help) Sex therapy and other masturbatory techniques
Group III	(Only interested in oral medication or assistive devices) Dopamine-like drugs, Kegel exercises, perineometer, (vaginal cones), or vagitone device
Group IV	(Requests for all other therapeutic options) Proceed to systematic workup (Chapters 11 and 34): A. Noctural vaginal/anal probe EMG monitoring (Psychogenic type) sex therapy + group III treatment B. Endocrine evaluation and vitamin-mineral levels Estrogen + androgen combination and dopamine C. Neurological testings and Sacral EMG (Neurogenic type) Lumbar dermatone transcutaneous stimulation (TNS) orgasmic pacemaker and nerve transplant
Group V	Vaginal probe pletysmography (+ bruxing and so on) A. Good circulation but poor muscle contraction Vibrator, Kegel exercises, and personal perineometer B. Poor circulation with good muscle control Laser orgasm (stimulations) C. Poor circulation and poor muscle contraction Orgasmic pacemaker ? Periodic intravaginal probe stimulation

Appendix C

Table 1
Patient's Goal-Oriented Management
(After Sexological History, Physical Exam
and Basic Laboratory Diagnostic Tests)

	Male sexual dysfunction
Group I	(Not interested in treatment, only information) Sex education/counseling and no further workup
Group II	(Not interested in medical treatment, but desires some therapy) Sex therapy (stuffing technique, use of rubber or constriction bands with reflexogenic erections)
Group III	(Only interested in oral medications or erective assistive devices) Dopamine-like drugs (Levo-Dopa), Yohimbine, dildo, and/or vacuum constriction device
Group IV	(Requests for all other treatments) Proceed to systematic workup (Chapter 35): A. Noctural penile tumescence and rigidity monitoring (Psychogenic type) sex therapy and Group III treatment B. Endocrine, mineral levels, and neuroreceptor diagnostic tests (Hormonal type) zinc + testosterone and vitamin B complex C. Neurological testing and cavernosus EMG (Neurogenic type) dopamine + vitamin B complex electrical stimulations (erection pacemaker), nerve "cellular" transplant
Group V	Intracorporeal cavernous chemoinjection and stimulation tests (mixed neurovascular type) A. (Full erection even without manual stimulation) Sex therapy + Group III, Group IV (C) therapy, or chemoerection B. (Full erection only after manual/vibratory stimulation chemoerection (prostaglandin E1) C. (Partial erection) use vacuum constriction device (VCD) If good response—chemoerection + VCD If poor response—penile prostheses or erection pacemaker D. Doppler-duplex or "color" ultrasonography (1) If good arterial circulation—perform cavernosometry venous leak—rubber band constriction? venous surgery (2) If poor arterial circulation—perform selective (pudendal) arteriography arterial insufficiency or obstruction—? Balloon/laser arterioplasty (dilatation) ? Bypass arterial surgery plus erection pacemaker or penile prostheses

Appendix D

Obstructive Sleep Apnea and Sexuality

I. Definition and Clinical Aspects

Obstructive sleep apnea (OSA) is the repeated cessation of airflow through the mouth and nose for at least 10 s despite active respiratory effort (*1*). It is believed to be caused by transient obstruction of the upper airway. These cases can be seen in SCI patients with incomplete C7 and recovered lesions, who are labeled as having "adult respiratory distress syndrome." Some of them have temporary tracheostomies as a form of treatment. However, the clinical clues of OSA are: history of loud, disrupted snoring during naps or nocturnal sleep and an occasional snort or gasp that is punctuated by breathing pauses (apnea) and brief awakening. Men are usually obese, impotent, and sometimes doze during sex, while females have frequent mood changes; are too tired to perform pre-sexual bowel/urinary preparation and foreplay, and both sexes fall asleep immediately after sexual intercourse (*1*).

II. Diagnoses

1. Polysomnography (electroencephalography, electroculography, and electromyography)
2. Upper airway cinefluoroscopy
3. Pulmonary function tests

III. Management

1. Elimination of cardiorespiratory problems and correction of anatomic abnormalities in the nose and face with associated endocrinopathy-hypothyroidism.
2. Avoidance of alcohol and cessation of smoking.
3. Weight reduction (to 10–15% lower than ideal body weight)
4. Nasal continuous positive airway pressure (NCPAP) via a nasal mash.
5. Surgery: uvulopalatopharynogoplasty, tonsillectory, adeniodectomy, and tracheostomy are rarely needed nowadays (*1*).
6. Sexual counseling (male and female/gay).
7. Sex therapy: use of vacuum constrictive devices and chemoerections.
8. Sexual SCI surrogate therapy.
9. Enlist family members support/cooperation.
10. Engage in lovemaking at least 2 h after meals or consume only a low-fat diet/light meal before sexual celebrations.

1. Quittel, L. M., Schidlow, D. V., and Goldberg, R.: (1990) Obstructive sleep apnea: effects on sexuality. *Med. Asp. Human Sexuality* **24**, 34–45.

Appendix E

Sex Clinics or Sexuality Resource Units of Spinal Cord Injury Centers Department of Veterans Affairs, USA

Chief, Spinal Cord Injury Service (SCI)
Department of Veterans Affairs Medical Center
Augusta, GA 30910

Chief, Spinal Cord Injury Service
Department of Veterans Affairs Medical Center
130 Kingsbridge Road
Bronx, NY 10468

T. O'Connor, RN
Spinal Cord Injury Service
Department of Veterans Affairs Medical Center
Castle Point, NY 12511

L. Rustad, PhD
Spinal Cord Injury Service
Department of Veterans Affairs Medical Center
10701 East Boulevard
Cleveland, OH 44106

J. F. Leyson, MD
Spinal Cord Injury Service
Department of Veterans Affairs Medical Center
East Orange, NJ 07019

M. Eisenberg, PhD
Department of Veterans Affairs Medical Center
Hampton, VA 23667

M. Blanchard, RN
Department of Veterans Affairs Medical Center
Hines, IL 60141

R. Bostick, PhD
Department of Veterans Affairs Medical Center
2002 Halcombe Boulevard
Houston, TX 77031

B. Rabin, PhD
Department of Veterans Affairs Medical Center
5901 East Seventh Street
Long Beach, CA 90801

Chief, Spinal Cord Injury Service
Department of Veterans Affairs
Seattle, WA 98208

B. Mueller, MD
Chief, Spinal Cord Injury Service
Department of Veterans Affairs Medical Center
1030 Jefferson Avenue
Memphis, TN 38104

Chief, Spinal Cord Injury Service
Department of Veterans Affairs Medical Center
1201 N.W. 16th Street
Miami, FL 33125

Chief, Spinal Cord Injury Service or M. Dunn, PhD
Department of Veterans Affairs Medical Center
3801 Miranda Avenue
Palo Alto, CA 94304

M. Spruill, PhD
Department of Veterans Affairs Medical Center
1201 Broad Rock Road
Richmond, VA 23249

R. M. Cayere, MD
Chief, Spinal Cord Injury Service
Department of Veterans Affairs
Medical Center
One Veterans Plaza (128)
San Juan, Puerto Rico
00927-5800

T. Serota, SW
Department of Veterans Affairs
Medical Center
1300 N. 30th Street
Tampa, FL 33612

K. Sherman, OT
Department of Veterans Affairs
Medical Center
1400 VFW Parkway
West Roxbury, MA 02132

J. Barracks, MD
Department of Veterans Affairs
Medical Center
St. Louis, MI 63125

Chief, Spinal Cord Injury Service
Department of Veterans Affairs
Medical Center
5000 West National Avenue
Milwaukee, WI 53295

Rodney Y. Torigoe, PhD
Department of Veterans Affairs
Medical Center
PO Box 50188
Honolulu, HI 96850

Appendix F

International Sexual Dysfunction Centers or Human Sexuality Programs (with Spinal Cord and Disability or Resource Units)

United States

Susan E. Knight, LCSW
Director, Sex and Disability Unit
University of California
814 Mission Street
Second Floor
San Francisco, CA 94103

Dr. Scott Manley
Director, Craig Hospital
Rocky Mountain Regional
Spinal Cord Injury Center
3425 S. Clarkson
Englewood, CO 80110

Dr. Joan Bardach
Director, Institute
of Rehabilitation Medicine
New York University
Spinal Cord Injury Center
400 E. 34th Street
New York, NY 10016

Chief, Rehabilitation Medicine
Service
Moss Rehabilitation Hospital
12th and Tabor Road
Philadelphia, PA 19141

Dr. A. Estin Commar
Director, Rancho Los Amigos
Hospital
Outpatient Services
7601 E. Imperial Highway
Downey, CA 90242

Dr. Don Olson
Director, The Rehabilitation
Institute of Chicago
345 E. Superior Street
Chicago, IL 60611

Dr. Dan Mayclin
Director, Rehabilitation Medicine
Santa Clara Valley
Medical Center
751 S. Bascom
Santa Clara, CA 95128

Joyce Salhoot, MSW
Director, The Texas Institute
for Rehabilitation and Research
(TIRR)
PO Box 20095
Houston, TX 77025

Dr. Sharon Satterfield
Director, Human Sexuality
Program
University of Minnesota
2630 University Avenue, SE
Minneapolis, MN 55414

Dr. Daniel Goldberg
Director, Dept. of Psychiatry
and Human Behavior
Jefferson Medical College
of T. Jefferson University
Sleep Lab, 2nd floor
1015 Chestnue Street
Philadelphia, PA 19107

Dr. Raul Schiavi
Director, Human Sexuality Program
The Mt. Sinai Medical Center
One Gustave Levy Place
New York, NY 10029

Dr. Sandra Leiblum, PhD
Director, Rutgers Medical School
University of Medicine and Dentistry of New Jersey
University Heights
Piscataway, NJ 08854

Dr. Theodore Cole
Director, Dept. of Physical Medicine and Rehabilitation
The University of Michigan Medical Center
Ann Arbor, MI 48109

The New York Hospital—Cornell Medical Center
Director, Erectile Disorders Program, Westchester Division
21 Bloomingdale Road
White Plains, NY 10605

Director of Training
Master and Johnson Institute
4910 Forest Park Boulevard
St. Louis, MO 63108

Dr. Barry McCarthy
Dept. of Psychology
The American University
5010 Wisconsin Avenue, NW
ste 304
Washington, DC 20016

Dr. Harold Lief
Director, Dept. of Psychiatry
The University of Pennsylvania
Philadelphia, PA 00000

Dr. John Money
Director, Medical Psychology (Human Sexuality)
Johns Hopkins University Hospital
Baltimore, MD 00000

Dr. John Rock
Harvard Medical School
Dept. of Obstet. and Gynecology
Boston, MA 00000

Dr. Paul Gebhard
Director, University of Indiana
Institute for Sex Research, Inc.
Bloomington, IN 00000

Dr. Clifford Sager
Director, New York Hospital
Cornell Medical Center
Family Psychiatry and Sex Therapy Program
New York, NY 00000

Dr. Milton Diamond
University of Hawaii at Manoa
J.A. Burns School of Medicine
Dept. of Reproductive Biology and Anatomy
Honolulu, HI 96850

G. H. Golden, MSW or K. F. Schepp, EdD
University of Vermont
Dept. of Psychiatry/Counseling and Testing Center
Burlington, VT 05041

Dr. P. M. Sariel and Ms. Sariel
Yale University Hospital Health Services
Box 1505A
Yale Station, CT 06520

Dr. Jose Florante J. Leyson
Director, Center for Sexual Dysfunction
Dept. of Veterans Affairs Medical Center
East Orange, NJ 00000

Shirley Nickols Fahey, PhD
University of Arizona
College of Medicine
B.S. Building, Rm. 2102B
Tucson, AZ 85724

Canada and Europe

Dr. A. Morales
Queen's University Victory 4
Kingston General Hospital
Dept. of Urology
Kingston, Ontario
K7L 2V7, Canada

W. Babchuk, MD
University of Manitoba
720 Bannatyne Avenue
Winnipeg, Manitoba
Canada, R3E 0W3

Paul Davis, MD
University of Alberta
9-112 C Clinical Science Bldg.
Edmonton, Alberta
Canada, T6G 2G3

John Lewis, MD
Memorial University of Newfoundland
School of Medicine
St. John's, Newfoundland
Canada, A1B 3V6

Heidi Leipold
Federal Center of AIDS
301 Elgin Street
Ottowa, Ontario, Canada

H. C. Still, MD
Dalhousie University
5599 Fenwick Street
Halifax, Nova Scotia
Canada, B3H 1R2

George Szasz
University of British Columbia
2075 Wesbrook Mall
Vancouver, B.C.
Canada, V6T 1W5

Dr. R. Gemme
Universite du Quebec
Dept. De Sexologie
Quebec, Montreal
Canada

Chief, Dept. of Rehab. Medicine
Univ. of Dublin Medical School
Dublin, Ireland

C. J. Mathias, MB
St. Mary's Hospital Medical School
Medical Unit (Univ. of London)
Paddington, London
W21PG, England

Chief of Rehabilitation
National Spinal Injured Centre
Stoke Mandeville Hospital
Aylesbury, UK

Dr. K. Loewit
Institute fur Medixinische Biologie and Genetik Der Universitat
Div. of Reproductive Biology and Sexual Medicine
Innsbruck, Austria

Dr. B. A. von Bargen
Dijkzigt Hospital
Dept. of Psychiatry
Rotterdam, Netherlands

Dr. G. S. Vassilchenko
Director, Moscow Scientific Research Institute of Psychiatry
Dept. of Sexual Pathology
Moscow, Russia

Dr. P. Lucisano
Ospedale Fatebenefratelli
I 00100 Roma, Italy

Professor Dr. Med. C. Van Emde Boas
Sex Clinic
Stadionweg 80
1077 SP Amsterdam, Holland

Dr. G. Tordjman
Redacteur en Chef
Chaiers des Sexologie Clinique
21 Blvd. Brune
75014 Paris, France

Piet Nijs, MD
University Hospital Gasthuis
St. Rafael-Herestratt 49
Leuven, Belgium B-3000

Major Briht Bergstrom-Walan, PhD
Swedish Inst. for Sex Research
Lasmakargatan, 14-15
Stockholm, Sweden 11144

Charo (M.R.) Verde, MD
Via Augusta 134-3o3a
Barcelona, Spain 08006

Orloff W. Miller, PhD
Pfalzgrafenstr, 44
6700 Ludwigshafen
West Germany

Caribbean and South America

Arletty Pinel, MD
Caixa Postal 54132
01296 Sao Paulo, SP, Brazil

Institute Superior de Siencias
Mediceo de La Havana
Calle 146 y Avenida 31, Playa
La Havana, Cuba

Escuela de Medicina (Luis Razetti)
Universidad Central de Venezuela
Cuidad Universitaria
Caracas, Venezuela

Miquel-Gonzales Manrique, MD
University of Puerto Rico
Medical Science Campus
PO Box 5067
San Juan, Puerto Rico 00936

Enrique A. Aviles-Aceves, MD
Av. Lopez Portillo
171 SM 69 M3
Cancun, Quintana R, Mexico 77500

Africa, Middle East, Asia, Australia, New Zealand, and South Pacific

Mrs. A. I. Odebiyi
University of Ife
Dept. of Sociology
and Anthropology
Ile-Ife, Nigeria, Africa

Lonny Myers, MD
Peace Corps
Box 208
Lilongwe, Malawi, Africa

Dr. Z. Hoch, Director
Pambam Med Ctr, Dept OB-GYN
Center for Sexual Therapy, Ed.
and Research
Technion-Israel Institute
of Technology
Hafia, Israel

Putu W. Mansa, MD
Jalan Timor No. 1
Denasar 80114
Indonesia

Chief of Urology or Rehab. Med.
University of the Philippines
Medical School
Diliman-Quezon City, Philippines

Josefina Leyson Poblete, MD
Dean, Cebu Institute of Medicine
79 F Ramos Street
Cebu City, Philippines

Chief, Dept. of Urology
Univ. of Hongkong Med. School
Hongkong, British Crown Colony
China

Man-Lun Ng, MD
Hongkong Sex Ed. Assoc.
PO Box 50419
Sai Ying Pun, Hong Kong

Dr. A. A. Khattab
Ains Shams University
Dept. of Pathology and Fertility
Sterility Clinic
Cairo, Egypt

Ishwarprasad S. Gilada, MD
RMO's Bungalo (Near L. Hostel)
J. J. Hospital, Bombay
Maharashtra, India 400008

Chief, Dept. of Urology
University of Tokyo Medical
Tokyo, Japan

Okamura Yasushi, MD
University of Occup.
and Env. Health
Iseigaoka 1-1, Yahatanishiku
Kitakyusha, Japan 807

Michael W. Ross, PhD
PO Box 395 Wentworth Bldg.
University of Sydney Union
Sydney, Australia NSW 2006

Wendy Ann F. Brumley, PhD
140 Church Street
Richmond 3121
Victoria, Australia

Chief of Urology
Pulse Beat Medical School
University of Whitwater Strand
Whiterstrand Hosp. Street
Johannesburg, So. Africa 2000

Athol Maurice Abrahams,
MB, ChB
6 Military Road, Lower Hutt
New Zealand

Raymond H. Hamden, PhD
United Arab Emirates
PO 18206
Washington, DC 20036

Chief, Dept. of Urology
Shanghai Medical College
No. 1
Shanghai, China

Chief, Dept. of Urology
University of Malaysia
Medical School
Kuala Lumpor, Malaysia

Paul Jagdish Singh, PsyD
PO Box 3669
Lautoka, FIJI Islands
South Pacific

Note: The majority of university hospitals and medical schools all over the world have sexual dysfunction units or programs run by either Dept. of Obstet. and Gynecology, or Dept. of Psychiatry. In the Third World countries, sexuality courses are called ethics and health education programs. Those hospitals or medical centers that have SCI or disability sexuality units, but are not included here, have not listed their services in major sexuality organizations or journals.

For a detailed list of certified sexologists worldwide, please write to: American Board of Sexology, 1050 Connecticut Avenue, NW, Suite 66138, Washington, DC 20035-9998.

Certifying Organizations

American Association of Sex Educators, Counselors and Therapists (AASECT)
435 North Michigan Avenue
Suite 1717
Chicago, IL 69611

American Board of Sexology (ACS)
1050 Connecticut Avenue, NW
Suite 66138
Washington, DC 20035-9998

International Council of Sex Education & Parenthood (ICSEP)
11 Dupont Circle, NW
Suite 220
Washington, DC 20016

Information

Sex Information and Education Council of the US (SIECUS)
80 Fifth Avenue
New York City, NY 10011

Fertility Reseach Foundation
1430 Second Avenue at 75th St.
New York City, NY 10021

Consortium of Sex Educators
Michael Plant, PhD
Department of Psychiatry
University of Maryland
School of Medicine
645 West Redwood Street
Baltimore, MD 21211

AIDS Education and Training
Centers Program
Bureau of Health Professions
5600 Fishers Lane
Room 4C-03
Rockville, MD 20857

Paralysis Society of America
(PSA)
Paralyzed Veterans of America
801 18th St., NW
Washington, DC 20006

Center for Spinal Cord Injury
Rigshospilat TH 2002
Blegdamsvej 9 DK — 2100
Copenhagen, Denmark

International Medical Society
of Paraplegia
Department of Rehabilitative Medicine
La Fe Hospital
Valencia, Spain

Japan Medical Society of Paraplegia
The Secretariat
San-in Rosai Hospital
Yonago-Shi, Tottoriken 683
Japan

Index

Note: Page numbers in italics indicate illustrations.

T

U

GPSR Compliance

The European Union's (EU) General Product Safety Regulation (GPSR) is a set of rules that requires consumer products to be safe and our obligations to ensure this.

If you have any concerns about our products, you can contact us on ProductSafety@springernature.com

In case Publisher is established outside the EU, the EU authorized representative is:

Springer Nature Customer Service Center GmbH
Europaplatz 3
69115 Heidelberg, Germany

Batch number: 10620078

Printed by Printforce, the Netherlands